# Child Health for All

# Dedication

This book is dedicated to the memory of
Janet Hollingshead, who passed away on
20 September 2000. She was a valued contributor to
the present edition of *Child Health for All*, as well as
to the 1st, and 2nd editions. As a social worker,
Jan was widely known and respected, and she will
long be remembered for her vigorous promotion of
the rights of children with disabilities.

# Child Health for All

## A Manual for Southern Africa

Third Edition

EDITED BY

MA Kibel and LA Wagstaff

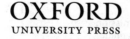

OXFORD
UNIVERSITY PRESS

# OXFORD
UNIVERSITY PRESS

Great Clarendon Street, Oxford OX2 6DP

Oxford University Press is a department of the University of Oxford.
It furthers the University's objective of excellence in research, scholarship,
and education by publishing worldwide in

Oxford New York

Athens Auckland Bangkok Bogotá Buenos Aires Calcutta
Cape Town Chennai Dar es Salaam Delhi Florence Hong Kong Istanbul
Karachi Kuala Lumpur Madrid Melbourne Mexico City Mumbai
Nairobi Paris São Paulo Shanghai Singapore Taipei Tokyo Toronto Warsaw

with associated companies in Berlin Ibadan

Oxford is a registered trade mark of Oxford University Press
in the UK and certain other countries

Published in South Africa
by Oxford University Press Southern Africa, Cape Town

## Child Health for All: A Manual for Southern Africa

ISBN 0 19 571928 X

First published 1991
Second impression 1993
Second edition 1995
Third edition 2001

Editor: Martha Evans
Medical proofreader: Claire Irving
Designer: Mark Standley
Indexer: Mary Starkey

Published by Oxford University Press Southern Africa
PO Box 12119, N1 City, 7463, Cape Town, South Africa

Set in 9 pt on 12.5 pt Utopia by Positive Proof
Reproduction by Positive Proof
Cover reproduction by The Image Bureau, Cape Town
Printed and bound by Creda Communications

The authors and publishers gratefully acknowledge permission
to reproduce material in this book. Every effort has been made
to trace copyright holders, but where this has proved impossible,
the publishers would be grateful for information which would
enable them to amend any omissions in future editions.

# Contents

# List of contributors

ADNAMS CM, BSc (Natal), BScHons (Cape Town), MBChB (Cape Town), FCPaeds (SA)
Senior Lecturer, Department of Paediatrics and Child Health, University of Cape Town

ALLWOOD CW, MB BCh (Cape Town), FF (Psych) (SA), MMed (Psych) (Wits), MD (Pretoria)
Professor and Head, Department of Psychiatry, University of the Witwatersrand

ARENS LJ, BSc (Cape Town), MBChB (Cape Town)
Part-time lecturer and Principal Medical Officer, Department of Paediatrics and Child Health, University of Cape Town; part-time Chief Medical Officer, Cerebral Palsy Schools and Centres, Cape Town

BECKETT G, BA (Speech and Hearing) (Witwatersrand), Hons (Psychology) (Cape Town), MA (Clinical Psychology) (Witwatersrand)
Part-time lecturer and consultant to Early Childhood Development Sector, Department of Speech Pathology and Audiology, University of the Witwatersrand; Second-Language Therapist, APPS

BLUMBERG LH, MB BCh (Wits), DCH (SA), DTM & H, DOH (Wits)
Clinical Microbiologist, SAIMR, Johannesburg

BRADSHAW D, MSc (UCT), DPhil(Oxon)
Unit Director, Burden of Disease Research Unit, Medical Research Council, Parow-Vallei

COETZER T, NDOT (Pretoria), Mphil MCH (UCT)
Part-time lecturer, Department of Occupational Therapy, University of Cape Town; private practitioner in Occupational Therapy, Cape Town

COOPER PA, MB ChM (Cape Town), DCH, FCP (Paeds) (SA), PhD (Wits)
Professor and Clinical Head, Department of Paediatrics, Johannesburg Hospital, University of the Witwatersrand

COOVADIA HM, MSc (Birmingham), MD (Natal), FCP (SA)
Professor and Head, Department of Paediatrics and Child Health, University of Natal

DAUBENTON JD, BSc MB BCh (Wits), MD (Cape Town), FCP DCH (SA)
Associate-Professor, Department of Paediatrics and Child Health, University of

Cape Town

DE VILLIERS F, BA (Unisa), MB ChB (Stellenbosch), MMed (Paeds), PhD (Wits), DCH (SA), MFGP (SA), DTM & H (Wits)
Professor and Head, Department of Paediatrics and Child Health, Medunsa

DONALD PR, MD (Stellenbosch), FCP (SA)
Associate-Professor, Department of Paediatrics, University of Stellenbosch

DROWER SJ, B Soc Sci (Hons) (PSW), PhD (Cape Town)
Associate-Professor, School of Social Work, University of the Witwatersrand

DU TOIT N, BA (Social Work), Hons (Medical Social Work)
Chief Social Worker and Regional Manager, Child Accident Prevention Foundation of South Africa, Red Cross Children's Hospital

GOODMAN M, BSc (Physio), PhD (Wits)
Emeritus Professor and Head, Department of Physiotherapy, University of the Witwatersrand

GREENFIELD DH, MB ChB (Cape Town), MCGP (Z), DCH (SA), DTM & H DPH (Wits)
Principal Medical Officer, Department of Paediatrics and Child Health, University of Cape Town

GUTHRIE TA, BSc (Hons) (Zimbabwe)
Senior Policy Researcher, Child Health Policy Institute, University of Cape Town

HOLLINGSHEAD J (deceased), B Soc Sci (Rhodes), BA (Hons) (Social Work) (Stellenbosch)
Formerly Chief Social Worker, Red Cross War Memorial Children's Hospital, Cape Town

HUSSEY GD, MB BCh, MMed (Com Health) (Cape Town), FFCH (SA), DTM & H, RCP & S (Eng), MSc, CTM (London)
Associate-Professor, Department of Paediatrics and Child Health, University of Cape Town

IRLAM J, BSc (Applied Mathematics) (Cape Town), BSc (Hons) (Medical) (Biomedical Science) (Cape Town), MPhil (Epidemiology) (Cape Town)
Director, Maternal and Child Health Information and Resource Centre, University of Cape Town

ISAÄCSON M, MB BCh, MD, DSc (Med), DPH, DTM & H (Wits)
Emeritus Professor of Tropical Diseases, School of Pathology, University of the Witwatersrand

JACKLIN L, MB BCh (Wits), MMed (Pretoria), FCP (Paeds) (SA), MSc (Med) Child Health (Wits)
Principal Paediatrician, The Memorial Institute for Child Health and Development, Department of Paediatrics and Child Health, University of the Witwatersrand

JACOBS ME, MB ChB DCM (Cape Town), FCP (SA)
Stella and Paul Loewenstein Professor of Child Health, Department of Paediatrics and Child Health, University of Cape Town

JEENA PM, MBChB, FCP (Paeds), FCP (Pulmonolgy)
Senior Lecturer, Senior Specialist, Department of Paediatrics and Child Health, University of Natal

KATZ B, BA (Speech and Hearing Therapy) (Wits), HDipEdAd (Wits)
Manager, Outreach Community Service, Sunshine Centre, Johannesburg

KIBEL MA, MB BCh (Wits), FRCP (Edinburgh), DCH RCP & S (London)
Emeritus Loewenstein Professor of Child Health, Department of Paediatrics and Child Health, University of Cape Town

KLUGMAN KP, BSc (Hons), MB BCh, MMed, PhD, DTM & H (Wits), MRCPath (London), FFPath (SA), FRSS Afr
Professor and Chairman of the School of Pathology, University of the Witwatersrand; Director of the MRC

Pneumococcal Diseases Research Unit; Director of the South African Institute for Medical Research

KROMBERG JGR, BA (Social Work), MA, PhD (Wits)
Honorary Professor, Department of Human Genetics, University of the Witwatersrand; Principal genetic Counsellor, Queensland Genetics Service, Australia

LACHMAN PI, BA, MB BCh (Wits), MMed (Paeds) (Cape Town), FCP (SA), DCH (SA)
Clinical Director, Women and Children Services Division; Deputy Medical Director, North West London Hospitals NHS Trust; Consultant Paediatrician, Northwick Park Hospital, Harrow

LEARY PM, MB ChB MD (Cape Town), FCP (SA), DObst RCOG, DA (London), DCG (London), DCH RCP & S (Eng), DA RCP & S (Eng)
Emeritus Associate-Professor, Department of Paediatrics and Child Health, University of Cape Town

LEWIS HA, DH, DHSM (Wits)
Honorary Lecturer, Department of Community Dentistry, Faculty of Health Sciences, University of the Witwatersrand

LOENING WEK, FCPaeds (SA)
Emeritus Loewenstein Professor of Child Health, University of Natal; Senior Specialist, Department of Health (National)

LOFFEL J, BA (Social Work), PhD (Wits)
Advocacy Co-ordinator for Johannesburg Child Welfare Society

LLOYD G, BA (UCT), Dip Spec Ed (orally impaired), M Ed (UNISA), PhD (Wits)
Education Manager, Sunshine Centre, Johannesburg

MOLTENO CD, BA (Hons) (Sociology) (Unisa), PhD (Cape Town), MD (Cape Town), MMed (Paeds) (Cape Town), FCP (SA), MB ChB DCH RCP (London)
Vera Grover Professor of Mental Handicap, Department of Psychiatry, University of

Cape Town

PETTIFOR JM, MB BCh, PhD (Wits), FCP (Paeds) (SA), DCH
Professor and Head, Department of Paediatrics and Child Health, University of the Witwatersrand

PHILOTHEOU A, BA (Hons), MB ChB (Cape Town)
Senior Lecturer, Department of Paediatrics and Child Health, University of Cape Town

POWER DJ, MD (Cape Town), MB BS DCH (London), DCH MRCP (UK), DCM MD (Cape Town)
Professor and Head, Department of Paediatrics and Child Health, University of Cape Town

RICHTER LM, BA (Psych), PhD (Natal)
Professor and Head, School of Psychology, University of Natal, Pietermaritzberg

ROBERTSON BA, MD (Cape Town), DPM (McGill)
Professor and Head, Department of Psychiatry, University of Cape Town

RUDOLPH MJ, BDS, MSc (Witwatersrand), MPH (Harvard)
Professor and Head, Division of Community Dentistry, Department of Community Health, Faculty of Health Sciences, University of the Witwatersrand

SALOOJEE H, MB BCh (Wits), MSc (Med) (Wits), FCPaeds (SA)
Senior Lecturer, Division of Community Paediatrics, University of the Witwatersrand; Principal Specialist, Chris Hani Baragwanath Hospital

SEMPLE F, BSc (Physio) (Wits)
Chief Paediatric Physiotherapist, Johannesburg Hospital

SCHOUB BD, MB BCh, MMed (Microbiol Path) MD, DSc, FRCPath, FRSSAf
Director, National Institute of Virology; Professor and Head, Department of Virology, University of the Witwatersrand

SWINGLER GH, PhD (Cape Town) FCPaeds (SA)

Senior Lecturer, Department of Paediatrics and Child Health, University of Cape Town

VAN COEVERDEN DE GROOT HA, MB ChB (Cape Town), FRCOG (London)
Emeritus Associate-Professor of Community Obstetrics, Department of Obstetrics and Gynaecology, University of Cape Town

VILJOEN D, MB ChB (Birm), MD (Cape Town), DCH (SA), FCPaeds (SA)
Professor and Head, Department of Human Genetics, SAIMR and University of the Witwatersrand

WAGSTAFF LA, D Sc (Med) (Hons), FRCPCH (UK) (Hon), MB BCh, DipPaeds (Wits), DCH, DObst, RCOG (London), FRCP (Edin)
Emeritus Loewenstein Professor of Community Paediatrics, University of the Witwatersrand

WEINBERG EG, MB ChB (Cape Town), FCP (SA)
Associate-Professor, Department of Paediatrics and Child Health, University of Cape Town

WOODS DL, MB ChB MD (Cape Town), FRCP (UK), DCH RCP & S (London)
Associate-Professor, Department of Paediatrics and Child Health, University of Cape Town

..................................................

We are grateful to the following who contributed to previous editions. Those whose original material is still largely retained, are included in the chapter headings of this edition:

BEATTY DW, MB ChB MD (Cape Town), FCP (SA)

BEETON H, DIP (OT) (US), BA (SA)

BOWIE MD, BSc (Natal), MB ChB MD (Cape Town), FRCP (Edinburgh), DCH RCP & S (London)

CARSTENS IL, BDS (Wits), HDDent (Wits)

CHIKTE UME, BChD (UWC), MDent (Wits), MSc (UCL), DHSM (Wits)

HANSEN JDL, MD (Cape Town), FRCP (London), DCH (London)

HAY IT, MB BCh (Pretoria), MRCP (London), MMed (Paediatrics) (Pretoria), DCH (London)

HOOGENDOORN L, State Registered Nurse and Midwife, Diploma in Paediatrics, Community Health Science (Cape Town)

HOUSEHAM KC, MB BCh (Cape Town), MD (Cape Town), FCP (SA), DCH (SA)

JENKINS T, MD (London), MRCS, LRCP, DRCOG (London), FRSSAP

JOUBERT G, BA, BSc (Hons) (Cape Town)

KIBEL SM, MB ChB (Cape Town), DCH (SA)

LABADARIOS D, BSc (Hons), MBChB, PhD, FACN

ROSEN EU, BMus, MB ChB (Paeds) (Cape Town), DCH (London), MPH (UC Berkley)

SCHALL R, BSc (Hons) (Cape Town), DipMath (Karlsruhe), PhD (Cape Town)

SCHOEMAN CJ, MB ChB (Pretoria), MMed (Paeds) (Cape Town), DCH (London), DCM (OFS)

SCHREIER AR, MA (SocWk), PhD (Wits)

URBAN M, MB BCh, BSc (Med) (Wits), MRCP (Paeds) (UK)

WAGNER JM, MB BCh (Wits), FRCP (London)

YACH D, MBChB, BSc (Hons) (Epidemiology) (Cape Town), MPH

..................................................

We are grateful to the following for their advice and assistance:

Dr J Kulig, Dr C Roberts and Dr H Zar

# Preface

Southern Africa has a kaleidoscope of communities, with a diversity of health care needs variously met or unmet by available services. The children of this vast subcontinent may be categorized as belonging to the developing or developed world, as privileged, deprived, or disadvantaged, as rural or urban, and as members of different nationalities and cultures. All these children should be given the opportunity to reach their full potential.

In a foreword to the first edition of *Child Health for All* in 1991, Professor John Hansen made reference to 'far reaching political and social changes, which were of fundamental relevance to child health in South Africa'.

The second edition in 1995 saw the dawning of democracy in South Africa and in the foreword the then Minister of Health Dr Nkosazana Dlamini-Zuma stressed the pivotal issue of child health in a progressive primary health care policy. South Africa has ratified the Convention on the Rights of the Child and there is political will and action and societal concern to meet the agreed commitments. Unfortunately, the major impediments to practical implementation of these rights remain poverty, unemployment, violence, and the increasing problem of human immuno-deficiency virus infection.

This new millennium edition aims to further promote and achieve 'child health for all in southern Africa'. The book has been compiled to meet the varying needs of the wide spectrum of health care personnel who provide child health care. While some may merely seek practical guidance and a broad outline of a subject; others may choose to study topics in greater depth. Information is included on promotive and preventive health care and community-based management of children with special needs. Attention is given to major determinants of child health, to the monitoring and measuring of child health, and to the provision of related services.

Broad practical guidelines are included as well as more in-depth information about selected topics such as immunization, nutrition, child development, children with special needs, tuberculosis, HIV/AIDS, and diarrhoeal disease. The book is not intended to replace but rather to complement standard clinical textbooks. References have had to be limited and some further recommended reading is listed.

Recently there have been significant developments in the delivery of child health care, in particular the integrated management of childhood illness (IMCI). The important role and functions of colleagues in the allied disciplines are being adapted to changing circumstances and also expanded considerably.

We welcome the new contributors, and, at the same time, wish to express our gratitude and thanks to those who have assisted previously. Their efforts contributed greatly to the success of earlier editions, and much of their work is still apparent in these pages.

We trust that *Child Health for All* will continue to serve our readers and the children of the subcontinent for decades to come.

The Stella and Paul Loewenstein Educational and Charitable Trust has enabled the production of this third edition, via a grant to O'Dowd Outreach, and thus have maintained a long-term commitment to promoting child health.

*Maurice Kibel and Lucy Wagstaff*
*Emeritus Loewenstein Professors*

# PART ONE

# Introduction

This part introduces the rights of the child and outlines the broad principles of the discipline of child health. These principles are elaborated on in later chapters. The conditions under which people live are basic to the spread and severity of infectious disease: water supplies, sanitation, housing, heating, ventilation, food supply, and storage all impact on the health of the child. In this section, the physical and psychosocial factors of the child's environments are also described.

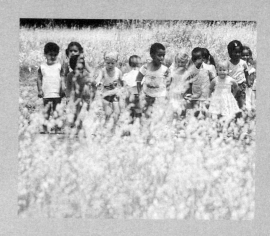

# 1    Introduction

**MA KIBEL &
LA WAGSTAFF**

Children are our most precious asset, and their well-being reflects the future of the nation. Children differ from adults in two important ways: they are growing and developing, and they are dependent on others for sustenance and protection. In order to grow, develop, and thrive, children need adequate nutrition, protection from the environment, essential health care, and an emotionally nurturing family setting. Deficiencies in one or more of these components are why millions of children around the world still die unnecessarily every year, and why untold millions fail to reach their genetically endowed potential.

Children have always been seen as vulnerable and in need of protection, but only recently have attempts been made to entrench the rights of children in law. The first such attempt was the Declaration on the Rights of the Child in 1959, which was adopted by the United Nations. But declarations are statements of general principles; no government is compelled to carry out principles. A convention, on the other hand, is a detailed international agreement, and its ratification means that a country commits itself to the items listed in it (McCurdie, 1992). Such a Convention on the Rights of the Child was adopted by the United Nations in November 1989, and has been ratified by all the nations of southern Africa.

The document is unique in its breadth, bringing together in one comprehensive code the legal benefits and stipulations concerning children, which were previously scattered through scores of other international agreements of varying scope and status. It applies to all persons under the age of 18 years, except where national law dictates that children attain their majority at an earlier age.

The rights enshrined in the Convention apply equally to all children, with no regard to race, colour, sex, language, religion, political or other opinion, national, ethnic or social origin, property, disability, birth or other status. Another fundamental principle is that the best interests of the child should be used as the touchstone for all decisions affecting children's health, well-being, and dignity.

## The three main areas of children's rights

The provisions of the Convention apply to three main areas of children's rights: survival, development, and protection.

- *Survival:* the first specific right mentioned is the inherent right to life. States must ensure, to the maximum extent possible, the survival and development of the child. The Convention recognizes the right of access to health care services (such as immunization and oral rehydration therapy), and to an adequate standard of living (including food, clean water, and a place to live). In addition, the child has the right to a name and a nationality.
- *Development:* to allow all individuals the chance to develop to their potential, the Convention contains provisions relating to the child's right to education, to rest and leisure, to freedom of expression and information, and to freedom of thought, conscience, and religion. It also stipulates that parents shall give due weight to the views of children, in accordance with their age and maturity.
- *Protection:* many of the Convention's provisions are designed to provide protection for children in a wide range of circumstances. Some deal with mentally or physically disabled children, others with refugees or orphans, or with children who are separated from their parents. It also recognizes that, in some cases, children need to be protected from their own parents, or may be in a situation where the parents are unable to take proper care of them.

The Convention also covers economic, sexual, and other forms of child exploitation, and requires that appropriate measures be taken to protect children from the use and sale of drugs. In addition, it sets out the rights of children in times of armed conflict, and of children who are in trouble with the law (UNICEF, 1990).

These new attitudes to children, admirable as they are, will only have meaning when they are enforced. The reality is that a large proportion of the world's children are growing up in circumstances of extreme poverty and disadvantage. Their future holds only the prospect of hunger, illness, poor education, unemployment, and lack of opportunities.

Wars and civil conflicts are taking a massive toll on children. In the past decade many millions have died, been disabled, or have been displaced from their families as a result of conflict (UNICEF, 1996). The use of children as fighters (made possible by the proliferation of lethal light weapons) is particularly reprehensible. Children have certain advantages as soldiers: They are easier to intimidate and they do as they are told. They are also less likely to run away than adults, and they do not demand salaries. Over 250 million children around the world work, and many are at risk from hazardous and exploitative labour (UNICEF, 1997). While much progress has been made in the prevention of certain infectious diseases by vaccination, the spectre of HIV/AIDS looms large, particularly in sub-Saharan Africa.

The children of the world's rural and urban poor pose the major challenges in child health, but these are not the only sectors that should command our attention. Because of unhealthy lifestyles, even modern, 'rational-purposive' societies, which enjoy all the benefits that affluence and technology can bring, are prone to a new set of ills. These include the dangers of overnutrition.

Children may also be categorized according to race or ethnic group. The southern African population is made up of black, white, coloured, and Asian groups. This only has scientific validity when related to genetically or culturally determined conditions. In South Africa race serves as an overall quasi-indicator of socio-economic status and until recently was misused in the political ideology and practices of the then government. Happily, racial classification is no longer

3

entrenched in the laws of South Africa, but racial differences remain regrettable realities. Race is referred to in this text as social class categories based on non-racial comparisons are not yet available. There are wide discrepancies between the health of the affluent and that of the poor, both rural and urban.

## Child health as a discipline

Health is defined in the constitution of the World Health Organization as a state of physical, mental, and social well-being and not merely as the absence of disease or infirmity. This definition has been strongly criticized. It defines the health of the individual rather than that of the community, and it fails to recognize that health problems may lie in society and not in the individual. It does not acknowledge that children with disabilities may be healthy (Colver et al., 1989). A child's health is perhaps better defined as a state of well-being and effective functioning that is satisfactory to the child and his or her environment. The discipline of child health is concerned with the realization of this optimal state of well-being and effective functioning. It embraces the health of children in the various developmental phases from conception to delivery:

- the prenatal and perinatal periods;
- infancy;
- the pre-school years (two to six years);
- later childhood; and
- adolescence and youth.

Any consideration of a child's health must always include the health of the mother, for the health of mother and child are intimately related. The mother or substitute child-care person has a fundamentally important role in maintaining and promoting the health of her child. Recognition of this is reflected in the thrust for female education, which has been shown to be an important determinant of child well-being. The mother–child dyad is crucially important as women and children are generally the first victims of poverty. Hence maternal and child health occupies a pivotal place in many communities.

## Aspects of child health

The discipline of child health embraces the following aspects:

*Comprehensive paediatrics:* This is the way all paediatrics should be practised. Comprehensive paediatrics is promotive, preventive, curative, and, where necessary, rehabilitative. In the assessment of the individual child it aims to include all these components of care. Where indicated, points of failure in the prevention of ill health as well as deficiencies in the facilities for effective management should be identified. The concept of prevention is central to the comprehensive approach.

*Community child health:* This aspect deals with the health of groups of children rather than with individual children. Community child health lies in the ambit of the community paediatrician, the community health specialist, and the health services administrator, but every professional working with children should have an understanding of the principles and methods used.

*Community paediatrics:* This term will be used to encompass paediatrics practised in a community setting, generally at the primary care level, by nurses, medical officers or family doctors. Paediatricians who provide consultant services and education in the community rather than in hospitals, and who are skilled in such community problems as the management of child abuse and handicap, are known as community paediatricians. The community paediatrician is a useful resource person, or participant, in community health.

*Ambulatory paediatrics:* This discipline had its roots in the United States in the 1960s, when the increasing superspecialization of paediatricians with the major focus being on in-patient care led to concerns that there were no generalists available to take an over-all view of the child and the family and little emphasis was being placed on the needs of the child who did not require admission to hospital (Heller, 1994). This discipline includes primary care paediatrics, communi-ty paediatrics, accident and emergency con-sultations, out-patients, daycare paediatrics, hospital at-home schemes, and community nursing services for children. As an academic discipline it has burgeoned in North America and Australia in recent years, and the field has been split up into many subdisciplines, such as adolescent health, child abuse, and learning disabilities. In the far less resource-blessed environment of Africa this concept is attractive for its potential to bridge the gap between the hospital and primary health care: a relatively small number of well-trained ambulatory paediatricians could do much to co-ordinate and improve services for children in a whole region.

# Methods of assessment

The aim of community child health is to improve the health of all children in a com-munity. The methods of assessment involve:
- assessment of the health status of the child in the community and the identifica-tion and formulation of the problems;
- selecting such problems for remedial action in terms of their priority;
- planning and taking remedial action to alleviate the problems; and
- evaluating the effects of such action.

# 1 ASSESSMENT OF HEALTH STATUS

## The definitive measures of child health

The dynamic process of physical, intellectual, and emotional growth offers a unique way to assess the well-being of individuals or groups of children. The definitive measures of child health may be taken as the extent to which all children in a community achieve optimal developmental progress in terms of their physical growth and intellectual and emo-tional growth.

## Measures of physical growth

Using weight- and height-for-age as the indi-vidual measures, the status of the community can be compared with international growth standards, such as those from the National Center for Health Statistics, by calculating the percentage of children deviating from the mean. This can be expressed in standard deviations (SDs) or Z-scores for weight, height, and weight-for-height (see Chapter 16: Malnutrition). The term 'expected', as used to refer to the 50th centile for age, should not necessarily be interpreted as the correct or ideal weight or height.

## Intellectual and emotional development

This is notoriously difficult to assess accu-rately for large numbers, but a convenient method involves a survey of the school achievements of a satisfactory sample of chil-dren. More sophisticated methods involve formal psychometric and other psychological testing, such as school readiness evaluation.

## 2 OTHER MEASURES OF CHILD HEALTH

Certain other methods can be used conveniently as indicators of child health because they have been shown to have marked effects upon the developmental processes themselves. They are thus indirect measures of child health.

### Health services for children

The provision of adequate health services for children may be assessed by examining:
- *Health service provision:* rate of provision of first contact care facilities; number of hospital beds for children per unit population; and the rate of provision of facilities for chronic conditions.
- *Health service use:* percentage of children under five years regularly attending child health clinics; rates of occupancy of children's beds in hospitals; and the duration of bed occupancy in above.
- *Outcome of health service use:* level of community protection by immunization procedures; specific hospital mortality rates; morbidity profiles; and therapeutic compliance.

### Nutrition

Assessment of the state of childhood nutrition in the community may involve several aspects:
- *maternal nutrition* This is related to fetal nutrition and may be evaluated by the distribution of maternal weight-for-height or the incidence of low birthweight;
- *fetal nutrition* Malnutrition of the fetus leads to growth retardation and in extreme cases to stillbirth. It may therefore be evaluated by the pattern of birthweight-for-gestational age and the stillbirth rate (see Chapter 11: The low birthweight infant);
- *nutrition of the infant and child* This may be assessed by the prevalence in the community of each category of malnutrition: underweight (less than 80 per cent of expected weight for age), marasmus (less than 60 per cent of expected weight for age), and kwashiorkor (any child with nutritional oedema). This is the Wellcome classification. More useful for statistical purposes is the use of SD scores, referred to earlier.
- prevalence of *specific nutritional deficiencies* e.g., iron, vitamin A, iodine (see Chapter 16: Malnutrition).

### Functioning of the family in the community

A picture of the quality of family functioning within the community may be obtained by studying factors such as:
- family income;
- social class;
- family size;
- mother's age;
- parents' marital state;
- parental education;
- identity of child's caretaker;
- marital disruption;
- domestic overcrowding;
- level of basic amenities (provision and use of); and
- postnatal separation of mother and infant.

### Illness in childhood

For a variety of reasons it is difficult to measure the frequency of episodes of acute illness among children in a community. Therefore, the following are often used as indicators:
- the age-specific incidence/prevalence of particular acute conditions, including notifiable infectious diseases;
- the age-specific incidence of chronic disease/disability; and
- comparison of morbidity patterns in first contact care with those of hospital admissions.

## Disability

The prevalence, types, and causes of disability are an essential part of the picture of child health in a community. These include:
- cerebral palsy;
- learning disability; and
- sight and hearing loss.

## Death

Death is the most commonly used index of child health because of its finality and the relative ease of its measurement. Measurements of mortality are as follows:
- stillbirth rate – the number of stillbirths per 1 000 total births;
- perinatal mortality rate – the number of stillbirths over 500 g and deaths during the first week of life per 1 000 total births and stillbirths;
- early neonatal mortality rate – the number of deaths in first week per 1 000 live births;
- neonatal mortality rate – the number of deaths under 28 days in a year per 1 000 live births;
- post-neonatal mortality rate – the number of deaths from 29 days to first birthday per 1 000 live births;
- infant mortality rate – the number of deaths in first year per 1 000 live births;
- under-five mortality rate – the number of deaths under five years per 1 000 live births;
- age-specific mortality rate – the number of deaths in the specified age range per 1 000 children in that age range (see Chapter 26: Epidemiology).

All the above rates can be broken down into causes of death. Ideally the following factors should also be considered:
- birthweight;
- birth order;
- gestational age; and
- maternal age.

These factors have profound effects on the death rates of children under five years.

The sources of information for the above assessment of child health status are:
- published data – reports of Public Health Authorities (e.g., Medical Officers of Health, State Health Departments, and the Hospital Departments of Provincial Administrations);
- surveys published in press – medical, educational, and sociological; and
- unpublished data – may be collected by surveys, which need not be large or costly. An alternative would be the use of rapid assessment techniques.

Once the picture of child health is as complete as available data and resources allow, problems can be identified, their possible remedies formulated, and their priorities assessed.

A very useful source of information on global child health is the *State of the World's Children* published annually by UNICEF.

A Situation Analysis of Children and Women in South Africa was sponsored by UNICEF and the National Children's Rights Committee, and was published in June 1993. This lists the following goals to be implemented by all countries, adapted appropriately to specific needs:

## Major goals for child survival, development, and protection

- Between 1990 and the year 2000, reduction of infant and under-five child mortality rate by one-third or to 50 and 70 per 1 000 live births respectively, whichever is less;
- Between 1990 and the year 2000, reduction of maternal mortality rate by half;
- Between 1990 and the year 2000, reduction of severe and moderate malnutrition among under-five children by half;

7

- Universal access to safe drinking water and to sanitary means of excreta disposal;
- By the year 2000, universal access to basic education and completion of primary education by at least 80 per cent of primary school-age children;
- Reduction of the adult illiteracy rate (the appropriate age group to be determined in each country) to at least half its 1990 level with emphasis on female literacy;
- Improved protection of children in especially difficult circumstances;
- Before the end of 1995, ratification of the United Nations Convention on the Rights of the Child by all countries.

# Supporting/sectoral goals

## WOMEN'S HEALTH AND EDUCATION

- special attention to the health and nutrition of the female child and to pregnant and lactating women;
- access by all couples to information and services to prevent pregnancies that are too early, too closely spaced, too late or too many;
- access by all pregnant women to prenatal care, trained attendants during childbirth, and referral facilities for high-risk pregnancies and obstetric emergencies;
- universal access to primary education with special emphasis for girls and accelerated literacy programmes for women;

## NUTRITION

- reduction in severe, as well as moderate, malnutrition among under-five year old children to half of 1990 levels;
- reduction of the rate of low birthweight (2,5 kg or less) to less than ten per cent;

- reduction of iron deficiency anaemia in women by one-third of the 1990 levels;
- virtual elimination of iodine deficiency disorders by 1995;
- virtual elimination of vitamin A deficiency and its consequences, including blindness;
- empowerment of all women to breast-feed their children exclusively for four to six months and to continue breast-feeding with complementary food well into the second year;
- dissemination of knowledge and supporting services to increase food production to ensure household food security.

## CHILD HEALTH

- global eradication of poliomyelitis by the year 2000;
- elimination of neonatal tetanus by 1995;
- a 90 per cent reduction in measles cases and a 95 per cent reduction in measles deaths, compared to pre-immunization levels;
- achievement and maintenance of at least 90 per cent immunization coverage of one-year-old children and universal tetanus immunization for women in the childbearing years;
- a halving of child deaths caused by diarrhoea and a 25 per cent reduction in diarrhoeal diseases;
- a one-third reduction in child deaths caused by acute respiratory infections; the elimination of guineaworm disease.

## References and further reading

COLVER A, ALLSOP M, and MCKINLEY I. 1989. *Measurement of child health: report of a working party of the community paediatric group.* London: British Paediatric Association.

DAVIE R, BUTLER N, and GOLDSTEIN K. 1972. *From birth to seven.* London: Longman.

HELLER DR. 1994. Stepping out in a new direction? *Ambulatory Paediatrics.* 70(4):339–42.

MCCURDIE J. 1992. *Children's rights. Developing justice series.* Cape Town: University of Cape Town.

MITCHELL RG. 1987. *Child health in the community.* Edinburgh: Churchill Livingstone.

MOLTENO CD, KIBEL MA, and ROBERTS M. 1986. Child health in South Africa. In: S Burman & P Reynolds (eds.). *Growing up in a divided society.* Johannesburg: Ravan Press.

NATIONAL CHILDREN'S RIGHTS COMMITTEE. 1993. *Children and women in South Africa: a situation analysis.*

POLNAY L & HULL D. 1993. *Community paediatrics* 2nd ed. Edinburgh: Churchill Livingstone.

UNICEF. 1990. *State of the world's children.* Oxford: Oxford University Press.

UNICEF. 1996. *State of the world's children.* Oxford: Oxford University Press.

UNICEF. 1997. *State of the world's children.* Oxford: Oxford University Press.

# 2

# Environmental influences on child health

MA KIBEL &
TA GUTHRIE

The environmental impact on the health of children is an issue that has gained recognition and importance internationally. The United Nations Convention on the Rights of the Child draws attention to the dangers and risks of environmental pollution and states that children have the right to be provided with clean drinking water and a generally clean and safe environment where they can grow up and play. The South African Constitution states that everyone has the right to an environment that is not harmful to his or her health or well-being.

It is within this 'rights' framework that we examine many aspects of the physical environment and its impact on child health. Environment is defined as the biosphere in which people and other organisms live. Pollution is the introduction into the environment of any substance or property (including radiation, heat, and noise) that has harmful effects on humanity or the environment, or that makes the environment less fit for its intended use.

## The physical environment

Clean water for drinking and washing, hygienic disposal of domestic and human waste, protection from the elements, and clean air are the essentials of a health-promoting physical environment. The availability of piped water supplies, water-borne sanitation, and electrification have made a huge impact on public health, and these amenities are now taken for granted in the urban environment of the developed world.

### WATER QUALITY AND ACCESSIBILITY

Large numbers of South Africans are still without access to clean drinking water and adequate sanitation, particularly within the rural areas (Genthe & Seager, 1996). Often a family's water supply is completely untreated and the water may have to be laboriously transported for long distances. This task is generally delegated to women, requiring them to expend considerable time and energy. Adverse effects on their nutritional status and the associated consequences for their babies are particularly significant during pregnancy and lactation. In

10

addition, the drain on a mother's time and energy may limit her ability to become involved in other activities, including child rearing and self-fulfilment in her community.

Sewage disposal in the modern sense may be non-existent, and pollution of water by sewage is still the major source of contamination. Under these conditions water- and food-borne infections flourish. Episodes of diarrhoea are common in the young child and constitute a major cause of death in infancy. Factors leading to the triad of diarrhoea, malnutrition, and infection are shown in Figure 2.1. Water and diseases have a complex relationship – diseases such as cholera, typhoid, dysentery, and intestinal parasites may be prevented not only by improving water quality but also by increasing its accessibility and quantity.

Health workers need to be aware of the implications of these water issues for bottle-feeding – the water used for the preparation of commercial milk formulae and the cleaning of utensils must not be contaminated.

Infections of the scalp, skin, and eyes (common problems in poor communities) are related to a lack of water for bathing. Bilharzia, a water-related disease dependent on an aquatic host, occurs when communities derive their water supply from untreated water, or live close to natural water bodies. Finally, insect vectors, which breed and bite near water, may be responsible for tropical diseases. The most important of these is malaria.

Appropriate technology has been developed to improve water collection and storage as well as sanitation.

The dramatic fall in mortality in the cities is largely a result of the increased availability of piped water, the improved disposal of sewage, and the general improvement in hygiene (and especially in food handling techniques). Where efficient chlorination systems exist with piped water supplies, the contamination of natural water with faecal coliforms becomes less important. Thus many rivers and river outlets are heavily contaminated, but the municipal water supplies are still of a high quality. The quality of water supplies can be assessed by counting indicator organisms such as faecal coliforms in water samples.

## Chemicals in water

Excessive levels of heavy metals and other elements, resulting particularly from industrial pollution, are a problem in some countries. Such pollution – with, for example, arsenic, cadmium, mercury, and lead – may be widely distributed to areas far removed from the source of the contaminants. These problems have only occasionally been reported in southern Africa so far, but the situation is being monitored.

Excessive levels of natural fluoride are found in some water sources, resulting in isolated cases of fluorosis. However, a far greater problem is the generally low level of fluoride in our water supplies, leading to dental caries being the most widespread and universal health problem among children (see Chapter 22: Oral health).

### FOOD CONTAMINATION

Contamination of the weaning foods given to young children is a major cause of diarrhoeal disease. Freshly cooked foods are generally acceptable in quality, but, in poor environments, high levels of pathogens can be detected in such food when it has been left standing for even half an hour.

## Pesticides in food

DDT is the best-known pesticide used in agriculture, forestry, and public health programmes; others include aldrine, dieldrine, HCH, and lindane. However, their use in

11

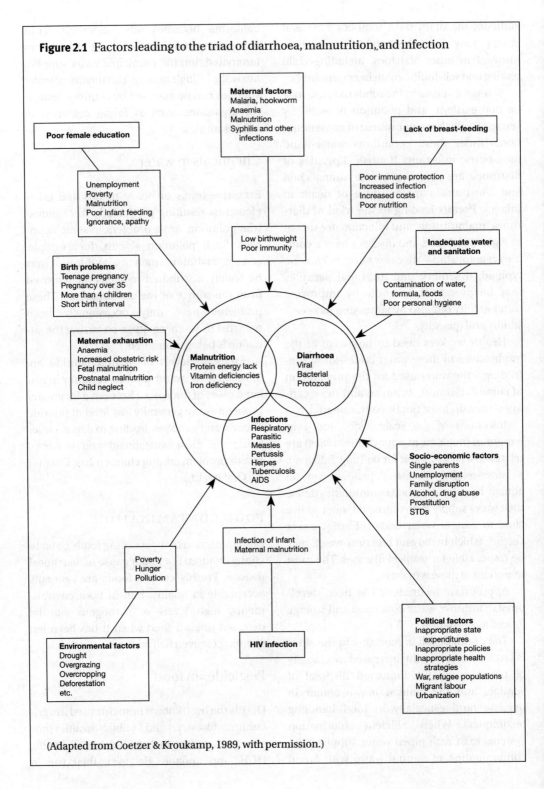

**Figure 2.1** Factors leading to the triad of diarrhoea, malnutrition, and infection

**Poor female education**

**Maternal factors**
Malaria, hookworm
Anaemia
Malnutrition
Syphilis and other
   infections

**Lack of breast-feeding**

Unemployment
Poverty
Malnutrition
Poor infant feeding
Ignorance, apathy

Poor immune protection
Increased infection
Increased costs
Poor nutrition

Low birthweight
Poor immunity

**Inadequate water and sanitation**

**Birth problems**
Teenage pregnancy
Pregnancy over 35
More than 4 children
Short birth interval

Contamination of water,
   formula, foods
Poor personal hygiene

**Maternal exhaustion**
Anaemia
Increased obstetric risk
Fetal malnutrition
Postnatal malnutrition
Child neglect

**Malnutrition**
Protein energy lack
Vitamin deficiencies
Iron deficiency

**Diarrhoea**
Viral
Bacterial
Protozoal

**Infections**
Respiratory
Parasitic
Measles
Pertussis
Herpes
Tuberculosis
AIDS

**Socio-economic factors**
Single parents
Unemployment
Family disruption
Alcohol, drug abuse
Prostitution
STDs

Poverty
Hunger
Pollution

Infection of infant
Maternal malnutrition

**Political factors**
Inappropriate state
   expenditures
Inappropriate policies
Inappropriate health
   strategies
War, refugee populations
Migrant labour
Urbanization

**Environmental factors**
Drought
Overgrazing
Overcropping
Deforestation
etc.

**HIV infection**

(Adapted from Coetzer & Kroukamp, 1989, with permission.)

12

many industrialized countries has been banned or severely restricted because of their potential toxicity and their ability to persist in the environment and accumulate in animals and humans. There are special concerns about children in terms of neurotoxicity from the use of DDT in rural areas. However, harmful effects have not yet been clearly delineated, and at present these dangers remain largely theoretical.

## Toxins and industrial chemicals in food

Food can deteriorate during storage because of fungal growth, and toxins produced by these fungi may have long-term effects. In children, aflatoxin has been incriminated as a cause of kwashiorkor, but the issue remains debatable. As far as industrial chemicals in food are concerned, the greatest worry centres around three substances – polychlorinated bipheniles (PCBs), lead, and cadmium. PCBs also occur in milk (including breast-milk) and are highest in fish.

### URBANIZATION

Urbanization refers to the move from rural areas to urban areas. Urbanization is intensifying world-wide, but particularly in developing countries, where people, driven by many factors (economic, social, and political), move from depleted rural agricultural areas to urban shanty-towns within and on the periphery of cities. In 1950, 17 per cent of people in developing countries lived in urban areas; by the year 2000 this figure is expected to have increased to 45 per cent. In southern Africa, these huge population shifts, combined with high rates of natural increase, have outstripped the available amenities resulting in gross deficiencies in urban housing (Von Schirnding & Aucamp, 1991). In such settings, environmental contamination and overcrowding ensure

optimal conditions for the transmission of micro-organisms by contact, droplets, dust, food, water, and insect and animal vectors.

Another serious consequence of urbanization is the accumulation of solid waste, such as plastic, tin cans, and glass. South Africa has an extremely high rate of production of plastic bags per capita, while having inadequate disposal and recycling mechanisms to cope with these quantities.

### HOUSING

Overcrowding and poor ventilation are major causes of airborne infections.

Apart from acute respiratory infections of viral aetiology these infections also include meningitis, streptococcal infections and their complications (rheumatic fever and acute nephritis), tuberculosis, and the vaccine-preventable diseases (measles, whooping cough, diphtheria, and *Haemophilus influenzae* type B). Damp and mould have been shown to be important factors in increasing the number of asthmatic attacks and acute respiratory infections in general.

Indoor pollution from wood, coal, or gas fires and paraffin burners is also an important cause of higher frequencies of respiratory infections in children (Mbuli et al., 1996).

It has been estimated that some 3,5 billion people still rely predominantly on biofuels (wood, dung, and crop residues) for domestic energy. This fuel is typically burned in open fires or simple stoves, often indoors, and rarely with adequate ventilation or chimneys. This leads to extremely high levels of air pollution, to which women and young children in particular are exposed for many hours a day.

### ENVIRONMENTAL TOBACCO SMOKE

Environmental Tobacco Smoke (ETS) is one of the most common indoor environmental pollutants to which children are exposed, often beginning before birth and continuing throughout childhood. The preliminary findings of the Birth-to-Ten study conducted recently in South Africa indicated that 64 per cent of children in South Africa are living with a tobacco smoker in their homes (Steyn et al., 1999).

Many studies have confirmed the effects of tobacco smoke on the health of children:

- increased incidence of asthma, pneumonia, and bronchitis;
- increased incidence of middle ear disease; and
- increased risk of sudden infant death (see Chapter 49: Sudden Infant Death Syndrome).

Maternal smoking during pregnancy is a further hazard to unborn children; it has been found to double the risk of Intra-uterine Growth Restriction (IUGR) and low birthweight, as well as increasing the risk of ectopic pregnancies and fetal and infant deaths (Horta et al., 1997). Also of importance is the fact that *non-smoking* pregnant women exposed to ETS (i.e., as 'passive smokers') place their babies at risk of low birthweight, a fact of which most women are unaware. Different smoking patterns exist between the different racial groups in South Africa, but overall it was found that 21 per cent of women smoked during pregnancy and 50 per cent of pregnant women were exposed to environmental tobacco smoke (Steyn et al., 1997).

With regard to active smoking by children and youth, increasing numbers of youth are smoking and beginning at earlier ages. Obviously these youths are exposed to the same health risks as adult smokers. However, there are differences in prevalence between countries, between rural and urban areas, between socio-economic groups, and between races and genders (Guthrie et al., 1999). The internal documents of the tobacco industry provide much evidence of their aggressive marketing campaigns, which target teenagers specifically. Banning of all tobacco advertising and promotional events by the industry is a powerful way to curb this influence over the youth.

## INDUSTRIAL POLLUTION

Atmospheric pollution with smoke has been recognized as a health hazard ever since the beginning of the Industrial Revolution. The most obvious effects of air pollution are seen in an increased incidence of lower respiratory infections, such as bronchitis and pneumonia, which are most marked at the extremes of life – in old people and in infants under one year. The motor vehicle is the principal source of major air pollutants in urban areas. In city centres, motor traffic accounts for practically all the carbon monoxide, about 60 per cent of the oxides of nitrogen and hydrocarbons, 10 per cent of the oxides of sulphur, and about half the particulate matter in the air.

The principal respiratory irritants are sulphur dioxide, oxides of nitrogen, and suspended particulate matter. Children are much more susceptible than adults because of their narrow airways and lower resistance to infection. Apart from the general effect on all children, those with heart and lung diseases are potentially more sensitive. Children with asthma also constitute a large group at risk.

Carbon monoxide in the atmosphere is absorbed and bound permanently to haemoglobin as carboxyhaemoglobin. Measurable effects may be observed when blood levels of carboxyhaemoglobin are as low as 2.5 per cent. Children with cardiovascular diseases may be at special risk in this respect. Raised carbon monoxide levels are also thought to be the pathway by which smoking adversely affects the fetus *in utero*; to be responsible for the postnatal growth failure; and for the higher incidence of cot deaths, which are a feature in infants of tobacco-smoking mothers.

## LEAD

The greatest concerns regarding motor car exhaust emission revolve around the release of alkyl lead into the atmosphere. In southern Africa petrol still contains this substance as an anti-knocking agent, although the levels have been reduced in recent years. About ten per cent of the lead released from exhausts is deposited within 30 to 50 metres of the road. The rest is distributed into the air and can be transported over considerable distances. The lead from petrol may thus be absorbed directly by inhalation, indirectly via its incorporation into dust and water supplies, or from deposition on the surface of plants. Dusty homes in the inner city areas are also a special risk for children as house and street dust may be heavily lead-contaminated. Peeling paint from old buildings often has a very high lead content and is a well-known source of poisoning. With increasing awareness, other sources of lead poisoning have come to light: for example, electric kettles, that have been poorly soldered, and pottery glazes.

The clinical effects of severe lead poisoning in children – generally an acute encephalopathy, with drowsiness, followed by convulsions and coma – have long been recognized, and are associated with levels of lead in the blood in the order of 50 microgrammes per decilitre (2,5 µmol/l) and higher. Over the past twenty years our understanding of the harmful effects of lead has changed substantially. A number of carefully conducted studies in several different countries have shown that lead has detrimental effects on learning ability and behaviour in children at levels previously considered safe. These effects are directly related to blood lead level (Vos et al., 1997). As more and more sensitive measures and better study designs have been used, the generally recognized level for lead toxicity has shifted downwards and begins well below 25 microgrammes per decilitre (1,21 µmol/l).

The great majority of these studies have been conducted in developed countries. There is as yet little information from the Third World on the environmental impact of lead or on its role in furthering disadvantage in childhood (Mathee et al., 1996). Higher rates of school failure are a consistent feature in disadvantaged communities, and many factors detract from satisfactory school performance in such communities. Family dysfunction, social problems, and ineffective school systems may be viewed as external adverse factors. Chronic undernutrition, particularly when initiated prenatally, and chronic iron depletion are additional factors that add to learning impairment. Lead toxicity could well have an additive effect to these other risk factors. The effects of lead may be small, but are important in the context of other aspects of disadvantage.

## INDOOR POLLUTION IN MODERN CITIES

While outdoor air quality has rapidly and significantly improved in many first world countries, complex questions are now being raised about the possible harmful effects of indoor environments in which the use of synthetic chemicals and modern technology play a large role. The term 'tight box children' has been used for children growing up in enclosed air-conditioned environments. 'Sick Building Syndrome' refers to a constellation of symptoms often encountered in the inhabitants of certain buildings – irritation of the eyes, nose, and throat; dry mucous membranes; skin rashes; fatigue; and other symptoms have been reported. A range of volatile organic compounds has been incriminated as causes of these symptoms. Other possible harmful pollutants of the indoor environment include asbestos, non-ionizing radiation, fungal intoxicants, and allergens of various types. Lastly, the role of radon 222 that is released

15

from traces of natural radium 226 in the earth's crust has been the cause of much concern. High levels of this radiation may accumulate in the cellars of buildings, with possible but as yet theoretical long-term harmful effects.

Many children in poorer communities are exposed to environmental and health hazards in the school setting itself. Schools are often badly designed, poorly equipped, and understaffed.

## The school environment

The school environment itself can be a health hazard, forming a setting for the transmission of a wide range of infections and health disorders. This is particularly true if there is overcrowding.

Factors that need to be kept in mind if the school is to be a healthy environment are:
- ventilation;
- adequate lighting;
- temperature control;
- access to safe water;
- adequate toilet facilities;
- appropriate waste disposal mechanisms;
- sanitary environments;
- the state of the buildings; and
- clean eating places.

The quality of the school environment and the effects on the health of children impacts directly on their learning ability. It is recognized that schools provide centres for the organization and provision of environmental and health care, for the education of children in healthy living, for community action, and, in addition, that they have a major role to play in the facilitation of socio-economic and human resource development of societies (Mathee & Von Schirnding, 1994).

## CHILDREN IN PROTECTED ENVIRONMENTS

Certain acute disorders are seen characteristically in children who grow up in better-off communities. It may be speculated that these result from overprotection from infection, which leads to the infective agents gaining entry at an older age. Infectious mononucleosis (IM) is such an example. Clinically apparent IM is unusual in poor, Third World communities, and it seems likely that among such children infection occurs at a much earlier age resulting only in non-specific symptoms or no obvious illness. Herpes virus type 6 is the causative agent of roseola infantum, a common exanthem in infants between the ages of six and 18 months. This virus has been found to be passed on from mothers to infants in the first week or two of life. It is only when infants are first infected at an older age that the symptom complex of roseola infantum develops. This relative protection of young infants in better-off homes from various infections may be the explanation for the emergence of several new diseases, such as the haemolytic-uraemic syndrome, Reye syndrome, Kawasaki disease, and the haemorrhagic shock and encephalopathy syndrome.

## ALCOHOL

No discussion on environmental hazards to children would be complete without some mention of alcohol consumption, which can adversely affect their health in a variety of ways.
- Regular intake of alcohol during pregnancy has adverse effects on fetal growth and development (Fetal Alcohol Syndrome).
- Consumption of alcohol has strong associations with traffic and other accidents, child abuse, crime, family disruption, and psychosocial problems.
- The effects of chronic alcoholism on the drinker's own health are well known.

16

- Finally, as in almost all countries, alcohol and drug abuse are major problems of youth across the entire social spectrum.

Wilson and Ramphele (1989) give some indication of the seriousness of the problem of alcohol misuse in South Africa. The problems associated with liquor are not of course peculiar to the poor, but the effects on families are more severe in disadvantaged settings – effects that are wreaking havoc in both urban and, more recently, in rural areas of southern Africa. Contrary to the stated view of the liquor industry that alcohol misuse is confined to less than ten per cent of drinkers, the weight of empirical evidence supports the view that this is a gross underestimate of the number of persons at risk for alcohol-related problems (see also Chapter 9: Fetal Alcohol Syndrome).

## ACCIDENTS

The motor car is a major environmental hazard to children in urban areas because it is the main cause of serious accidental injury. In South Africa traffic accidents are now the leading cause of death after the age of one year, the rates being three times higher than in the United Kingdom.

Children are especially vulnerable to injury for several reasons (see Chapter 40: Childhood injuries). Children's height places them at a disadvantage in seeing on-coming traffic, and young children may find it hard to localize the sound of an approaching car. They are also easily distracted so they are developmentally incapable of adapting to a high traffic density environment. Poorly designed streets and the absence of pavements, both features of overcrowded, poor communities, are also conducive to traffic accidents.

Accidents in and around the home are also far more common in poor and overcrowded environments. The relative under-electrification of large areas of the subconti-

nent makes household heating costly, inefficient, and potentially injurious. Lack of electricity in the home means that hazardous forms of heating, such as open fires and paraffin burners, must be used. Burns and poisoning from paraffin are thus common accidents in these settings. As in all countries, the frequency of accidents is class related.

Technology has introduced many new hazards to the modern home, in the form of labour-saving appliances and toxic chemical preparations and medicines. Despite popular belief, accidents are not simply chance occurrences. Stresses within the family play a part, and mothers of injured children are more likely to be single or separated from their husbands, or to have physical or mental illness.

## CHILD VICTIMS OF VIOLENCE

The number of violent crimes perpetrated against children also create an unsafe physical environment. Many children are caught in the cross-fire between gangs or in drive-by shootings, as well as being subjected to many other violent crimes. The South African Child Protection Unit reported in 1998 a total of 37 352 crimes against children, of which 21 204 were sexual offences (including rape, molestation etc.); 8 613 were murder and assaults; 2 254 were abductions and kidnappings; and 5 281 others. It is difficult to obtain statistics for children who are victims of gun-shot wounds, and to ascertain whether the firearms responsible were licensed household firearms or other. In Cape Town, for the period 1992 to 1996, at least 1 736 children were victims of firearm-related incidents. A total of 322 (18,5 per cent) died (Wigton, 1998).

## Conclusion

This chapter has looked at the impact of the physical environment on the health of children.

Children have the right to a safe and healthy environment, and failure to address the issues raised in this chapter represents a violation of these rights. Governments, communities, and children should together commit to the protection and improvement of the environment, for the sake of the children and future generations.

## References and further reading

BRUCE N. 1999. Indoor air pollution. *Urban Health and Development Bulletin.* 2 (2):21–9.

COETZER PWW & KROUKAMP LM. 1989. Diarrhoeal disease – epidemiology and prevention. *South African Medical Journal.* 76:465–72.

EBRAHIM GJ. 1991. *Social and community paediatrics in developing countries.* London: Macmillan.

GENTHE B & SEAGER J. 1996. *The effect of water supply, handling and usage on water quality in relation to health indices in developing communities.* CSIR.

GUTHRIE T et al. 1999. Tobacco and child health, youth smoking patterns and control interventions in the SADC, CHPI and MRC.

HORTA BL, VICTORA CG, MENEZES AM, HALPERN R, and BARROS FC. 1997. Lowbirth weight, preterm births and intrauterine growth retardation in relation to maternal smoking. *Paediatric and Perinatal Epidemiology.* April; 11(2):140–51.

MATHEE A & VON SCHIRNDING YER. 1994. Towards environment and health promoting South African schools.

MATHEE A et al. 1996. Surveys of blood lead burdens among school children and newborns in greater Johannesburg. *Urbanisation and Health Newsletter.* 29:43–9.

MBULI et al. 1996. Exposure characterisation and potential health impacts of domestic fuel use in homes in Khayelitsha, Western Cape. *Clean Air Journal.* 9(5):11–15.

STEYN K et al. 1997. *Smoking in urban pregnant women in South Africa.* MRC.

STEYN K et al.1999. The cardiovascular disease risk factors in five-year-old urban children in South Africa. *The birth to ten study.* MRC.

VON SCHIRNDING YER & AUCAMP PJ. 1991. Urbanisation and environmental health. *South African Medical Journal.* 79:414–15.

VOS DE H, BARTEN FJ, MORALES BC. 1997. *Proceedings of the conference: urban childhood.*

WILSON F & RAMPHELE M. 1989. *Uprooting poverty: the South African challenge.* Cape Town, Johannesburg: David Philip.

WIGTON A. 1998. Firearm-related injuries in Cape Town. Children and Youth. 1992–1996. CHPI, UCT.

# 3

# Psychosocial factors in child health

## LM RICHTER

Donald Winnicott, the famous British paediatrician, once said that there is no such thing as a baby. What he meant, and his observation is profound, is that a baby is not something separate from other human beings; rather, an infant or young child is always part of a community of others and is attended by caregivers, most typically by their mothers. This illustrates the point that human beings are born into psychosocial contexts that have evolved, biologically and culturally, not only to safeguard the health and well-being of infants and young children, but also to provide the essential elements of experience necessary to stimulate the maturation of uniquely human capacities – language, the emotional reciprocity necessary to co-operate with other human beings, and mental faculties capable of creative abstract reasoning. Of course, these goals are not always reached; babies can be born with defective biological systems for a multitude of reasons, and pathological psychosocial environments sometimes fail to provide infants with the experiences necessary to fulfil their human potential. These children and their families need special understanding and care, and issues specific to them are discussed in detail

in the chapters in Part 13: Child mental health.

Psychosocial factors that influence children's health and development make up an ecological system in which features interact with each other to produce effects that, in turn, interact with other features and other outcomes (Bronfenbrenner, 1979). For this reason, it is not possible to speak about strong or linear determination between the child and any one environmental feature taken out of context. For instance, it is not appropriate to say that teen motherhood will have an invariable effect on a child, such as always to produce poorer cognitive or social development. What can be done, though, is to sketch a general map of environmental features and describe the ways in which they may affect the health and well-being of young children.

## Macro-environmental influences

At the most general level, political and economic factors determine how people live, the activities on which they base their livelihood, the health hazards to which they are exposed,

19

their access to health care, and so on. For this reason, malnutrition is a major problem in the poor developing regions of the world, such as South Asia where approximately 60 per cent of under-five-year-old children are malnourished, as well as amongst the poorest groups of people (usually immigrants, refugees, migrant labourers, and minority groups) in industrialized countries (UNICEF, 1993). In these situations, which are frequently characterized by political intolerance and economic instability, large numbers of children grow up in households with little certainty that they will have sufficient food. They also tend to be exposed to a large number of infectious agents in housing settlements with inadequate water and sanitation, as well as being subjected to social stresses that threaten traditional family and household systems for caring for young children.

Culture also has its effects on the macrosocial system. One well-known cultural effect is the preference for male children in many parts of the world. This value influences child care practices and the allocation of household resources in such a way that the health and nutrition of boys is protected at the expense of girls. Fortunately, male preference is not a cultural value of people in southern Africa. It is important to realise that cultural values are not divorced from economic issues. In fact, cultural practices sometimes become established as a result of adaptations to economic conditions, such as subsistence, and economic conditions sometimes result from cultural practices. Following the previous example, when male children in many Asian societies marry, their wives come to live in the husband's home and the labour of the new wife benefits the household. On the other hand, daughters leave home when they marry, usually after an ill-afforded dowry has been paid to her husband's family. Thus a cycle of cultural and economic conditions comes into being – one that doesn't encourage families to invest in the well-being of their daughters. Some African customs require that the husband pay 'lobola' (a negotiated number of cattle or the financial equivalent) to the family of the bride. This has a range of related implications. It may also be the practice to give priority to the father's dietary needs or wishes.

Housing settlements or neighbourhoods also affect the development of children. That environments in which children grow up differ is very apparent in the strong contrasts between rural and urban areas. However, even within urban areas in South Africa, affluent suburbs border on traditional townships and squatter settlements, and inner-city poverty exists only blocks away from high-tech hospitals and tertiary educational institutions. The health and psychosocial outcomes of children growing up in these neighbouring but contrasting sites can vary dramatically. Several studies of neighbourhood effects in the United States (Garbarino, 1985) have shown that 'good' neighbourhoods bolster the coping strategies of stressed and disorganized families, and help to maintain prosocial behaviour in children. 'Poor' neighbourhoods (for example, those with derelict housing and high crime rates), on the other hand, continually undermine the values and socialization goals of intact and well-functioning families. In a study of Sowetan families, for example, children from poor areas with high crime rates were found to show more emotional disturbances, although children with well-functioning and coping caregivers were less affected than other children (Barbarin & Richter, 1999).

These macro-social factors influence children's health and well-being both directly and indirectly. They impact on children directly by determining the physical environment in which children grow up in terms of housing, sanitation, pollution, the safety of the surroundings, the quality of health care, the education that is available to children and their families, and the amount and kind of contact children have with social institutions, like libraries, clubs, and so on. Among the most obvious macro-social impacts on children are the traumatic effects that result from children being dislocated from their families and communities during war and civil strife. However, these macro-social factors also impact on children indirectly by affecting family life and the quality of care provided for small children.

Both structural and functional aspects of households and family life are related to socio-economic and political forces. For example, the size of a family and whether or not the father is routinely present in the household are frequently related to economic security, the availability of housing, and migrant labour patterns. Similarly, how parents handle stress and conflict, whether they engage in anti-social behaviour, and how much time and energy they have for their children, are factors that are associated with income levels, distance from work, membership of a discriminated minority, and so on.

Macro-environmental factors are very important influences on children, and tend to exert their effects in one of two general directions. Materially and socially privileged environments protect children from many hazards to their health and development, and when problems occur they usually offer opportunities for compensation and intervention. On the other hand, impoverished and disadvantaged environments contain many threats to the well-being of children and they seldom have facilities or resources for dealing with problems when they do occur. For example, relatively more babies of low birthweight are born to poor women in developing countries, but there are fewer intervention programmes for the stimulation of mental and motor development, and fewer counselling facilities are available for caregivers in these settings than in health facilities catering for the middle classes in developed countries.

Poverty, whether absolute or relative, generally places children at risk. The risks begin to operate right from conception because many of the environmental influences to which the child will be exposed contain harmful or disadvantaging elements – the intra-uterine environment of an undernourished mother who may have conceived too young or too often, a crowded home environment without clean water, a family broken up by migrancy or social stress, a school without desks or qualified teachers, a neighbourhood ruled by gangs of violent youths, an economy offering few, if any, poorly paid jobs to under-educated and unqualified young people, and so on. Many of the harmful effects of poverty are believed to emanate, not from the operation of any one of these negative environmental features, but from their combined effects and enduring nature. Negative environmental influences frequently occur simultaneously and the resulting effects on children are therefore compounded. In addition, for many children in poverty there is little respite. Usually, there are only limited opportunities for children to catch up through naturally occurring or formal intervention and rehabilitation.

The ubiquitous negative effects of poverty on children, as well as the major social interventions designed to remedy them (for example, Head Start in the USA), are often conceptualized in terms of two mistaken notions (Richter, 1994). Firstly, the idea of the *culture of poverty* suggests that categories of people in society are poor, not because they are trapped in the web of prejudicial social or political organize, but because they have acquired values and patterns of behaviour that contribute to their situation – for example, they lack ambition, and are short-sighted and fatalistic. Moreover, just as they acquired these value orientations from their parents, they pass on these self-defeating attitudes to their own children, thereby creating transgenerational poverty and marginalization.

The second popular misconception of poverty can be described as the *poverty of culture*, or the idea that certain classes and cultures, specifically those other than the middle-class of developed countries, are deficient in terms of the stimulation they offer to young children. That is, they don't talk enough to their young children, don't buy them challenging toys, and don't prepare them for school or support the values of education. It is very ethnocentric to assume that Western middle-class environments and values are the universal standard for the optimum development of children. It is a notion that ignores the diversity of social and physical environments of children living in poverty as described, for example, in Pamela Reynolds's observations of children in Crossroads (1989). It also ignores the fact that poverty is created and maintained through socio-political structures that pit the rich against the poor and create conflicts between minority family environments and social institutions.

What is clear is that most parents, at least those who don't suffer from some form of serious psychopathology, rear their children as best as they can under the prevailing circumstances. Parents also rear children to be equipped for the world as they (the parents) understand and experience it. If infant mortality is a major problem in a community, one is likely to find many social and cultural practices, supported by local belief systems, to prevent childhood illnesses and to protect children from perceived harm. For example, in South Africa, many women believe that babies should not leave the household for the first ten to 30 days of their lives so that they are shielded from potential threats to their health and well-being, both physical and spiritual. For the same reason, young babies are frequently wrapped in abundant blankets when they are taken out of the home or are given over the counter and traditional remedies to ward off illnesses and misfortune.

# Family and household influences

Families and households, at least in terms of their significance for young children, vary along both structural and functional dimensions. On a structural level, they differ in terms of size and density, whether they are extended or nuclear, female or male-headed, what the age of primary caregiver is, and so on. The functional dimension refers to who does what in the household or family, and how. For example, the father might discipline the children, while the mother is indulgent on disciplinary matters; both parents decide jointly on the household budget, parents spend time playing with children when they get home from work, etc. Structural dimensions often determine the parameters of family functioning; for example, the structure of a single-parent, female-headed household in which the mother is the major breadwinner will determine how much time she has available for relaxed play with her children.

It is not very clear how structural and functional aspects of households and family life specifically influence child health and development outcomes, particularly since they, like macro-social determinants, are a level removed from children's day-to-day experience. The many characteristics of family structure and function are also likely to interact with each other. For example, a very crowded household, which has been found to have a negative impact on children in some studies, may contain many compensatory features which override the negative influences of excessive noise, lack of privacy, and so on, leading to the opposite results in other studies. Such a household may consist of several potential caregivers so that young children are exposed to a highly stimulating social environment; or else several adults may be breadwinners, all contributing to the economic status of the household, thus increasing its resources and facilities.

Two concepts that have been found helpful in understanding family and household effects on children are *stress* and *social support*. Stress is linked to negative child outcomes, probably as, among other things, it decreases the time parents have available for small children, and increases parental irritability and anti-social inclinations, making it more likely that they may abuse alcohol or act aggressively. Social support, on the other hand, has been found in many studies to mitigate the adverse effects of stress, probably through material assistance, role and work sharing, and advice, as examples. It is likely that structural and functional aspects of families and households exert their effects on children through increasing or decreasing stress and social support levels available to major caregivers.

Some child care circumstances are thought to inevitably give rise to adverse effects, like teen parenting, disrupted or broken families, and children growing up outside the home, family, and school environments. However, even in these cases, the social and cognitive outcomes of children depend on the unique circumstances of each case. A teenage girl may be a conscientious and devoted mother because the birth of her baby leads to the reciprocal love relationship for which she may have been wishing; a marital separation or divorce may be a positive resolution of problems occasioned by an abusive father and husband; a child may take to the streets in an effort to deal constructively with seemingly insoluble difficulties at home or school.

# Micro-environmental influences

What becomes clear from the above is that the most critical level of analysis for child health and development is the micro-envi-ronment of the child, consisting of the household, the family, and the child's relationships with caregivers. It is the nature of these proximal factors that creates the day-to-day experiences of children and is thereby most closely related to children's survival and developmental outcomes. While poverty and its associated negative physical and social environmental features may place children at risk, whether that risk is actualized is, to a great extent, dependent on the nature of the micro-environment of the child. The health and well-being of a baby born to a single mother living in an informal settlement with no visible means of support is crucially dependent on the psychological and social resources of the proximal caregiving environment of the child. Factors that are important to this caregiving circle are: the emotional state of the mother and her responsiveness to her baby, the social support she receives from caring others around her, the protection offered to the child by household practices, and so on.

Parenting, or the more general term 'caregiving', refers to the motives and actions of adults in their attempts to rear and socialize their small children. These factors comprise a crucial domain of influence over a child's experiences and exposures and most caregivers, except those who suffer pathological personality defects or major depression, endeavour in all ways to ensure the survival and well-being of their children. Socio-economic and other stresses can be detrimental to these motives and actions through the struggle, fatigue, and demoralization that many poor and disadvantaged women endure. Emotional withdrawal associated with pervasive low-level depression is one of the most common forms of psychological distress found among economically deprived communities who suffer chronic stress. As a consequence of their emotional retreat and isolation, caregivers may not engage in the usually ceaseless examination of young infants that is part of routine care. This surveillance is necessary to ensure that changes in infant state, feeding, appearance and so on, which may be indicative of illness, are reacted to and acted upon. When mothers and other caregiving women are overwhelmed by their social and economic circumstances, they lose the energy normally required for investment in child care. They often feel helpless and hopeless and lose any sense of confidence that they can do something about their child's health and development.

A consciousness on the part of caregivers about the importance of their perceptions and behaviour to children's health and development, as well as a belief in their capacity to fulfil children's physical and emotional needs has been found, in several studies, to be the axis around which optimal child care takes place (Tinsley & Holtgrave, 1989). These caregiving convictions, which entail a sense of pride in themselves and a belief in the meaning and coherence of their lives are, in turn, a reflection of the wider social relationships in which caregivers participate.

The implications of this model for intervention on behalf of children are the importance of affirmation, support, and encouragement for caregivers. We should also be wary of health care attitudes and practices which deplete caregivers' confidence and devalue their accomplishments under conditions of hardship that are barely imaginable. In many ways, education and 'modernity' are juxtaposed to 'traditional' in such a way that people are unsure, and even ashamed, of their cultural and common-sense skills necessary for the adequate care of their infants and young children. When this happens, the health services can become a site of humiliation rather than comfort.

## References and further reading

BARBARIN O & RICHTER L. 1999. Adversity and psychological functioning of children growing up in black townships of South Africa: Effects of community danger and socio-economic status. *Journal of Orthopsychiatry.* 69:319–27.

BRONFENBRENNER U. 1979. *The ecology of human development.* Cambridge: Harvard University Press.

GARBARINO J. 1985. Habitats for children: An ecological perspective. In: J Wohlwill & W Van Vliet (eds.). *Habitats for children: The impact of density*, pp 125–43. New Jersey: Lawrence Erlbaum.

GARBARINO J. 1992. The meaning of poverty in the world of children. *American Behavioral Scientist.* 35:220–37

REYNOLDS P. 1989. *Children in Crossroads: Cognition and society in South Africa.* Cape Town: David Philip.

RICHTER LM. 1993. Many kinds of deprivation: Young children and their families in South Africa. In: L Eldering & P Leseman (eds.). *Early intervention and culture: Preparation for literacy – the interface between theory and practice.* The Hague: UNESCO.

RICHTER LM. 1994. Economic stress and the family. In: A Dawes & D Donald (eds.). *Childhood and adversity: Psychological perspectives from South African research*, pp 28–50. Cape Town: David Philip.

TINSLEY B & HOLTGRAVE D. 1989. Maternal health locus of control beliefs, utilization of childhood preventive health services, and infant health. *Journal of Developmental and Behavioral Paediatrics.* 10:236–41.

UNICEF. 1993. *The progress of nations.* New York: UNICEF.

WORLD BANK. 1993. *World development report 1993: Investing in health.* New York: Oxford University Press.

PART TWO

# Normal growth and development

This part briefly outlines the physical, psychomotor, and emotional aspects of normal infant and child development. Puberty and adolescence are dealt with in later sections.

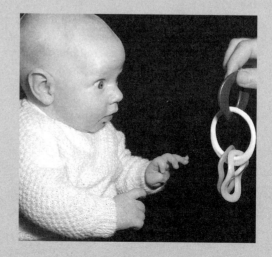

# 4

# Physical growth and development

F DE VILLIERS

## Physical growth

Health workers at all levels, from community workers to specialist paediatricians, should know the patterns of normal growth and the factors that influence these. The child is a creature constantly changing in size, shape, emotions, and abilities. Nowhere is this more obvious than in the field of physical growth.

Various ailments and anomalies may affect growth and development. A normal rate and pattern of growth on the other hand, are important indicators of the well-being of the child.

Physical growth and development in children can be divided into various stages. The embryonic period refers to the first eight weeks of development after fertilization of the ovum. The fetus develops from nine weeks after conception until birth – birth occurring (under normal circumstances) at an average of 280 days after conception. The neonatal period extends from birth to 28 days of age.

Infancy refers to the remainder of the first year of life, with early childhood spanning the pre-school period between one and six years. Puberty and adolescence, which follow later childhood, will be dealt with separately.

Each of the stages has one or more typical characteristics relating to growth and development that set it apart from the others, but there are no sharp dividing lines between the various developmental periods. Even puberty with the obvious physical changes that accompany secondary sexual development lacks a clear-cut differentiation from the pre-adolescent period.

Infancy is the period of fastest growth and thereafter growth is relatively slow and steady throughout childhood. During these stages function becomes increasingly co-ordinated and intellectual skills are developed.

Measurement of physical growth is important in the monitoring of growth and development. The measurement of weight (or for the punctilious, mass), height (or recumbent length in those younger than three years) and head circumference are most common and useful. Health workers should use every opportunity to monitor growth when a child presents for health care. The findings are recorded on a growth chart and appropriate action should follow (see Chapter 20: Child health cards – The Road to Health Chart). Growth monitoring is essential and expected standard practice.

Evaluation of the normality of a given measurement depends on a comparison of that value with values for normal children of the same age. Normal values are presented in the form of percentile charts that express the range of normal values for age from birth through various ages to maturity. An understanding of percentile charts is crucial if they are to be put to the best use in the promotion of child health.

# Derivation and interpretation of growth charts

Most growth charts are derived from cross-sectional studies. A large number of healthy children from a given population are weighed, and their heights (or recumbent lengths) and head circumferences determined in a standardized fashion by trained investigators. Their ages are also determined exactly. The measurements (e.g., weight) are sorted in age categories. In each category the measurements are sorted from lowest to highest. They are then divided into 99 equal intervals (with an equal number of measurements in each interval, but not with an equal weight difference in each interval). Each interval represents a percentage of the measurements. The lowest limit of the first interval then represents the first centile (or percentile) value, the lowest limit of the next (second) interval the second centile, and so on.

It is clear that if a child's weight falls on the 3rd centile, then 3 per cent of normal children of that age weigh the same amount or less. Similarly, if a child's weight falls on the 50th centile, 50 per cent of children weigh that much or less (and 50 per cent of normal children weigh more than that). Most children who are malnourished will fall below the 3rd centile, although some will not. Similarly, many obese children will weigh more than the 97th centile, but some will weigh less.

When centile (or percentile) values are calculated for a population or group, there is no assumption that the values are distributed in

a certain way (unlike most statistical distributions). On the contrary, the values are derived from the measurements obtained in the investigation. The percentile rank means that the equivalent per cent of values in the study falls on or beneath that numerical value. In other words, if a child's weight is on the 10th centile, then 10 per cent of children weigh the same or less.

For practical purposes cut-off points had to be established. In South Africa the 3rd and 97th centiles are used (in some other countries, e.g. USA, the 5th and 95th centiles are used). By convention then, if a child's weight falls between the 3rd and 97th centile, it is to be interpreted as a normal weight. If the weight falls below the 3rd centile, the child is malnourished or failing to thrive. And if it falls above the 97th centile, it is interpreted as obesity. Additional information (e.g., the child's medical history, nutritional history, or previous growth measurements) may modify this diagnosis.

Major centile divisions are indicated on most charts. They are usually the 3rd, 10th, 25th, 50th (median), 75th, 90th, and 97th centiles. If there is a discrepancy of more than two major centile divisions between two measurements (e.g. weight and height), this may cause concern.

It should always be remembered that the division between what is normal and what is abnormal is arbitrary. If there is doubt as to the significance of a particular value in clinical practice, the trend of previous measurements should be taken into account. In all instances the rate of growth, when available, is more informative than an isolated measurement.

The composition of the population on which these growth charts are based is of vital importance. The values used most widely are those of the National Center for Health Statistics, the NCHS centiles. Although they are based on a population of normal North American children (and there are consequently those who object to their use elsewhere), it is generally accepted that these values represent the important international reference standards.

Some believe that a national reference of growth is better than an international one. Clearly local genetic and environmental factors have an effect on growth, and a national reference shows whether children are different from or similar to their peers in the same area. This may be important when deciding local priorities, such as deciding which children need intervention. However, most national growth references have been lower than international growth references and it has been argued that their use obscures some of the malnutrition problem to the detriment of the children.

In South Africa, weight-for-age charts are generally based on NCHS centiles and form part of the Road to Health Chart that is or should be issued to every mother for her baby. Such charts also provide for recording other useful health-related data (see Chapter 20: Child health cards – The Road to Health Chart). Regular growth monitoring is important for all children in any circumstances. It has particular application in disadvantaged communities where early detection of weight faltering or other unsatisfactory progress facilitates prompt and appropriate intervention.

Over the past half century, there has been a tendency to earlier maturation and increased adult size in developed countries (the secular trend in height). Newer growth charts, such as the Tanner-Whitehouse charts, or more recently, those of the Child Growth Foundation in the UK, have been introduced to reflect such changes. Classification systems are discussed further in Chapter 16: Malnutrition.

## Technical statistical issues

- The word 'parameter' should not be used to mean a growth measurement. It is a quantity that is a constant and not a changing variable. Weight or height measurements are constantly changing. Therefore, they are not parameters.
- The concept of 'normal distribution' is statistical rather than biological. There is a symmetrical distribution around the mean, and the curve reflects a complex mathematical formula. If any biological variable is 'normally distributed', it is an accident. The use of 'normal distribution' was popularized by statisticians who found that calculations were easier if they assumed that a population was normally distributed. Now we live in an era of powerful macrocomputers (even our personal computers are more powerful than university computers in the 1960s), and it is no longer useful or necessary to assume that biological variables are normally distributed when they are not.
- The Wellcome classification of malnutrition uses the term 'expected weight' to refer to the 50th centile. This is also an incorrect application of a mathematical term. 'Expected' refers to the mean or average when using a mathematical formula. The mean is not the same as the median or the fiftieth centile. The term 'expected weight' is thus completely wrong in this context. A further unfortunate consequence has been the misguided assumption that every child is therefore expected to be on (or close to) the 50th centile. The term 'expected weight' should be replaced by the correct term, which is 'median'. Therefore, the 3rd centile is the equivalent of 80 per cent of the median, and the marasmic line is the equivalent of 60 per cent of the median.

# Weight

Weight is the measurement most often used to determine physical growth. Children should be weighed undressed, using an accurate standardized scale. Ideally, with regular weighing and charting the trend can be assessed, rather than just an individual value. Weight-for-age reflects the immediate nutritional status of the child. The infant should be weighed monthly, as growth during this period is extremely rapid. In the older child weight gain is slower and less regular. Beyond the age of two years the average annual increase in weight will be in the region of 2 to 2,5 kg until the adolescent growth spurt. For the second and third years the child should be weighed at least twice a year, and more frequently in communities where there is a high incidence of malnutrition. Weight is a poor indicator of general growth in the older child and adolescent, as it may reflect the amount of body fat present rather than any increase in lean body mass or physical size.

# Height or length

In children under the age of three years the length is measured in the recumbent position, while after three years height is measured standing. Accurate measurement is essential and scrupulous attention to technique is important if height is to be a useful measurement of growth. The normal potential for growth is genetically determined and for this reason a consideration of parental height is important. Initially the newborn infant of a short mother and tall father is likely to be small.

The factors that control the weight of a fetus and newborn are mostly concerned with the mother's health and nutrition during pregnancy, although genetic anomalies in the baby may have an effect. After birth the factors that control growth are genetic since small parents tend to have small children and large parents, large children. Therefore, looking at the child's birthweight to establish which centile the child will grow along is not useful; values obtained after three or six months of age are more likely to be helpful.

The combined parental genetic endowment for growth manifests itself by between two and five years. Growth charts that take into account the mid-parental height are available, although they are not used for routine screening purposes. Reduced height-for-age indicates a chronic illness, a longstanding growth problem such as that caused by malnutrition or an hormonal deficiency.

Height is a valuable growth measurement in the older child. During the early school years there is a slow increase in height, with an average annual gain of around 5 cm.

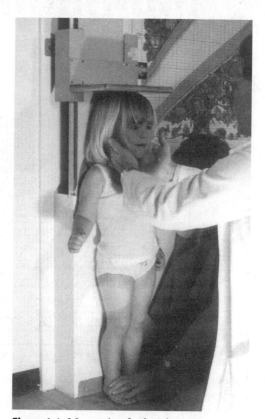

**Figure 4.1** Measuring for height

**Figure 4.2** NCHS charts for boys

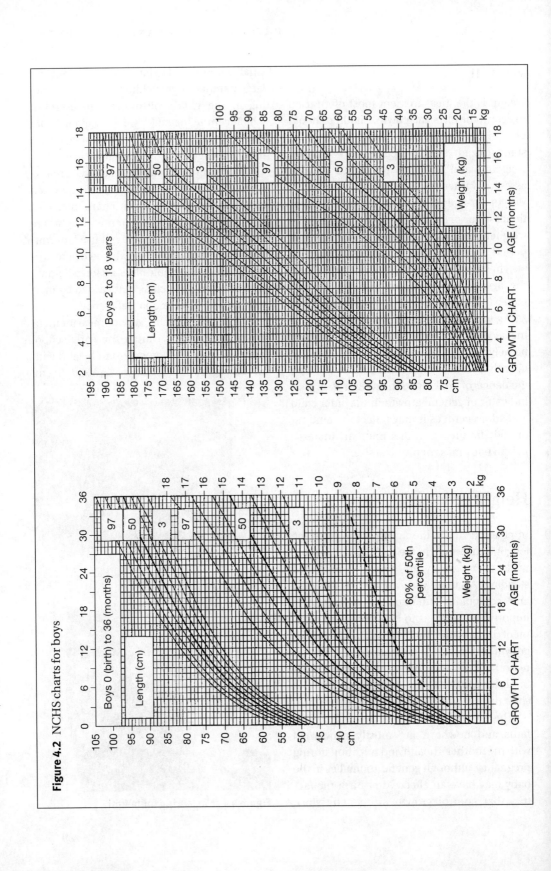

**Figure 4.3** Boys' height velocity charted against age

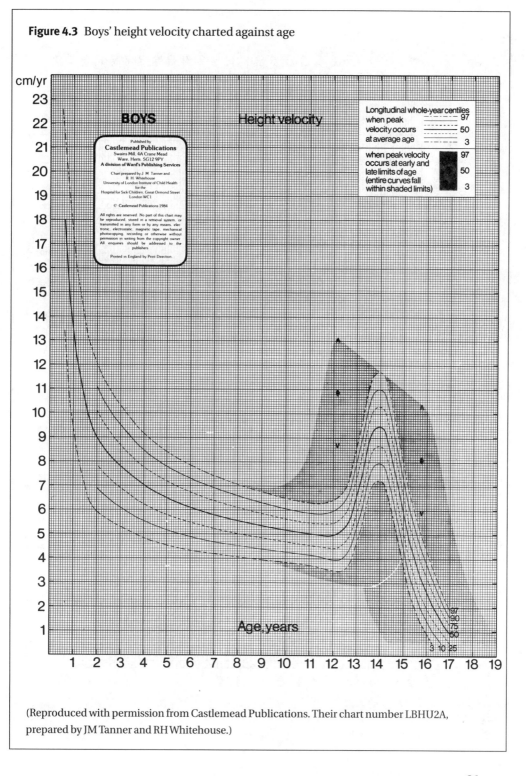

(Reproduced with permission from Castlemead Publications. Their chart number LBHU2A, prepared by JM Tanner and RH Whitehouse.)

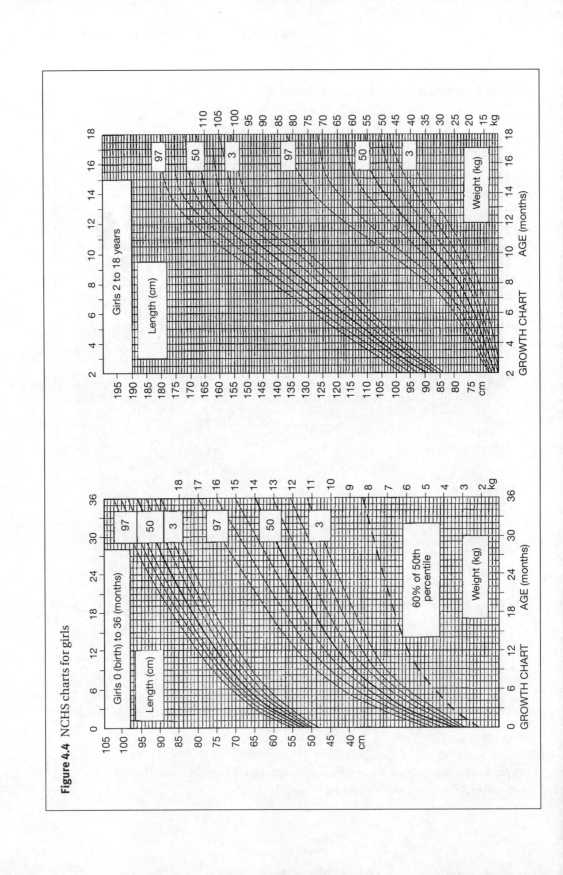

**Figure 4.4** NCHS charts for girls

**Figure 4.5** Girls' height velocity charted against age

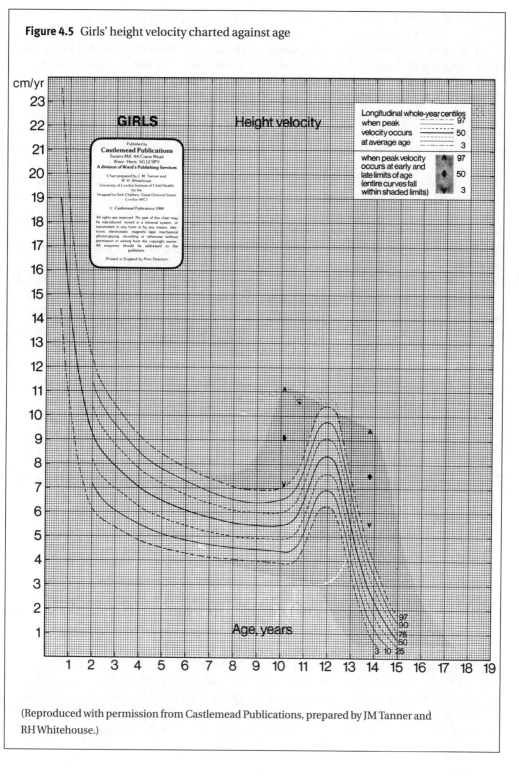

(Reproduced with permission from Castlemead Publications, prepared by JM Tanner and RH Whitehouse.)

Velocity of growth is an important concept. In growth charts (Figures 4.2 and 4.4) the total height appears to increase in a near linear steady fashion with a further increase in later childhood and adolescence. However, if the rate of increase is plotted against age (Figures 4.3 and 4.5), it becomes obvious that after the initial growth of infancy the rate of growth remains static until the dramatic increase before puberty. Puberty is heralded by this rapid acceleration of rate of growth. A delay in acceleration of growth often causes concern to both the child and parents. In most cases it is simply a constitutional delay and the ultimate height reached, albeit somewhat later than the average, will be within the normal range.

The shape of the growth curve in girls differs from that in boys (Figure 4.4). In girls the growth spurt begins earlier, peaks at a lower level and ceases earlier than in boys. The total growth velocity in boys is greater than that in girls during the period of rapid adolescent growth.

# Head circumference

The maximum circumference of the cranium is measured. This measurement reflects brain growth, which peaks during the first year of life. For practical purposes brain growth is complete after the first three years. Microcephaly, or a head circumference below the 3rd centile, usually reflects either a familial trend or a cerebral insult affecting brain growth prenatally or in early childhood. It is very unlikely to be due to malnutrition. Macrocephaly, or a large head circumference above the 97th centile, is most often due to hydrocephalus, which is not the result of an abnormality of physical growth, but rather the abnormal accumulation of cerebrospinal fluid. On rare occasions excessive physical growth of the whole body (macrosomia) may result in macrocephaly. Crossing of head growth centiles alerts the clinician to probable abnormalities, and for this reason regular monitoring is particularly indicated in those infants who are at risk for cerebral disorders.

## Z-scores

Centiles have been explained. The mean of a group of values is the arithmetical average. The median is the value obtained by the middlemost individual, which is the same as the 50th centile. The standard deviation is a statistical measurement of dispersion, or distance from the mean. The standard deviation is the basis of z-scores. A measurement that is 1 standard deviation bigger than the mean has a z-score of 1, a measurement 1 standard deviation smaller, a z-score of -1, and a measurement with no standard deviation, i.e. the same as the mean, a z-score of 0. In order to apply z-scores to measurements, they should be normally distributed. This is not the case with weight, which is skewed. Therefore the mean and median differ, and the area under the curve between a z-score of -1 and 0 is different from that between a z-score of 0 and 1. Applying z-scores to weight measurements is therefore, strictly speaking, incorrect.

However, this has been done in several computer software packages, and published studies have used z-scores. It should be noted that this may lead to an underestimate of undernutrition and an overestimate of overnutrition. It has no place in the assessment of an individual child. It makes the comparison of studies of growth in different populations easier, but at the cost of statistical assumptions of which researchers are often not aware. There is a risk of incorrect conclusions.

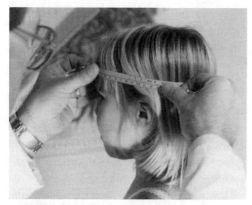

**Figure 4.6** Measuring head circumference

The above-mentioned growth measurements are those most commonly measured during the physical examination of the child or routine screening at a clinic. If all are normal it is unlikely that there is a problem related to physical growth. Other measurements such as the mid-arm circumference or skinfold thickness can be obtained, but are used primarily as tools either in mass screening programmes or research projects. The weight-to-height ratio may be a useful indicator of malnutrition in the older child and may be used in famine conditions to assess the magnitude of the problem. The age of the child need not be known, but normal values cannot distinguish between normal and proportionately reduced growth.

# Discrepancies in measurements

There may be a discrepancy between weight, height, and head circumference measurements in a child. This is most often simply because of poor measurement of height. However, when the weight centile is considerably below the height centile, this is generally attributed to acute malnutrition. Although this may be true, there may also be a causative medical condition. In either case

## Growth spurts and catch-up growth

A growth spurt means an increase in growth velocity. It tends to refer to height. Growth delay or growth lag refers to a decrease in the rate or velocity of normal expected growth. It refers to all three growth measurements. Catch-up growth is an increase in growth rate in order to return to the size that would have been attained if growth lag had not occurred. It refers to weight and height, but not usually to head circumference.

the condition may actually be sub-acute, or even chronic. However, when both weight and height are decreased, the condition is chronic. The term 'symmetrical growth retardation' should be reserved for the neonate, and not applied to infants or children.

# Obesity

Obesity may be diagnosed if the child's weight is above the 97th centile, if the child's weight exceeds his or her height by two major centile divisions, or if the child's weight has crossed two major centile divisions in a six month to one year period (without the child entering puberty). If the height is below the 50th centile and the weight increased, be on the alert for endocrine causes of the obesity. Obesity is discussed in greater detail in Chapter 16: Malnutrition.

# Body proportions

With growth there is not only an increase in size but also a change in body proportions. At birth, the head and trunk account for 70 per cent of the total length. In infancy the head grows at a relatively rapid rate, but by two years of age the ratio has decreased to 60 per cent. During childhood, growth is mostly linear and by ten years the sitting height is 52 per cent of the total height. When the sitting height is more than 50 per cent of the total, the body proportions are said to be infantile. Adult proportions are attained during adolescence. Early development of adult proportions occurs in conditions characterized by sexual precociousness. On the other hand, retention of infantile body proportions in the older child may indicate either a constitutional delay in the onset of puberty, or an endocrine disorder such as hypothyroidism.

# Changes in general appearance and normal postural variations

There is a gradual transition from the generally rounded infant to the leaner toddler and pre-schooler, the latter tending to have a relatively lordotic stance and hence fairly prominent abdomen, but both these characteristics disappear by the age of five to six years.

Other normal postural variations may cause unnecessary concern. Both in-toeing and out-toeing gaits are common in the first two years of life and almost always resolve within a couple of years without treatment.

The appearance of flat feet in young infants results from the normal fat pad occupying the medial arch of the foot. Persistent flat feet are of no significance if normal arches are apparent when the child stands on tip-toe and the feet are pain-free.

Genu varum (bowlegs) is common in infancy and, unless severe or associated with abnormalities such as rickets or Blount's disease, will correct with growth.

Genu valgum (knock knees), when noted in the slightly older pre-schooler is also usually innocent and transitory.

Benign postural scoliosis corrects with full flexion when the child bends forward from the waist.

# Organ development

Together with the increase in body size and change in body proportions, the rate of growth and development in various organ systems varies with age and sex.

Lymphoid tissue (i.e., lymph nodes, adenoids, tonsils, and similar tissue) increases steadily in mass during childhood, reaching a peak at around 11 to 12 years. Small cervical and inguinal lymph nodes are often normally palpable in this age group, and it is normal to have large tonsils. The spleen, which also forms part of the lymphoid system, is relatively large at birth and increases in size steadily during childhood to become twelve times its original size in adult life. The thymus is also relatively large at birth and, for this reason, is often seen prominently in the chest radiographs of young infants. It does increase in size during childhood but only by a factor of three, leading it to become a relatively small organ in the chest cavity.

In general, most other organs undergo their major growth in infancy and early childhood. The brain, for example, grows rapidly during the first 18 months and relatively slowly thereafter.

The reproductive organs, however, undergo rapid growth predominantly during later childhood and adolescence. The testes have two major growth spurts, first in early infancy when they are relatively large, and again in adolescence when there is marked enlargement. The ovaries increase in weight from birth until the age of 12 to 15 years. Primordial follicles, from which ova originate, are prominent in the ovary of the newborn infant but have decreased by 90 per cent at maturity. The uterus is relatively large at birth but involutes markedly during the first weeks of life. There may be mild oestrogen-withdrawal uterine bleeding in the newborn, while residual circulating maternal hormones can cause transitory gynaecomastia in either sex. The weight of the uterus at birth is not regained until the age of 10 or 11 years.

## Dentition and teething

Teeth are generally a good indicator of a child's age. This can be helpful when there is uncertainty about exact age. However, teething should not be regarded as having any significance as a developmental milestone, nor is it a cause of significant illness. The first teeth appear between five and nine months. The lower central incisors erupt first, followed by the upper central and lateral incisors until, at one year, most children have between six and eight teeth. A further eight teeth follow during the second year, including the first deciduous molars and canines. By two-and-a-half years a total of 20 deciduous teeth have erupted in most children (see Chapter 22: Oral health).

The jaw develops during the latter part of the pre-school period to accommodate the permanent teeth. The first permanent teeth, the first molars, usually erupt during the seventh year of life. Thereafter the deciduous teeth are replaced in more or less the same sequence as initial eruption. They appear at a rate of about four teeth per year. During the school-going years the facial bones and sinuses develop rapidly to assume adult proportions at maturity.

## Sinuses

Development of nasal sinuses occurs after birth with the maxillary and ethmoid sinuses becoming visible radiologically at between one and two years of age. The sphenoidal and frontal sinuses are undeveloped in the newborn and are not visible until five or six years of age. Further development of the sinuses, which is often asymmetrical, continues well into adolescence.

## Factors influencing growth and development

During the period of embryonic and fetal growth through to early infancy, factors such as adequate nutrition, placental development, and maternal care play an important role in determining the rate of growth. Growth during this period is independent of hormonal influence, except for gonadal differentiation into a male or female fetus.

From early infancy to adolescence, factors such as nutrition, chronic disease, and endocrine function determine the rate of growth. Adequate nutrition is cardinal to optimal physical growth and a lack of nutrition will result in severe impairment. Emotional deprivation may also inhibit growth.

Growth hormone is necessary for the increase in cell numbers, while thyroid hormone stimulates cell multiplication in addition to increasing cell size. Intact endocrine function is essential for normal growth.

## References and further reading

DATTANI MT & PREECE MA. Physical growth and development. In: AGM Campbell & N McIntosh (eds.). *Forfar and Arneil's textbook of pediatrics*, 5th ed. New York: Churchill Livingstone.

# 5.

# Neurodevelopment

CD MOLTENO &
CM ADNAMS

Development may be defined as a progressive series of orderly coherent changes in skills and abilities, which can either involve structural differentiation or are behavioural in nature. *Neurodevelopment* focuses on emerging motor, sensory, language, cognitive, and social skills in infants and children.

Development is largely predictable, although the rate varies in individual children. It is a result of both maturation, an intrinsic unfolding of characteristics in the individual (dependent upon the genetic endowment), and the process of learning, which stems from contact with the environment.

*Suboptimal development* may result from biological and environmental factors, or a combination of both. Biological factors usually relate to genetic or acquired conditions that interfere with neurological function, while environmental factors include poor psychosocial influences such as poverty, lack of environmental stimulation, and the opportunity to practise skills.

For descriptive purposes, development is divided into six modalities: gross motor, fine motor, sensory, language, cognitive, and personal and social. Cognitive and sensory development will be dealt with in Chapters 6 (Emotional and cognitive development) and 57 (Sensory impairment).

In health practice, development is assessed on four of these modalities (see Table 5.1). Cognition is evaluated by psychometric tests.

## Gross motor development

A number of important locomotor changes take place during infancy and childhood.

- General physiological flexor hypertonus gives way to extensor facility. The neonate, having spent nine months in the fetal position, assumes a posture of semiflexion in all these joints. Gradually, over a period of six months the infant attains the ability to extend all its joints, the process spreading cephalo-caudally and proximo-distally.
- Muscle tone increases. The neonate is generally low-toned although the full term infant has more tone than the premature infant. Over a period of six months the tone increases progressively. This may be tested by observing the degree of head lag on pull-to-sit, the position of the head and limbs in ventral suspension, and by passive movement of the limbs.

38

- Primitive reflexes are assimilated. Primitive responses such as the Moro, grasp, rooting, sucking, and walking reflexes are present during the first three months of life and then gradually disappear over the next few months. However, the foot grasp and primary walking may still be present in a normal infant until nine months.
- Mass action of the limbs gives way to voluntary movement of one limb at a time.
- Postural development matures. This involves both righting and equilibrium reactions. Righting reactions enable the infant to maintain a normal position of the head in space as well as to align head, neck, trunk, and limbs. The equilibrium reactions are automatic responses to changes in posture and act to restore balance.

These processes are translated into motor milestones in the following way: increasing head and trunk extension in the prone position enables the infant to lift up the head and then raise both head and chest. At first the weight is supported on the elbows and later on extended arms. Extension also allows the infant to roll over from the prone to supine position. Rolling over from supine to prone requires hip flexion and body derotative righting (the ability to rotate the hips without automatic rotation of the shoulders). In order to sit alone, there must be an end to the total patterns of flexion or extension that characterize early infancy – sitting requires simultaneous flexion of the hips and extension of the back. This ability is facilitated by the symmetrical tonic neck reflex. This reaction, together with forward protective extension of the arms, also allows for the crawling position. The next step is the ability to pull up to stand. Once the child has lateral, forward, and backward protective extension as well as all the equilibrium reactions, standing and walking are possible. Early walking is characterized by a high guard position of the arms. The guard is gradually lowered and after it has been dropped, reciprocal arm movements occur, which enable the child to run.

# Fine motor development

The grasp reflex predominates in the neonate and the hands are held in a fisted position most of the time. By two months of age this should be disappearing, allowing the hands to be held open. Over the next three months visually guided reaching matures, requiring an interaction between hand, eye, and mouth. Initially, when visually tracking an object held in front, the infant's arms extend forward and the mouth opens. Later the hands will bat at the object, usually without connecting with it. When they do strike the object, it is grasped and brought immediately to the mouth. The action, which is called obligatory mouthing, is then terminated. As the reaching becomes more accurate the object is still brought to the mouth, but the mouthing becomes more exploratory. By nine months the object will be mouthed and then taken out of the mouth and inspected.

At six months the infant is able to transfer an object from one hand to the other, usually via the mouth. Reaching should be equally good with either hand. Until seven months there is a midline barrier as far as hand use is concerned. The infant is not able to reach across the midline and cannot retain an object in each hand simultaneously, but this becomes possible by eight months. However, it is not usually until after a year that bimanual manipulation becomes important. Initially when a five- or six-month-old infant reaches for an object a total (palmar) grasp is used. Over the next few months the grasp becomes more radial and the object is held between thumb and proximal phalanx of the index finger. By 12 months the pincer grasp has matured and there is apposition of the thumb

**Table 5.1** Developmental milestones in the first 10 years of life

| Age | Gross motor | Fine motor/vision | Hearing and speech | Personal/social | Warning signs |
|---|---|---|---|---|---|
| Newborn | Ventral suspension: head droops, hips flexed, limbs hang downwards; Moro reflex; Palmar/plantar grasp reflexes | Hands fisted; closes eyes to sudden bright light | Stills to sound, startle s to sudden loud sounds | Alternates between drowsiness and alert wakefulness | Hyper-/hypotonia, asymmetrical reflexes; excessive head lag; poor sucking |
| 6 weeks | Some head control; prone: head to side, buttocks moderately high; Moro reflex, ventral suspension | Stares; follows horizontally to 90° | Startle response | Smiles at mother | No visual fixation or following; asymmetry of tone or movement; floppy, excessive head lag; failure to smile; poor sucking |
| 3 months | Pull-to-sit: little/no head lag; prone: support on forearms, lifts head, buttocks flat, rolls over | Follows through 180° Holds rattle when placed in hand | Coos, chuckles | Excited when sees mother; reacts to familiar situations | |
| 6 months | Pull to sit: braces shoulders and pulls to sit; sits with support; prone: lifts head and chest well up; supports on extended arms | Reaches for and grasps toy; transfers toy from one hand to the other | Initiates 'conversation' | Takes everything to mouth; responds to mirror image | Floppiness; failure to use both hands; squint; failure to turn to sound; poor response to people |
| 9 months | Sits without support, attempts to crawl; pulls to stand | Immediately reaches out; holds a cube in each hand | Vocalizes deliberately; babbles | Stranger anxiety; holds bottle/cup | Unable to sit; hand preference; fisting; squint; persistence of primitive reflexes |
| 10 months | Pulls to stand | Picks up small object between thumb and index finger | Shakes head for no; waves bye-bye | Plays peek-a-boo with mother | |
| 12 months | Bear walks; walks around furniture lifting one foot and stepping side-ways; may walk alone | Pincer grasp; releases object on request | Knows own name; 2–3 words with meaning | Finger feeds; pushes arm into sleeve | Unable to sit or bear weight; abnormal grasp; failure to respond to sound |
| 15 months | Walks alone – uneven steps, arms out for balance | 2-cube tower | Jabbers with expression | Holds and drinks from cup; attempts feeding with spoon, spills most | |
| 18 months | Walks well, arms down, pulls a toy, throws a ball; climbs onto chair | 3-cube tower; scribbles | 2-word utterances | Handles spoon and cup; indicates wet nappy | Failure to walk; no pincer grip; inability to understand simple commands; no spontaneous vocalization; mouthing; drooling |
| 24 months | Runs; up and down steps two feet per step | 6 cube tower; train with cubes; imitates vertical line; hand preference usually obvious | Short phrases; uses pronouns | Spoon feeds without spilling; clean and dry by day | Unable to understand simple commands; tremor; incoordination |
| 36 months | Rides a tricycle; up steps one foot per step and down two feet per step | 9 cube tower, bridge with cubes; copies circle | Knows name and sex; talks incessantly | Toilet trained; dresses without supervision | Ataxia; using single words only |
| 48 months | Up and down stairs one foot per step; stands on one (preferred) foot for 3–5 seconds and hops on preferred foot | Copies cross; gate with cubes | Full name, home address and (usually) age; recognizes colours | Eats with spoon and fork; washes and dries hands; dresses and undresses; make-believe play | Speech difficult to understand because of poor articulation or omission or substitution of consonants |
| 60 months | Walks easily on narrow line; can hop on each foot separately | 6–10 cube steps; copies square and triangle; draws a man with full features | Fluent speech; full name, age (usually) | Uses knife and fork competently; undresses and dresses alone; chooses own friends | Emotional immaturity |
| 72 months | Sits up without help of hands; walks backwards along straight line (10 paces) | 10 cube steps; copies ◇ and ⊠ | Word definition (5); compositions – door, shoe, spoon; knows birthday, address | Cooperative play - leadership and division of labour | Clumsy, poor posture, stutter |
| 7–8 years | Jumps 25 cm feet together; throws ball up and catches | Writes name; draws a man, facial features, limbs correct, align to body, hands | Talks sentences of 10 syllables | One special friend; dresses, undresses completely without help | Poor pencil grip; School refusal |
| 9–10 years | Runs downstairs; skips with rope | Writes 3-word sentences | Produces all speech sounds incl. s, z, ng | Takes full responsibility for personal care | Speech sound difficulty; Failure to progress at school |

and terminal phalanx of the index finger. While the pincer grasp is developing, the infant will characteristically isolate and explore with the index finger, but once the grasp has become mature, the infant can release an object on request, and mouthing should be infrequent. Children of this age frequently enjoy throwing toys out of the cot. From 15 to 18 months play becomes increasingly bimanual and manipulative skills develop. These can be tested by block construction, puzzles, and formboards. During the next three years perceptual skills and sensory motor integration develop to lay the foundation for those activities that are required for schooling. Handedness appears after one year of age, but may change over the next few years.

## Language

The newborn infant cries and is able to produce only a few throaty sounds. By eight weeks vowel sounds appear and these are used to vocalize pleasure. Thereafter the infant initiates sounds to which the mother responds with sensitive timing. This synchrony is referred to as 'vocal contagion'. At 20 weeks guttural sounds are produced, while by 32 weeks syllables are being combined (babbling, such as baba, mama, dada). Soon after this, early concept formation can be demonstrated by object permanence. The infant can retrieve a hidden object such as a block placed under a cup. Gradually the babbling sounds achieve meaning so that by one year the baby has two to three meaningful 'words'. Language development slows down for the next few months, but between 15 and 18 months the child shows the beginning of symbolization (inner language) by demonstrating definition by use (e.g., understanding of the use of a brush or telephone is indicated by gesture). This heralds a new acceleration of language development and by 18 months two-word utterances commence. At two years the child is capable of short phrases and uses pronouns. A three-year-old has an extensive vocabulary and chats incessantly. Immature articulation is common at this stage, but by five years articulation errors have usually disappeared and the child uses full sentences.

## Personal and social development

The mother and child relationship is established by means of the bonding and attachment process. Bonding commences immediately after birth and assures the acceptance of the infant by the mother. The development of the infant's attachment to its mother is more gradual. Bowlby's theory of attachment emphasizes the first three years of life, during which the infant establishes a relationship with another person. During the first three months of life the relationship is characterized by the mother's response to the infant's cues. Thereafter they both interact with reciprocal vocal and affectionate exchanges. Between five and seven months the infant establishes a preference for the primary caretaker (usually the mother). From then until three years of age the relationship matures and an understanding of cause and effect in the interaction with the mother develops.

The role of the father is also important, while interaction with siblings and peers extends the social relationships. A two-year-old plays alone or, if with other children, in parallel fashion. Group activities commence after three years and usually involve two or three children. By the age of five years group play is common, although the size of the group remains relatively small (three to five members). The play becomes symbolic in that the children identify themselves as people, such as postmen, teachers, or shopkeepers.

# Detection of developmental problems

Developmental delays or disabilities are detected at two different levels. Firstly there is *developmental surveillance*, which simply involves taking a developmental history based on milestones or the use of a questionnaire (see Chapter 21: Health surveillance). Some developmental milestones applicable to the first three years of life are given in Table 5.1. This should be selectively applied at every paediatric consultation, whether it takes place in a child health clinic, an office, or a hospital (either as outpatient or inpatient). *Developmental screening* refers to a procedure that is rapidly applied and gives a pass/fail result. Screening is usually carried out at specific ages on total child populations. Where facilities are limited, a single developmental screening at nine months for all children should be aimed for as the minimum requirement. At this age the focus should also be on hearing and vision screening and the detection of squints.

The children flagged at surveillance or screening are referred for *developmental assessment*. In ideal circumstances this is carried out by a team coordinated by a paediatrician, and consisting of a physiotherapist, occupational therapist, speech therapist, psychologist, and social worker as core members (see Chapter 55: Intellectual disability). Referrals to other medical specialists should be arranged as indicated. Assessment not only arrives at a diagnosis but also outlines a management programme which includes counselling and liaison with community-based facilities.

## References and further reading

HARRISON VC (ed.). 1999. *Handbook of Paediatrics,* 5th ed. Cape Town: Oxford University Press.

ILLINGWORTH RS. 1985. *Development of the infant and young child: Normal and abnormal.* Edinburgh: Churchill Livingstone.

SHERIDAN MD. 1980. *Children's developmental program – From birth to five years: The STYCAR sequences.* NFER Publishing Co.

# 6

# Emotional and cognitive development

## BA ROBERTSON

The principles of emotional and cognitive development are as follows:

- Each individual is born with latent psychosocial resources and an unstoppable drive to develop them. Examples of such resources are the capacity for attachment, the capacity for independent functioning, and the capacity for organizing experiences. The process of realizing these resources continues throughout life and leads to the formation and growth of the personality.
- There is a normal progressive sequence in the realization of psychosocial resources, although its rate and intensity differs between individuals.
- The successive realization of these resources occurs when they are needed, in response to life-challenges, many of which are common to everyone. Examples of common life-challenges are the mother's gradual withdrawal of her total care of the infant, sending the young child to school, the onset of puberty, and leaving school. The resources become either fully or partially realized and, in some cases, may be distorted.
- Life-challenges stir up a mixture of positive and negative feelings in the individual. The challenge is met successfully by a very individualized blending of positive and negative feelings, with a predominantly positive outcome. However, complete suppression of the negative side is inappropriate and unhealthy.

## Emotional and cognitive resources

The primary *emotional resources* that are latent in each normal newborn child become manifest in the drive *to love* and *to work*. The hallmark of the mentally healthy adult is the capacity for love and for work. In this context 'love' refers to both self-esteem and the capacity for meaningful and appropriate relationships with others. 'Work' refers to the ability to use one's knowledge and skills creatively and effectively. Play and learning are the childhood precursors of adult work skills.

Although *aggression* is sometimes considered to be a separate emotional resource, it is probably best understood as an integral component of love and relationships. Aggression is constructive and adaptive when it assists the child to overcome those obstacles that come in the way of the drive to love and to work. It is

43

then known as assertiveness. When drives are thwarted or the child deprived of being loved and nurtured, aggression becomes destructive and is referred to as maladaptive or hostile aggression.

*Cognitive resources* in the newborn child refers to the emerging ability to think and to reason. Children's emotional and cognitive resources develop in a progressive, sequential manner, which, although unique to each child, follows a pattern common to all.

# Normal emotional development

## THE DEVELOPMENT OF THE CAPACITY FOR LOVING

The childhood stages in the development of the capacity for loving are summarized in Table 6.1. The approximate age-period for each achievement is given, although in reality there are considerable individual differences as well as overlap between successive stages. This profile is based on Erikson's psychosocial theory of development.

**Table 6.1** Stages in emotional development

| | |
|---|---|
| • Basic trust | 0–18 months |
| • Autonomy | 18–36 months |
| • Assertiveness | 3–6 years |
| • Socialization | 6–12 years |
| • Personal and sexual identity | 12–20 years |
|    through the peer group | 12–16 years |
|    through intimate relationships | 16–20 years |

The baby who experiences warm nurturing and care during the early months develops a sense of well-being and *trust* in the world that will serve as the basis of trust for future relationships. Rapid development of language and motor skills during the second year of life makes toddlers want to start managing for themselves, both physically and emotionally.

Increasing success in this area leads to a sense of *autonomy*.

Between three and six years of age the child learns to become *assertive* but co-operative with his or her little circle of family and friends. Without this skill the child is ill-prepared to meet the demands of larger society as experienced in the classroom, the peer group, and in early contacts with the community. This relatively quiet and orderly state of development comes to an end with puberty, which heralds the onset of the more turbulent stage of adolescence.

## FROM PLAY TO LEARNING TO WORK

The main achievements of each stage in the childhood development of the ability to work are given in Table 6.2. The profile is adapted from the developmental lines described by Anna Freud.

**Table 6.2** Stages in work-related ability

| | |
|---|---|
| • Transitional play | 0–18 months |
|   – body play | |
|   – play with 'transitional' object | |
|   – play with cuddly toys | |
| • Constructive and symbolic (fantasy) play | 18–36 months |
| • Task orientation | 3–6 years |
| • Formal learning | 6–20 years |
|   – primary school | |
|   – secondary school | |

The baby's initial preoccupation with his or her own and the mother's body gives way to play with transitional objects that are usually soft materials associated with mother. This is the way the infant negotiates the transition from the mother's to his or her own world, which soon begins to be peopled with cuddly dolls and animals. The emerging ability of the infant to play out with toys fantasies about their interactions with one another is called symbolic play, and develops in relation to the child's peers through the stages of solitary, parallel, and co-operative play.

At the same time the child is exercising and developing perceptual and motor abilities through activities like filling and emptying containers, and opening and shutting doors. This leads on to building and moulding activities and to the expression of ideas and fantasies through drawing and painting. Interest develops not only in the play and activity themselves, but also in the product that has been created. This is the crucial stage of task orientation, the ability to focus on activities that have aims other than simple self-gratification. It is an important component of school readiness and prepares the child for the formal learning requirements of primary school. Ultimately, with entry into secondary school the young teenager should be well on the way to taking personal responsibility for his or her own education.

# Normal cognitive development

Piaget describes the development of the ability to assimilate information, to reason, and to accommodate oneself to the external world according to the profile in Table 6.3 (Hobson, 1985).

Neonatal reflexes give way to early goal-directed behaviour as the infant tries to repeat random movements and actions. Gradually actions such as grasping become co-ordinated with hearing and sight until more complex sensorimotor functions like the co-ordination of hand movements and the manipulation of objects in the environment become possible. Meanwhile the infant learns that an object continues to exist even when out of sight.

In the next stage on the way to fully understanding causal relationships the child begins to link present experiences to past ones and to classify perceived differences such as colour, which is the commencement of symbolic thinking. Language and fantasy play develop rapidly once the capacity for symbolic thought has been established. Early attempts at explaining new experiences and new observations of the environment are pre-logical, or 'intuitive', and are egocentric, animistic, and magical in nature.

The development of a capacity for concrete concepts, such as conception of mass, spatial relationships, and similarities, allows the primary school child to achieve a true understanding of causality and gives the ability to categorize and classify at an advanced level. In Piaget's final stage of cognitive development the adolescent moves from the actual to the possible, from the concrete to the abstract, and from child to adult reasoning and thinking.

**Table 6.3** Stages in cognitive development

| | |
|---|---|
| • Sensorimotor stage | 0–18 months |
| – neonatal reflexes | 0–1 month |
| – co-ordination of hearing, sight, grasping | 1–4 months |
| – co-ordination of hand movements | 4–8 months |
| – object permanence | 8–12 months |
| – complex goal-directed behaviour | 12–18 months |
| • Pre-operational stage | 18 months–7 years |
| – symbolic stage: emergence of symbolic thought, language, and play | 18–36 months |
| – intuitive stage: egocentricism, animism, and magical thinking | 3–7 years |
| • Stage of concrete operations | 7–11 years |
| – mastery of concrete concepts such as causality, conservation of mass and classification | |
| • Stage of formal operations | 11–20 years |
| – the ability to make and manipulate | |
| – abstract concepts | |

# General characteristics of the mentally healthy child

Child mental health is an evolving process, which is characterized by continuous progress in all areas of personal development and adaptation to the family and community.

Child mental health is characterized by:

- adequate self-esteem;
- warm, appropriate relationships with family members;
- ability to relate to peers;
- adaptive aggression (assertiveness); and
- capacity for appropriate play, task-orientation or learning.

In particular there should be:

- appropriate mood responses;
- the ability to communicate effectively;
- a balance between dependent and independent functioning;
- appropriate physical and emotional control;
- adequate frustration tolerance;
- adequate problem-solving ability; and
- good social judgement.

## References and further reading

ERIKSON E. 1963. Eight ages of man. In: *Childhood and Society*, 2nd ed. New York: WW Norton.

FREUD A. 1965. *Normality and pathology in childhood*. New York: International Universities Press.

HOBSON RP. 1985. Piaget: On the ways of knowing in childhood. In: M Rutter & L Hersov. *Child and adolescent psychiatry*, 3rd ed. Oxford: Blackwell Scientific Publications.

RUTTER M, TAYLOR E, and HERSOV L (eds.). 1994. Influences on development. In: *Child and adolescent psychiatry*, 3rd ed. Oxford: Blackwell Scientific Publications.

## Individual differences in emotional and cognitive development

The rate and intensity of the developmental process varies from child to child. Some of the factors that contribute to individual differences are:

### Sex
Girls develop more rapidly than boys. Boys are more active, aggressive, and vulnerable to physical hazards.

### Temperament
The temperament shown by individual infants seems to remain fairly stable throughout life. Temperament has the following nine components:
- activity level;
- rhythm of biological functions;
- approach or withdrawal to new situations;
- intensity of emotional reactions;
- threshold of sensory responsiveness;
- adaptability;
- quality of mood;
- distractibility; and
- attention span and persistence.

### Intelligence

### Family influences
Some of the important family influences are the personality and adjustment of the parents; marital and family relationships and functioning; child-rearing patterns and discipline; and separation and loss.

### Socio-cultural differences
These include types of schooling and living environments as well as broader issues such as social disadvantages, structural violence, urbanization, social mores, and the breakdown of traditional ways of life.

# PART THREE

# Genetics

This part sets out the developments in human genetics in the context of child health. With the decrease in infectious disease, genetic disorders are becoming increasingly important, and now contribute to the burden of community disease. Furthermore, the consumption of alcohol during pregnancy is an important cause of malformation and intellectual disability. This is discussed in some detail.

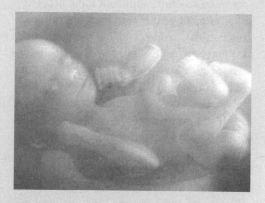

# 7

# Inherited disorders and congenital abnormalities

JGR KROMBERG &
T JENKINS

Genetic disorders assume greater relative importance as infectious and environmentally induced diseases are brought under control. As long as the infant mortality rate (IMR) remains at 100 or higher there is little justification for the allocation of scarce resources for the combat of inherited disorders. The emphasis in such societies will be on introducing and sustaining immunization programmes, improving the care of women at delivery in order to reduce the incidence of birth asphyxia, combating iodine deficiency, improving nutrition, and educating the population in basic health and hygiene matters. Some would argue that all societies are entitled to enjoy, as 'inalienable human rights', safe water to drink, sufficient food, access to some form of health care including protection against communicable disease, and assistance in controlling fertility. The poor, (historically disadvantaged) sectors in southern Africa, with IMRs in some rural areas higher than 100, have different priorities in health and may still have to grapple with the classic Third World diseases. However, as living standards improve, families tend to limit the number of their children and they are also desirous of genetic services.

In recent years there has been a dramatic increase in the knowledge about genetic disorders. In 1958 there were only 412 disorders that were recognized as being caused entirely by defective genes. In 1971 this number was 1 876, by 1986 it had increased to 3 907 and by 1994 it was 6 678. Congenital malformations, mild and severe, including those due to genetic causes, occur in four to five per cent of all live births and are, in addition, the cause of many stillbirths and neonatal deaths. It has been estimated that one person in ten will experience a genetic disorder at some time of life, and in developed countries at least 20 per cent of the beds in paediatric wards will be taken up by children with genetic disorders. Scientists have suggested that every person carries approximately three or four mutant genes which, when present in double dose, could cause a defect in their offspring.

## Congenital abnormalities

Clinical geneticists and genetic counsellors are called upon to deal with families into which a child with congenital abnormalities has been born. These are disorders that may occur as a

48

result of environmental conditions *in utero,* or may also be caused by predisposing genetic factors in the mother, fetus or both, in conjunction with the environmental factors. For example, if a mother with a certain predisposition (not yet defined at the genetic level) takes excessive alcohol or certain drugs, or has an infection, particularly in the first trimester of pregnancy when organogenesis is occurring in the developing fetus, various abnormalities, including an intellectual defect, may ensue. Similarly, if a woman has a family history of twins she may be at risk of having twins herself, but if she then takes fertility drugs because of failure to conceive, she has an even higher risk of multiple births. In the case of neural tube defects, such as spina bifida, a woman with a positive family history can take folic acid supplementation peri-conceptually and this will lower the recurrence risk. In some cases, therefore, where some of the causative factors are understood, there are means available for preventing the congenital defect occurring or recurring. Simple guidelines suggest that all women should avoid alcohol, drugs, and X-rays when they are planning a pregnancy, as well as during the pregnancy itself, and should have a good healthy balanced diet and, if necessary, vitamin and folic acid supplementation throughout the period. Couples with questions such as 'Will my next child have the same problem as the first one?' can be counselled by their medical practitioner or referred to a genetic counselling clinic (see Chapter 8: Genetic services) for an expert opinion.

# Monogenic inheritance

## AUTOSOMAL DOMINANT INHERITANCE

About 1 000 disorders are known to follow a dominant pattern of inheritance (see Table 7.1) and, individually, most of them have

## Modes of inheritance

The majority (80 per cent) of the serious birth defects are hereditary and it is therefore important for the paediatrician to have a basic knowledge of the genetic principles that determine their modes of inheritance. These may be divided into three major groups:
- the monogenic and unifactorial or Mendelian disorders, caused by a single gene. All the dominant, recessive, and X-linked disorders are included in this group;
- the polygenic or multifactorial disorders, caused by a combination of genes at two or more loci interacting with environmental agents; and
- the chromosomal disorders, either numerical or structural.

prevalence rates of less than one in 5 000. They may be easily identifiable at birth, as is the case with achondroplasia, or they may only become obvious in the third or fourth decade of life, as in Huntington's disease.

**Table 7.1** Some common dominantly inherited disorders

| | |
|---|---|
| Achondroplasia | Neurofibromatosis |
| Apert syndrome | Osteogenesis imperfecta |
| Cataracts | Polycystic kidneys |
| Ectodermal dysplasia | (adult type) |
| Familial hypercholesterolaemia | Polydactyly |
| Huntington's disease | Porphyria |
| Marfan syndrome | Retinitis pigmentosa |
| Myotonic dystrophy | Tuberous sclerosis |
| | Waardenburg syndrome |

A dominantly inherited disorder is caused by a gene that manifests itself phenotypically in a single dose even though it is paired with a normal functioning allele. Males and females are affected equally by these disorders and a person who carries such a gene has a 50 per cent (or a one in two) chance of passing it on to his or her offspring (see Figure 7.1). Each pregnancy carries the same risk, regardless of the outcome in previous pregnancies. New mutations can, however, occasionally occur and in these cases the gene will have mutated in the ovum or sperm that gave rise to the child; parents in such a case will be normal. In some conditions new mutations are very common. For example, 80 per cent of cases of achondroplasia are caused by new mutations, while new mutations are thought to be extremely rare in Huntington's disease. In cases of new mutations the siblings of the affected child will not be at increased risk, but the offspring of the affected child will run a one in two risk of inheriting the mutant gene. New mutations are more likely to occur in the gametes of older men than among younger controls.

The expression of the phenotype in the case of many dominantly inherited conditions differs among family members. The phenomenon is known as variable expressivity, and it may make the condition almost unrecognizable to the unsuspecting doctor. Waardenburg syndrome provides a good example; the symptoms include white forelock, early greying, heterochromia irides or 'steely' blue eyes, increased intercanthal distance (often mistaken for hypertelorism), and profound deafness. Some affected relatives may have only the deafness, others only a white forelock or a brown segment in a blue iris, while others may have the full-blown syndrome.

The gene for a dominant condition may also be non-penetrant, and the condition may be observed, for example, in the first and third generation, but may miss out a member of the intervening generation, even though that member carries the gene. One such condition is post-axial polydactyly, which is very common in the South African black population. Penetrance is said to be incomplete in these cases and if 20 out of 100 people who possess the gene show no effects from having it, then the penetrance is said to be 80 per

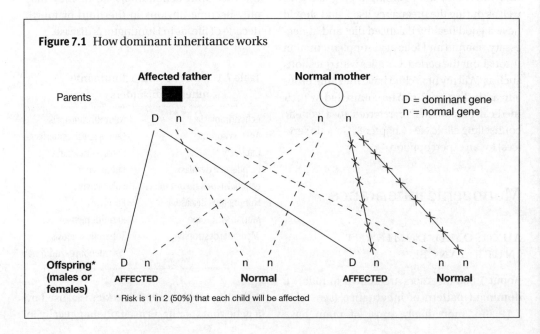

**Figure 7.1** How dominant inheritance works

Parents

Affected father

Normal mother

D    n

n    n

D = dominant gene
n = normal gene

**Offspring*** (males or females)

D    n
AFFECTED

n    n
Normal

D    n
AFFECTED

n    n
Normal

* Risk is 1 in 2 (50%) that each child will be affected

cent. It is not known what determines incomplete penetrance.

The characteristics of dominantly inherited conditions are:
- only the relatives on one side of the family are affected;
- one in two children of an affected person will, on average, be affected;
- when one of the affected person's parents is affected, the siblings will have a one in two risk of being affected;
- in most instances there is variability in the expression or severity of the disorder;
- males and females are affected in equal proportions; and
- new mutations can occur, in which case the normal parents will not have an increased risk of having another affected child.

## AUTOSOMAL RECESSIVE INHERITANCE

About 500 recessively inherited disorders are known, and taken together these occur in about 2,5 per 1 000 live births. Their individual prevalence in a population may be as high as one in·3 000 births, and some of the better-known conditions are listed in Table 7.2. Many of these disorders are caused by a recognizable biochemical defect, such as a gross reduction in the level of the hexosaminidase isoenzyme A in children with Tay-Sachs disease, and, in the case of cystic fibrosis, a defective transmembrane regulator. These conditions tend to have different prevalence rates in different populations. In South Africa the black population has an increased rate of oculocutaneous albinism; the Indian and Greek populations have increased rates of beta-thalassaemia; the Jewish population is at increased risk for Tay-Sachs disease, and the whites, in general, for cystic fibrosis. Screening and prevention programmes can be offered to high-risk populations in some cases.

**Table 7.2** Some common recessive conditions

| | |
|---|---|
| Adrenogenital syndrome | Mucopolysaccharidosis (some) |
| Albinism (oculocutaneous) | Phenylketonuria |
| Ataxia telangiectasia | Retinitis pigmentosa (some) |
| Cystic fibrosis | Sickle-cell anaemia |
| Deafness (some types) | Spinal muscular atrophy |
| Epidermolysis bullosa (some) | Tay-Sachs disease |
| Galactosaemia | Thalassaemia (alpha and beta) |
| Microcephaly (some) | |

Recessive conditions are caused by the presence of a double dose of the mutant gene, which in a single dose usually causes no problem. Occasionally the carrier of a single dose of the gene for a recessive disorder may show minor symptoms, as is the case in carriers for thalassaemia who may have a mild anaemia. The affected individual is said to be homozygous for the mutant gene, while the carrier is said to be heterozygous. Couples who both carry the same recessive gene have a one in four chance of having offspring with a severe recessive disorder (see Figure 7.2).

Screening for carriers, and prevention by prenatal diagnosis and selective abortion is offered to high-risk populations in South Africa, such as the Jewish population for Tay-Sachs disease, and the Greek and Indian populations for beta-thalassaemia. Screening for relatives of a child with cystic fibrosis is also available and prenatal diagnosis is possible using molecular techniques. The site of some of these genes is also known. For example, the Tay-Sachs gene is on chromosome 5 and the cystic fibrosis gene on chromosome 7.

Populations in which there are numerous consanguineous marriages are also at higher

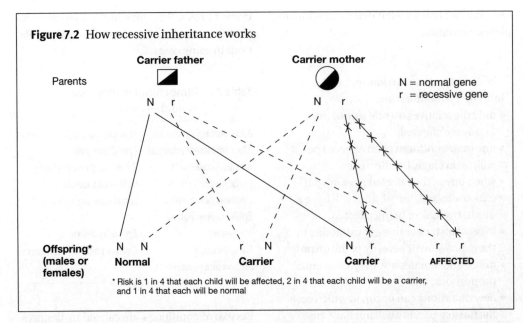

**Figure 7.2** How recessive inheritance works

Parents

Carrier father

Carrier mother

N = normal gene
r = recessive gene

N    r

N    r

Offspring*
(males or
females)

N    N
**Normal**

r    N
**Carrier**

N    r
**Carrier**

r    r
**AFFECTED**

* Risk is 1 in 4 that each child will be affected, 2 in 4 that each child will be a carrier,
and 1 in 4 that each will be normal

risk of producing recessive disorders. If a couple are first cousins they share one-eighth of their genes and there will be a theoretical risk of 1 in 16 that they will produce a child with a severe recessive disorder (see Figure 7.3). For example oculocutaneous albinism occurs at a high rate amongst the Tswana partly because first cousin marriages were, until recently, the preferred mating pattern. Physical and/or mental abnormalities affect about 25 per cent of the offspring of incestuous matings.

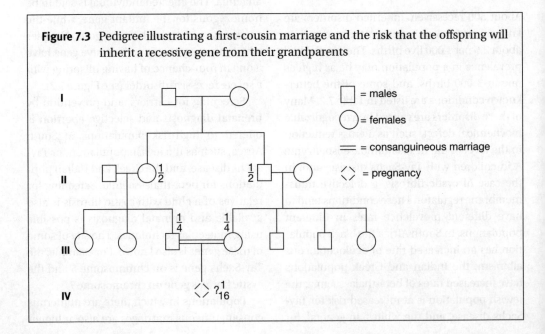

**Figure 7.3** Pedigree illustrating a first-cousin marriage and the risk that the offspring will inherit a recessive gene from their grandparents

I

II    $\frac{1}{2}$    $\frac{1}{2}$

III    $\frac{1}{4}$    $\frac{1}{4}$

IV    $?\frac{1}{16}$

= males
= females
= consanguineous marriage
= pregnancy

The characteristics of autosomal recessive disorders are:
- it is unlikely that a previous relative, other than an older sibling, will be affected;
- one in four siblings will on average be affected;
- the risks to the children of an affected person are low and are determined by the frequency of the gene in the population;
- there is an increased consanguinity rate among the parents of affected children, particularly when the gene is rare; and
- males and females are affected in equal numbers.

## X-LINKED INHERITANCE

This mode of inheritance results from genes on the X chromosome and the majority are recessively inherited, with dominants being rare. About 100 disorders fall into this category and their combined frequency is 0,5 to 1,5 per 1 000 births. Some of the common disorders in this group are listed in Table 7.3. Individually they may occur as often as one in 2 500 boys.

**Table 7.3** Some common X-linked conditions

| | |
|---|---|
| Glucose 6 phosphate dehydrogenase deficiency | Mucopolysaccharidosis (Hunter type) |
| Haemophilia A and B | Muscular dystrophy (Duchenne and Becker) |
| Hydrocephalus (Aqueduct stenosis) | Ocular albinism |
| Incontinentia pigmenti | Retinitis pigmentosa (some) |
| Microphthalmia | Testicular feminization |

Because the abnormal gene is on the X chromosome, only boys, with the X carrying the mutant gene or the gene deletion, will ordinarily manifest the disorder. A girl who carries the defective gene on one of her X chromosomes usually has a normal gene on her other X chromosome and she is, therefore, phenotypically normal, even though she is a carrier. Such females have a 50 per cent chance that their male children will be affected and a 50 per cent chance that their daughters will be carriers (see Figure 7.4). Males who have the mutant X-linked gene produce daughters who are all carriers, but their sons, who must inherit their father's Y chromosome, will be normal.

The best-known condition in this group is haemophilia A. Female carriers of the gene may be detected by their reduced factor VIII activity levels, especially when compared with the level of factor VIII-related antigen or by molecular studies. Prenatal diagnosis, however, can only be achieved by molecular analysis of fetal DNA if the family has a mutation identified, or has been found to be informative on linkage studies, or by fetoscopy and fetal blood sampling. Another option is fetal sexing and termination if the fetus is an at-risk male. This last option is seldom used where good treatment for haemophilia is available. The added risk of developing AIDS from infected blood products has in recent years made some at-risk couples reconsider their decisions about prenatal diagnosis for haemophilia.

Duchenne muscular dystrophy is another example in this category and the defective gene situated on the long arm of the X chromosome has been found to be extremely large. About 60 per cent of the mutations are due to a deletion that can be relatively easily detected. If a deletion is not evident a detailed family work-up is necessary and linked DNA markers are used to follow the segregation of the mutant gene. DNA from the affected males is generally essential for both the success of the family study and for comparison when prenatal diagnosis for at-risk fetuses is requested. Blood specimens

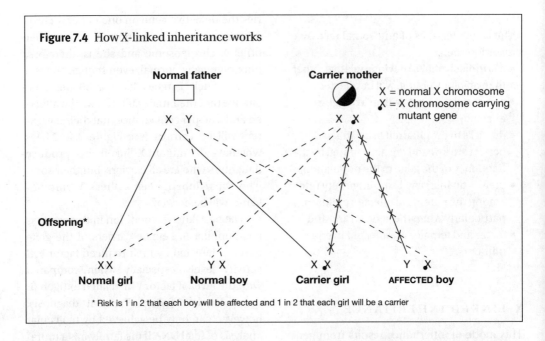

**Figure 7.4** How X-linked inheritance works

Normal father

Carrier mother

X = normal X chromosome
X̣ = X chromosome carrying mutant gene

X  Y

X  X̣

Offspring*

X X          Y X          X X̣          Y  X̣
**Normal girl**   **Normal boy**   **Carrier girl**   **AFFECTED boy**

* Risk is 1 in 2 that each boy will be affected and 1 in 2 that each girl will be a carrier

from these males, who have shortened life spans (often only about 20 years), should, therefore, be collected and stored for possible future use. New mutations occur in less than one-third of cases. In many instances it is difficult to be sure if the mutation occurred in a gamete producing the affected child or in an earlier generation, and genetic counselling can, therefore, be complicated.

## Polygenic inheritance

This mode of inheritance is called polygenic because genes at two or more loci, rather than at a single locus in one or both parents, are responsible for the defect or for a predisposition towards the development of the defect. Individuals who have such genes and are exposed to certain environmental influences (not clearly defined) at crucial stages of their pregnancies may then have children with one of several common and well-known abnormalities. Because these defects are caused by a combination of

The characteristics of X-linked recessive conditions are:
• the affected person is almost always male;
• only male relatives are affected (there are very few exceptions;
• such relatives are affected through carrier females;
• there is never male-to-male transmission;
• all the daughters of affected males are carriers; and
• carrier females have a 50 per cent chance of passing the gene to their male offspring, and female offspring have a 50 per cent chance of being carriers.

genetic and environmental factors they are also called multifactorial. Some of these disorders are indicated in Table 7.4 and their combined prevalence is about 22 to 24 per 1 000 births.

**Table 7.4** Common polygenic disorders and their prevalence*, sex ratio, and recurrence risk

| Disorder | Prevalence | Sex ratio M:F | Recurrence risk** |
|---|---|---|---|
| Neural tube defects (anencephaly, spina bifida, some hydrocephalus) | 1:900 | 1:2 | 1:30 |
| Cleft lip and palate | 1:700 | 2:1 | 1:25 |
| Talipes equinovarus | 1:700 | 2:1 | 1:30 |
| Congenital heart disease (some) | 1:200 | 1:1 | 1:20–1:30 |
| Diabetes (some types) | 1:500 | 1:1 | 1:20 |
| Congenital hip dislocation | 1:200 | 1:3 | 1:20 |

\* The prevalence varies in different populations
\** For normal parents after one affected child

The neural tube defects represent well-known examples of this group of disorders. They are most prevalent in people of Celtic origin, which includes the Welsh, Scots, and Irish, in whom the incidence is about one in 200 births, but they also occur in about one in 600 black infants in South Africa. In Britain they occur more commonly in the winter months, and are found more frequently in the lower socio-economic groups, in the first and fourth child in a family, in mothers who are diabetics, and in mothers who have had high body temperatures as a result of fevers or saunas at about six weeks of gestation. Folic acid supplementation pre- and post-conception for two months can reduce the occurrence and recurrence rate, which is normally about one in 30. After a couple have had two affected children the risk increases to one in ten, and an affected person has a risk of about one in 30 of producing an affected child. Prenatal diagnosis is available by measurement of alpha-feto protein in the amniotic fluid at 16 to 17 weeks gestation, and by ultrasound scans.

The environmental factors responsible for these multifactorial conditions are generally not well understood. Congenital heart defects are, however, associated with maternal rubella or diabetes, increased maternal age, increased maternal alcohol consumption, with drugs such as lithium (used in bipolar mood disorder), and with the anti-epileptic drugs. Clefts can be associated with anticonvulsants and also with steroids, barbiturates, caffeine, and valium taken during the pregnancy. The drug, dose, timing during gestation, and genetic predisposition all play a part in determining the effect of the drug and the malformation that might ensue.

Many of the conditions included in this group also occasionally appear in conjunction with other defects as part of a syndrome. For example, congenital heart disorders are found in about 40 per cent of children with Down syndrome and in other chromosome disorders such Turner syndrome. Facial clefts are found in chromosome abnormalities such as trisomy 18, and the recurrence risk would then be very low (less than one per cent). Neural tube defects may be associated with polydactyly and kidney abnormalities in the Meckel syndrome, which is an autosomal recessive disorder with a one in four recurrence risk. As a general rule, if the condition is an isolated case and there is no family history and no associated abnormality the rules of polygenic inheritance will apply, but if the condition is part of a syndrome an entirely different mode of inheritance (and risk of recurrence) will need to be considered.

# The chromosomal disorders

The incidence of all chromosome abnormalities at birth is 0,5 per cent. The great majority of these disorders have a very low risk of recurrence. However the great majority of hereditary disorders show no recognizable chromosome abnormality. Since the chromosomal disorders are difficult to treat, but often easily detectable on amniocentesis, they need to be recognized before birth whenever possible.

The most common condition in this group is Down syndrome (or trisomy 21), which occurs once in every 700 births in most populations. The affected child has decreased intelligence, generalized hypotonia, a characteristic facial appearance, and various minor physical features that appear to be due to the trisomy of the distal part of the long arm of chromosome 21. The extra chromosome material may be maternal or paternal. The affected person has a high risk (probably one in three) of producing a Down child. A strong correlation with maternal age has been shown, but correlation with paternal age is still being investigated. The extra chromosome is a separate entity in about 90 per cent of cases (and the recurrence risk is then only one per cent), but in five per cent of cases it is attached (translocated) – usually to chromosome 14 – and then a translocation type Down syndrome is said to exist. It represents a new mutational event in about half the cases, but is inherited from a parent carrying a balanced translocation in the other half. This latter group has a high recurrence risk of about one in ten if the mother is the carrier, and one in 40 if the father carries the translocation. A further five per cent of cases have the mosaic type in which some cells have the extra chromosome 21 and the others do not. These affected children have a similar clinical picture to the other two types. Chromosome studies should therefore be carried out on every child with Down syndrome, so that high-risk families are identified, counselled, and offered prenatal diagnosis and selective abortion.

The two other viable trisomies, Edward syndrome (trisomy 18) and Patau syndrome (trisomy 13) have an incidence of about one in 3 500 births and one in 7 000 births respectively. These syndromes have such severe abnormalities that a short life span of three months to three years results. The recurrence risk is low – less than one per cent.

The majority of sex chromosome abnormalities involve too few or too many sex chromosomes. The best known is probably Turner syndrome, when only one X chromosome is present in a female instead of two. This syndrome occurs in approximately one in 2 500 females. Various minor physical abnormalities result, including short stature and sterility. Mental retardation is present in only about five per cent of cases. Recurrence risks are low. Other abnormalities in this group include Klinefelter syndrome (XXY) with a prevalence rate of one or two per 1 000 males and the rarer triple X (XXX) and XYY syndromes.

Structural changes, chromosome rearrangements, and deletions generally cause severe intellectual disability and physical abnormalities. If a translocation is found in a child the parents should have their chromosomes analysed, and if a balanced translocation state is found in one of them all the siblings and other close relatives of the affected member should be tested, so that carriers can be detected and offered genetic counselling. In this way the future births of severely handicapped children may be prevented.

It has long been observed that there are more intellectually disabled males than females and the Renpenning or fragile X syndrome is probably partly responsible. In this condition an abnormality or fragile section on the distal part of the X chromosome can generally be detected when the lymphocytes are cultured in a folate deficient medium. Males who have this defect are usually intellectually disabled and have large testes and a fairly characteristic facies with a large jaw and large ears. Females are generally of normal intelligence, although occasionally mildly retarded. Reports suggest that this condition might be nearly as common as Down syndrome.

## Indications for chromosome studies

Indications for chromosome studies include:

- intellectual disability of unknown aetiology;
- multiple congenital anomalies;
- ambiguous genitalia, hypogonadism, primary amenorrhoea;
- recurrent (three or more) miscarriages occurring before 12 weeks of gestation (10 per cent of this group have a chromosome defect);
- unexplained stillbirths or neonatal deaths; and
- family history of chromosome translocation.

## Congenital anomalies

There are many different causes of congenital anomalies and these causes are frequently unknown. The known causes include teratogens, such as infections, drugs, alcohol, and radiation, which may harm the developing fetus. A deformity caused by intra-uterine positioning, for example, due to oligohydramnios (reduced intra-uterine fluid) may mimic club foot, but this deformity can be passively corrected whereas club foot can not. Constrictions of body parts displaced through holes in the amnion may lead to limb abnormalities.

The major *infections* include rubella, cytomegalovirus, hepatitis, HIV (AIDS), toxoplasmosis, and syphilis. In the case of rubella

the risk to the fetus is 60 per cent if a primary infection occurred in the first month of gestation, 25 per cent if it occurred in the second month, 8 per cent in the third month, and small in the second trimester. The chief malformations associated with rubella infection are listed in Table 7.5. Apparently normal at-risk infants should be examined carefully (including audiometry) to exclude minor degrees of damage. Malformations that may occur in association with the other infections are also shown in Table 7.5.

**Table 7.5**  Congenital infections causing defects in the fetus

| | |
|---|---|
| Rubella | Cataract, deafness, congenital heart defects |
| Cytomegalovirus | Microcephaly, chorioretinitis, hepatosplenomegaly |
| Hepatitis | Biliary atresia, hepatic damage |
| HIV (AIDS) | Immune deficiency, minor dysmorphic features |
| Toxoplasma | Chorioretinitis, microcephaly, hepatosplenomegaly |
| Syphilis | Facial and other bony abnormalities, keratitis |

Various drugs can cause congenital abnormalities in the fetus if they are taken early in a pregnancy. Thalidomide is the best known and it is associated with limb abnormalities. Since it has been withdrawn from the market the most important teratogenic drugs are probably warfarin (used to treat rheumatic heart conditions necessitating valve replacement), which causes a high fetal and perinatal loss and bony abnormalities in some of the survivors, the anticonvulsants and retinoids. The anti-epileptic drugs (e.g., phenytoin and valproate) can cause congenital heart disease, clefting, neural tube defects, mental retardation, and behavioural problems. Lithium, used in treating bipolar mood disorder, may cause fetal heart defects. Vitamin A analogues (e.g., retinoids), used for skin disorders, are associated with a pattern of defects similar to the Di George sequence.

Congenital disorders can also result from inadequate or inappropriate maternal diet. Excessive alcohol taken in the first trimester of pregnancy, or even one binge at a crucial stage of fetal development, can result in infants with the Fetal Alcohol Syndrome: abnormal facies, reduced somatic and brain growth, microcephaly, mental retardation and heart defects (see Chapter 9: Fetal Alcohol Syndrome). Cigarette smoking in pregnancy may cause growth retardation in the fetus.

There is an increase in the prevalence of congenital abnormalities in the offspring of diabetic women, especially in those with vascular complications. The defects include sacral agenesis, proximal femoral deficiency, and caudal regression syndromes. However, if the diabetes is under good control, the risk of fetal abnormalities is reduced.

Iodine deficiency in the pregnant woman is associated with goitre, intellectual disability of varying degrees, nerve deafness, and hypothyroidism in the child.

Radiation in pregnancy has been thought to produce fetal defects. However, if an excessive amount of radiation has been used on the pregnant (first trimester) woman's abdomen the result will often be fetal loss. If the fetus is retained the risk is only about one in 1 000 for mental retardation, childhood cancer, and malformations, and the background risk for every pregnancy is higher than this.

# Prevention of genetic and congenital disorders

In some cases genetic disorders can be prevented before they occur (primary prevention), and in others a recurrence can be prevented (secondary prevention). Where at-risk populations are identified, members of these groups can be screened for a particular disorder. These groups include:

- the older mother (more than 35 years), who is at increased risk of producing a child with Down syndrome, trisomy 18 and 13, Klinefelter, or the triple X syndrome. The risk for any chromosome abnormality is one in 180 when maternal age is 35 years, one in 60 at 40 years and one in 20 at 45 years. These women can be offered prenatal diagnosis and selective abortion;
- the Jewish population who are at risk for Tay-Sachs disease, a severe neurodegenerative disorder, which causes the death of the child by four years of age. One in 25 Ashkenazi Jews carries the gene for this recessive condition, and every Jewish couple of childbearing age should be tested so that the carriers can be identified. If two carriers marry they can be offered prenatal diagnosis;
- the Greek and Indian populations are at risk for beta-thalassaemia, a severe recessively inherited anaemia. About one in six Greek Cypriots and one in 12 inhabitants of the Greek mainland, as well as one in 40 of the South African Indian population, carry the gene. Carrier couples can be identified by means of a relatively simple blood test and pregnancies monitored by DNA analysis, or else by fetal blood sampling and globin chain synthesis;
- pregnant women found to have raised serum alpha-feto protein (AFP) levels at 16 weeks gestation are at risk of having a child with a neural tube defect. On the other hand, reduced maternal levels of AFP and oestriol (as well as increased levels of human chorionic gonadotrophin) at 16 weeks are associated with Down syndrome and other chromosome abnormalities in the fetus. In these cases amniocentesis is indicated.

Pregnant women may also have a first trimester scan to assess fetal nuchal fold thickness. An abnormally thick fold may indicate a chromosome or other anomaly and chorionic villus sampling or an amniocentesis for prenatal diagnosis should be performed. Similarly fetal scans in the second trimester can detect abnormalities which may need to be diagnosed by amniotic fluid analysis.

The occurrence or recurrence of a genetic or birth defect may be 'prevented' by either environmental manipulation or by prenatal diagnosis with selective abortion. As previously noted, the risk of a recurrence of a neural tube defect in a family may be reduced if vitamin and folate supplementation is given peri-conceptionally, especially in the lower socio-economic groups. Other environmental manipulation methods include: routine rubella vaccinations prior to pregnancy; altering the drug regimen of patients with disorders such as epilepsy (where phenytoin is the teratogen), bipolar mood disorder (where lithium is the culprit) or heart conditions (when women are treated with warfarin); and warning women not to take saunas in the first trimester (which can be associated with neural tube defects in the fetus).

Prenatal diagnosis for detection or prevention of recurrences of genetic disorders can be achieved by the following methods:

- *amniocentesis* – usually performed at 15 to 16 weeks gestation for chromosome abnormalities, the neural tube defects and some metabolic and other disorders. In experienced hands the risk of miscarriage associated with the procedure is 0.7 per cent and the reliability rate 99.9 per cent, so this is a safe and useful procedure;
- *chorionic villus sampling* – performed at 9 to 11 weeks gestation for all the disorders that can be detected on amniocentesis with the exception of neural tube defects. The miscarriage rate is about five per cent, so this procedure should only be used in

high-risk cases such as cystic fibrosis, Duchenne muscular dystrophy, thalassaemia, Tay-Sachs disease, or haemophilia;
- *sonar scans* – performed by an expert during the second trimester and serially if necessary – can sometimes detect microcephaly, hydrocephaly, achondroplasia, and severe forms of osteogenesis imperfecta (where fractures occur *in utero*), and heart and kidney defects;
- *fetal blood sampling* – cord blood can be collected from the at risk fetus for chromosomal, haematological and other studies where necessary. Thalassaemia, haemophilia, severe clefting syndromes, oculocutaneous albinism and chromosome abnormalities suspected on sonar can be diagnosed in this way.

## DNA studies

With our increasing understanding of the molecular basis of disease it is now possible to study the DNA directly from blood, chorionic villi or amniotic cell specimens, to diagnose certain disorders prenatally. These disorders include: cystic fibrosis, Huntington's disease, Duchenne muscular dystrophy, haemophilia, thalassaemia, and other rarer conditions. Most of these disorders are heterogeneous at the molecular level, even though they might appear to be relatively homogeneous at a clinical level. Beta-thalassaemia, for example, is due to 85 different mutations within and around the beta-globin gene, all of which cause some form of beta-thalassaemia. Different populations have characteristic mutation profiles, which often narrow down the number of molecular lesions responsible for a particular disorder in a specific group.

The DNA analysis for prenatal diagnosis falls into two groups: those disorders for which closely linked markers are identified and the diagnosis is made by tracking a marker with the disorder in a particular family; and those for which the gene has been cloned and some of the disease- causing mutations identified. In many cases it is essential that blood samples be collected from at least both parents and an affected child, and also from normal children if possible. In exceptional families with no living affected members, prenatal diagnosis may nevertheless be offered if the parents have the common mutation. For example, in the case of cystic fibrosis, where 68 per cent of the North American cases have an identifiable mutation caused by the deletion of three base pairs resulting in the loss of a single amino acid, it is possible to offer prenatal diagnosis without investigating samples from living affected family members. Generally, however, if an affected member is terminally sick it is very important that a blood sample be collected and 'banked' so that information from the individual is available for use by other at-risk family members in the future.

Couples who choose to have these molecular studies should present before becoming pregnant, so that the family work-up, which can take three or four weeks, is completed in sufficient time to offer appropriate counselling prior to a pregnancy, and the appropriate method of prenatal diagnosis can be selected and organized.

Progress in the field of human genetics has been dramatic in the past decade and new information is continually becoming available. The clinical geneticist has the responsibility of keeping colleagues informed so that new techniques become practical options, to the benefit of affected families and society as a whole.

## References and further reading

CARTER CO. 1975. *An ABC of medical genetics.* London: Lancet.

CONNOR JM & FERGUSSON-SMITH MA. 1997. *Essential medical genetics,* 5th ed. Oxford: Blackwell.

HARPER PS. 1998. *Practical genetic counselling,* 5th ed. Bristol: John Wright.

KROMBERG JGR, BERSTEIN R, JACOBSON MJ, ROSENDORFF J, and JENKINS T. 1989. A decade of mid-trimester amniocentesis in Johannesburg. *South African Medical Journal.* 76:344–9.

KROMBERG JGR & JENKINS T. 1982. Common birth defects in South African blacks. *South African Medical Journal.* 62:599–602.

MCKUSICK VA. 1994. *Mendelian inheritance in man,* 11th ed. Baltimore: Johns Hopkins University Press.

SMITH DW. 1982. *Recognizable patterns of human malformation,* 3rd ed. Philadelphia: WB Saunders.

# 8    Genetic services

T JENKINS &
JGR KROMBERG

Genetic services are fairly recent arrivals on the medical scene. Although individual doctors have undoubtedly been aware of inherited disorders since the start of the century and have cared for affected patients and their families, medical genetics did not come of age until after the Second World War. The first genetic clinics were founded at the University of Michigan in the United States in 1941 and at the Hospital for Sick Children, Great Ormond Street, London in 1946. There are now more than 40 such genetic counselling centres in the United Kingdom, more than 450 in the United States and a dozen or so in South Africa.

Genetic services are provided in different ways by a variety of professionals in various settings. The major providers in South Africa are the university departments of Human Genetics, and the Genetics Services Division of the Department of Health. However, general practitioners, obstetricians, paediatricians, and other specialists in private practice frequently give genetic advice and deal with the genetic questions of their patients. These providers usually only refer their patients to a genetic counselling clinic when the disease is very rare or they are unsure of how to manage an unusual situation.

## What are genetic services?

Genetic services are now an integral component of the health care systems of most developed countries, although many medical practitioners feel that medical genetics is an esoteric speciality that caters only for the needs of a small number of patients with exceptionally rare diseases for which little (if anything) can be done. Inherited disorders are, however, already assuming greater importance in many countries, including some in the developing world.

In most countries that have well-developed genetic services the State has assumed the main responsibility for initiating and funding them. There have, however, been some strikingly successful prospective prevention programmes, which were initiated and carried through by particular communities. The Tay-Sachs disease prevention programmes introduced by highly motivated members of the Jewish community in Baltimore, and more recently in other centres in the United States and Canada, are outstanding examples.

The university-based and the State Department of Genetic Services, together with vol-

## The objectives of a genetics service

The objectives of a genetic service are:
- to diagnose, treat, and prevent genetic disease;
- to provide expert advice, help, and support for affected individuals and their relatives (genetic counselling);
- to provide high-quality laboratories capable of carrying out appropriate cytogenetic and biochemical investigations;
- to help train health care workers for practice in the field;
- to increase public awareness of inherited disorders;
- to initiate primary prevention programmes; and
- to reduce the burden for society.

- comprehend the medical facts, diagnosis, prognosis, and how best to manage the disorder;
- appreciate the genetics of the disorder and the risk of recurrence;
- understand the options for dealing with the risks (for example, of another pregnancy with or without prenatal diagnosis, adoption, foster care, artificial insemination by donor, or childlessness);
- choose and instigate an appropriate course of action; and
- make the best possible adjustment to their situation.

In South Africa many families, referred generally by obstetricians and other specialists, started to use genetic counselling in the 1970s, and, by the end of the 1980s about 2 000 families were being seen annually by the South African Institute for Medical Research geneticists in Johannesburg, in association with the University of the Witwatersrand, and at the Universities Of Cape Town, Stellenbosch, Natal, Pretoria and Orange Free State, and the Medical University of South Africa.

The main reasons for referral to a genetic counselling clinic are:
- birth defects (e.g., neural tube defects, cleft lip and palate, congenital heart disease and multiple congenital abnormalities);
- known genetic disorders (e.g., Down syndrome, cystic fibrosis, Duchenne muscular dystrophy, haemophilia, and metabolic disorders);
- mental retardation and/or seizures;
- visual or hearing impairment;
- a history of multiple miscarriages, stillbirths or neonatal deaths; and
- an increased risk of a disorder due to ethnic origin (e.g., Greeks have an increased risk for thalassaemia, Ashkenazi Jews for Tay-Sachs disease), consanguineous marriages, exposure to drugs, alcohol, chemicals, radiation, or the

untary organizations, fulfil the objectives of a genetic service in various ways, and they will be briefly described here.

## ACADEMIC DEPARTMENTS OF HUMAN GENETICS

These departments are generally based in medical schools or teaching hospitals and provide comprehensive genetic services, which include: genetic counselling clinics, laboratory investigations, education of the medical and lay public, and research on genetic disorders.

## GENETIC COUNSELLING CLINICS

As knowledge of genetic disorders grew, people began to demand genetic counselling, and so clinics were set up in major centres around the world. The aims of genetic counselling were defined by the World Health Organization in 1974, and these were specified as helping individuals or families to:

advanced age of the woman (women aged 35 years and over are at increased risk for chromosome aneuploidies and sex chromosome abnormalities in their offspring).

The counsellors at genetic counselling clinics generally use a non-directive counselling approach, so that patients can be given the facts and encouraged to make their own decisions about future family planning and reproduction.

Genetic counselling clinics in South Africa are run by the academic departments of Human Genetics at most of the universities and can be contacted through these major departments. In Durban, clinics are run by the Department of Paediatrics at Addington Hospital.

## LABORATORY SERVICES

A range of laboratory tests, depending on the expertise and interests of the staff in each department, are offered. Cytogenetic, serogenetic and molecular laboratories generally offer routine diagnostic services, as well as tests for very rare conditions. Enquiries should be made in advance about these rare disorders before a service is offered to patients.

## EDUCATION AND INFORMATION SERVICES

The staff of academic departments provide education on human genetics to medical personnel, including students, specializing medical practitioners, general practitioners, and other health care professionals, including nurses, physiotherapists, occupational therapists, speech therapists, and medical social workers. Lectures are given to the lay public including scholars, women's groups, and service organizations. Leaflets and articles have been produced on specific disorders for patient education. Articles have been pub-

lished in the popular press, and television programmes have been prepared to inform the general public about genetic disorders. The Southern African Inherited Disorders Association (SAIDA) provides an information service, a biannual newsletter and updates on the field.

## DEPARTMENT OF HEALTH

The Human Genetics division has four main objectives: to prevent genetic and congenital disorders; to formulate policy regarding genetic services; to educate the population about genetic disorders; and to help affected individuals and their families cope with their situation. To achieve these aims genetics nurses are employed at provincial level to serve the different regions of South Africa. These genetics nurses provide a communication and liaison service between the genetic counselling clinics and the public, arrange for specific tests to be done prior to counselling, offer long-term support and follow-up, and also provide a referral service to appropriate community resources. They can be contacted through the Provincial Department's offices in Cape Town, Kimberley, Port Elizabeth, Bloemfontein, Durban, Pietermaritzburg, Johannesburg, and Pretoria (where the head office is situated).

The Department also runs selected small-scale screening programmes in specific areas of the country. These include maternal serum alpha-feto protein screening for the detection of neural tube defects and newborn screening for phenylketonuria and hypothyroidism. Their screening by amniocentesis of high-risk pregnant women for prenatal diagnosis of chromosome defects and their Rhesus factor prenatal screening are countrywide programmes. Some screening for cystic fibrosis and other conditions in high-risk families, using the new molecular technique, is funded by the Department.

A genetic disorders surveillance programme is being undertaken by Genetic Services and the staff also attempt to stimulate new services and to co-ordinate existing ones. Education plays a large part in their prevention programme, and booklets on many dierent genetic disorders are available in several local languages.

## THE SOUTHERN AFRICAN INHERITED DISORDERS ASSOCIATION (SAIDA)

This association is a lay/medical organization that aims to:
- educate the medical and lay public on inherited disorders;
- oer fellowship and support to those with genetic disorders and their families; and
- encourage and support research into the causation, treatment and prevention of inherited disorders.

SAIDA was founded in 1973 and members include families with many different genetic disorders as well as interested lay people and medical personnel throughout the country. A newsletter, which reports new developments in the field (*SAIDA News*), is produced twice annually.

Leaflets on various conditions and on genetic counselling have been produced and radio programmes undertaken to increase public knowledge in the field. SAIDA provides an information and referral service for the many people from all over the subcontinent who contact the association for help with inherited conditions. Support groups have been set up or stimulated for 14 different disorders and a (now independent) toy library was initiated in the 1970s for handicapped children with specific needs. Funds have been made available for international experts to visit South Africa, and for South Africans to attend international congresses overseas.

The specific needs of members have also been met in various ways. Membership of SAIDA is open to all and is recommended to those who wish to maintain an interest in inherited disorders.

## INHERITED DISORDERS AND PUBLIC HEALTH

Are inherited disorders 'insignificant' causes of ill health in the developing segments of the populations of southern African countries? Can they justifiably be ignored when planning health services? Would genetic services in these countries be a luxury, diverting valuable, scarce resources from areas of health care with higher priorities?

There is, undoubtedly, very little epidemiological data on which rational decisions can be made. It is probably reasonable to assume that inherited disorders are as common in developing communities as they are in any other population, but when infant mortality rates (IMRs) are higher than around 100 per 1 000 live births, inherited disorders must assume less relative importance. Some workers have suggested that the IMR must get down to 50 before genetic disorders can be considered. IMRs are still around 100 in most southern African countries, but are as low as ten in the more affluent sections of the South African population. The rate in Soweto (prior to the HIV/AIDS epidemic) was as low as 26. As more people in all communities aspire to a markedly improved standard of living, they may expect genetic services to be available to them should they ever need them. In addition, the principle of equity in health care cannot be ignored.

It is debatable whether prospective prevention programmes for inherited disorders are feasible in developing countries. Even in some First World countries the utilization rates for amniocentesis among women aged 35 years or older are still below 50 per cent. Among the disadvantaged black people in the United

States the rate is significantly lower than in the more privileged groups. Rural dwellers have a lower rate of utilization of genetic services than those living in the urban areas.

The hereditary anaemias (sickle cell anaemia and the thalassaemias) constitute a huge public health problem in some developing countries, although in African countries south of the Cunene/Zambezi rivers, the problem is relatively minor. The enormous burden caused by the haemoglobin disorders is because they are both common and chronic. Sickle cell anaemia carries a very bad prognosis in tropical Africa but, as primary health care improves, the number of surviving homozygotes will increase, and with an expected average of one or two hospital admissions per year the burden on the family as well as on society will increase. Beta-thalassaemia in some of the Mediterranean countries and beta- and alpha-thalassaemia in Asian countries are already costing those countries enormous sums of money for blood transfusion therapy and desferrioxamine infusions to minimize iron overload. Greece has shown that its beta-thalassaemia prevention programme (screening to identify carriers and then monitoring all 'at-risk' pregnancies) is cost effective. It costs about US$1 million annually – the same sum that is consumed in treating the 200 cases born in a single year. The life expectancy of thalassaemia patients is now over 25 years in Greece and Italy. Screening programmes have not been introduced in the developing countries (India is a good example) and prenatal diagnosis is not generally available. Blood transfusion services cannot cope with the demand for blood for hypertransfusion therapy and desferrioxamine is too expensive for general use. The increasing prevalence of HIV infection in the developing countries makes blood transfusion more hazardous. Prenatal diagnosis is often not available but the wealthy can afford to pay often for investigations to be carried out in the United Kingdom, or the USA.

# Effective strategy

Genetic services in which the emphasis is on carrier detection, followed by prenatal diagnosis and selective abortion, is the only effective strategy for dealing with the hereditary anaemias in developing countries. Even now, plans should be made for this eventuality and pilot schemes introduced without delay. They should probably be organized at academic hospitals or other tertiary care centres where the necessary laboratories, genetic counselling clinics, and public education programmes can all be established in order to deal with the problem.

The technology already exists for the DNA diagnosis of sickle cell anaemia and most of the thalassaemia syndromes. By using the polymerase chain reaction (PCR) to amplify the part of the gene that encompasses the specific mutation, or else a closely linked restriction enzyme site, diagnoses can now be made quickly and accurately without resorting to the time-consuming family studies which were needed barely two or three years ago. Once established, PCR can be used for other purposes as well – for example, to assess the distribution of parasites in mosquitoes or the incidence of multiple infections by multiple pathogens in a population.

Genetic services can reasonably be expected to improve primary health care by encouraging people through counselling to make responsible decisions on every aspect of life and health, thereby contributing to effective development. It is envisaged that genetic services can be integrated with family planning programmes, as appeals to individuals to restrict family size or to space their children ought to be accompanied by help to ensure that the children who are born are healthy.

# Primary health care perspective

Inherited disorders, however, already constitute a significant health burden in many countries, including some in the developing world. Unless plans are made now for the introduction of pilot genetic services, the public health burden arising from some of these disorders will become overwhelming when the IMR is reduced.

There is no need to wait for specialist medical geneticists to be available in large numbers. The average doctor and primary health care worker (including nurses and auxiliaries) can quickly master the basic principles of genetics and can be trained to counsel patients. The Department of Health in South Africa has shown that a good nurse can become proficient in genetic counselling for the common disorders with a two-week intensive course and an 'apprenticeship' period of a few months.

Genetic services should not be seen as part of the 'high-tech' medicine available only at the tertiary health care facilities. Genetic services, if they are to make the contribution to the health of a country that they are capable of making, must be in the front line, in the community itself. Their doctors and other health care workers will then fulfil the role suggested by the great German physician and 'father of pathology', Rudolf Virchow, over 100 years ago: they will serve as 'advocates for the poor'. The introduction of genetic services will, it is predicted, help to strengthen scientific medicine and improve the primary health care infrastructure of the community.

## References and further reading

BEIGHTON P & BOTHA MC. 1986. Inherited disorders in the black population of southern Africa, parts I, II, and III. *South African Medical Journal.* 69:247–9, 293–6, 375–8.

CONNOR JM & FERGUSSON-SMITH MA. 1997. *Essential Medical Genetics*, 5th ed. Oxford: Blackwell.

EMERY AEH. 1979. *Elements of Medical Genetics*, 5th ed. Edinburgh: Churchill Livingstone.

JARPER PS. 1998. *Practical Genetic Counselling*, 5th ed. Oxford: Butterworth-Heinemann.

JENKINS T. 1990. Medical genetics in South Africa. *Journal of Medical Genetics.* 27:760–79

WEATHERALL D. 1991. *The New Genetics and Clinical Practice*, 3rd ed. Oxford: Oxford University Press.

# 9 Fetal Alcohol Syndrome

**D VILJOEN**

Fetal Alcohol Syndrome (FAS) is the most common preventable form of mental retardation world-wide. Lemoine first reported the disorder in French literature in 1968 and Jones & Smith (1973) were credited with coin-ing the term 'fetal alcohol syndrome'. FAS causes a range of disorders, is found in all ethnic groups and populations, and is most prevalent in impoverished communities. In South Africa, epidemiological studies have

## Terminology

The Institute of Medicine Report (1996) suggests the following terminology for use in relation to alcohol-related teratogenesis. These terms cover a wide spectrum of severity and a range of disorders and are applied to *children born to mothers following heavy alcohol consumption during pregnancy, which they either admit or for which there is direct evidence.*

- **Fetal Alcohol Syndrome (FAS)**
  This applies to a child who has growth retardation together with central nervous system anomalies and characteristic facial dysmorphology.
- **Alcohol-related birth defect (ARBD)**
  This refers to a child with some of the commonly reported alcohol-related structural organ anomalies, but not the full clinical phenotype usually required for a confident diagnosis of FAS (See Table 9.1).
- **Alcohol-related neurodevelopmental defect (ARND)**
  The neurodevelopmental deficiencies common to alcohol-related teratogenesis are present, but without sufficient structural anomalies or phenotypic criteria for a confident diagnosis of FAS.

The term 'Fetal Alcohol Effects' (FAE) is considered misleading as the diagnosis is often applied loosely to children of mothers who have consumed minimal amounts of alcohol during pregnancy, and who have a few phenotypic or behavioural anomalies as seen in cases of alcohol-related teratogenesis. The term has been abandoned in favour of the better-defined terms of FAS, ARBD, or ARND.

shown that rural populations in the Western Cape Province are particularly affected and have FAS rates exceeding those reported in other world communities. FAS, and alcohol abuse generally, are the consequences of many socio-economic and cultural factors. All of these will need to be addressed in the formulation of preventative strategies in order to reduce the tremendous social and economic burdens of the disorder in South Africa.

# Clinical manifestations and diagnosis

The clinical features of FAS are due to the teratogenic effects of alcohol on the embryo and fetus. The diagnosis is mainly based on several clinically derived phenotypic and neurodevelopmental features, as there are no biological markers for the disorder. The optimal age for the recognition of FAS-associated features is between three and ten years of age. A confident diagnosis based on clinical features alone can be problematical in the neonate or adolescent and adult.

The principal clinical features of Fetal Alcohol Syndrome (FAS) comprise a triad of signs:

## GROWTH DEFICIENCY

All the body measurements may be affected, both pre- and postnatally. In typical cases, these are usually all less than the 10th centile for age and sex and either a reduction in head circumference or a reduction in both weight or height together, are needed for a confident diagnosis. These measurements remain deficient throughout life, with the exception of pubertal girls with FAS, in whom body mass approaches or may frequently exceed the 50th centile.

## CENTRAL NERVOUS SYSTEM INVOLVEMENT

The growth of the brain, particularly the frontal lobes, is deficient in FAS. Microcephaly, partial or complete agenesis of the corpus callosum, and cerebellar hypoplasia are structural anomalies frequently encountered. Impaired fine motor skills, neurosensory hearing loss, poor hand–eye co-ordination, and poor tandem gait are other usual findings. The average IQ is 63 with a wide range, from profound mental retardation to a level where individuals can function adequately in mainstream schools. Behavioural anomalies are frequent, generally inconsistent with the developmental level, and not able to be explained by the familial background or environment alone. Learning difficulties (with specific deficits in mathematics), poor school performance, deficits in receptive and expressive language, short concentration spans, poor memory, hyperactivity, and poor judgement are some of the characteristic findings in children with FAS.

## FACIAL FEATURES

Characteristically the mid-face is hypoplastic in FAS. The timing and dose of maternal alcohol consumption determines the degree of facial dysmorphology, which includes shortened palpebral fissures (less than the third centile), flattened nasal bridge (with epicanthic folds), shortened nose with upturned nares, a long smooth upper lip with thin vermilion border, and micrognathia. The mid-face may be flattened, and minor ear anomalies are usual.

Other organ system anomalies, which are commonly associated with FAS, are listed below in Table 9.1. These, too, are timing- and dose-dependent as far as maternal alcohol ingestion is concerned.

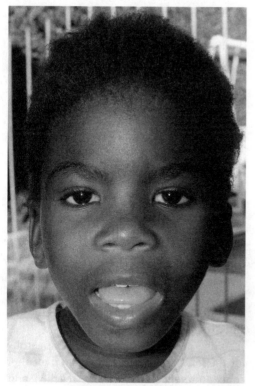

**Figure 9.1** Photograph of a child affected with Fetal Alcohol Syndrome

**Table 9.1** Alcohol-related birth defects (ARBD)

| Organ system | Defect |
|---|---|
| • Cardiac | Atrial septal defect; ventricular septal defect; tetralogy of Fallot; aberrant great vessels |
| • Skeletal | Radio-ulnar synostosis; digital and flexion contractures; shortened fifth digits; camptodactyly; hypoplastic nails; pectus excavatum; hemi-vertebrae; scoliosis; Klippel-Feil anomaly |
| • Renal | Aplastic, hypoplastic, dysplastic and horse-shoe kidneys; hydronephrosis; ureteral duplications |
| • Ocular | Strabismus, retinal vascular anomalies, refraction errors |
| • Auditory | Conductive and neurosensory hearing loss |
| • Other | Neural tube defects, cleft lip and palate, many others |

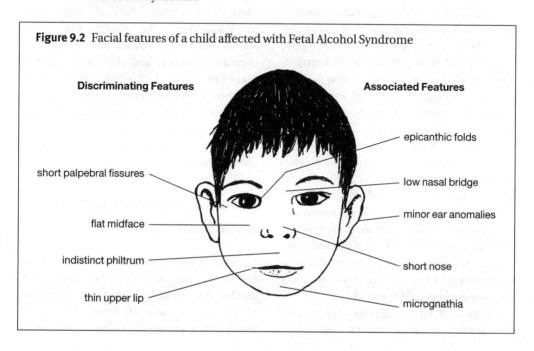

**Figure 9.2** Facial features of a child affected with Fetal Alcohol Syndrome

Discriminating Features

- short palpebral fissures
- flat midface
- indistinct philtrum
- thin upper lip

Associated Features

- epicanthic folds
- low nasal bridge
- minor ear anomalies
- short nose
- micrognathia

# Maternal drinking history

A maternal history of (usually heavy) alcohol ingestion during the index pregnancy is a prerequisite for a confident diagnosis of ARND or ARBD. Drinking in the father does not affect the pregnancy directly, but has a profound influence on maternal drinking habits. In 85,7 per cent of FAS affected cases in the Western Cape, the partner of the mother was found to be a heavy drinker. For a diagnosis of FAS, either a history of heavy drinking or strong clinical clues that maternal alcohol abuse occurred during pregnancy is required.

In the high-risk Western Cape communities, alcohol consumption during pregnancy occurred in 40,5 per cent of gravid women with a prevalence of heavy drinking of 23,8/100. Comparable figures for women in the USA are 20 per cent and 1/100. First-world figures for pregnancy-related alcohol consumption usually approximate those quoted for the USA, whereas the national averages for developing nations have not been determined.

Alcohol exposure during pregnancy is universally under-reported due to the stigmatization of the drinking mother and her guilt, knowledge of 'wrong-doing', fear of retribution from the father of the child, and possible exposure to litigation in some instances. A skilled interviewer well trained in extracting valid information must therefore preferably undertake an accurate assessment of substance abuse during pregnancy. The interview should be conducted in a non-threatening, quiet environment. The woman undergoing evaluation should be assured of anonymity, total confidentiality, help to overcome her problem, and the empathy and interest of the interviewer. Appropriate referral of the alcohol abuser and her partner, who invariably also abuses alcohol, is essential.

Heavy drinking *during pregnancy* is usually defined as at least five standard drinks taken more than twice a month, or an average of at least two standard drinks per day. A single standard drink contains 15 ml of absolute alcohol (AA), which is equivalent to 150 ml of wine (a large wineglass), 340 ml of malt beer (one can) or 30 ml of spirits (just exceeding one standard tot). Care should be taken in assessing the containers in which alcohol is bought when interviewing women as, for instance, beer may be purchased in 340 ml containers (i.e., a can or 'dumpy'), 375 ml bottles, and 750 ml bottles (quarts). In the rural areas of the Western Cape three or four women customarily drink together at home by sharing quarts of beer or two-litre containers of wine. These receptacles are passed from person to person during the 'party', thereby making the assessment of exact quantities drunk by each person difficult to determine.

Binge drinking is particularly dangerous for the fetus in that very high blood alcohol concentrations (BACs) can be reached and maintained. Animal experimentation has demonstrated that teratological effects are more pronounced with a high BAC. Investigations in the Western Cape have shown that binge drinking over weekends is common practice, and that on average in excess of 12 standard drinks per week are imbibed in one or two sessions by women who have previously produced children with FAS. Sustained BACs in excess of 200 mg per decilitre have been demonstrated in some of these mothers.

# Alcohol consumption in South Africa

In 1997, the retail sector of the liquor industry calculated that the annual per capita pure alcohol (i.e., absolute alcohol) consumption in the country was 4,9 litres. This placed South Africa at near the mean for per capita alcohol consumption amongst all nations. Approximately half the South African population is currently under 20 years of age, and this group does not contribute appreciably to the overall national consumption of alcohol. Furthermore, a large amount of beer is brewed at home in traditional settings and this is not included in the industry census of alcohol consumption. These factors would require a revised per capita consumption of alcohol amongst adults and may place South Africa amongst the heavier per capita alcohol-consuming nations of the world.

Two historical factors that have had a major impact on alcohol consumption and its abuse in South Africa are the 'dop' system and the existence of beerhalls. The 'dop' or 'tot' system is the part-payment of farm workers' wages in the form of alcohol. The custom was introduced from Europe more than 200 years ago and continues to be employed in certain European countries to this day. The 'dop' system was made unlawful in 1928 by an Act of Parliament, but the practice continued on a minority of farms in the Western Cape until recently. It is now strongly discouraged by the large wine-producing co-operatives and advocacy groups within the liquor industry. Non-complying farmers are penalized by such institutions. However, the long-term effects of the 'dop' system have helped engender a custom of abusive drinking amongst farm workers who became 'dependent' on the farmer. Alcohol dependence and full-blown alcoholism gained a hold on many individuals who did not have ready access to rehabilitation programmes. The poverty and lack of recreational outlets for farm workers have further entrenched the abuse of alcohol and culminated in the common practice of weekend binge drinking.

Beerhalls are particularly associated with the mining industry. In addition the construction by the former Nationalist government of beer halls situated between places of work and 'black' residential townships encouraged alcohol abuse, particularly among men living in 'hostels' and separated from their families and womenfolk. A culture of heavy drinking amongst male partners has also led to black women using and abusing alcohol more frequently, and thus deviating from traditional tribal customs of minimal alcohol use until after the child-bearing years.

Findings of increased prevalences of FAS in socio-economically deprived communities are therefore to be expected.

Several additional studies in South Africa have now demonstrated that the very high rates of road- and work-related accidents are frequently linked to alcohol abuse, as are instances of child and woman abuse, and violent crime. Thus the costs of alcohol abuse, both to the user's family and to the State, are enormous.

## Prevalence of FAS

The frequency of FAS in all the South African provinces has not been determined. Epidemiological studies are currently underway in Gauteng, and will shortly begin in the Eastern Cape Province. In the Western Cape, two epidemiological investigations undertaken in 1997 and 1999 in a small rural agricultural setting have revealed prevalence rates of 48/1000 and approximately 75/1000 (some data still to be analysed), respectively. When compared with other populations and subgroups in world populations, FAS is likely to be confirmed as a widespread public health problem in South Africa (see Table 9.2 below). It is estimated that as many as 10 000 to 12 000 new cases may be born annually, thereby constituting the single most common serious birth defect. A total of 80 000 babies with serious congenital anomalies are born in South Africa each year.

**Table 9.2** Prevalence of Fetal Alcohol
Syndrome (per 1 000)

| | |
|---|---|
| • USA (Abel & Sokol, 1991) | 0,33–2,2 |
| • France (Dehaene et al., 1991) | 1,2 |
| • Sweden (Olegard et al., 1979) | 1,33 |
| • Certain sectors of the Native | |
| • American Indian population (May 1991) | 8 |
| • An isolated Canadian Indian community (Robinson et al., 1987) | 125 |
| • Western Cape | 48–75 |

# Prevalence of ARND and ARBD

An attempt to estimate the prevalence of ARND in Seattle, USA, concluded that the rate was 9,1 per 1 000 live births, a figure in excess of three times that of true FAS prevalence in that community.

No estimates of ARBD have been calculated thus far, but they are probably in the order of three times that for FAS. Thus, ARBD and ARND are likely to be approximately six times more common than FAS, raising the total South African health burden from 10 000 to 12 000 children affected with FAS to 60 000 to 72 000 total individuals affected by alcohol teratogenesis annually. The lifetime costs of a FAS-affected individual in the USA exceeds half a million US dollars and, although disease-specific cost estimations have not yet been undertaken in South Africa, it is likely that this amounts to several billion Rands annually.

# Prevention of FAS

A National FAS Awareness Programme was launched nationally (November 1998) with the aim of reducing the burden of FAS in highly susceptible communities.

Current awareness of FAS in the Western Cape is high and local prevention workshops, community upliftment programmes, campaigns against the 'dop system', life skills programmes, educational thrusts, and new labour laws are currently being introduced. Specific prevention programmes need to be designed, piloted, tested for cost-effectiveness, and introduced to high-risk communities. A national FAS surveillance programme is currently being designed to aid in prevention activities.

Some aspects of prevention of FAS deserve special mention as these problems can begin to be addressed immediately. One is a need to alleviate poverty particularly in rural communities. Another is to improve maternal nutrition prior to and during pregnancy. Community education on the dangers of alcohol abuse is an additional urgent requirement.

In the long term, state-funded rehabilitation programmes, together with affordable and accessible in-patient and outpatient treatment facilities, need to be built and adequately staffed.

# References and further reading

ABEL EL & SOKOL RJ. 1991. A revised conservative estimate of the incidence of FAS and its economic impact. *Alcoholism: Clinical and Experimental Research.* 15:514–24.

DEHAENE P, SAMAILLE-VILLETTE C, BOULANGER-FASQUELLE P, SUBTIL D, DELAHOUSSE G, and CREPIN G. 1991. Diagnostic et prevalence du syndrome d'alcoolisme foetal en maternite. *Presse Medecine.* 20:1002.

IOM – INSTITUTE OF MEDICINE REPORT (USA). Division of biobehavioral sciences and mental disorders. Committee to study fetal alcohol syndrome (1996) *Fetal alcohol syndrome: Diagnosis, epidemiology, prevention and treatment.* Stratton KR, Howe CJ, and Battaglia FC (eds). Washington, DC: National Academy Press.

MAY PA. 1991. Fetal alcohol effects among North American Indians. *Alcohol Health and Research World.* 15(3):239–48.

OLEGARD R, SABEL KG, ARONSSON M, SANDIN B, JOHANSSON PR, CARLSSON C, KYLLER-MAN M, IVERSEN K, and HRBEK A. 1979. Effects on the child of alcohol abuse during pregnancy. *Acta Paediatrica Scandinavia.* 275(suppl [Stockholm]): 112–21.

PARRY CDH & BENNETS AL (eds.). 1998. *Alcohol policy and public health in South Africa.* Cape Town: Oxford University Press.

ROBINSON GC, CONRY JL, and CONRY RF. 1987. Clinical profile and prevalence of fetal alcohol syndrome in an isolated community in British Columbia. *Canadian Medical Association Journal.* 137:203–7.

STREISSGUTH A. 1997. *Fetal alcohol syndrome: A guide for families and communities.* Maryland: Paul Brookes Publishing Company.

# PART FOUR

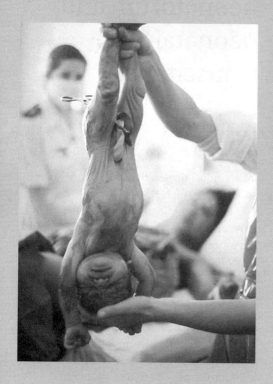

# Newborn

Perinatal disorders account for a full 56 per cent of infant deaths in South Africa. Pre- and perinatal events and the quality of perinatal care often have a crucial impact on later child development and well-being. Two clinical issues of special importance in this regard are addressed in this section – neonatal asphyxia and low birthweight. Ethical issues that emerge from the management of such infants in the developing world are also discussed. Perinatal care is reviewed fairly comprehensively, and a training programme, which is now widely used, is described. The reader is referred to general paediatric texts for additional important areas, such as neonatal jaundice, syphilis, and other infection.

# 10 Asphyxia neonatorum and neonatal resuscitation

## PA COOPER

Birth asphyxia is the cause of 20 per cent or more of all neonatal deaths in most southern African public sector hospitals. In addition, while figures from developed countries indicate that less than 10 per cent of children with cerebral palsy are a result of birth asphyxia, local studies suggest that this number may be substantially higher.

Many obstetric risk factors that predict newborns who may suffer from birth asphyxia have been identified, while other cases are preceded by a clinical or biophysical diagnosis

## Equipment needed for neonatal resuscitation

- An area should be set aside for resuscitation close to the place of delivery.
- A flat, firm surface heated by an overhead radiant warmer is recommended. Good lighting is essential.
- Suction apparatus should be provided with a low pressure adjustment to avoid damage to the delicate mucosa.
- Suction catheters should range in size from 5,0 to 10,0 Fr.
- Oxygen supply without a metered blender – 100 per cent oxygen is not considered toxic when administered for short periods.
- Suitable resuscitation bags and face masks for premature and full-term infants. The Laerdal Infant Resuscitator is ideal but

other less expensive systems such as the Samson-Blease may be satisfactory in the presence of normal lung compliance.
- Laryngoscope with straight blades 0 and 00.
- Endotracheal (ET) tubes – non-cuffed, marked in centimetres. Sizes 2,5; 3,0; 3,5; and 4,0 should be available.
- Umbilical catherization set with 3,5; 5,0; and 8,0 Fr. umbilical catheters (feeding tubes may also be used), cord ligatures, and clamps.
- The emergency drug tray should contain:
  - Adrenaline 1 in 1 000
  - Sodium bicarbonate 8,4 per cent
  - Dextrose 50 per cent
  - Naloxone (Narcan – adult strength vials)
  - Rapid blood glucose test strips
  - Neonatal maintenance fluid and a plasma volume expander

of 'fetal distress'. However, many asphyxiated infants are not predicted by prenatal complications or peripartum events. Thus all those involved in the delivery of newborn infants need to be trained adequately in the diagnosis and management of birth asphyxia.

Asphyxia can be defined as a lack of oxygen at tissue level, but this is not an easy definition to use in practice. A newborn who fails to maintain adequate cardio-respiratory function within one minute of birth should be considered to have birth asphyxia.

## Evaluation of the infant

The Apgar score should be properly estimated wherever possible. However, the two most important components of the Apgar score are the assessment of respiration and heart rate: if the infant is not breathing and the heart rate is more than 100, a diagnosis of mild to moderate asphyxia should be made (also referred to as primary apnoea based on animal experimentation); if the infant is apnoeic and the heart rate is less than 100, the infant is likely to be severely asphyxiated (secondary apnoea).

An attempt should be made to resuscitate all neonates showing any signs of life. Included in this category are babies, apparently stillborn, but where the fetus was thought to be alive immediately prior to delivery. Infants with congenital abnormalities should also be resuscitated since the full prognostic implications can rarely be predicted in the delivery room.

## Management

The mouth and nose should be gently cleared. Deep and vigorous suctioning is harmful and contraindicated except in the case of meconium stained liquor. In the case of mild to moderate asphyxia, tactile stimulation from drying the infant and nasal suctioning is often suffi-cient to promote respiratory effort, but many infants need bagging with oxygen before respiration is initiated. The mask should cover the mouth and nose and seal well.

If improvement does not occur or in cases of severe asphyxia when the heart rate persists below 100 per minute, endotracheal intubation of the infant is indicated wherever this is practically possible. Intubation should be via the mouth and should be performed by someone experienced in neonatal intubation. Ventilation should commence at a rate of 40 to 60 breaths per minute. Chest movement and air entry should be assessed. If, after initial ventilation, the heart rate remains below 60 beats per minute then chest compressions are needed. This is performed by using two fingers of one hand or both thumbs on the sternum with the hands encircling the chest. Compressions are given at a rate of 90 per minute and it is important to ensure that the sternum is depressed by two to three cm. When chest compressions are performed, three compressions are given for every one breath, i.e., 90 compressions and 30 breaths per minute in a synchronized fashion.

When meconium is present in the amniotic fluid, it is imperative that it be removed from the airway prior to the first breath. In vertex vaginal delivery or delivery of the head at Caesarian section the mouth and nose should be cleared of all traces of meconium by careful suctioning prior to the delivery of the chest. Following delivery, the mouth, nose, and posterior pharynx should be thoroughly suctioned. A large bore catheter (at least 8 Fr.) is necessary. Asphyxiated infants requiring ventilation who are also meconium stained should be intubated and direct suctioning of the endotracheal tube performed (using the ET tube as the suction catheter) prior to positive pressure being initiated – bag and mask should not be used in this situation unless no one experienced in endotracheal intubation is immediately available.

77

Where opiates have been given to the mother within six hours of delivery it should be presumed that this is contributing to the asphyxial state. This should be reversed with naloxone (0,1 mg/kg), which can be given intramuscularly or intravenously if an intravenous drip has been established.

## Drugs and fluids

The initial approach to resuscitation depends on effective oxygenation and ventilation, not on drugs. *The most common cause of the infant's failure to improve is inadequate ventilation, ineffective cardiac massage, or both.* Thus always check that adequate ventilation and cardiac massage are being performed effectively prior to drug administration.

- *Adrenaline:* 0,01–0,03 mg/kg intravenously or via the endotracheal tube for bradycardia or asystole.
- *Sodium bicarbonate:* A 4,2 per cent solution is prepared by diluting the 8,4 per cent ampule with an equal volume of water and then 2 ml/kg is given slowly over two to five minutes intravenously for severe metabolic acidosis.

Other drugs such as glucose, calcium, and isoprenaline are very rarely indicated in the resuscitation of the neonate, though additional glucose may be needed later if the rapid blood glucose measurement is low. Volume expansion with plasma, plasma volume expanders, or blood may be needed if excessive bleeding has occurred.

## Prognosis following birth asphyxia

It is important to counsel parents after a baby has been resuscitated successfully. The degree of asphyxia as indicated by the Apgar scores,

### When to stop resuscitation

Resuscitation should be abandoned when:
- The heart rate has remained less than 100 beats per minute for 10 minutes or
- There is no spontaneous respiration by 30 minutes

Infants meeting these criteria will rarely be normal survivors if they are admitted to the intensive care unit for ongoing ventilation.

the time taken to spontaneous respiration, and pH measurements are all useful in assessing the severity of the asphyxial insult, but should not be used to predict long-term prognosis.

Infants who are likely to suffer long-term sequelae following birth asphyxia will invariably manifest with abnormal neurological signs in the early neonatal period. This is described as hypoxic-ischaemic encephalopathy (HIE) and can be classified as mild, moderate, or severe. Infants with mild HIE will usually be normal at follow up; those with moderate HIE have a 20 to 50 per cent chance of later handicap; those with severe HIE have a high mortality rate and, if they survive, usually have major disability.

Thus careful documentation of the severity of HIE is essential in order to make a reasonable prognosis for an asphyxiated infant. It is important to note also that handicap following birth asphyxia invariably includes motor dysfunction (cerebral palsy) with or without intellectual disability and/or epilepsy. An intellectually disabled child *without* cerebral palsy is unlikely to be a result of birth asphyxia.

## Conclusion

Birth asphyxia remains a major cause of neonatal morbidity and mortality, particularly in the developing world. Prevention of birth asphyxia prior to delivery and effective resuscitation of those infants who are asphyxiated are important perinatal priorities. At the present moment only vigorous supportive therapy is available in the management of infants who have suffered a severe asphyxial insult. More specific therapies, however, may become available in the years to come.

## References and further reading

ESPINOZA MI & PARER JT. 1991. Mechanisms of asphyxial brain damage, and possible pharmacologic interventions, in the fetus. *American Journal of Obstetrics and Gynaecology.* 164: 1582–91.

LOW JA. 1993. The relationship of asphyxia in the mature fetus to long-term neurological function. *Clinical Obstetrics and Gynecology.* 36: 82–90.

# 11

# The low birthweight infant

## DL WOODS

The range of infant weight at birth is wide, with the majority of infants falling between 2 500 and 4 000 g. 'Low birthweight infants' are defined as being those infants weighing less than 2 500 g at birth. Their incidence in a given community is expressed as a percentage of all live births in that community during a specified period, and it is termed the low birthweight rate (LBWR).

There are many reasons why an infant might be born with a weight of less than 2 500 g (WHO, 1961). These LBW infants can be divided into *preterm* deliveries (defined as being those born before 37 weeks of gestation) and those born *underweight for gestational* age (i.e., with weights below the 10th percentile). In addition, some are both preterm and underweight for gestational age. There are two major categories of infants born underweight for gestational age, and these are clinically distinguishable at birth. Prolonged intra-uterine growth restriction affects weight, length, and head circumference, with all these values being below the 10th percentile at delivery. Where there is soft tissue wasting in the last weeks of pregnancy, birth weight will be disproportionally low compared to length and head circumference.

These infants have suffered starvation during the last weeks of pregnancy. While the phrase 'small for gestational age' (SGA) is often used instead of 'underweight for gestational age' (UGA), the latter is preferred, as the definition is based on weight. Many UGA infants are also wasted.

In affluent communities most LBW infants are born preterm, while among the underprivileged, the majority of LBW infants are full-term babies born underweight for gestational age. Common causes of LBW deliveries in a developing community include preterm labour, low maternal weight, poor maternal calorie intake or excessive physical labour during pregnancy, smoking and alcohol abuse, and multiple pregnancies. In an affluent community the cause of newborn UGA is usually a medical complication of pregnancy, such as hypertension. Primary placental causes of LBW are rare. Occasionally the causes of LBW are severe congenital abnormalities, chromosomal defects, or chronic fetal infections. The latter, and particularly syphilis (which is still common in some communities) may result in an infant being born both preterm and underweight for gestational age. The main causes of LBW are given in Table 11.1.

**Table 11.1** Common causes of low birtweight deliveries

......................................................................

- Maternal:
  preterm labour;
  low maternal weight;
  poor calorie intake during pregnancy;
  excessive physical labour during pregnancy;
  smoking;
  alcohol abuse; and
  maternal illness, such as hypertension
- Fetal:
  multiple pregnancy;
  congenital abnormalities;
  chromosomal defects; and
  chronic intra-uterine infections.

......................................................................

## Epidemiology

The LBWR provides a useful measure of maternal and child health, socio-economic status, and the general standard of living of a community (Louw et al., 1995). In affluent communities the LBWR is usually less than seven per cent while the rate in poor communities is often above 30 per cent. Therefore a high LBWR usually indicates a deprived community. In developing countries, there may be seasonal fluctuations in the LBWR, reflecting the availability of food and the amount of hard manual labour by pregnant women who are involved in such tasks as collecting water, carrying fuel wood, and working in the fields. Serial LBWRs may be used to monitor changes in a community and to evaluate the effects of an intervention programme.

## Morbidity and mortality

It is important to identify LBW infants at delivery as they are at increased risk of clinical problems in the newborn period and therefore may need special nursing and medical care.

The neonatal death rate is greatly increased in infants weighing less than 2 500 g at delivery. The lower the birthweight, the higher the incidence of neonatal morbidity and mortality. The specific problems to which such infants are prone depend on the underlying cause of the low birthweight. Preterm infants have immature organs and often develop hypothermia, hypoglycaemia, hyaline membrane disease, recurrent apnoea, jaundice, and periventricular haemorrhage. Term infants who are born growth retarded or wasted suffer from the effects of prenatal undernutrition and hypoxia, and may have hypoglycaemia, hypothermia, meconium aspiration, and hypoxic-ischaemic encephalopathy.

## Longer term effects of low birthweight

Low birthweight infants also face an increased risk of problems during later childhood. Postnatal growth may be impaired, especially if the infant suffered prolonged intra-uterine growth restriction. Postnatal development may be abnormal, particularly if there were severe perinatal complications such as hypoxia and hypoglycaemia. Many low birth weight infants return to poor families and thus also experience nutritional and educational deprivation. The risk of non-accidental trauma may also be increased in these families. Intra-uterine growth restriction in underweight women starts from early in pregnancy and may be an adaptation to a nutritionally hostile environment (Woods, 1989). There is increasing evidence that low birthweight renders the individual prone to diabetes, hypertension and heart disease in adulthood (UNICEF, 1999).

Optimal management of the low birthweight baby depends on determining the category and cause and preventing or treating associated complications. Clinical examination includes assessment of gestational age and carefully measured parameters of size. Specific investigations and treatment may be indicated.

The single most important strategy to decrease the neonatal mortality rate of a deprived community would be to reduce the LBWR. This would require improved living conditions and maternal nutrition, control of smoking and alcohol abuse, avoidance of heavy manual labour during pregnancy, and better family spacing. Antenatal care alone probably has a limited effect on lowering the LBWR.

# Kangaroo Mother Care

Kangaroo Mother Care (KMC) is the preferred 'baby-friendly' way of caring for newborn infants, especially newborns who have low birthweight. The infant (naked except for a nappy and a woollen cap) is placed in an upright position between the mother's breasts to keep it warm. KMC involves almost constant skin-to-skin contact between the infant and the mother. Numerous studies have documented that KMC is both safe and effective. It is often preferable to incubator care as it promotes bonding and breast-feeding. By colonizing the infant with the mother's own skin flora, the risk of infection is also reduced. Small infants can be moved out of an incubator earlier (when they weigh about 1 700 g)

with KMC. This reduces hospital expenses and lessens the demands on nursing staff. In poor communities with limited neonatal care facilities, KMC greatly reduces neonatal mortality. It also enables the mother to keep her infant warm in cold conditions. Even infants in a neonatal ICU can be often be given KMC when their parents visit. This allows the mother to contribute to the care of her infant. KMC is often life saving in poor communities and it is a better way of caring for infants in affluent communities.

## References and further reading

BELIZAN JM, LECHTIG A, and VILLAR J. 1978. Distribution of low birth weight babies in developing countries. *American Journal of Obstetrics and Gynaecology.* 132:704–5.

LOUW HH, KHAN MBM, WOODS DL, POWER M, and THOMPSON MC. 1995. Perinatal mortality in the Cape Province: 1989–1991. *South African Medical Journal.* 85:352–5.

UNICEF. 1999. *The Progress of Nations.* New York: UNICEF.

WHO. 1961. Public health aspects of low birth weight. *WHO Technical Report Services* No. 217.

WOODS DL. 1989. The constraint of maternal nutrition on the trajectory of fetal growth in humans. In: MN Bruton (ed.). *Alternative life-history styles of animals.* Dordrecht: Academic Publications.

# 12

# Perinatal services

DH GREENFIELD &
HA VAN COEVERDEN
DE GROOT

*'Stress has been laid on the importance of health education and preventive policies. But these must not be dissociated from professional competence. People do not take note of what is taught by people who are not competent.'*

RG Hendrickse (in Philpott, 1979).

Perhaps nowhere in medicine is this more true than in perinatal care. Good care given to the pregnant woman and her newborn baby greatly improves the chances of the woman later accepting the preventive and promotive services that are available. It is therefore of practical importance to keep this in mind when considering perinatal services, particularly in view of the fact that much of this work must inevitably be done by health personnel other than doctors.

For the purposes of this discussion, perinatal care will be defined as 'the care of pregnant women and their newborn babies'.

## The components of a perinatal service

The following are the main components of a perinatal paediatric service:

- the facilities;
- the personnel;
- communication.

## The aims of perinatal care

The overall objective is to ensure that at the end of every pregnancy there is a healthy baby and a healthy mother.

### Specific objectives

- To care for the pregnant patient in such a way that problems may be detected early and appropriate treatment given at the appropriate time, so that the effects on the baby are eliminated or reduced to a minimum. This applies to both pregnancy and labour.
- To prevent and, where appropriate, treat problems occurring in the mother and her newborn baby.
- To establish successful breast-feeding, and so ensure a healthy growth pattern.
- To ensure bonding between the baby, the parents and the family.
- To use the contact with the mother to provide basic health education.

83

## THE FACILITIES

## Type

*Permanent buildings* may be facilities that are only staffed at certain times or where there may be a full-time service.

*Mobile clinics* are provided where the population density in an area is low. These clinics may be a more appropriate and less expensive means of delivering a service than a permanent building with resident staff. The advantages are that a service can be given to even remote communities, and on a regular basis.

It is a particularly useful type of facility for providing antenatal and postnatal care, for family planning, and for providing care for the baby.

Wherever a part-time service is provided, it must be backed up by an accessible 24-hour facility for deliveries, and for dealing with emergencies.

## Level of care available

*Primary care at a level 1 centre.* The essence of any health care service is to ensure that at least primary health care is available for all the people. In the context of perinatal care, primary or level 1 care involves:
- access to antenatal care for the assessment of the maternal and fetal condition, and the screening for and management of easily treatable and preventable problems;
- facilities for adequate monitoring during labour and the treatment of emergencies which may arise;
- the management of normal deliveries;
- facilities for the resuscitation of the newborn baby;
- the emergency management of a sick neonate, and a mother who is ill after delivery;
- phototherapy and facilities for bilirubin monitoring if resources allow;

- the availability of transport for the mother or baby with 'problems' to a centre where there are better facilities.

This is a service that is run by nursing staff who have training and experience in midwifery. There may or may not be a visiting doctor.

The type of health care provided at this level essentially provides for the management of normal patients. The high-risk patients should be identified by routine screening procedures and referred to another health care centre where there are facilities for dealing with the problems which have been identified.

*Secondary care at a level 2 hospital* will involve:
- the monitoring and management in pregnancy of patients who have some risk factors;
- facilities for instrumental deliveries and caesarean sections;
- neonatal facilities such as phototherapy, oxygen therapy up to a limit (40 per cent), and antibiotic therapy;
- basic laboratory facilities – e.g., 'bubbles' test, urine microscopy, blood counts, total serum bilirubin, Gram stain, and reasonable access to facilities for bacteriological culture and biochemical tests.

At this level of care, there should be a doctor available 24 hours per day.

*Tertiary care in a level 3 hospital* is usually found in university teaching hospitals and includes intensive care units and extensive laboratory facilities. The medical staff would include specialist obstetricians and paediatricians, who are available for 24 hours per day.

## Relationships of the levels of care to each other

A service of this nature should be developed on a regional basis, where a single health authority is responsible for all the health services within a circumscribed geographical area.

A regional service (from the point of view of a perinatal service) should have a base hospital with a number of satellite delivery units. These satellite units would normally be level 1 facilities, and the base hospital a level 2, or on occasions a level 3 facility. It is often necessary for a facility to provide services normally only present in a higher level facility – e.g., it may be necessary to estimate total serum bilirubin levels, and provide phototherapy at a level 1 facility.

Communication and transport between the various health centres is essential. This will be discussed later in the chapter.

## Siting of the facilities

Primary care centres should be sited in such a way that everybody has ready access to one of them.

'Base hospitals' (level 2) should be readily accessible by transport from the primary care facilities, and similarly level 3 hospitals accessible from either primary or level 2 units. It is clear, therefore, that the siting of level 2 units in particular should be in a larger centre, usually a regional town, which is easily reached by road.

## Equipment that is needed in such a service

This will depend on the level of care to be provided, and will not be discussed in detail here, but will be alluded to when considering the problems to be dealt with (see Chapter 10: Asphyxia neonatorum and neonatal resuscitation).

## Outpatient or 'maternity' villages

When a patient has to go to a hospital distant from her home for delivery, perhaps because

of elective caesarean section, she needs to have accommodation at or near the hospital. It is, therefore, useful to have such accommodation available close to the hospital for waiting mothers who only need to attend antenatal clinic once or twice a week, and are not sufficiently ill to warrant admission. The patient is then close enough to be admitted in early labour. This is particularly important in rural areas.

## Domiciliary service

It is very difficult to provide an antenatal care service at the patients' homes. Such a service is not economical in its use of personnel and other resources.

Home deliveries are a reality in many communities, either because of lack of health care facilities or because of the dictates of local tradition and culture. In southern African urban environments, the majority of births take place in health centres. However, in rural environments many patients still deliver at home. Medical and nursing staff are seldom present at these deliveries, the mothers being attended by a traditional birth attendant, who may be a family member. Where people can be identified as traditional birth attendants, assistance may be offered and given in order to improve the quality of care that they provide.

A domiciliary postnatal service is recognized as being an important function of a perinatal service, where it can be provided, as in an urban environment. It enables women, who have had normal deliveries and who have normal babies, to be discharged from the hospital within a few hours of delivery, and still have the advantage of follow-up by the staff of the health service. This has considerable advantages for the baby, as the mother then has support and encouragement to establish breast-feeding, problems with the baby can be detected early, and appropriate management instituted. At the same time the health of the mother can be attended to while she has the support of her family.

## THE PERSONNEL

### Utilization of the available personnel

As has already been mentioned, all personnel should be deployed in such a way as to make maximum use of their skills. For example, the basic nursing tasks should be done by a nursing assistant with training in basic nursing care, rather than by more highly trained members of the staff. This does not imply that highly trained members of staff should consider themselves 'above' doing the more routine tasks, but rather that they should be available primarily for tasks in which they have training and expertise. *Maximize the use of people's talents and skills.* In particular, their skills and expertise should be used for teaching and for handling the more difficult problems. Similarly the doctor should be delegating many of the traditionally 'doctors' tasks' to nursing personnel, while providing the latter with teaching and 'back-up' support.

### Education and perinatal personnel

Continuing education is a priority at all levels of the service. In order to maintain their levels

### Categories of personnel

*Nursing staff* are the most important staff members in such a service because:
- there are insufficient doctors to be able to see the number of patients attending such a service;
- the majority of the patients who attend the service do not present with problems which need a doctor's level of expertise;
- the nurse is usually 'closer' to the community than the doctor and often has a better understanding of that community and its problems.

All levels and categories of nursing staff can and should be used to the maximum capacity of their competence. This is important as such a service releases more skilled and experienced personnel to deal with the more difficult problems.

*Doctors* who are competent in managing both obstetric problems and problems in the newborn baby must be available. Each region needs at least one such doctor, who should be available not only for clinical work, but also for teaching and for visiting the various health centres in the region. These visits should be arranged in such a way that the doctor is available to see the 'problem' patients, as well as to discuss both the problems experienced by the staff in the health centre and the problems arising from patients referred into hospital. This is a very important part of the communication between the peripheral health centre and the base hospital.

*Lay community health workers* should also be involved, particularly in encouraging people to make use of the services which are available for antenatal care and delivery. They can be very effective in ensuring the establishment of breast-feeding, supporting new mothers, and in providing basic domiciliary postnatal care, where such a service does not exist.

There should be regular liaison between the community health workers and the staff in the formal health service (and particularly the staff in the health centres).

of knowledge and skills, it is important for the doctors in the service to ensure that they are engaged in a continuing medical education programme relevant to the service that they are providing. At the same time, as a leader in the health team, the doctor also has a major responsibility as a teacher, encourager, and facilitator, and should be involved in maintaining and improving the knowledge, skills, and attitudes of those working in the service.

The same principles apply to all staff members and at all levels of the service. Thus professional (state registered) nurses should be responsible for ensuring their continuing professional education, while also teaching colleagues who are working under their leadership.

## COMMUNICATION

Communication falls into two main sections. The first is related to transport, while the second has to do with interpersonal communication within the service.

## Transport

At any time during the pregnancy, labour or the puerperium/neonatal period, the mother or her baby may have to be transferred to another health care facility within the service. On many occasions this is an emergency situation which can affect the lives of mother, baby, or both.

There is also a need to transport supplies.

The following must be regarded as basic necessities:

- *a vehicle* will be needed. The type of vehicle will depend on local circumstances. A multi-purpose vehicle is the most useful in rural areas. Circumstances will dictate whether this will be stationed at the health centre or at the base hospital;
- *access roads* to all health care facilities;
- *public transport* may be used when patient transfer is not urgent.

## Interpersonal communication

Even more important than transport is that people within the service should be able to talk to each other.

*Telephone or radio*: It is essential for staff in both peripheral health centres and base hospitals to be able to contact each other for advice and to discuss problems, both clinical and administrative, or to arrange for transport for patients, should this be needed. This is usually done by means of the telephone, although a radio communication system may be needed.

*Interunit visits*: A second essential form of communication is that staff from the base hospital should visit the clinic and vice versa. This is extremely important for the following reasons:

- *person-to-person contact* – the people in the various parts of the health service need to get to know each other. This greatly facilitates the discussion of problems over the telephone;
- *assessment of clinical problems* – staff from the base hospital visiting a peripheral health centre should be prepared to see clinical problems which have been gathered by the resident staff. The staff from the hospital should not be expected to see 'normal' patients, but should be used for problem solving and problem discussion. Patients should be seen by the person from the hospital and the person from the health centre together. This will also help the education process;
- *education* – every contact between hospital and health centre staff should be used as a teaching/learning experience. Staff working in peripheral centres should be constantly kept up to date and enabled to improve their standard of care. This forms an integral part of the work of the visiting staff from the base hospital.

87

In addition, staff from peripheral centres should regularly be brought into hospital for in-service training, refresher courses, etc. Part of this continuing education needs to be specifically oriented towards skills training, as well as to improve knowledge.

Staff working in health care facilities often have to deal with problems that would normally be dealt with by doctors. Their knowledge and skills therefore need to be maintained at a high level in order to cope with these problems effectively.

An exchange of staff between the hospital and the health centre often gives a feeling of being involved in a single health unit and of being part of the same health team. It is not only the peripherally based staff who benefit from this contact. The staff at the base hospital learn about the problems that are experienced in the health centres, and how these are handled.

## Protocols for management and referral criteria

Staff working in the peripheral units need to have clear guidelines for the management of problems on the principle that primary care units should only be dealing with 'normal' patients in the antenatal clinic, in labour, and with normal newborn babies. By implication, any patient who shows an abnormality should be referred to the base hospital. In order to avoid unnecessary referrals and delays in referral, guidelines for diagnosis and management need to be worked out and discussed with the staff working in the peripheral units.

*Regular audit:* A regular and frequent assessment of the quality of the service must be provided. This is done by means of:

- *perinatal mortality and morbidity meetings.* These should take place as soon as possible after the problem has arisen, but in any event at least monthly. The aim is to try to detect problems in the health care provided so as to learn from mistakes made. In this way the quality of health care may be improved. There is, however, a danger of these meetings becoming 'witch hunts', and this should be avoided. Nevertheless, when management has been incorrect, this must be clearly stated so that similar problems can be avoided in the future. These discussions should be primarily educational activities. The good management and the good outcomes should also be fed back as an encouragement to the staff:

- *record keeping and writing of notes.* The writing of notes is an essential part of any health service. This is often seen as a rather unimportant task by staff working in a busy peripheral health centre, but brief concise notes, in which the problems are identified and documented, and management specified, form a basic component of good health care. Simple problem-oriented records should be used. Part of the audit of the health service should be a regular, random assessment of the notes in patients' records. Part of the record keeping is the collection of accurate but simple statistics with regard to deliveries, problems, deaths, etc.;

- *assessment of patients who have been referred to hospital.* The essence of good management of problem patients in a primary care situation is the stabilization of the patient prior to transfer. Therefore, by assessing the condition of the patient on arrival at the hospital to which she has been referred, it is possible to gain a good idea of the quality of the care given at the health centre from which the patient has come;

- *effects of the service on the health of the community.* In the context of perinatal care, this means the effect on:
  - *The perinatal mortality rate* (the number of stillbirths and neonatal

88

deaths occurring in the first seven days of life per 1000 total births). This is the simplest statistic to obtain, and gives a good idea of the quality of the service. The ratio of stillbirths to neonatal deaths is not only a measure of the service, but also a marker of the socio-economic status of the community;

- *Perinatal morbidity*. There are a few conditions that can be fairly easily monitored, and which will give an indication of the standard of care and also of the neonatal problems in the community. For example, the incidence of asphyxia neonatorum is a marker of the quality of care given during labour, and of the quality of resuscitation. The incidence of low birthweight babies reflects the socio-economic status of the community, and also to some extent the usage of the service.

# The problems that affect the fetus and newborn baby

## During pregnancy

- Maternal disease, especially hypertensive disease and diabetes mellitus;
- obstetric problems
  - preterm labour and preterm rupture of the membranes,
  - multiple pregnancy,
  - abnormal lie,
  - antepartum haemorrhage;
- intra-uterine growth retardation;
- intra-uterine infections, of which syphilis is the most important;
- congenital abnormalities; and
- blood group incompatibilities.

## During labour

- Fetal hypoxia with fetal distress;

- prolonged labour, both first and second stages (resulting in fetal hypoxia);
- trauma – usually associated with difficult and assisted deliveries.

## Early neonatal period

- Asphyxia neonatorum and perinatal hypoxia;
- low birth weight, which may be caused by intra-uterine growth retardation, preterm delivery or both;
- hypothermia;
- metabolic problems
  - hypoglycaemia,
  - metabolic acidosis, usually related to perinatal hypoxia or infection;
- respiratory distress;
- neonatal jaundice;
- tetanus;
- convulsions;
- apnoea;
- congenital abnormalities; and
- surgical problems.

# The requirements to deal with these problems

## During pregnancy

- A good history and clinical examination are essential;
- urine testing;
- blood pressure estimation;
- assessment of fetal movement – 'kick chart';
- blood tests. There are two tests that are important in caring for the fetus:
  - serological tests for syphilis (VDRL or RPR). The treatment of syphilis in the mother is a priority in perinatal care in southern Africa, as there is a high prevalence of this disease in pregnant women;
  - blood grouping (ABO and Rh) of the mother during pregnancy, and of the

89

baby after delivery. Rh blood group problems are no longer common because of the use of human anti-D serum. However, significant numbers of babies are born with an ABO incompatibility. Babies born to mothers who are group O and/or rhesus negative should therefore be carefully watched for the development of jaundice, particularly in the first 24 to 48 hours after delivery;

- ultrasonography. This is useful for:
  - determining the gestational age of the fetus, when done before 22 weeks gestation;
  - detecting certain congenital abnormalities, which, if known before 22 weeks gestation, gives the option of termination of the pregnancy; or will enable the parents and health workers to prepare for the problems at birth;
  - confirming abnormal lies and multiple pregnancy;
  - confirming the presence or absence of fetal movement;
  - localizing the placenta.

    Ultrasonography can be useful in certain circumstances, but tends to be overused, and the results, particularly with regard to gestational age when done in the second half of pregnancy, can be misleading. It is also an expensive and operator-dependent facility, which is not available in the peripheral health centres. However, when it is used appropriately, it can provide very valuable information about the fetus;
- cardiotocography. This is useful for determining fetal heart rate patterns when fetal hypoxia is suspected. Its main uses are in stress tests, and in monitoring the fetal heart in labour. This facility is usually only available in level 2 or 3 facilities, and experience is needed in interpreting the results.

# During labour

Careful monitoring of the first stage of labour is essential in order to prevent fetal hypoxia or injury.

In the first stage of labour the following are monitored:

- maternal condition. This requires monitoring the blood pressure, pulse rate, temperature, and urinary output, as well as urinalysis;
- fetal condition. This requires careful monitoring of the fetal heart rate pattern and the state of the amniotic fluid;
  - the fetal heart rate pattern can usually be accurately monitored by being listened to with a *fetal stethoscope*;
  - a *'Doptone'* may be used when the fetal heart is difficult to hear;
  - *cardiotocography* may also be helpful when the fetal heart is difficult to hear or in a high-risk labour, as the fetal heart rate pattern can then be monitored continuously;
  - *fetal scalp blood sampling* may be performed in certain circumstances. The pH is measured, using fetal acidosis as a marker of fetal hypoxia. Fetal scalp blood sampling should not be done unless the mother is known to be HIV negative, as this procedure increases the risk of maternal to child transmission of the virus.
- progress of labour. This involves clinical assessment only, but it is most important that it is done carefully and conscientiously.
  - Cardiotocography and fetal blood sampling are available in virtually all level 3 hospitals. Many level 2 hospitals, however, now also have a cardiotocograph;

The two most important features of the monitoring of the first stage of labour are the accurate use of the partogram (composite labour graph), and the correct interpretation of the findings. These will reduce the dangers of perinatal hypoxia and undetected cephalopelvic disproportion by enabling the problems to be detected early.

The partogram *must* be used in *all* facilities providing obstetric care.

In the second stage of labour, in a level 1 unit, the only facilities needed are those required for performing and repairing an episiotomy, or repairing a perineal tear.

In a level 2 hospital, obstetric forceps or a vacuum extractor should be available, provided there are suitably experienced doctors or midwives.

Most, if not all, level 2 hospitals should have the facilities for doing a caesarean section under general, epidural or spinal anaesthesia.

## EARLY NEONATAL PERIOD

### Facilities for resuscitation

In the Peninsula Maternal and Neonatal Service in Cape Town, approximately 20 per cent of the newborn babies who are referred to hospital from the primary care centres (Midwife Obstetric Units) are referred because of asphyxia neonatorum or problems related to it. It is imperative that EVERY health care person who delivers babies must be fully competent to resuscitate a newborn baby.

### Neonatal jaundice

There should be reasonable access to means of monitoring and treating this condition. The minimum requirements would be a way of estimating serum bilirubin levels and giving phototherapy at the base hospital.

### Congenital abnormalities

Babies with these problems should be managed and transferred according to protocols laid down within the particular service.

## Other problems

Almost all the other problems that may arise in the neonatal period can be dealt with by ensuring:

- the provision and maintenance of a warm environment;
- that the baby is fed (intravenously if necessary);
- an adequate supply of oxygen;
- the prevention and, if necessary, the treatment of infection.

The technology should be appropriate at all levels of care. In particular, the technology should not exceed the skills of those who are expected to use it.

# On the newborn's discharge

Perinatal paediatric care does not end when the mother and her baby have been discharged home. Every effort must be made to ensure that this baby develops normally. The following matters must, therefore, be dealt with:

- an arrangement must be made for the baby to be seen within the first month after discharge, in order to assess growth, and to enable the mother to discuss any problems that she may have. At present this is usually done at the local authority clinic in the urban areas, but in many rural areas it is done at the same clinic in which the child was born. Special follow-up arrangements, or referrals, must be made for babies in whom a non-urgent problem has been detected. As far as possible the implications of the problem should be explained to the mother;
- the baby should receive BCG vaccination and the first dose of oral poliomyelitis vaccine prior to discharge. The mother should be told when the next immunization visit will be and where she must attend;

- the Road to Health Chart must be properly filled in and given to the mother, and its use explained;
- the whole question of future pregnancies should be discussed with the mother (and her husband/partner if possible). One of the main tasks of the health worker is to encourage the development of a healthy family. One of the ways to achieve this is to ensure appropriate family spacing, and if the couple are satisfied that their family is complete, to arrange for either tubal occlusion or vasectomy – whichever is the more acceptable.

# The place of a perinatal service in the overall health service

Perinatal care is an integral part of an overall health service. Just as the labour ward forms part of the service of a hospital, so also should maternal and neonatal services be integrated into the total health service. For this to work efficiently, health services must be regionalized and each regional health service placed under a single regional authority, responsible to central government. All those concerned with health care services in a region must be represented at regional authority level.

The regional authority must identify the health problems in its region, establish priorities, implement strategies to deal with the problems, and evaluate the effects of the service on the health of the community. This does not mean that some organizations will have to withdraw their services, but rather that all organizations in the region should cooperate with each other within a single service. Thus, the local authority clinic may also become a maternity centre and a primary health care centre, if those changes would benefit the community.

A regionalized, single authority health system is far more sensible than the situation where the local authority provides an immunization centre ('child health clinic'), another organization provides maternity and newborn services, and yet another provides a service for sick children. The decisions about where services are provided, which services should be provided, and by whom, should be made by the regional health authority after discussion and in collaboration with all those who are providing health services in that region.

## References and further reading

FROST O. 1975. Community obstetrics in an urban situation. *South African Medical Journal.* 49:1309.

LARSEN JV & MULLER EJ. 1978. Obstetric care in a rural population. *South African Medical Journal.* 54:1137.

MALAN AE. 1975. Regionalisation in perinatal care. *South African Medical Journal.* 49:1363.

PHILPOTT RH (ed.). 1979. Maternity services in the developing world – what the community needs. Proceedings of the Seventh Study Group of the Royal College of Obstetricians and Gynaecologists, London.

VAN COEVERDEN DE GROOT HA et al. 1978. The Midwife Obstetric Unit. *South African Medical Journal.* 53:706.

VAN COEVERDEN DE GROOT HA et al. 1981. The selection of patients at the Groote Schuur Maternity Hospital. *South African Medical Journal.* 59:824.

VAN COEVERDEN DE GROOT HA. 1982. Community perinatal care. *South African Medical Journal.* 61:30.

VAN COEVERDEN DE GROOT HA et al. 1982. The Peninsula Maternity and Neonatal Service. *South African Medical Journal.* 61:35.

VARIOUS. 1978. Papers presented at the Seminar on Maternal and Child Health Care Delivery, Durban, 1977. *South African Medical Journal.* 53:821–38.

# 13 The Perinatal Education Programme

## DL WOODS

Each year about one million infants are born in South Africa with a relatively high perinatal mortality rate of about 30 per 1 000 deliveries. Many of these deaths could be prevented if effective and appropriate care were given to all newborn infants. In order to achieve this goal, a massive education programme is needed to make continuing training available to both nurses and doctors. Unfortunately, in-service courses and occasional lectures by visiting tutors are expensive, often unsuited to the needs in rural areas, and have not proved adequate to meet the ever-growing need for perinatal education.

A correspondence course in perinatal care has therefore been designed to meet these needs. It was written by a team of paediatricians, obstetricians, and midwives after wide consultation with colleagues to ensure a well-balanced approach to the diagnosis and management of common and important disorders. This innovative method of self-education, called the Perinatal Education Programme (or PEP), is cheap, comprehensive, and appropriate to the needs of a developing country. In addition it requires few teachers and does not disrupt staffing as the students do not have to leave their regular

posts. The responsibility for gaining the knowledge, skills, and attitudes needed to provide better perinatal care is placed on the student rather than the teacher.

PEP consists of two manuals, one on maternal care and another on newborn care. Each manual comprises 15 theory units that address important clinical problems. The units in the Newborn Care manual deal with resuscitation, assessing size and gestational age at birth, care and feeding of both well and high-risk infants, hypothermia, hypoglycaemia, jaundice, respiratory distress and oxygen therapy, infection, trauma, bleeding and congenital abnormalities. A final unit addresses communication with patients and between colleagues in an integrated, regionalized health care system. Similarly, the Maternal Care manual addresses all the important topics in caring for women during pregnancy, labour, and the puerperium.

A question-and-answer method of teaching based on problem solving is used to lead the student step-by-step through the required information. The causes, prevention, clinical presentation, complications, and management of each problem are examined and the most important lessons are stressed. Case studies at the end of each unit help students integrate their newly acquired knowledge into everyday clinical practice. Flow diagrams summarize many of the approaches to specific problems such as the management of hypoglycaemia. In addition, illustrated skills workshops teach the practical procedures needed to apply the theoretical knowledge. Important attitudes and concepts such as a regionally based, integrated perinatal service with doctors and nurses working together as a team are emphasized. A multiple-choice test before and after each unit allows students to monitor their progress through the programme.

PEP therefore provides a learning opportunity for all clinical staff working in clinics and level 1 and 2 hospitals. It is also suitable for training students in medical schools and nursing colleges. As the manuals are modular, individual units can be integrated into other courses. On completion PEP forms a useful work manual in the clinic, labour ward, or nursery.

Students are advised to study the Programme in groups, which are co-ordinated by a locally elected group leader. Each group meets for a few hours every two to four weeks to discuss the unit studied since the previous meeting.

This system of co-operative learning is proving to be most effective. The multiple-choice tests are written and marked by the group leader or the students themselves at these meetings. In addition, the group leader invites a suitable colleague to assist with the skills workshop. Each manual provides a course lasting about 12 months.

When students have completed one of the manuals they can write a formal multiple-choice examination. Successful students receive certificates. Students who pass both the maternal and newborn care examinations receive a pin-on PEP badge. It is hoped that state recognition of the course, salary increases, or job promotions might in future also reward the successful students.

Students are encouraged to use their new knowledge in their work situations and also to involve colleagues in the new management protocols. A few students within a hospital or group of clinics can rapidly improve the standard of care provided by many of their peers and thereby raise the standard of perinatal care delivered by the service.

An initial field study of 114 midwives in both urban and rural services showed a 30 per cent increase in cognitive knowledge after studying one of the PEP manuals. This is similar to the improvement found in expensive, in-service courses currently offered by teaching hospitals. Two subsequent prospective, controlled doctoral studies documented that PEP significantly increased cognitive knowledge and clinical skills, altered attitudes, and improved the standard of care provided to women and their infants. These unique studies prove the value of self-directed courses in training health care workers.

By the end of 1998 over 25 000 doctors, nurses, medical, and nursing students had completed one or both manuals. It is hoped that within a few years all doctors and nurses who care for pregnant women and newborn infants will take the opportunity of using PEP to improve and expand their clinical abilities and, as a result, help to provide better perinatal care to all communities in southern Africa.

In 1999 the first supplement to PEP was published. This manual addresses the problems of HIV and AIDS in the pregnant woman and her newborn infant. Again a field study showed that the HIV/AIDS manual improved cognitive knowledge by 30 per cent. It is hoped that this manual will allow all midwives to improve their management of patients with this major perinatal problem.

Further information on the Perinatal Education Programme can be obtained from the Editor-in-Chief, P O Box 34502, Groote Schuur, Observatory, 7937.

## References and further reading

THERON GB. 1999. Effect of the maternal care manual from the perinatal education programme on the quality of antenatal and intrapartum care rendered by midwives. *South African Medical Journal.* 89:336–42.

THERON GB. 1999. Improved cognitive knowledge of midwives practising in the Eastern Cape Province of the Republic of South Africa through the study of a self-education manual. *Midwifery.* 15:66–71.

WOODS DL. 1999. An innovative programme for training in maternal and newborn care. *Seminars in Neonatology.* 4:151–7.

# 14

# Ethical issues in neonatology in southern Africa

PA COOPER

## Equitable distribution of resources

The organization of neonatal care in southern Africa has, as in many other countries, developed in an unstructured way, often depending on local circumstances or the availability of resources and personnel. However, existing services are being rationalized and proper forward planning is essential.

While parts of southern Africa are providing reasonable primary and secondary levels of neonatal care, especially in the urban and peri-urban areas, this is by no means true for the whole region. Basic level 1 care is not being offered and/or utilized in many areas and level 2 care is frequently either unavailable or the facilities are lacking in terms of equipment and trained personnel. Thus the priorities in neonatal care over the next decade from both an ethical and social standpoint will revolve around ensuring the provision of adequate primary care for the entire population and providing an equitable distribution of level 2 facilities of an acceptable standard for all infants in need of such care. This will require significant investments in

Neonatal care is usually stratified according to the level of care provided (see also Chapter 12: Perinatal services):

**Level 1 (primary) care:** This should be provided for all newborn infants and includes such things as measuring weight, adequate care of the umbilical cord, vitamin K administration, as well as detection of conditions such as jaundice and administration of phototherapy.

**Level 2 (secondary) care:** This is usually required for infants who have neonatal problems related to such conditions as birth asphyxia, prematurity, infections, and congenital abnormalities. These infants may require intravenous fluids, antibiotics, incubators, oxygen administration, and other appropriate management.

**Level 3 (tertiary) care:** This level of care is required for infants needing neonatal intensive care and, for practical purposes involves the provision of assisted mechanical ventilation. This level of care is expensive in terms of personnel and resources.

facilities, equipment, and personnel in order to upgrade existing services and to provide new services where these do not exist. It is thus unlikely that level 3 neonatal services in public sector hospitals will be expanded during this period.

Tertiary neonatal care in public sector hospitals is located largely within teaching hospitals, though some regional hospitals are able to provide such a service. These level 3 units not only provide tertiary care for their own delivery service, but act as referral centres for the surrounding region as well. Inevitably there is great pressure on these facilities with many more infants requiring tertiary care than can be provided for. As a result of such pressure, private sector hospitals, again mainly in the larger urban areas, have increasingly developed neonatal intensive care facilities on a fee-for-service basis. The result has been the emergence of a three-tiered system:

- Those with adequate means to pay themselves or through medical insurance have been able to 'purchase' level 3 neonatal care in the private sector for any condition deemed warranted by the paediatrician caring for the infant in consultation with the parents.
- Those born in a public sector hospital with level 3 neonatal facilities or referred from another hospital at a time when a level 3 bed was available. Most public sector level 3 units have policies regarding non-admission of certain categories of newborns (see below).
- The majority of infants in southern Africa falling into neither of the above categories have minimal or no access to level 3 care. The inevitable result is that the overwhelming majority of such infants in need of level 3 care die.

As mentioned above, developing level 1 and 2 facilities over the next decade should be considered as priorities and will provide the greatest 'return' in terms of improvements in neonatal mortality and morbidity. Nevertheless, the role of level 3 neonatal facilities in both private and public sector hospitals needs to be carefully examined so that optimal use is made of these expensive resources. Regionalization of perinatal services is often advocated as an efficient means of optimizing financial resources; however, it is an ethical imperative as well!

# Decision making in the neonatal unit

Ethical issues regarding the treatment of newborns with life-threatening conditions in the (Western) medical literature have usually revolved around the best interests of the individual patient. In the United States in particular, the autonomy of the individual rather than the needs of the community have been stressed, but even where debates have occurred in industrialized countries concerning the place of neonatal intensive care in the management of extremely premature newborns or those with gross malformations, the ethical principles discussed have seldom gone beyond the quality of individual life and the impact on the family. Only recently is it being recognized in these countries that the doctor's obligation to the patient can be limited by constraints set by society as a result of limited resources.

Neonatal intensive care in southern Africa has long been limited by available resources as illustrated in the section above. At the level of individual units, policies that place restrictions on the admission of certain categories of patients are usually in place. For example most public sector hospitals offering level 3 care have a general policy of not ventilating infants with a birthweight below 1 000 g, although variations may occur depending on local circumstances. This is applied with the aim of providing such scarce resources for the greatest number of infants since infants below 1 000 g would occupy ventilators for prolonged periods of time at the expense of larger infants with a better prognosis. For example, the ventilator time required to produce one survivor with a birthweight below 1 000 g would produce two survivors with birthweights between 1 000 and 1 500 g who need ventilatory support, four survivors with birthweights between 1 500 and 2 500 g and ten survivors with birthweights above 2 500 g. Furthermore, neonatal intensive care is not usually offered to larger infants considered to have a poor prognosis or likely to survive with major mental disabilities and, when such circumstances become apparent after an infant has already been admitted to the intensive care unit, such therapy may be withdrawn.

While such issues should be discussed with the parents of infants about whom such difficult decisions may have to be made, the ultimate decision is usually made by medical and nursing staff in accordance with the general guidelines of the unit. Parental expectations of treatment may differ from the policies of the unit and it is believed that it is inappropriate for parents to be able to countermand decisions that avoid inappropriate life support because of the major ramifications this would have for other infants in need of intensive care.

Thus the realities of neonatal intensive care in a developing country may require the needs of the community to be considered above the needs of an individual infant so that limited resources can be used optimally. However, since staff changes are frequent and conditions within the health services may change over time, it is essential that such policies are regularly discussed in the neonatal unit. It is important, too, that issues such as these become the subject of public debate.

## References and further reading

CAMPBELL AGM & DUFF RS. 1979. Deciding the care of severely malformed or dying infants. *Journal of Medical Ethics.* 5:65–7.

LOUW HH & KHAN MBM. 1989. *Perinatal mortality: The Province of the Cape of Good Hope,* 1988. Proceedings of the 8th Conference in Priorities in Perinatal Care in South Africa, Mpekweni.

OSBORNE M & EVANS TW. 1994. Allocation of resources in intensive care: A transatlantic perspective. *Lancet.* 343:778–80.

WAINER S & KHUZWAYO J. 1993. Attitudes of mothers, doctors and nurses toward neonatal intensive care in a developing country. *Pediatrics.* 91:1171–5.

# PART FIVE

# Nutrition

Early nutrition is of crucial importance not only to the infant's development but also to the child's later well-being, adult size, and, probably, longevity. Dietary needs and related issues are discussed, and malnutrition is addressed in some detail.

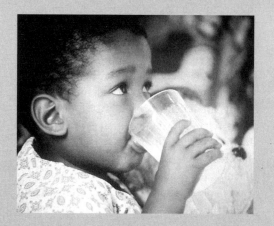

# 15

# Infant and child nutrition

JM PETTIFOR, H SALOOJEE,
D LABADARIOS, H MARÉ &
M PENTZ

## Dietary requirements

Normal growth and development requires food that will supply sufficient energy, protein, essential fatty acids, minerals, vitamins, and trace elements. Generally if the diet provides adequate amounts of energy and protein, then vitamin, mineral, and trace element deficiencies are unlikely to occur except in special circumstances. During childhood, there are two periods during which the child is most at risk of developing nutritional deficiencies; the first is during infancy, when requirements per kilogram of body weight are the highest, and the infant is dependent on others for feeding, and the second period is during adolescence, when the pubertal growth spurt raises requirements, and food fads, dieting, and irregular eating habits may become the dietary pattern. Protein, energy, vitamin, mineral, and trace element requirements are reflected in Table 15.1 (see definitions related to dietary intakes used by the Institute of Medicine).

Breast milk or properly constituted milk formula feeds in sufficient amounts are generally able to supply these requirements for the first four to six months of life. Most mixed diets that are adequate in quantity and frequency will provide an infant's needs as outlined in the tables, and complicated calculations in prescribing diets are, in general, unnecessary. Reference to these tables and others detailing food composition can be useful when:

- infants and children fail to thrive or show specific nutritional deficiency signs that cannot be adequately explained by the history of the child's food consumption;
- diets consist of one food source only (for example, only a cereal); and
- fad or weight-loss diets are being consumed or prescribed.

Table 15.1 illustrates the relatively greater food requirements of the younger child and infant whose rapid growth is associated with increased vulnerability to nutritional deprivation. Energy and protein requirements per kilogram of body weight diminish with increasing age as a result of a slowing of the growth rate. During the weaning period 60 ml/kg/day of cow milk would supply the required amount of protein (2 g/kg/day). It would, however, be very deficient in energy, supplying only 156 kJ/kg/day, and therefore an additional energy source in the form of carbohydrates or fat is necessary. An infant or child who is (or who should be) on a mixed diet should not drink more than 500 ml of cow milk per day. Possible consequences of exceeding this amount are:

- insufficient intake of other foods because of the volume of milk consumed;
- delay in the child acquiring familiarity with, and a taste for, other foods; and
- development of iron deficiency because of inadequate iron intake, or associated occult blood loss from the bowel (cow milk enteropathy).

The values provided in this table are drawn from the Dietary Reference Intakes of the Institute of Medicine, where available, otherwise the Recommended Dietary Allowances have been used.

A satisfactory intake of energy and iron after the age of four to six months depends on the introduction of mixed feeding. Weaning or transitional diets bridge the gap between breast milk being adequate as the sole source of nourishment and the infant's ability to handle food in adult form.

The quality of protein consumed is also important. Cereal proteins in general are lacking in the essential amino acid lysine, and maize (corn) is additionally deficient in tryptophan. Mixing of a cereal such as maize or sorghum porridge, rice, or bread with animal

> ## Definitions used by the Institute of Medicine for Dietary Reference Intakes (DRI)
>
> **EAR** (Estimated Average Requirement): The intake that meets the estimated nutrient need of 50 per cent of the individuals in a defined group.
>
> **RDA** (Recommended Dietary Allowance): The intake that meets the nutrient need of almost all (97 to 98 per cent) individuals in that group.
>
> **AI** (Adequate Intake): An intake that in the judgement of the DRI Committee appears to sustain a normal nutritional status in a group.

protein (e.g., milk, meat, fish, or egg) *or* with a high-protein vegetable (e.g., beans, peas, peanuts, or lentils) will ensure an improvement in the quality of cereal protein. In South Africa, a mix of beans and porridge (maize samp) is a traditional food whereby there is healthy complementing of essential amino acids. Adequacy of protein and energy intake will be reflected in a normal rate of growth as shown on a weight-for-age chart. Table 15.1 also shows the vitamin, mineral, and trace element requirements throughout childhood and adolescence. During puberty and adoles-

**Table 15.1** Protein and energy requirements

| Age | Energy kJ/day | Protein g/day | Calcium mg/day | Thiamine mg/day | Riboflavin mg/day | Niacin mg/day | Folate µg/day | Vitamin A µg/day | Vitamin C mg/day | Vitamin D µg/day | Iron mg/day |
|---|---|---|---|---|---|---|---|---|---|---|---|
| 0–6 mo | 2717 | 13 | 210 | 0,2 | 0,3 | 2 | 65 | 375 | 30 | 5 | 6 |
| 7–12 mo | 3553 | 14 | 270 | 0,3 | 0,4 | 4 | 80 | 375 | 35 | 5 | 10 |
| 1–3 y | 5500 | 23 | 500 | 0,5 | 0,5 | 6 | 150 | 400 | 45 | 5 | 10 |
| 4–8 y | 7100 | 30 | 800 | 0,6 | 0,6 | 8 | 200 | 500 | 45 | 5 | 10 |
| 9–13 y | 9200–11300 | 45–46 | 1300 | 0,9 | 0,9 | 12 | 300 | 800–1000 | 50 | 5 | 18 |
| 14–18 y | 8800–11800 | 46–56 | 1300 | 1,0–1,2 | 1,0–1,3 | 14–16 | 400 | 800–1000 | 60 | 5 | 18 |

cence there are gender differences in the
Reference Intakes for a number of vitamins
and trace elements. For example, adult females
require greater iron intake on account of menstruation and pregnancy.

# Infant feeding

Breast milk is widely accepted as the food of
choice for young infants. Its nutritional value
and the various advantages of breast-feeding,
both for mother and baby, should be well
known to health workers. In Table 15.2 the
composition of breast milk and cow milk is
compared.

**Table 15.2** Composition

| Nutrients (g/dl) | Cow milk | Breast milk |
| --- | --- | --- |
| Protein | 3,3 | 1,2 |
| Whey : Casein ratio | 19:81 | 65:35 |
| Carbohydrate (Lactose) | 4,8 | 7,0 |
| Fat | 3,7 | 3,8 |
| *Minerals* (mg/dl) | | |
| Ca | 123 | 33 |
| P | 96 | 15 |
| Na | 58 | 15 |
| K | 138 | 55 |

Desirable features of *breast milk* and breast-
feeding include the following:
- *A lower mineral and electrolyte content:*
  Breast-feeding babies are less prone to
  hypocalcaemia in the newborn period
  and to hypernatraemia later in infancy
  when exposed to excessive fluid loss as
  may occur in extremes of heat or in association with diarrhoea or vomiting.
- *A predominance of whey protein*, which is
  more digestible.
- Easily absorbed *cholesterol and polyun-
  saturated long-chain fatty acids.*

- The presence of several *active enzymes
  such as lipase and amylase*, which aid the
  digestion of fats and proteins.
- *Carrier proteins:* Specific carrier proteins
  synthesized in the human breast enhance
  the absorption of many vitamins and trace
  elements, as well as of iron. The bio-avail-
  ability of iron in breast milk is five to ten
  times higher than in cow milk, and this
  compensates for the normally low iron
  levels (0,2–0,4 mg/dl). The binding of iron
  as lactoferrin not only increases iron
  absorption but also exerts a bacteriostatic
  effect through a reduction of the free iron
  on which bacteria depend.
- *Antimicrobial and antiviral factors:* These
  provide passive immunity against a wide
  range of pathogens. Colostrum in particular has a very high concentration of
  immunoglobulins, and early suckling
  should be encouraged for this and other
  reasons, such as stimulating uterine con-
  tractions, stimulating milk production,
  and enhancing bonding. The mammary
  gland may well be regarded as part of the
  immunological system. The absorption,
  migration, and continuing function of
  immunocompetent maternal cells may
  explain why breast-fed babies not only
  have fewer gastrointestinal infections but
  also fewer respiratory and urinary tract
  infections. Breast-feeding avoids the possible risks of contaminated or unhygienic
  artificial feeding. Morbidity and mortality
  rates of bottle-fed children are five to ten
  times higher in developing communities
  and are comparable with observations in
  England early this century when bottle-
  feeding was introduced.
- *Contraceptive effects:* Frequent suckling
  induces prolactin levels high enough to
  suppress ovulation. As a family spacing
  strategy, it has application at a community
  rather than an individual level. In the
  developing world suckling prevents more

pregnancies than all other contraceptive techniques combined.

- *Prevention of allergy/atopy:* Delaying the introduction of foreign proteins (e.g., cow milk and eggs) for at least the first three months of life has been advocated as a means of preventing the development of allergies. If there is a family history of allergy, this period may be extended by a few months. It is postulated that relative gut immaturity allows large particle protein absorption to trigger an allergic response. It appears probable that exclusive breast-feeding delays rather than prevents atopy.

- *Economics:* Every child health worker should know the cost of 'artificial' infant feeding (e.g., milk formulae, essential equipment for preparation and administration – bottles, teats, methods of sterilization, etc.). This should be related to local circumstances, such as family income and facilities. The 'cost' to the mother/family of breast-feeding (e.g., resuming employment or education) also deserves attention. In general it can be stated that, as a method, breast-feeding is more economical than artificial feeding.

## VARIATIONS IN THE COMPOSITION OF BREAST MILK

- The lactating mother of a premature infant initially produces breast milk with a higher protein content, thus meeting the special growth needs of her preterm newborn.

- Mothers may express concern that their breast milk looks blue and watery. This is normal fore-milk and is followed by milk of a higher fat content. It has been postulated that this might have a regulatory effect on infant intake.

- The quality and quantity of human milk will be adversely affected only if the maternal diet provides less than 60 per cent of the recommended daily energy intake (supplementary feeding for deprived pregnant and lactating women is a cost-effective child health promotion measure – see Chapter 19: Global strategies for child health). The greatest benefit is derived from pre-delivery maternal feeding, which enhances fetal growth and postnatal survival in situations of severe energy deprivation.

Seasonal variations and excessive manual work may cause variations in the vitamin content and quantity of breast milk. For example, the vitamin D content may be very low in winter. It should be noted however that the vitamin D content of breast milk even in summer months is inadequate to maintain vitamin D sufficiency in the young infant unless sunlight exposure is also assured. Vitamin A- and K-deficient diets are also reflected by low levels of these vitamins in breast milk.

## PRACTICAL ISSUES RELATED TO BREAST-FEEDING

- Put the baby to the breast as soon after birth as possible.

- *Extra water and sugar:* Do not give healthy breast-fed babies extra water. The practice of giving the normal newborn water with or without sugar after birth or until 'the milk comes in' is not necessary, as it may introduce infection and is counter-productive to the establishment of breast-feeding, both in terms of milk production stimulated by suckling, and in developing a different feeding technique. Extra water is only indicated to replace exceptional fluid loss as occurs with high environmental temperatures, pyrexia, and tachypnoea. When there is diarrhoea and/or vomiting, both fluid and salts should be replaced using an oral rehydration solution. Extra sugar may be required to counteract hypoglycaemia in sick or low birthweight infants.

## Breast-feeding guidelines

To check infant attachment, look for:
- chin touching breast;
- mouth wide open;
- lower lip turned outward; and
- more areola visible above than below the mouth.

All these signs should be present if the attachment is good.

- *Feeding techniques:* Infants' feeding techniques with breast *suckling* and bottle *sucking* differ greatly. In suckling, the nipple is drawn well into the mouth and the gums close over the collecting sinuses of the areola. Engorgement of the breast may prevent this action, and cracked nipples will result from the baby's sucking and biting. *Unnecessary bottle-feeding* for breast-feeding infants should be avoided – one reason why babies may 'refuse the breast' is the different technique required for suckling and sucking. The following are other issues related to breast-feeding:
- *Breast milk jaundice:* The transmission in breast milk of maternal progesterone and the presence of various enzymes may inhibit bilirubin conjugation, resulting in jaundice persisting after the first week of life. It generally clears from the age of two weeks, and is not an indication to withhold breast-feeding. There is some evidence that the mild hyperbilirubinaemia may actually have a protective 'antioxidant' function. It is nevertheless necessary to consider other possible causes of prolonged jaundice such as infection, excessive haemolysis, or hypothyroidism. Pale stools should indicate the need for the exclusion of obstructive jaundice and in particular biliary atresia.

- *Constipation:* Ascertain precisely what the mother means. Infrequent stools, even at intervals of four or five days, are a normal variant if *soft*. Reassure the mother, and avoid potentially harmful 'remedies' such as enemas and laxatives.
- *Frequent stools or 'diarrhoea':* Watery, frothy, yellow, stools that are not particularly offensive may be associated with *transitory lactase insufficiency*. If the baby is well and thriving, as endorsed by satisfactory weight gain, the mother can be reassured. Empathize about the frequent nappy changes! Advise the mother to protect the buttocks with a simple cream and not to stop breast-feeding.
- *Refusing the breast:* If this should happen:
  - attempt to ascertain the cause: See above for infants' feeding technique; inappropriate introduction of bottles; engorged breasts create problems for both mother and infant;
  - encourage regular and frequent satisfactory breast emptying. This is better performed by the suckling infant than a breast pump;
  - advise and enable early feeding by rooming-in of infants. There is much in favour of demand rather than 'clock-watching' feeding. A baby whose cheek is 'pushed' to latch on to the breast may exhibit a normal rooting reflex and turn away;
  - inform, advise, encourage, and support mothers to promote breast-feeding;
  - breast-fed babies should be offered the breast whenever the infant appears hungry. The frequency of feeding should not be regulated by the clock.

## PROMOTING BREAST-FEEDING

Most health workers promote breast-feeding with enthusiasm, dedication, and determination. To achieve results, awareness of the many determinants of successful breast-feeding are important. Health service practices, role models, and emotions pertaining to breast-feeding call for careful consideration. Breast-feeding should continue for as long as possible (up to two years), even though the infant is consuming a mixed diet by that stage.

Respect the mother's feelings and right to choose, particularly if her circumstances allow safe alternatives to breast-feeding. There is little or no conclusive evidence that the substitution of breast milk by infant formulae of correct quantity and quality is measurably detrimental. A problem is the example or role model seen by the underprivileged or impoverished. If, for whatever reason, a mother does not breast-feed she should still receive the health worker's care and concern. Don't preach and be judgmental, and try to avoid fanaticism!

## BABY-FRIENDLY HOSPITALS

WHO and UNICEF have drawn up a code of practice for hospitals, setting out *Ten steps to successful breast-feeding*. Hospitals following the code are designated baby friendly. The South African national breast-feeding policy is based on this joint WHO/UNICEF statement.

## ATTITUDES AND FEELINGS ABOUT BREAST-FEEDING

The breast may be perceived exclusively as a sex symbol. There may be fears that breast-feeding will permanently alter breast size or shape, which may or may not happen! The demands consequent on lactation tend to mobilize fat stores laid down during pregnancy, and thus may improve or return the figure

## Ten steps to successful breast-feeding

Every facility providing maternity services and care for newborn infants should:

- have a written breast-feeding policy that is routinely communicated to all health care staff;
- train all health care staff in skills necessary to implement this policy;
- inform all pregnant women about the benefits and management of breast-feeding;
- help mothers initiate breast-feeding within half an hour of birth;
- show mothers how to breast-feed and how to maintain lactation even if they should be separated from their infants;
- give newborn infants no milk feeds or water other than breast milk, unless indicated for a medical reason;
- allow mothers and infants to remain together 24 hours a day from birth;
- encourage natural breast-feeding frequently and on demand;
- do not give, or encourage, the use of artificial teats or dummies to breast-fed infants. Do not encourage the use of nipple shields either; and
- promote the establishment of breast-feeding support groups and refer mothers to these on discharge from the hospital or clinic.

to its former state. The mother may experience breast-feeding as very pleasurable and rewarding, or she may perceive it as primitive and repulsive. She may feel trapped and ruled by a demanding infant and thus forcibly removed from the mainstream and her career.

The father may be a valuable support person, or he may feel jealous and excluded. He may indeed be neglected by a harassed, weary mother, and disturbed by a restless, crying infant. The father's presence at the delivery, if this is culturally acceptable, and subsequent rooming-in of baby with mother, may well add to effective family functioning and more successful breast-feeding.

Lifestyles are drastically changed by the arrival of a new family member. Grandparents and other relatives may be helpful or interfering. Community support groups may provide invaluable advice and support, or be dictatorial and domineering.

## CONTRA-INDICATIONS TO BREAST-FEEDING

These are few:
- *Drugs excreted in breast milk:* While most medications can be safely taken by the lactating mother, serious adverse effects in the infant have been described in the case of the following: gold salts, indomethacin, phenindione, lithium, oestrogens, antineoplastics, and ergotamine. Chloramphenicol and tetracyclines are also contra-indicated. Before prescribing drugs for any breast-feeding mother it is wise to check updated information sheets.
- *Severe illness in the mother* whose own well-being would then be compromised by breast-feeding.
- The acutely *psychotic mother* who may harm her infant.
- *AIDS:* This issue is still controversial. Evidence exists that HIV is transmitted in breast milk, and increases the likelihood of the infant becoming HIV infected from the mother by about one-third. However, the consequences of *not* breast-feeding in underprivileged societies may far outweigh this increased risk. Each case should be judged on its merits, and the parents counselled accordingly. Whether or not the infant should be breast-fed will depend on the home circumstances (can the family

afford the purchase of a milk formula, is there a supply of clean water, etc.). A recent study from Durban, which still needs confirmation, suggests that *exclusive* breast-feeding may actually lessen the transmission of HIV. The study suggests that mixed feeding (breast-feeding plus other foods) may allow the virus present in breast milk easier passage through the gastrointestinal mucosa.

## NON-CONTRA-INDICATIONS

- *Tuberculosis in the mother* (unless she herself would be jeopardized by breast-feeding): With active open maternal infection or infected household contacts the infant should be treated with isoniazid and rifampion for three months. A tuberculin test should then be done, and if negative, a BCG should be given.
- *Epilepsy in the mother:* Unfounded fears that this could be transmitted to the infant or that injury may result because of a fit should be allayed. The latter risk is present whenever the mother handles the baby. Anti-epileptic drugs generally do not pass into the breast milk in sufficient quantities to harm the child.

## BREAST-FEEDING PATTERNS IN SOUTH AFRICA

Breast-feeding is a well-established practice in the black population of South Africa, even in the urban environment. However, the early introduction of other foods, such as soft porridge or herbal teas, is a traditional practice. In the townships around large towns and cities, many infants receive both breast milk and a breast-milk substitute. Thus the emphasis of education programmes should not be on the importance of starting and maintaining breast-feeding, but rather on the harmful effects of the early introduction of foods other than breast milk. Some of these harmful effects include the introduction of pathogenic bacteria, the change in bacterial flora in the gastrointestinal tract, reduction in milk production, reduced iron absorption, and possibly an increase in the incidence of atopy and allergy. A possible further disadvantage is an increase in mother-to-infant transmission of HIV infection.

## ARTIFICIAL FEEDING OF YOUNG INFANTS

If an infant under the age of four months is not breast-fed, resort must be made to bottle- or cup-and-spoon feeding. Bottle-feeding is generally more convenient for the mother but cups and spoons are easier to clean. The latter are therefore favoured in developing countries where bottle-feeding often leads to diarrhoea and malnutrition.

There are a wide variety of breast milk substitutes that provide the infant's nutritional requirements if given in recommended strengths and quantities.

The recommended quantity of milk in early infancy prior to the introduction of mixed feeding is 150 ml/kg/day.

## BREAST-MILK SUBSTITUTES

A variety of *commercial infant formulae* have been designed to match as closely as possible the nutritional composition of breast milk. Thus the mineral load of cow milk is reduced, the fatty acid spectrum may be changed by the substitution of vegetable oils, the proportion of whey to casein may be altered, and necessary carbohydrates are added in the form of lactose, sucrose, or maltodextrose. Supplements of vitamins and iron that are needed are also added.

In practice, the majority of healthy infants can handle and will thrive on simple cow milk formulae or on any of the more modified

preparations. A reasonable choice may therefore be made on the basis of convenience and cost.

There is, however, a stated rationale for the composition and production of these very different formulae.

- *Special premature baby formulae* can be useful for the very low birthweight newborn (less than 1 500 g), who has additional protein, energy, and vitamin requirements. Special premature baby formulae, (e.g., PreNan and S26 Preeme) accelerate early growth, but the long-term effects are still uncertain. A powdered breast-milk fortifier is also available to increase the mineral, protein, and energy content of breast milk for the feeding of very low birthweight infants.
- *Starter formulae* to replace or complement mother's milk. These are:
  - whey protein predominant (e.g., Nan, S26). This has a reputed advantage for the smaller infant;
  - casein protein predominant (e.g., Lactogen I, SMA, Similac). This is deemed suitable for the larger full-term infant. As casein is more slowly digested, such infants are likely to feel satisfied for a longer period. These feeds may thus be useful in the 'hungry crying' but not underfed baby;
  - pre-acidified milk (e.g., Pelargon). This is said to be advantageous in inhibiting bacterial pathogens and aiding digestion. It may also be less likely to be used in the family tea!
- *Follow-up formulae* are designed to be part of early mixed feeding. The full protein of cow milk is now particularly advantageous as a complement to the carbohydrate cereal intake. In addition, the fat and the calcium, as well as added iron, of full-cream milk provide a more adequate dietary intake during this period of transition feeding (e.g., Lactogen II, Infagro).

## NON-COW MILK INFANT FORMULAE

These are commonly based on soya protein isolate bean preparations, such as Infasoy, Mulsoy.

Specific indications are intolerance to cow milk, which may imply either allergy/sensitivity to cow milk protein or lactase deficiency.

Allergy to cow milk is frequently overdiagnosed and held accountable for a wide range of minor or vague symptoms. The real incidence of cow milk allergy is probably less than two per cent of infants in the first year of life. When suspected, a firm diagnosis can be made by observing symptoms after three milk withdrawals and subsequent milk challenge tests. In such situations, the use of a soya isolate preparation is probably not appropriate as many infants with cow milk protein allergy are also soya protein intolerant.

If cow milk allergy is confirmed, a protein hydrolysate (AL110) feed should be substituted.

Intolerance to lactose because of lactase deficiency may result from bowel mucosal damage associated with malnutrition or diarrhoea. Lactose may be detected in the stools whilst the infant is on lactose-containing feeds. The stools are typically loose and frothy with an acid reaction to litmus paper (pH less than 6), and contain reducing sugars (positive Clinitest® reaction >½%).

Lactose-free feeds are prescribed to tide the baby over a temporary enzyme deficiency, usually of short duration of about ten days. Congenital lactase deficiency or acquired deficiency later in life – common in blacks – call for appropriate long-term dietary management.

## SPECIALIZED FEEDS

These may be required for rare conditions such as inborn errors of metabolism, fat malabsorption, or the less common types of carbohydrate intolerance.

## MARKETING OF COMMERCIAL 'BABY FOODS'

Not surprisingly, there is keen competition in the profitable infant formula market. In the past this led to aggressive advertising likely to overwhelm and mislead a non-discerning public. The South African code of ethics on the marketing of breast milk substitutes is based on World Health Organization recommendations, and addresses this issue. Copies are obtainable free of charge from the Department of National Health, Private Bag X828, Pretoria, 0001, Republic of South Africa. In essence, the major companies producing and distributing 'breast milk substitute preparations' have become voluntary signatories, thus committing themselves to state unequivocally (and legibly) that breast milk is the food of first choice for babies and to act accordingly.

People in positions of influence ought to consider the effects of their actions and attitudes in relation to breast or artificial feeding.

## IMPLICATIONS OF ARTIFICIAL FEEDING OF INFANTS

The economics of infant feeding have been considered earlier in this chapter. Availability of clean water and facilities for heating and storage are determinants of success or failure, as are knowledge, understanding and the ability to maintain hygienic practices. Increased morbidity and mortality are the high price of poor feeding practices. Comparative costs of commonly used formulae are shown in Table 15.3.

Both overdilution and underdilution may be harmful. The former, often necessitated by economic constraints, results in undernutrition while the latter, possibly the result of misguided zeal, may lead to hypernatraemia or obesity.

Oral thrush is more likely to occur in bottle-fed babies. This calls for attention to

**Table 15.3** Daily cost of feeding a 4 kg baby at 150 ml/kg (lowest to highest cost in cents)

|  | 1980 | 1982 | 1986 | 1990 | 1995 | 2000 |
|---|---|---|---|---|---|---|
| Formula 1 | 18–33 | 26–49 | 33–75 | 71–114 | 143–206 | 173 |
| Formula 2 | 16–33 | 22–45 | 33–72 | 74–112 | 194–214 | 193 |
| Formula 3 | 18–33 | 21–44 | 33–68 | 108–112 | 216–343 | 197 |
| Cow milk | 30–35 | 34–37 | 51–58 | 155–194 | 177–263 | 200 |

teat cleaning or the possibility of contamination because of maternal monilial vaginitis.

Maternal attitudes and practices may range from casual and haphazard 'topping up' of bottles throughout the day to obsessive fanaticism whereby the infant is expected to take exact and carefully measured feeds at strictly controlled intervals. All mothers using an artificial feeding method should be clearly informed about the correct and hygienic preparation of feeds.

## WARNINGS

The following may not be used as breast-milk substitutes:

- *skimmed milk*. Although this a useful source of protein and a valuable addition to cereals in weaning diets, the removal of fat results in a low-energy content and a lack of linoleic acid, an essential fatty acid;
- *creamers and dairy blends*. These are totally unsuitable for infant feeding. They are

## Points from the code of ethics

- Objective and consistent information about infant and young child feeding should be provided.
- Any information or educational material in whatever form that is aimed at pregnant women or the mothers of infants and young children should direct attention to the benefits and superiority of breast-feeding and to measures to promote lactation.
- Health, financial, and other undesirable implications of the inappropriate or improper use of infant formulae should be stated.
- Instructions on the correct use of infant formulae should be given specifically when needed. Such preparations should not be idealized either by pictures or text.
- There should be no direct advertising,

e.g., posters and pamphlets in clinics, nor general supplies of breast milk substitutes to mothers, pregnant women or the general public.

- Gifts or any other form of inducement to promote breast milk substitute sales should not be given to potential buyers or company staff. Health care personnel are similarly obligated not to be thus compromised.
- No facility of a health care system should be used for the purpose of promoting infant formula or other products within the scope of this code. This code does not, however, preclude the dissemination of information to health professionals. The use by the health care system of 'professional service representatives', mothercraft nurses' or similar personnel provided or paid by manufacturers or distributors is not permitted by the code.

deficient in protein, and contain saturated fatty acids and high levels of minerals. These products are generally cheaper than milk, which they physically resemble. Special efforts are thus called for to prevent their misguided use. Labels carry the warning 'Not suitable for infant feeding'.

- *fresh cow milk.* The American Academy of Pediatrics recommends that fresh cow milk should not be fed to infants less than 12 months of age, because of the risk of cow milk-induced colitis and iron-deficiency anaemia.

## SUPPLEMENTATION

Full-term infants in the first six months of life, whether exclusively breast-fed or artificially fed on a breast-milk substitute, generally do not need mineral or vitamin D supplements. Although breast milk is deficient in vitamin D, exposure of breast-fed infants to sunlight for short periods (approximately 30 minutes a day) effectively maintains an adequate vitamin D status and prevents vitamin D deficiency.

If, for social or other reasons, an infant is unlikely to get enough sunlight exposure, a vitamin D supplement of 400 IU/day should be provided until the child is walking (approximately until one year of age).

Once complementary foods have been introduced into the diet (from four to six months of age), iron supplements (such as ferrous sulphate or gluconate – 1 ml/kg/day) should be provided as it is difficult to ensure an adequate iron intake unless an iron supplement or iron-fortified foods are consumed.

Natural cow milk is both iron- and vitamin D-deficient. Therefore, supplements should be provided if cow milk forms a substantial part of the diet.

Premature infants are particularly prone to rickets and iron deficiency, because of their limited transplacentally acquired stores

**Table 15.4** Supplements

| | |
|---|---|
| Vitamin K at birth: | 1–2 mg |
| Vitamin D – 400 IU | Prems 800 IU/day from first week |
| Iron | Minimum of 1 mg/kg/day (starting from third month; prems from second month) continuing until the age of one year |
| Fluoride: 0,25 mg/day. | Zymoflor tablets 0,5 mg (see text) |

and their rapid postnatal growth. All low birthweight infants and twins should receive vitamin D 800 units/day for the first six weeks, and 400 units/day thereafter; and they should also receive iron supplementation from the age of one month.

Fluoride is a valuable protective measure against dental caries (see Chapter 22: Oral health). Requirements vary with the local fluoride content of water, the age of the child, and other sources such as supplemented toothpastes.

# Weaning

This term has two meanings. It can either mean the stopping of breast-feeding or the introduction of a transitional diet. The latter interpretation, namely the process of letting the infant gradually become accustomed to a full adult diet, is preferable for several good reasons.

Weaning normally extends from not earlier than four months to about one year of age. During this period exclusive milk feeding will not meet the quantitative and qualitative (e.g., iron) nutritive requirements. However, breast-feeding, even extended into the second year of life, can still make a useful contribution to the protein and energy intake of the child. An exception to this is the child who becomes addicted to the breast and refuses solid foods with consequent failure to thrive. In these circumstances the breast should be offered only after, and not in place of, other feeds.

It is generally advised that weaning foods be introduced in small amounts one at a time, starting with cereals, porridge with milk, puréed vegetables or fruit, and progressing to a mixed diet in mashed form. While commercial baby food may be chosen for convenience, eating from a nutritious family pot is a good and less costly alternative.

When breast-feeding ceases, full-cream cow milk, preferably fortified with vitamins and iron, should be an important part of the diet of the young child (not more than 500–600 ml/day), but the present high cost of milk products often place them beyond the reach of disadvantaged families.

The weaning period is associated with the following risks:

- *susceptibility to infections* because of declining levels of protection from maternally transmitted antibodies and increased *exposure to infections* because of greater mobility, contact with more people, and unsatisfactory hygiene in preparing, storing or giving mixed feeding;
- *dietary inadequacies* because of non-availability or ignorance of satisfactory weaning diets. It is important to remember the small size of the infant's stomach and therefore to give at least three meals per day with in-between snacks such as milk, bread, or fruit. It should be noted that weaning foods may be bulky but of low energy density, e.g., maize-meal porridge, and thus may satisfy the child's hunger without providing adequate energy or nutrients.

A one-year-old would have to eat ten cups of soft porridge per day to meet normal energy requirements. A two-year-old in a developing country needs to eat twice the weight of food of a pure staple diet as a two-year-old eating a high-quality Western mixed weaning diet. Growth failure from the second six months of life is commonly observed in less advantaged communities and may be the result of several factors, including frequent infections with increased energy requirements and associated loss of appetite, infrequent meals, and low energy density of weaning foods.

The weaning diet of the Third World child can be greatly improved by adding small amounts of animal protein or by mixing vegetable proteins with the basic cereal. Energy intake can be increased greatly by the addition of a fat (e.g., margarine, oil, or peanut butter) or sugar. It is in fact easier to meet the protein requirements than the energy requirements in a young child. Table 15.5 is a weaning meal with satisfactory protein and energy content:

**Table 15.5** An adequate weaning meal

|  | Energy | Protein |
|---|---|---|
| Maize-meal porridge (1 cup = 200 mls/100 gm) | 300 kJ | 2 g |
| Full-cream milk powder (2 teaspoons = 10 g) | 110 kJ | 1,7 g |
| Sunflower oil or margarine (1 teaspoon = 5 g) | 190 kJ | – |
| Sugar (1 teaspoon = 5 g) | 85 kJ | – |

The fat, milk powder, and sugar supplements have a small volume but virtually double the energy and protein content in a more easily consumed feed.

It is noteworthy that the developing-world toddler should be encouraged to eat as much as possible, while the mother of a First World toddler should guard against overfeeding of very refined and high-energy density foods.

# Dietary issues in later childhood

The concept that the correct nutrition in childhood has implications in terms of disease prevention in later life is becoming important. Nevertheless, there is a lack of data on what toddlers and pre-school children eat and what they should eat. A number of questions in terms of total energy needs, fat, and fibre in the diets of this age group still need definite answers.

Parental education on nutrition and appropriate support are necessary for the prevention of malnutrition among toddlers and pre-schoolers. Parents should be aware, for instance, that the rate of growth of this age group is slower than in the first year of life. In nutritional terms a slower growth rate implies less need for food, which manifests as a decreased appetite. A decreased appetite concerns parents, who respond by trying to force-feed the child, with ensuing feeding problems. Similarly, during the pre-school years there is a greater increase in height relative to weight. This transforms the chubby toddler into a leaner, taller pre-schooler, a transformation that is often misinterpreted.

It is widely believed that this period in the life cycle is of great importance in establishing healthy eating habits for adult life. Although this concept still has to be proven, it is nevertheless a sensible one and parents should ensure that the child consumes a nutritionally adequate diet and develops good eating habits. This can be achieved by serving meals consisting of a variety of foods of appropriate portion size in an atmosphere conducive to eating and allowing sufficient time to complete the meal. Other factors of importance include balancing rest and physical activity in relation to meal times, introducing new foods gradually, refraining from forcing the child to eat, refraining from using food as a punishment or as a reward, encouraging table manners, as well as the use of appropriate utensils. It is often insufficiently appreciated that anatomical considerations make it necessary for young children to eat five to six daily meals, including in-between meals in mid-morning, mid-afternoon and at bed time.

# Nutritional requirements

Table 15.1 lists the recommended intakes of various nutrients for different stages of childhood and adolescence. Assessment of nutrient intakes is difficult and is plagued by problems of inaccuracies of recall and by the lack of complete information on the nutrient content of various foods. The Institute of Medicine is currently revising its recommendations for Dietary Reference Intakes for North American adults and children and is publishing its recommendations. Attention needs to be drawn to the fact that the recommendations are specifically designed for the North American population and that the recommendations may not be strictly applicable to communities and populations in other countries with very different life styles and dietary patterns. The institute has defined three different terms, which it uses to define the Dietary Reference Intakes. These terms are listed on page 101. It is important to know how to interpret these terms. When the nutrient intakes of a cohort of children are being assessed, the Estimated Average Requirement (EAR) is the figure against which the mean or median intake of the group should be compared. However, if a particular child's intake is being assessed, then the intake should be compared against the Recommended Dietary Allowance (RDA) or the Adequate Intake (AI) for the particular nutrient. The Institute of Medicine differentiates between the RDA and AI, in that the RDA has been calculated with more certainty as better scientific data is available. The AI is the institute's best estimate of the intake which will maintain normal nutritional status based on less than complete information.

Dietary intakes may be assessed by several different methods (24 hour recall, food frequency questionnaires, food diaries, and weighed intakes). The method depends largely on the type and accuracy of information needed. It should be remembered that nutrient intakes vary from one day to the next and in most communities differ between weekdays and weekends, thus assessments should not be based on the measurement over one day only. Further, nutrient intake assessments must be culturally sensitive, as foods and the preparation of these foods vary markedly between cultures and communities.

Apart from encouraging the maintenance of breast-feeding for as long as possible, there is no one particular food that must be eaten or avoided in ensuring adequate nutrition. However, certain aspects should not be overlooked. Although milk forms an important part of a child's diet, it should be limited to no more than 600 ml per day; furthermore, although staple foods should be eaten daily, their bulky nature after preparation should be taken in to consideration in terms of satiety. Similarly, large amounts of fruit and vegetables may cause abdominal discomfort and diarrhoea. During the phase of transition from a mainly liquid diet (breast milk) to that of a more adult diet, toddlers may often consume large volumes of fruit juice or other liquids at the expense of more solid foods, thus reducing energy intake and resulting in poor weight gain and growth. This behaviour is more common in children who are bottle-fed, and should be guarded against. The importance of fat in the diet should not be overlooked, both in terms of adequate energy provision as well as a source of essential fatty acids. In general, disadvantaged communities tend to have a low intake of fat and the addition of fat or oil to cereals or other staples in appropriate quantities for the child's age will ensure sufficiency of energy intake.

In affluent communities the main concern is that unhealthy eating in early childhood increases the child's risk of developing degenerative diseases in later life. However, in the absence of any reliable evidence for this concept, as well as the absence of any documented dietary recommendations for the under-five-year olds, it would be unwise to apply adult dietary recommendations to this age group. The 'Muesli-Belt Malnutrition' phenomenon in toddlers (poor weight gain and loose stools) because of low-fat, high-fibre diets attests to the dangers of such an approach. Nevertheless, there is general agreement that in this age group salt and sugar intake should be moderate and that obesity should be avoided by early intervention and sound dietary practices; fat and fibre intake should be gradually adjusted between one and five years so that by the end of the fifth year of life the same recommendations as for adults are met. In practice, this means that dietary fibre should be gradually increased to 30 g/day and the percentage of energy from fat decreased to 30 per cent or lower. Unfortunately it is not always practical to implement these guidelines.

The need for micronutrient supplementation in children is as hotly debated a topic as it is in adult nutrition circles. However, there is probably general agreement that provided the diet is sufficiently varied and provides appropriate amounts of energy and protein, then micronutrient supplementation is unwarranted and micronutrient deficiencies are unlikely. Nevertheless, particular attention must be paid to micronutrient deficiencies in children whose diets are limited in the variety of foods, or are mainly vegetarian in composition.

# Common nutritional problems

## THE CHILD 'WHO WILL NOT EAT'

Curiosity and independence typically characterize the behaviour of the toddler: increasing mobility, development of various skills, and manipulation of the environment all form an integral part of this behaviour pattern. It is not surprising therefore that some toddlers do go through phases of being reluctant or refusing to eat. This may also form part of a manipulative strategy to seek parental attention or it could be because of food dislikes. There may also be parental misconception that the child is not eating enough, eating less than previously, or eating less than other children. Alternatively, refusal to eat may be associated with minor illnesses or restrictive therapeutic diets. In the absence of organic disease, the problem generally resolves itself. Parental education and minor dietary modifications are usually all that are necessary. It is essential that the health professional establishes that the child is growing adequately by assessing the child's growth pattern prior to reassuring the child's caregiver. Parents should recognize that appetites vary from day to day, some food wastage by the child is inevitable and experimentation with food is part of the toddler's normal development. Parents should not become overly concerned about long-term adverse effects. It is unwise to engage in counter-productive practices such as force-feeding and punishment or emotional isolation or reward to remedy the problem. Instead, toddlers should be offered foods that they like and that are also eaten by the family. Further, parents should ensure that the child's meals are appropriately spaced, that the child is not too tired or sleepy before meals, that the child is not drinking excessive fluids and that if breast-feeding is still practised or in-between meals are provided that they do not induce satiety before the main meals. However, persistent negativism, multiple food dislikes, or bizarre food habits such as pica, hyperphagia, polydipsia, or rumination that continue for longer than a few days warrant expert attention.

## TODDLERS' DIARRHOEA

Toddlers' diarrhoea is the frequent passage of loose stools (usually more than three a day) in an otherwise healthy toddler, who is thriving. It is probably the most common cause of chronic or persistent diarrhoea in the healthy toddler. Typically the consistency of the stools varies considerably, they often contain mucus, and the parent often comments on the presence of apparently undigested food particles (peas, carrots, mealies etc.). Although the diarrhoea may be quite copious and unpleasant, it does not have a detrimental effect on growth or weight gain. Toddlers' diarrhoea typically has an insidious onset around four to six months of life, and may continue until the child is three years of age.

If the child's weight gain and linear growth are satisfactory, there is no need for extensive investigations. However, pathogens such as Giardia lamblia or chronic bacterial pathogens, and lactose intolerance should be excluded. Parents should be reassured that the problem is self-limiting and that the child is not ill. It has been suggested that an increase in fat intake is helpful. It is important that the child is not placed on exclusion diets (unless under the supervision of an appropriate dietician) as these often induce weight loss or a faltering in weight gain and have not been shown to be effective in the management of the condition.

## POOR WEIGHT GAIN

Weight gain is the single most important evidence of satisfactory food intake. The reader is referred to Chapter 16: Malnutrition for information on the assessment of poor weight gain or failure to thrive. The most common reasons for poor weight gain are that the child does not eat sufficiently or eats the wrong types of food. Insufficient intake may be because of:

- illness or ill health;
- economic disadvantage;
- inadequate knowledge of the correct intake; or
- parental neglect and/or abuse.

The commonest age for poor weight gain is between 6 and 24 months, at the time of weaning and during a period when the child is often exposed to upper respiratory and gastrointestinal infections. Weight gain should be monitored frequently during this period (see Chapter 36: Integrated management of childhood illness) and any episode of inadequate or faltering weight gain should be an opportunity for the health professional to discuss feeding practices and nutrient intakes with the caregiver. Parents should also be educated about nutrition support groups within the community and feeding schemes that may exist. Apart from the provision of the appropriate type and quantity of foods, poor dietary habits may also contribute to the problem. For instance an excessive intake of one type of food may lead to the insufficient intake of other types of food; children who drink excessive amounts of milk/juice and only nibble on snacks often lose interest in food, and poor eating habits may develop. Parents need to be reassured that, provided the correct foods are given, withholding of food and snacks and limiting the intake of milk/juice will do no harm and that the child will eat when hungry.

In the case of parental neglect or abuse, the child is commonly the youngest in the family and born within 18 months of the next oldest sibling. Although poor weight gain within these situations can occur within families of all socio-economic groups, it is more common in single-parent families, those of low socio-economic status, and those with financial instability. It is not uncommon for the children of such families to have a history of recurrent poor weight gain from one year or even before six months of age. The situation may be aggravated by parents leaving their children in the care of often young and inexperienced child minders, who may be responsible for a large number of children without appropriate facilities or staff.

In the absence of parental neglect, abuse or poor dietary practices, failure to thrive may be indicative of underlying disease that will need further investigation.

## LACTOSE INTOLERANCE

Although lactose intolerance may rarely be due to a primary deficiency of intestinal lactase, the more frequent causes in children are secondary to bowel mucosal damage that result in temporary loss of lactase in the brush border of the intestinal mucosal cells. Lactose intolerance typically presents with watery acidic diarrhoea, secondary to the inability to hydrolyse dietary lactose (found in breast milk and cow milk and its products) to glucose and galactose. The retained lactose acts as an osmotic agent preventing fluid from being absorbed from the intestinal lumen. Bacterial flora in the large bowel metabolize the non-absorbed lactose to lactic acid and glucose and galactose, further aggravating the diarrhoea. Lactose intolerance is common in children suffering from severe protein energy malnutrition, may follow acute gastroenteritis and is a complication that may follow intestinal resection. Typically lactose containing foods (cow milk and its products) should be removed from the diet for periods ranging from 10 days to a month or more, while the intestinal mucosa recovers and intestinal lactase reappears. In certain situations, such as in the breast-fed infant or the child with severe malnutrition, removal of lactose containing feeds (stopping breast-feeding) may be unnecessary as long as extra fluids are given to compensate for the increased faecal fluid loss.

In older African children and adults, lactose intolerance associated with abdominal pain and excessive gas formation is a common finding if large lactose loads are given orally. However, the symptoms are generally very mild or actually absent if only small lactose loads are taken. Thus, this progressive genetically determined lactase deficiency does not generally preclude the drinking of milk in small volumes. The use of sour milk or yogurt should also be encouraged as the lactose levels are lower than those found in fresh milk.

## FOOD INTOLERANCE AND ALLERGY

The term 'food intolerance' is used to refer to reactions to food or food ingredients that do not involve a known immune mechanism. Such reactions include abdominal discomfort and pain, diarrhoea, and headaches. 'Food allergy' indicates that an immune response is involved in the reaction to food. Food intolerance includes normal reactions to large amounts of specific foods (e.g., caffeine in multiple cups of tea/coffee), irritants in foods (e.g., diarrhoea associated with highly spiced foods), and digestive impairment (lactose intolerance). Food allergy occurs in cow milk protein sensitivity, gluten enteropathy, and allergic responses to egg protein, peanuts, fish, or soya protein. Intestinal symptoms associated with food

allergy may include vomiting, diarrhoea, and malabsorption. If food intolerance or allergy is suspected, the suspected food allergen should be withdrawn for a period, followed by observation on the reintroduction of the presumed offending agent. Elimination diets should only be considered under carefully controlled situations. Only one food should be removed at a time, because unless carefully monitored, weight loss and malnutrition may develop on account of a reduction in energy and nutrient intake.

## References and further reading

FOOD AND NUTRITION BOARD. 1997. *Dietary reference intakes for calcium, phosphorus, magnesium, vitamin d, and fluoride.* Washington: National Academy Press.

FOOD AND NUTRITION BOARD. 1998. *Dietary reference intakes for thiamin, riboflavin, vitamin b6, folate, vitamin b12, pantothenic acid, biotin, and choline.* Washington: National Academy Press.

KUZWAYO PMN. 1991. *Infant and child nutrition – A manual for health workers.* Cape Town: College Tutorial Press.

PRENTICE AM, COLE TJ, FORD GA, LAMB WH, and WHITEHEAD RG. 1987. Increased birth weight following prenatal dietary supplementation of rural African women. *American Journal of Clinical Nutrition.* 46:912–25.

UNICEF. 1992. *The state of the world's children.* Oxford: Oxford University Press.

UNICEF. 1993. *The state of the world's children.* Oxford: Oxford University Press.

# 16         Malnutrition

H SALOOJEE &
JM PETTIFOR

Adequate nutrition is a basic human need that remains unmet for vast numbers of children throughout the world, despite the general improvement in food production, health conditions, and available educational and social services. Children are particularly vulnerable to nutritional inadequacies because of their rapid growth and their dependence on others.

An estimated 174 million children under five years of age in the developing world are malnourished, over 800 million people still cannot meet basic needs for energy and protein, more than 2 000 million people (a third of the world's population) experience micronutrient deficiencies, while hundreds of millions suffer from diseases caused by unsafe food or by unbalanced food intake. In 1995, malnutrition was associated with 6,6 million of the 12,2 million deaths in the under-five age group in developing countries. This represents 55 per cent of young child mortality. Not recognized for a long time is that 83 per cent of these malnutrition-related deaths are the result of mild or moderate malnutrition rather than severe malnutrition. These children betray no outward signs of malnutrition to the casual observer and are therefore frequently missed by aid agencies.

Although the word malnutrition is often associated with lack of food (i.e., undernutrition), it actually refers to a number of nutritional disorders. Undernutrition is only one of these. They can be categorized as:

- *undernutrition:* the condition that results from not eating enough;
- *dietary deficiency:* the condition that results from a diet that lacks sufficient amounts of a particular nutrient, such as a vitamin or mineral;
- *secondary malnutrition:* the condition that results from the inability to successfully utilize the food that is eaten because of some other factor, such as illness or diarrhoea; and
- *overnutrition:* the condition that results from consuming too many calories.

This chapter focuses mainly on undernutrition. Another name that is often used for this type of malnutrition is protein-energy malnutrition (PEM). The term PEM is generally used to describe both severe forms of clinical malnutrition (kwashiorkor and marasmus) and the more common forms of growth faltering or growth impairment (often termed mild or moderate malnutrition). However, the term PEM does not include specific or isolated deficiencies, such as of iron, iodine and vitamin A, which are separate major public health problems.

## Prevention

Malnutrition is frequently part of a vicious cycle that includes poverty and infection. These three factors are interlinked so that each contributes to the presence and permanence of the others. UNICEF has highlighted the dependence of infant well-being, growth, and the prevention of malnutrition (see Figure 16.1) on a combination of factors that affect household food security, child care, and the prevention of infections. All three aspects must be addressed if the prevalence of undernutrition in a community is to be decreased. Socio-economic and political changes that improve health and nutrition can break the cycle; as can specific nutrition and health interventions.

Figure 16.1 conceptualizes the influence of the various levels of government and society on the factors that promote or prevent malnutrition in the young child. In most countries, available resources are adequate and can improve the nutritional status of the

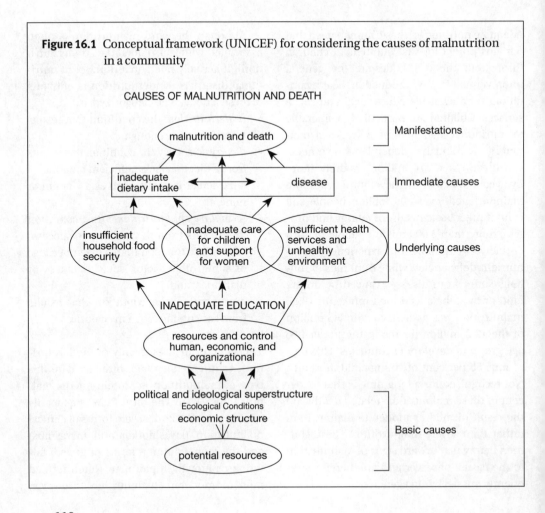

**Figure 16.1** Conceptual framework (UNICEF) for considering the causes of malnutrition in a community

population and reduce illness spells; that is, if the population can be motivated to take health-related actions and have the active support of the health delivery sector at a community level.

The strategies for preventing malnutrition are well known and include:
- Promoting exclusive breast-feeding for the first 4–6 months of life, and its continuation into the second year;
- Improving complementary feeding of children aged 6–24 months;
- Preventing childhood infections, such as diarrhoea and measles;
- Improving the availability of food in the household (food security);
- Providing environmental sanitation and personal hygiene;
- Making health services available; and
- Improving the status and education of women in society.

At the World Summit for Children in 1990 one of the goals was to reduce severe and moderate protein-energy malnutrition in pre-school children to half of 1990 prevalence levels by the year 2000. Although this goal was reaffirmed at the International Conference on Nutrition, it has not been achieved, the real decline being less than one-fifth of that necessary to reach this goal. With the spread of HIV it is unlikely to be attained in the next decade.

# Assessing nutritional status

Both clinical examination and anthropometry should be used to assess the nutritional status of a child. Anthropometry has particular application in community studies, while in the individual child, monitoring the rate of growth is a key factor in health surveillance and promotion. The clinical assessment of the degree of undernutrition is a poor substi-

tute for anthropometric evaluation. Many children look completely normal; it is only when they are measured and the results compared to norms that the degree of stunting or wasting is appreciated.

## ANTHROPOMETRIC MEASUREMENTS

The three most commonly used anthropometric indices to assess nutritional status in children are weight-for-age, height-for-age and weight-for-height. The advantages and disadvantages of the three indices and the information they can provide is summarized below:

### Weight-for-age

This is the most frequently used index in South Africa because weighing scales are available in most clinics. A single value simply shows whether or not the child's weight falls within the normal reference range. Although approximately five per cent of normal children have weights-for-age on or below the fifth centile, this reference standard is commonly used as a cut-off level below which the child is diagnosed as underweight. The advantages of using this index are that it can measure either recent (acute) or long-term (chronic) undernutrition (although it is unable to distinguish between the two). The major disadvantage of this index is that it does not take height into account. A 'healthy' child who is genetically shorter than his/her peers would be expected to weigh less and thus may fall below the normal reference range of weight-for-age.

### Height-for-age

Deviations in length or height become obvious more slowly than weight changes. Thus, this measurement of growth faltering reflects chronicity. Low length-for-age is termed 'stunting'. A decrease in the national stunting rate is usually indicative of improvements in overall socio-economic conditions of a country. The world-wide variation of the prevalence of low height-for-age is considerable, ranging from 2 per cent to 64 per cent among less developed countries. In South Africa, 23 per cent of children under five years of age are stunted, while only nine per cent are underweight for age (see Table 16.3).

## Weight-for-height

This is the current internationally accepted index and the recommended measurement to diagnose severe malnutrition (wasting). An added advantage is that it can be used even when exact ages are not known. The findings indicate whether or not the body is proportional and may confirm that the child is thin or overweight. If weight-for-height is normal the child may be either 'normal' or stunted. A low weight-for-height is termed 'wasting'. Wasting in individual children and population groups can occur rapidly, depending on seasonal changes in food availability or disease prevalence. However, wasting may also be the result of a chronic unfavourable condition.

Provided there is no severe food shortage, the prevalence of wasting is usually below five per cent, even in poor countries. Typically, the prevalence of low weight-for-height shows a peak in the second year of life. It is not as sensitive as weight- and height-for- age in detecting PEM; lack of evidence of wasting in a population does not imply the absence of nutritional problems – stunting and other deficits may be present.

'Overweight' is the preferred term for describing high weight-for-height. Although there is a strong correlation between high weight-for-height and obesity, as measured by adiposity (i.e., skinfold thickness), greater lean body mass can also contribute to high weight-for-height.

## Skull circumference

This measure is commonly used in paediatric practice, but mainly for purposes other than the assessment of nutritional status. In the newborn infant, disproportionate sparing of the head circumference suggests recent weight loss, while reduction of skull circumference in keeping with a reduction in weight and length centiles suggests prolonged intrauterine malnutrition.

## Mid-upper arm circumference

Arm circumference measurement can be done very quickly, and is often used in emergency situations when nutritional status information is needed quickly for large groups of people (e.g., in targeting food aid during natural disasters and conflicts). Arm circumference is measured using a measuring tape or simple techniques such as the Shakir strip (cut from X-ray films and marked with colour zones). A cut-off of 13,5 cm (or 12,5 cm to detect severe marasmus) is used. Many mild to moderate cases of malnutrition will not be detected by this tool. The MUAC detects loss of subcutaneous fat and muscle as occurs in wasting.

## Skinfold thickness

The use of this measure is generally restricted to research studies. Although the triceps area is usually measured, other sites can also be assessed. Skinfold thickness measures subcutaneous fat. This fat is believed to be a good indicator of total body fat. It is measured using skinfold-thickness calipers.

# The international reference population

Diagnosing a child with impaired growth relies on some means of comparison with a 'reference' child of the same age and sex. It is customary to compare an individual's anthropometric measurements with those of the National Center for Health Statistics (NCHS) growth reference, the so-called NCHS/WHO international reference population. The international reference growth curves were formulated in the 1970s by combining growth data from two distinct data sets consisting of healthy well-nourished US children. Although it was originally planned to serve as a reference for the USA, the WHO adopted the reference curves of the NCHS for international use in the late 1970s, as there was growing evidence that the growth patterns of well-fed, healthy pre-school children from diverse ethnic backgrounds were very similar. Genetic differences do occur, but these variations are relatively minor compared with the large world-wide variation in growth related to health and nutrition.

The suitability of these curves for international purposes has recently been challenged. It is felt that the current international reference is flawed, both technically and biologically, and interferes with healthy nutritional practices in infants and young children. In particular, the original data set included many infants who were formula-fed and who were supplemented with solids in the early months of life, rather than being exclusively breast-fed for four to six months. As a result, an international project is underway to develop a single new international growth reference that represents the best standard of optimal growth of young children from birth to five years. The sample is being drawn from seven diverse geographic sites around the world.

Country- or ethnicity-specific reference charts are proposed by some clinicians. These are useful to compare an individual child with her/his peers, but are not helpful if the degree of malnutrition is to be compared to international standards. Further, with widely differ-ent socio-economic situations in various communities, separate growth charts could not be designed for all possible situations.

# Comparisons to the reference standard

When a comparison is made between a child's measurements and the reference standards, the relationship between the two values is expressed in one of three ways:
- centiles;
- percentage of the median; and
- standard deviation units, or z-scores.

Each of these three methods is based on making comparisons to the centre point of the reference population measurements. This centre point can be addressed as the 50th centile, the median, or the mean. In all three cases, these centre points represent the 'average' healthy measurement for the reference population.

## CENTILES

To understand centiles, imagine, for example, the weight measurement scores for all the 12-month-old boys in the reference population being put in order from the lowest to the highest values. After they are in order, the weight measurement that represents the point where half the boys are heavier and half are lighter is found. This point is the 50th centile. In addition to the 50th centile, the measurement points that correspond with the 5th, 10th, 25th, 75th, 90th, and 95th centiles have been calculated for each of the measurement indexes (weight-for-age, length-for-age and weight-for-length) for boys and girls.

The measurements of an individual child can be compared to the reference standards using the centiles. A child whose measurement equals the reference measurement at the 50th centile is also heavier/taller than half of the reference population and lighter/shorter than half of the reference population. A measurement that puts a child near the 5th centile means that the child is lighter/shorter than 95 per cent of the reference children of the same age. Although the 5th centile is usually used to separate the well nourished from the poorly nourished, it must be emphasized that children whose measurements correspond to the 5th centile are not necessarily at risk. They may just be petite and healthy.

## PERCENTAGE OF THE MEDIAN

This statistic indicates where a child is in relation to the median of the reference population. The median is the value that splits the data set into two equal halves (which also makes it the value found at the 50th centile). If a child's measurement is exactly the same as the median of the reference population, the child would be '100 per cent of the median'. A child who weighs 6 kg when the reference median is 10 kg would be 60 per cent ($6/10 \times 100$) of the median. Cut-off values of 80 or 90 per cent of the median value are widely used to indicate malnutrition (see Table 16.1).

## THE STANDARD DEVIATION AND Z-SCORE CLASSIFICATION SYSTEM

(See also Chapter 4: Physical growth and development.)

The problem with the use of centiles is that:
- they are not continuous variables and thus children are diagnosed as being above or below a particular centile; and
- it makes comparison between different populations and communities difficult as there is no indication of the degree of spread of the measurements because all that is referred to is the position of the

average on the centile chart, or the percentage above or below a particular centile value.

To overcome these problems, z-scores have been introduced. The z-score is a continuous variable, which is based on the number of standard deviations (SD) above or below the mean reference value in which the individual child or population sample is situated. Standard deviation indicates how far measurements are spread out from the mean. One standard deviation score above and below the mean will include 68 per cent of any 'normal' population, while two standard deviations around the mean includes 95 per cent of the population. Thus, an individual can be defined as having a z-score of -2 when his/her weight is 2 SD below the reference mean. A similar calculation can be made from a population sample, which might have a mean z-score of -1,5 ± 1,2, which implies that the sample mean is 1,5 SD below the mean reference value and there is a scatter of 1,2 SD around this mean.

# Classification systems

The WHO Global Database on Child Growth and Malnutrition uses a z-score cut-off point of less than -2 standard deviations (SD) to classify low weight-for-age (underweight), low height-for-age (stunting), and low weight-for-height (wasting) as moderate undernutrition, and less than -3 SD to define severe undernutrition. The cut-off point of more than +2 SD classifies high weight-for-height as overweight in children (see Table 16.1).

Another classification in common use is the Wellcome classification, based on weight-for-age. This classification is shown in Table 16.2. It is useful to differentiate the clinical forms of severe malnutrition, but does not differentiate the underweight category.

**Table 16.1** Definitions of commonly used anthropological measurements

| Term | Description |
| --- | --- |
| Underweight | Weight-for-age < -2 SD of NCHS/WHO reference values, or <80% of median weight-for-age |
| Stunting | Height-for age < -2 SD of NCHS/WHO reference values, or <90% of median height-for-age |
| Wasting | Weight-for-height < -2 SD of NCHS/WHO reference values, or <80% of median weight-for-height |
| Severe malnutrition | Severe wasting < -3 SD of reference (<70% weight-for height), or severe stunting < -3 SD of reference (<85% height-for-age), or the presence of oedema of both feet, or clinically visible severe wasting |
| Overweight | Weight-for-height > +2 SD of NCHS/WHO reference values |

**Table 16.2** Wellcome classification of infantile nutrition (Source: Lancet, 1970)

| | 60–80% of standard* weight | Less than 60% of standard* weight |
| --- | --- | --- |
| No oedema | Underweight<br>– nutritional dwarfing<br>– growth retardation | Marasmus |
| Oedema | Kwashiorkor | Marasmic kwashiorkor |

\* Standard refers to the 50th percentile (median) and the term is used in preference to 'expected' weight

# Epidemiology

The WHO Global Database on Child Growth collates anthropometric data on under-five-year-olds in developing countries, and allows an accurate description of the magnitude and geographical distribution of PEM. The database confirms that more than a third of the world's children are malnourished. Globally, it was estimated that 226 million children are stunted, 183 million children underweight, and 67 million wasted (UNICEF, 1998).

Data on the nutritional status of South African children from a national survey done in 1994 is included in Table 16.3. It shows that rural children have a higher prevalence of malnutrition than urban children. While black children have the highest prevalence of stunting, Indian and 'coloured' children have a higher prevalence of underweight and wasting. The more severe kwashiorkor and marasmic syndromes make up one to four per cent of the pre-school population in poverty-stricken areas. With the increased prevalence of HIV disease in young children, marasmus and wasting are becoming more common.

The relative absence of wasting and the high prevalence of stunting in South Africa suggest that the main problem is chronic socio-economic underdevelopment, rather than a severe or immediate lack of food. The recent emphasis

**Table 16.3** Indicators of nutritional status in children aged less than five years from 1990–1998

| | %<br>underweight | %<br>stunted | %<br>wasted |
| --- | --- | --- | --- |
| World | 30 | 37 | 11 |
| Sub-Saharan Africa | 32 | 41 | 9 |
| South Africa (all) | 9 | 23 | 3 |
| Urban South Africa | 7 | 16 | 2 |
| Rural South Africa | 11 | 27 | 3 |

(Sources: UNICEF, 1997, South African Vitamin A Consultative Group [SAVACG] 1996)

of the National Nutrition and Social Development Programme of the National Department of Health on social development is therefore appropriate. Nevertheless, between 11 and 17 million South Africans have an unreliable supply of food, with 38 per cent of African households often or sometimes going hungry.

## Aetiology

### STUNTING

In South Africa this is the major form of undernutrition, and develops mainly in children under three years of age. The causes and aetiology of stunting are less understood than its timing and consequences. In particular, there is poor understanding of why and how stunting occurs in some settings extensively but not others. Environmental factors are predominantly thought to be responsible in poorer regions. Contributors to stunting include the following:

- poor nutrition (lack of energy, macronutrients, and micronutrients);
- infection (injury to gastrointestinal mucosa, systemic effects, and immunostimulation); and
- suboptimal mother–infant interaction (poor maternal nutrition and stores at birth and inferior behavioural interactions).

### SEVERE MALNUTRITION

In South Africa, maramus is frequently found in infants less than six months of age, while kwashiorkor occurs predominantly in the six-month to two-year-old age group. Studies in various settings have consistently identified some common risk factors. Severely malnourished children are more likely to have young mothers, low birthweights, tendencies of less feeding frequency, less access to breast-feeding, and less support by both parents.

Moreover, the parents of severely malnourished children have lower educational levels and lower income jobs compared with those of normal children. Rural living, poor health, the use of unprotected water supplies, lack of fuel, and lack of personal hygiene have also been identified as risk factors for marasmus.

## Pathogenesis

Deficiency of energy, protein, or type II nutrients, i.e., nutrients that cause growth failure (e.g., sulphur, phosphorus, zinc, potassium), causes stunting and wasting. The primary cause of marasmus is inadequate energy intake, or excessive energy requirements. The pathogenesis of kwashiorkor is more controversial. It is now accepted that it is not solely due to a low protein intake, but is associated with oxidant damage in the face of depleted anti-oxidant protection. In kwashiorkor, the deficiency is likely to be due to one or several type I nutrients, i.e., nutrients that cause clinical signs, particularly those involved with anti-oxidant protection (e.g., glutathione). The oxidative stress comes mainly from infection, although others have suggested sources that include ingested aflatoxin, mycotoxins, bacterial endotoxins, and small-bowel overgrowth.

## Clinical aspects of malnutrition

### UNDERWEIGHT AND STUNTING

Failure of growth as judged by inadequate weight or height gain is common to all the syndromes of malnutrition. In the mildest forms this may be the only sign that can alert the clinician or health worker. If weight and height are proportionately reduced, recognition depends on measuring and charting these anthropometric measurements.

124

A common pattern of growth in disadvantaged children in South Africa, and indeed throughout the developing world, is one of normal weight gain during the first six months of life, largely associated with successful breast-feeding. Thereafter, the proportion of children falling below the 5th weight-for-age centile increases. The prevalence of underweight-for-age and stunting increases rapidly after 6 to 12 months of age (at the time of the introduction of supplementary foods into the diet of the breast-fed infant).

It is postulated that slower growth may result from specific eating practices coupled with an increased incidence of infections. Township children of working parents who spend long hours away from home may depend almost entirely on a single large evening meal during which they cannot eat enough food to meet growth as well as maintenance requirements. Bulky low-energy-dense diets also add to this problem. There is a strong probability that growth is limited by multiple, simultaneous nutrient deficiencies in many populations.

Most stunting occurs before the age of three years, and stunted children usually become stunted adults, as catch-up growth is difficult to achieve. The results of becoming and remaining stunted are increased risk of morbidity, mortality, a delay in motor and mental development, and decreased work capacity. Thus, any programme aimed at reducing the prevalence of malnutrition in a community should be targeted at the six-month to two-year-old child in order to prevent growth faltering in this age group.

Severe stunting at age two years is significantly associated with later deficits in cognitive ability. Test performance is related to the timing of stunting, largely because children stunted very early also tend to be severely stunted. Deficits in children's scores are smaller at age 11 years than at age 8 years, suggesting that adverse effects may decline over time. (Mendez & Adair, 1999) Educational outcomes are blurred by numerous interfering variables such as quality and duration of schooling, home and community environment, and other socio-economic factors.

## KWASHIORKOR

This is a clinical syndrome characterized by pedal oedema, with a weight greater than 60 per cent of that expected for age. It is possible to have kwashiorkor with a weight-for-age above the 5th centile (i.e., more than 80 per cent of that expected for age). This generally reflects acute nutritional imbalance precipitated by an illness such as measles or gastroenteritis in a child with a previously reasonable energy intake. Kwashiorkor mainly occurs in children aged from 6 to 30 months.

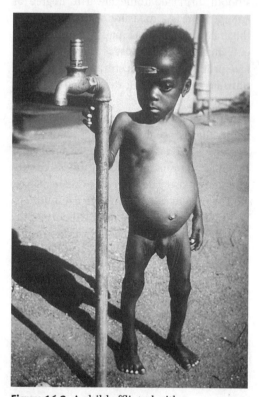

**Figure 16.2** A child afflicted with kwashiorkor

The facial appearance in kwashiorkor is often characterized by big cheeks and a dull expression of misery. Sparse, fine, or depigmented hair indicates chronic protein insufficiency. Eye signs include extreme dryness of the conjunctiva (xerophthalmia) and corneal ulceration due to vitamin A deficiency. Cracking of the lips (cheilosis) and angular stomatitis are common, as is a smooth tongue.

Skin lesions occur, particularly in areas of irritation such as the buttocks and perineum and on surfaces exposed to the sun. On dark skins the rash is pigmented, while on white skins it appears red. There may be scaling with subsequent depigmented areas and sometimes ulceration. Lesions similar to those seen in pellagra might also be noted. Open and weeping lesions are poor prognostic signs.

The liver is infiltrated by fat, resulting in smooth, firm hepatomegaly. The degree of enlargement is a measure of the severity of the malnutrition. There may be jaundice, and petechiae and ecchymoses (bruises) due to a low prothrombin concentration. Ascites is unusual and often indicates a need to search for other pathologies, e.g., TB peritonitis. Other findings include overwhelming bacteraemia that is usually associated with gram-negative bacteria. Severe hypoglycaemia and hypothermia may also occur, unless careful attention is also paid to feeding and heat loss.

The mental state may range from unhappy irritability to severe apathy, which, together with reduced activity/energy expenditure, impairs interaction with caregivers and the environment. There is associated deprivation of stimulation, a reduction in immediate exploratory/learning experiences and related developmental disadvantage.

The debate on the long-term effects on cognitive ability continues. It is virtually impossible to separate out the effects of environmental deprivation, nutritional deficiencies and possible direct nutritional insult to the brain. If adverse circumstances persist there is likely to be reduced adult stature and mental ability. Children with PEM can make a complete recovery if they are given proper care both immediately and later.

Over the past five decades the case fatality from severe malnutrition has remained unchanged and is typically 20 to 30 per cent, with the highest levels (50 to 60 per cent) being among those with kwashiorkor. A likely cause of this continuing high mortality is faulty case-management. Even with the best of care, acute kwashiorkor still carries a significant mortality of between 5 per cent and 10 per cent. Death usually results from overwhelming bacteraemia or other unrecognized infections. Poor prognostic features include infection, water and electrolyte disturbances, hepatomegaly, hypothermia, hypoglycaemia, severe dermatosis, xerophthalmia, and raised serum bilirubin.

## MARASMUS

Marasmus, characterized by wasting and emaciation, reflects extreme energy deprivation. In South Africa, marasmus occurs maximally between the ages of three months and one year. If there is also oedema the term 'marasmic kwashiorkor' is used. A child may move overnight from one category to the other, with accumulation or loss of oedema. The prevalence of maramus has increased in many communities with the increasing number of HIV positive children in these settings.

## PELLAGRA

Pellagra can also be classified under malnutrition because nicotinamide deficiency results from a low intake of the precursor amino acid, tryptophan. Maize is deficient in tryptophan, and adults who use this staple as the sole source of protein will develop pellagra. On the other hand, rapidly growing infants on the same diet may manifest protein inadequacy, and present with kwashiorkor. In South Africa, voluntary fortification of maize with niacin and riboflavin has considerably reduced the prevalence of pellagra. Clinically, pellagra presents in children with dermatitis and diarrhoea, although dementia is described in adults. The dermatitis is typically worse in sun-exposed areas of the body (characteristically the face, neck and arms) and appears as reddened hyperpigmented areas. A glossitis (i.e., inflammation of the tongue) may also be present.

# Management of severe malnutrition

In 1999, the WHO produced a standardized protocol manual to help health workers in the management of severely malnourished children and reduce the high mortality associated with the condition (WHO, 1999). The WHO strategy for the management of the child with severe malnutrition is divided into three phases. These are:

- *Initial treatment*: life-threatening problems are identified and treated, specific deficiencies are corrected, metabolic abnormalities are reversed, and feeding is commenced;
- *Rehabilitation*: intensive feeding is started to recover lost weight, emotional and physical stimulation are provided, the mother or caregiver is trained to continue care at home, and preparations for discharge of the child are made; and
- *Follow-up*: following discharge, the child and the child's family are followed up to prevent relapse and assure the continued physical, mental, and emotional development of the child.

The WHO guidelines have introduced some novel recommendations for the management of severely malnourished children. These include:

- a similar dietary approach being proposed for both marasmus and kwashiorkor;

- the use of specially prepared feeds (F-75 and F-100). F-75 (75 kcal or 315 kJ/100 ml) is used during the initial phase of treatment, while F-100 (100 kcal or 420 kJ/ 100 ml) is used during the rehabilitation phase once appetite has returned;
- the use of pre-mixed sachets of minerals (containing potassium, magnesium, and other essential nutrients) and vitamins which are mixed with the diet. This replaces the need for the provision of individual minerals and vitamins separately; and
- a modified low-sodium oral rehydration solution (ReSoMal) for rehydration of malnourished children.

While the WHO recommended feeds and mixes may represent a 'gold standard', their widespread use in less developed countries may be problematic because of resource constraints (costs, availability, etc.). Studies are underway to evaluate their use and effectiveness in these settings.

The WHO guidelines for routine treatment consist of 10 steps together with prescriptive actions.

A typical time-frame for the management of a child with severe malnutrition is shown in Table 16.4.

Table 16.4  The ten essential steps in managing severe malnutrition

1   treat/prevent hypoglycemia;
2   treat/prevent hypothermia;
3   treat/prevent dehydration;
4   correct imbalance of electrolytes;
5   treat infections;
6   correct deficiencies of micronutrients (vitamins and minerals);
7   start cautious feeding; then
8   rebuild wasted tissues (catch-up growth);
9   provide stimulation, play, and loving care; and
10  prepare for follow-up after hospital discharge.

## GENERAL PRINCIPLES

Children with malnutrition are often seriously ill, and often have an infection, when they first present for treatment. Severely malnourished children should, wherever possible, be referred to hospital. Initial treatment begins with their admission and lasts until the child's condition is stable and their appetite has returned. This usually occurs in three to five days. Failure to respond within 10 days requires additional measures.

Recently admitted malnourished children are ideally kept in a special area where they can be constantly monitored. Because of their increased susceptibility to infections, they should, if possible, be isolated from other patients. The child should not be positioned near a window or in a draught and should be kept clothed and covered. Washing should be kept to a minimum. Intravenous infusions should be avoided except where essential, e.g., severe dehydration or septic shock.

## INVESTIGATIONS

The following investigations should be considered in severely malnourished children who are admitted: haemoglobin and blood culture, glucose, urine dipstix and microscopy, tuberculin testing, and a chest x-ray. Serum electrolytes and protein and HIV testing should only be done for specific reasons.

## Hypoglycaemia

Malnourished children are at risk of developing hypoglycaemia (glucose < 3 mmol/l). Blood glucose monitoring (e.g., with Dextrostix) at the time of admission and during the first few days should be routine. Feeds should be provided at frequent intervals, at least every two to three hours, day and night, to prevent hypoglycaemia.

## Electrolyte imbalance

Severely malnourished children have deficiencies of potassium and magnesium, which may take two weeks or more to resolve. Oedema is partly a result of these deficiencies. Total body sodium is increased although the plasma sodium may be low. Giving high sodium loads to the child could potentially be

**Table 16.5** Treatment for children with severe malnutrition (WHO, 1999)

| | |
|---|---|
| • Vitamin A | 50 000–200 000 IU, depending on age, given orally on day 1 (if clinical signs of vitamin A deficiency, second dose given on day 2 and third dose at least two weeks later) |
| • Folic acid | 5 mg on day 1 and 1 mg daily thereafter for 5 days |
| • Potassium | 6–8 mmol/kg/day 6 hrly until discharge |
| • Iron | elemental iron 3 mg/kg/day daily for 3 months (only after acute infections have subsided, i.e., in rehabilitation phase) |
| • Multivitamin syrup | 5 ml daily |
| • Zinc (zinc sulphate) | 1 mg/kg/day for one week (zinc and castor oil cream is used for excoriated buttocks) |
| • Magnesium (magnesium hydroxide) | 1–2 mmol/kg/day for one week |

fatal. Diuretics are contraindicated in managing the oedema. High potassium supplementation (8 mmol/kg/day) may reduce mortality and morbidity in kwashiorkor.

## Infection

Bacterial infections, often with gram-negative organisms, are common and difficult to detect in children with malnutrition. Malnourished children may fail to respond appropriately to infection with fever and inflammation and may only display apathy or drowsiness. Hypoglycaemia and hypothermia are both signs of severe infection. Routine administration of broad-spectrum antibiotics to children with severe malnutrition, irrespective of clinical signs of infection, is most probably the single most effective measure to reduce the high case-fatality rate due to malnutrition in developing countries (Gernaat et al., 1998). Ampicillin and gentamicin given IM or IV for five to seven days should be prescribed. Nevertheless, an attempt to identify the site/s of infection should always be made. A urinary tract infection may, for example, be identified in about 30 per cent of severely malnourished children. Measles vaccine should be administered on admission to all children over six months who have not received it previously.

## Dietary treatment

Successful treatment regimens recognize that nutrient needs differ importantly between the acute phase of resuscitation and the phase of dietary rehabilitation. The objectives of the resuscitation phase are to provide an intake of energy and protein adequate to satisfy requirements for maintenance without promoting tissue deposition, while infections are treated, fluids and electrolyte balance re-established, and specific nutrient deficiencies corrected. During the rehabilitation phase, generous amounts of energy (and protein) are provided with other nutrients to promote net tissue deposition.

Feeding should begin as early as possible after admission. The only reasons for delaying the introduction of feeds might be in a severely toxic or shocked child. In South Africa, the initial feed is often a low solute breast-milk substitute (such as S26 or Nan) at 100–120 ml/kg/24hour. This volume should be given orally or by nasogastric tube every three hours throughout the day and night. If lesser amounts than this are given, tissues will continue to be broken down and the child will deteriorate. If the amount is exceeded the child may develop a serious metabolic imbalance. Patience and coaxing are needed to encourage the child to complete each feed. If the child's appetite improves, treatment has been successful. This usually occurs after two to seven days; however, in some children with complications it may take longer. The WHO recommends the use of F-75 for this stage of management.

Once the child's appetite has returned and the oedema is settling, larger volumes of a higher solute feed (such as Lactogen or SMA) may be introduced, and as the child improves, so porridge and other nutritious foods should be started. The WHO recommends the use of F-100 during this phase of rehabilitation.

Children less than two years can be fed exclusively on liquid or semi-liquid diets. Full-cream milk is excellent for the rehabilitation phase as well as being a valuable long-term complement to maize. It is usually appropriate to introduce solid foods for older children. During rehabilitation, feeds should be given every four hours, night and day, with a gradual increase in volume. Most children take between 150 and 220 kcal/kg (630–920 kJ/kg) per day. During the first few days of rehabilitation, children with oedema may not gain weight despite an adequate intake. This is the result of oedema fluid being lost while tissue is being restored.

Milk has been proven to be superior to a maize-based diet in the treatment of kwashiorkor in terms of mortality, weight gain, clinical sepsis, and improvement in intestinal permeability (Brewster et al., 1997). Local foods may need to be fortified to increase their energy and nutritional content. They are also relatively deficient in minerals and vitamins. Oil, mineral, and vitamin mixes and dried skimmed milk are all suitable additives. Porridge with peanut butter or samp with beans and margarine may be suitable, affordable, and locally available options.

## Micronutrient deficiencies

Table 16.5 lists the supplements prescribed for children with severe malnutrition. Doses administered will depend on preparations locally available.

Where available, the WHO recommended adding prepackaged mineral and vitamin supplementation mixes to feeds. They provide the child with most of the essential nutrients needed.

### REHABILITATION

It has been shown that physical and psychological stimulation, as well as care and affection, are necessary during the rehabilitation phase to prevent retardation of growth and psychological development (Elizabeth & Sathy, 1997). Structured play and other activities promote the development of language and motor skills. Toys can be made using locally available materials. Attention to the mother's needs is vital, as it is unrealistic to expect her to cope if she is exhausted, depressed, and possibly undernourished. Kind support and encouragement are called for.

Preparation for discharge and follow-up should begin soon after admission. Health workers need to assess the home environment and should help the mother and family in identifying feasible ways of providing for the child's nutritional needs. Nutrition education involves not only the imparting of necessary information but also the motivation of people to change their behaviour if and as needed. Cultural factors and taboos influence feeding practices and eating patterns. It is difficult, if not impossible, for a young mother to ignore her elders or her ill-informed peer group. Ascribing blame to the mother of a malnourished child is seldom, if ever, appropriate and is more likely to be unhelpful. Specific instructions such as five meals per day or snacks between meals are better than a general directive to improve the diet.

### DISCHARGE

Discharge should be considered when weight gain has been established, appetite has improved, and the child is again active and smiling. The WHO guidelines suggest that the child is ready for discharge once the child reaches 90 per cent of median reference weight-for-height. This milestone is usually reached after one month. However, a two-month period is needed for complete immunologic recovery. Children discharged after one month to high disease-exposure environments often relapse, because they are still immunodepressed. For this reason, home management of severely malnourished children after about one week of inpatient care can have economic and practical advantages over other methods. (Khanum et al., 1994).

Finally, it is important to create referral systems that are able to track at-risk children as they leave the hospital and move back to the community. There should be long-term follow-up with the provision of comprehensive health care for the whole family.

## Malnutrition and HIV

HIV-infected children with no access to antiretroviral therapy are stunted, under-weight, and wasted compared to same-age uninfected children. Stunting is a frequent early finding in perinatal HIV infection. Both HIV infection and HIV-associated signs and symptoms, not maternal immuno-logical or socio-economic circumstances, place children at risk for growth retarda-tion. The harmful effect of HIV on growth appears to be linked with the level of post-natal HIV viraemia.

The triad of HIV infection, nutritional status, and immune function are closely related, each factor affecting the others. The dominant effect in this three-way relation-ship is the effect of HIV infection on nutri-tional status. Until the advent of anti-retro-viral drugs, this manifested primarily as wasting. Recently, more complex metabolic abnormalities have become apparent, par-ticularly fat redistribution syndromes, hyper-lipidaemia and hypercholesterolaemia.

As for the converse effect of nutritional state on HIV disease progression, there is good evidence that clinical outcome is poorer in individuals with compromised nutrition. Strategies to improve nutritional status, both quantitatively and qualitative-ly, may have a beneficial effect on the clini-cal and immunological course of the dis-ease. Effective macronutrient supply improves survival in severely malnourished individuals and may benefit less severely affected individuals. Micronutrient defi-ciencies appear to be involved in modifying clinical HIV disease and may be associated with enhanced mother-to-child transmis-sion of virus, particularly in developing countries. Intervention trials in this setting are currently under way.

# Other nutritional deficiencies

### VITAMIN A

The impact of vitamin A supplementation on reducing child mortality is comparable to, if not greater than, that of any single immu-nization against a childhood disease. Vitamin A deficiency has increasingly been recog-nized as significantly increasing children's risk of dying from common diseases such as measles and diarrhoea. In countries where vitamin A deficiency is a particular problem, such as the Far East, ensuring that children receive adequate vitamin A can reduce mor-tality by 23 per cent. This effect is related to the underlying nutritional deficiency and is not a physiological effect of pharmacological doses. In addition, the benefits for maternal mortality are now being recognized.

Marginal vitamin A status of public health importance and/or overt vitamin A deficien-cy has been reported, apart from South Africa (33 per cent), in Lesotho (13 per cent), Namibia (20 per cent), Swaziland (50 per cent), and Zambia (66 per cent) in the under-five population.

The outstanding clinical features of vita-min A deficiency are night blindness, xeroph-thalmia (dry conjunctiva), and, in severe cases, keratomalacia (softening of the cornea). Vitamin A deficiency is the most important cause of preventable blindness in children. Delayed growth, especially stunting, has been reported in children with clinical signs of vita-min A deficiency. Vitamin A administration to children with measles reduces the complica-tions and duration of hospital stay. Vitamin A deficiency also increases the prevalence of iron deficiency, probably through impairing iron absorption and mobilization.

The present challenge is to get vitamin A, through supplementation or food fortifica-tion, to the more than 55 million children world-wide who are suffering from clinical and subclinical deficiency and who have not received any supplements. One recognized way of doing this is to build on existing measures and initiatives. WHO and UNICEF recommend that high-dose vitamin A capsule supplementation be included in routine immunization activities and events such as national immunization days (NID) in all countries where the under-five mortality rate is greater than or equal to 70 per 1 000. The progress made on vitamin A distribution, particularly through NIDs, has been remarkable. Currently, there are 35 countries where over 80 per cent of young children routinely receive at least one dose of vitamin A, and many of these nations seemed likely to achieve the goal of eliminating vitamin A deficiency by the year 2000.

Although South Africa has a high prevalence of vitamin A deficiency, it does not have a programme in place. From 1997, in some African countries, including South Africa, Namibia, and Zimbabwe, a few manufacturers started adding vitamin A, iron, and vitamins of the B complex to maize meal, with the purpose of supplying at least 25 per cent of the RDA values of these micronutrients.

## IODINE

Severe iodine deficiency *in utero* can cause profound intellectual disability. Milder deficiencies also take an intellectual toll. This deficiency still occurs in certain mountainous areas, resulting in a high prevalence of goitre and hypothyroidism; in southern Africa this form of thyroid disorder is rare in children, although it has previously been reported from Swaziland, Mpumalanga, and Lesotho.

Iodized salt is the best source of iodine. The reduction in iodine deficiency, the world's leading cause of preventable mental retardation, is a global success story. UNICEF

estimates that more than 60 per cent of all edible salt in the world is now iodized. Mandatory iodization of table salt was introduced in South Africa in 1995.

## IRON

Iron deficiency affects people of all ages and is the most common nutritional problem in the world today. Anaemia on account of iron lack is found in about a third of the population of most developing countries, while iron deficiency without anaemia occurs in about another third. In children under five years of age, the prevalence of anaemia may be as high as 50 per cent in developing countries. Depleted iron stores or deficiency has been reported in up to 36 per cent of children of all population groups in South Africa, while the prevalence of anaemia in primary school children can be as high as 83 per cent.

The transplacental passage of iron, particularly in the last trimester of pregnancy, is usually sufficient for the normal full-term purely breast-fed infant for the first four to six months of life. Delayed introduction of mixed feeding, diets poor in available iron or containing phytate and low vitamin C, or failure to provide the necessary supplements accounts for the commonly occurring hypochromic microcytic anaemia of later infancy. In the coastal areas of South Africa blood loss associated with hookworm infestation aggravates the problem.

There is good evidence that tissue and enzyme iron depletion and decreased iron stores precede the development of anaemia, and probably account for symptoms such as poor appetite, irritability, and pica, which are unrelated to haemoglobin values. There is substantial evidence that anaemia in children is associated with decreased physical and mental development (lowering IQ by about nine points), impaired immune function, and reduced capacity of leucocytes to kill micro-organisms. Iron supplements improve the cognitive scores of deficient groups of children. However, long-term iron supplementation does not appear to increase growth in children.

Much greater efforts need to be dedicated to effective promotion of the increased consumption of iron-rich foods and of enhancing factors. Efforts to remedy iron deficiency have been disappointing thus far. It is recommended that lean meat or fish be introduced to infants at six to nine months to provide haem-iron. Recent evidence suggests that a weekly oral dose of iron is as effective in managing iron deficiency as a similar daily dose. Iron-fortified cow milk formula significantly reduces the prevalence of anaemia in infants. Fortified wheat flour and maize have also successfully reduced anaemia rates in school children, but this is not done in South Africa.

## ZINC

In contrast to the clinical presentations of deficiencies of other micronutrients of public health importance, those of zinc deficiency are neither unique nor pathognomonic. Deficiency of zinc, which is essential for DNA and protein synthesis, leads to growth failure and delayed secondary sexual maturation. Zinc may also play a major role in brain function and in normal immune function.

Breast milk provides modest and steadily decreasing quantities of zinc but with relatively favourable bioavailability. Those at greatest risk for zinc deficiency are older infants and young children whose diets do not include animal products. In many communities the quantity of zinc is not low in absolute terms, but its bioavailability is poor. The high phytic acid content of vegetable products, especially grains and legumes, is regarded as the principal culprit. Excessive zinc losses in diarrhoeal fluids may contribute to zinc deficiency.

Zinc supplementation in children in developing countries is associated with sub-stantial reductions in the rates of diarrhoea and pneumonia, the two leading causes of death in these settings. Malaria is notable among other infectious diseases for which there is strong preliminary evidence for a beneficial effect of zinc.

In those communities where vegetable food staples are relatively low in zinc, quite possibly the result of mineral losses during refining, fortification with zinc (and, typically, iron) is a logical long-term strategy. More information is needed on the quantity and frequency of supplementary zinc dosing. Consideration also needs to be given to the routine inclusion of zinc in iron supplements provided to children, and to the simultaneous inclusion of other micronutrients in zinc supplements.

## VITAMIN D

Vitamin D deficiency leading to rickets and/or symptoms of hypocalcaemia is not uncommon in the first year of life, even in sunny South Africa. Deficiency is more prevalent in Cape Town than Johannesburg due to Cape Town's greater latitude. Vitamin D deficiency is primarily a disease of the two extremes of life, owing to a lack of sunlight exposure.

In South Africa dietary sources of vitamin D are generally insufficient to meet daily requirements as few foods are fortified. The exception to this is the fortification of all infant breast milk substitutes, thus young infants being fed infant formulae are protected. The same cannot be said for breast-fed infants, as breast-milk generally contains insufficient vitamin D to meet the infant's requirements. Thus all breast-fed infants should either be given vitamin D supplements (400 IU/day) or adequate sunlight exposure (30 minutes/week if the infant is only wearing a nappy).

Once a toddler is mobile and walking, the incidence of vitamin D deficiency rickets falls rapidly, as the child now is able to play out of the house in the sunlight. The exceptions to this are the toddlers living in inner city apartments. High crime rates and a lack of safe parks and green areas mean that young children seldom go outside, thus they are at risk of becoming vitamin D deficient.

Rickets remains a serious public health problem in a number of developing countries. It has been estimated that in Tibet and China over 50 per cent of infants have clinical signs of rickets. In Ethiopia, infants with rickets have a 13-fold increase in the incidence of pneumonia and the mortality rate is 40 per cent in those who develop pneumonia. In other developing countries, such as South Africa, Bangladesh, and Nigeria, rickets also occurs in children older than those usually at risk of vitamin D deficiency. Studies are suggesting that low dietary calcium intake plays an important role in the pathogenesis of the disease in this group of children. Typically the diets are mainly cereal-based (maize) and lack milk or milk products.

Treatment of rickets consists of vitamin D 1 000–2 000 IU/day for a month, and milk for the improvement of calcium intake. Giving vitamin D – 400 IU/day for the first year of life (800 IU for premature infants and twins) – best prevents rickets. Sensible but not excessive exposure to sunlight should be advocated. Sunshine through glass windows is ineffective.

# Child nutrition programmes in South Africa

## INTEGRATED NUTRITION PROGRAMME (INP)

Since 1994 official policy has been to develop an Integrated Nutrition Programme. The programme called for the transformation of existing interventions and for the institutionalization of a multisectoral approach, including the education, welfare, public works, and labour sectors. However, lack of resources and limited skills within the government to implement intersectoral and participatory programmes has strained development. The INP has three components: a health-facility-based component (e.g., growth monitoring); a community-based component (e.g., improving household food security); and a nutrition promotion programme (e.g., breast-feeding promotion).

The intention of the programme is to combat undernutrition through addressing the root causes rather than relying on food hand-outs. Thus, community-based programmes aimed at job creation, food production, and the development of infrastructure are supported.

## THE PRIMARY SCHOOLS NUTRITION PROGRAMME (PSNP)

The President of South Africa introduced this programme in 1994, in an attempt to address hunger in school children. Five million children (in 14 549 schools) who were deemed 'needy' by the provincial health departments were to get a daily snack and drink. The meal varied from province to province. The programme should not be seen as a nutrition programme, but rather as an education programme, as the major impact has been on improved attendance at school by pupils and better attention spans rather than improved nutritional status. Unfortunately, fraud and poor management have hindered the implementation of this programme in some regions, with as many as 30 per cent of eligible children not receiving any feeding.

## THE PROTEIN-ENERGY-MALNUTRITION SCHEME

This is a national programme that aims to address the problem of malnutrition in children, by providing food supplements to those children who fulfil certain anthropometric criteria. The programme is administered by local authorities and thus its implementation has had variable success. One of the major criticisms of the programme by some nutritionists is the provision of breast-milk substitutes as one of the food supplements. The programme is also criticized because it is often administered in isolation, so parents or caregivers are not being referred for community support.

Other programmes introduced by the Department of Health include the draft national breast-feeding policy and a commitment to the creation of 'baby-friendly' hospitals. A food fortification policy is also being developed.

# Obesity

Childhood obesity is rapidly emerging as a global epidemic that will have profound public health consequences as overweight children become overweight adults. As many as 250 million people world-wide may be obese (seven per cent of the adult population) and two to three times as many may be considered overweight. The prevalence of obesity seems to be increasing in most parts of the world. This change appears to be related more to a reduction in energy expenditure than to an increase in caloric intake.

In the developing world, obesity is emerging first in urban middle-aged women, then in men and younger women. There is also increasing concern about the potential consequences of the nutritional transition where many black South Africans, who may have been nutritionally deprived during childhood, have moved from undernutrition to extreme overnutrition without having achieved optimal nutritional status.

There is no internationally acceptable index to assess childhood obesity nor an established cut off point to define overweight in children. The most common definition of obesity in childhood is weight in excess of 20 per cent above ideal weight for age and gender and skinfold thickness in excess of the 85th centile for age and gender. Use of the body mass index (BMI) to define adult obesity has been recommended by the WHO, and this measurement is regarded as being appropriate for children too, but the reference curves are still under development.

Aside from calorie excess and inactivity, genetics and environment predispose a child to be obese. Children with obese mothers, low family incomes, and lower cognitive stimulation have significantly elevated risks of developing obesity. There is strong evidence for a role of genetic factors in the aetiology of childhood obesity. There is also increasing evidence that responsiveness to dietary intervention is genetically determined.

The severity of obesity and the age at which it occurs appear to be significant indicators of whether childhood obesity will persist into adulthood. At any age, severe obesity is more likely to persist, and obesity present in adolescents is much more likely to persist than obesity in young children.

The health consequences of obesity in adults are well established, including greater rates of hypertension, non-insulin dependent diabetes mellitus, and heart disease. In children, short-term risks for orthopaedic, neurological, pulmonary, gastrointestinal, and endocrine conditions are largely limited to severely overweight children. The social and psychological burden of paediatric obesity, particularly during middle childhood and adolescence, may have lasting effects on self-esteem, body image, and career opportunities. Reviews of the long-term morbidity and mortality linked with childhood obesity suggest that the risks of cardiovascular disease and all-cause mortality are elevated among those who are overweight during childhood.

135

The major issues that confront the clinician in relation to childhood obesity are identifying children at risk, deciding the goal and focus of therapy, and determining how to maintain weight loss. The goals of therapy depend on the child's age and the severity of obesity-related complications. Any treatment plan for overweight children and adolescents should include three major components: diet, exercise, and family-based behaviour management. It is most likely to be successful if realistic goals are set.

Assessment of the family's readiness to change represents the first focus of therapy. There needs to be a commitment by the family to making changes in the home and family environment to help reduce cues and opportunities associated with calorie intake and inactivity (e.g., reduction in time spent watching television or playing computer games), and to increase cues and opportunities for physical activity. Other components of successful programmes include self-monitoring, goal setting and contracting, parenting skills training, skills for managing high-risk situations, and skills for programme maintenance and relapse prevention. Therefore, any programme or treatment plan must include the caregivers, who in most cases are also overweight or obese.

Food preferences are influenced early by parental eating habits, and when developed in childhood, they tend to remain fairly constant into adulthood. Children and adolescents should not be placed on restrictive diets because adequate calories are needed for proper growth and development. A safe rate of weight loss of about 0,5 kg a week is achieved through moderate reduction of energy intake (about 20–25 per cent decrease). Adherence to exercise programmes may be improved by making the activity enjoyable, increasing the choice over type and level of activities, and providing positive reinforcement of even small achievements. Current behavioural treatments for childhood and adolescent obesity produce long-term weight control in up to one-third of participants. Nevertheless, when the right family dynamics exist – a motivated child with supportive parents – long-term success is possible.

Three key settings for implementing childhood obesity management support programmes have been identified in developed countries: the family, the school, and primary care. Educating parents on eating and lifestyle behaviour may significantly reduce the prevalence of obesity in their children. Classroom lessons on nutrition and physical health improve measures of fitness and body fat levels. However, maintaining these programmes in the school curriculum in the long term has proved difficult owing to competition for school time, the need for teacher supervision, and costs. Obesity prevention and control programmes delivered through primary care has received limited formal assessment, and its potential role seems to be unappreciated and underused at present.

## References and further reading

BREWSTER DR, MANARY MJ, MENZIES IS, HENRY RL, and O'LOUGHLIN EV. 1997. Comparison of milk and maize based diets in kwashiorkor. *Archives of disease in childhood.* 76:242–8.

ELIZABETH KE & SATHY N. 1997. The role of developmental stimulation in nutritional rehabilitation. *Indian Pediatrics.* 34:681–95.

GERNAAT HB, DECHERING WH, and VOORHOEVE HW. 1998. Mortality in severe protein-energy malnutrition at Nchelenge, Zambia. *Journal of Tropical Paediatrics.* 44:211–17.

KHANUM S, ASHWORTH A, and HUTTLY SR. 1994. Controlled trial of three approaches to the treatment of severe malnutrition. *Lancet.* 344:1728–32.

LANCET. 1970. Classification of infantile malnutrition. *Lancet.* ii:302–3.

MENDEZ MA & ADAIR LS. 1999. Severity and timing of stunting in the first two years of life affect performance on cognitive tests in late childhood. *Journal of Nutrition.* 129:1555–62.

SOUTH AFRICAN VITAMIN A CONSULTATIVE GROUP (SAVACG). 1996. Anthropometric, vitamin A, iron and immunisation coverage status in children aged 6–71 months in South Africa. *South African Medical Journal.* 86:354–7.

UNICEF. *State of the world's children.* 1988. New York: Oxford University Press.

WORLD HEALTH ORGANIZATION. 1999. *Management of severe malnutrition: A manual for physicians and other senior health workers.* Geneva: WHO.

# PART SIX

# Adolescence

The health care of young people is a much neglected field, particularly in developing countries, yet there is no age group in which the potential for prevention is greater. Preventive actions to diminish risk-taking behaviour in all adolescents, and to reach those who are truly dysfunctional, require innovative strategies. A necessary requirement will be personnel with appropriate training in adolescent health and health care.

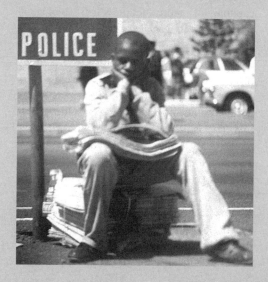

# 17

# Growth and pubertal development in adolescence

## A PHILOTHEOU & E ROSEN

A child enters adolescence as a dependent, sexually, and physically immature being, and leaves as a mature, independent adult with a unique personality. It is a process of becoming independent, and is accompanied by dramatic biological and physiological changes. Although the terms 'puberty' and 'adolescence' are often used interchangeably, both refer to different processes. Puberty involves a set of biological events, and is defined as that period of human development when sexual maturation takes place, after which both males and females are capable of reproduction. This biological process is a universal feature of human life, and is relatively unchanged from culture to culture, although the social and cultural interpretation of it may vary.

The nature of adolescence on the other hand is determined by the socio-cultural context. The World Health Organization defines adolescence as the period between the ages of 10 and 19 years, youth as being between 15 and 24 years, and uses the term 'young people' to refer to those between the ages of 10 and 24. Adolescence is the time when social, psychological, and cognitive maturation occurs, and when abstract thought becomes conceptualized. (These aspects are discussed in Chapter 53: Adolescence and its related psychology and psychiatry.)

Sexual maturation and the growth spurt that accompanies it proceed through various developmental stages in adolescents, and have a powerful influence on their cognitive and psychological behaviours. Knowledge of the events that occur at puberty – in its restricted sense, the period of attainment of physical adulthood – helps the clinician to understand deviations from the path of normality and individual differences in maturational timing.

Events at puberty can be divided into:
- hormonal changes;
- sexual maturation;
- physical growth (change of growth velocity); and
- skeletal maturation.

## Hormonal changes

Significant alterations occur in concentrations or patterns of secretion in the hypothalmic-pituitary-gonadal axis and in the growth hormone IGF-I (insulin-like growth factor I) system. At about six to eight years of age, secretion of androgenic steroids from the adrenal gland increases, heralding in some way a change in the sensitivity of the negative feedback system of the gonadostat. Firstly, a significant rise occurs in the mean concentration of FSH (follicle-stimulating hormone) and LH (luteinizing hormone) being secreted in a pulsatile fashion during the sleep period before there is any obvious increase in size of the gonads. Then puberty progresses with the development of secondary sexual characteristics as the concentration of sex steroids continues to rise during waking periods as well as during sleep. By mid-puberty, the amplitude and duration of pulses of growth hormone secretion increase significantly, and the sex steroid-induced increase in IGF-I reaches maximal concentrations coincidental with peak height velocity in both males and females.

## Sexual maturation

All adolescents go through the same process of pubertal maturation, and acquire secondary sex characteristics in a consistent pattern. The range of time over which these changes occur can be considerable, but it may take as little as 18 months or as long as five years to progress from pre-pubertal state to full reproductive capacity.

On average, male genitalia begin to develop only a few months later than female breasts, and complete sexual maturation is reached at about the same time in both sexes. In boys, the growth spurt, voice change, and facial hair occur late in puberty, leading to the impression that boys develop later than girls.

In girls, secondary sex characteristics involve breast development, changes in, and growth of, the vagina and labia, the appearance of pubic and axillary hair, and a change of general body appearance.

In boys, the changes are growth of the testes, penis and scrotum, the appearance of pubic, axillary, and facial hair, and the deepening of the voice. Assessment of the adequacy of pubertal maturation is most easily done by observing the stages of genital, breast, and pubic hair development, a method known as Tanner staging, depicted in Figures 17.1 and 17.2. Recording the progression from prepubertal stage to adult development is applicable worldwide if the pattern rather than the quantity or texture of pubic hair is taken into account. Measurement of testicular length or estimation of testicular volume by the Prader orchidometer allows for the early detection of the onset of puberty (length >2,5 cm, volume >4 ml), and corresponds to the appearance of breast buds in girls.

## Physical growth

The adolescent growth spurt is characterized by three phases: the prepubertal 'dip', which prolongs the height deceleration initiated in childhood, then the phase of maximal growth, when height velocity reaches peak levels, and finally the phase of decreasing growth velocity, heralding epiphyseal fusion and attainment of adult height (see Figures 4.3 and 4.5, Chapter 4: Physical growth and development).

The pubertal process begins at an approximately similar age in boys and girls, the main difference being the timing of the adolescent growth spurt. Girls start their pubertal growth spurt two years earlier than boys, and consequently are shorter than their male counterparts at the time of growth take-off. The peak growth velocity in girls is reached between breast stages 2 and 3. In contrast, boys start growing later in the sequence of pubertal development, and the peak growth velocity does not occur until mid- to late puberty (genital stages 4–5, testicular volume 12 ml or longest axis 3,6 cm).

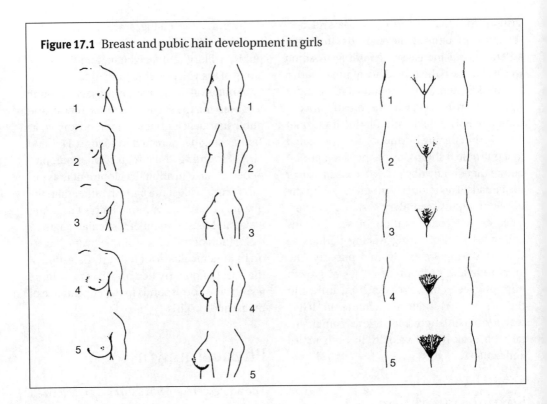

**Figure 17.1** Breast and pubic hair development in girls

## Skeletal maturation

The increase in statural growth during adolescence is accompanied by changes in epiphyseal maturation. These changes can be quantified by the radiological examination of the hand and wrist, either by comparing them to appropriate standards (Greulich & Pyle atlas) or by assessing a number of small bones separately and obtaining a cumulative maturity score (Tanner and Whitehouse method).

Skeletal age provides a measure of the proportion of total growth attained, and permits an estimation of the additional growth expected before skeletal maturation is complete. Simply dividing the current height by the percentage of final height attained provides an estimate of the final adult height, although this calculation probably does not apply to abnormal clinical states.

## General considerations

In terms of the reference population studied, the use of cross-sectional versus longitudinal data and the cut-off points – 3rd or 5th, 97th, or 95th centiles, or standard deviation scores, there has been a lack of standardization in growth chart design.

Rural black children have been consistently found to be shorter and enter puberty at a later age, but well-off black children living in urban areas are indistinguishable from their European or North American counterparts in this respect. Universal charts, particularly those based on longitudinal data, can thus be used with a reasonable degree of reliability and relevance.

Failure to achieve sexual maturation and growth acceleration at an age similar to that of one's peers – whether advanced or delayed – is frequently accompanied by psychological dis-

**Figure 17.2** Genital and pubic hair development in boys

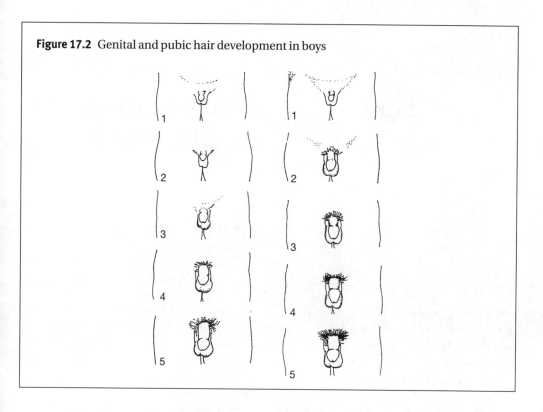

tress in the adolescent. The routine use of growth charts incorporating the centile distribution of secondary sexual characteristics will help establish the extent of an adolescent's deviation from the mean and whether any discordance is present between growth and puberty maturation. In addition, many types of laboratory data – haemoglobin, haematocrit, alkaline phosphatase, IGF-I, hormonal levels – cannot be interpreted without knowledge of the subject's maturity.

The discipline to monitor and record growth and sexual development patterns – obtained with courtesy and sensitivity – is an important practice habit for primary care physicians involved in the care of adolescents. Most patients need only comprehensive assessment and reassurance rather than an indiscriminate battery of unnecessary, expensive, and often confusing investigations.

## References and further reading

BROOK CGD & STANHOPE R. 1989. Normal puberty: Physical characteristics and endocrinology. In: CGD Brook (ed.). *Clinical paediatric endocrinology*. Oxford: Blackwell Scientific Publications.

FRIEDMAN HL. 1993. Promoting the health of adolescents in the United States of America: A global perspective. *Journal of Adolescent Health*. 14:509–19.

MARSHALL WA & TANNER JM. 1961. Variations in the pattern of pubertal change in girls. *Archives of the diseases of childhood*. 44:291.

MARSHALL WA & TANNER JM. 1970. Variations in the pattern of pubertal change in boys. *Archives of the Diseases of Childhood*. 45:13.

# 18    Health care services for adolescents

A PHILOTHEOU

As increasing attention is being paid to the well-being and needs of children, it is essential to ensure that the sharpening focus will include adolescents. This is an age group in which there is vast potential for comprehensive health promotion. Adolescence is a time of exploratory behaviour when fateful choices about eating, smoking, alcohol, drugs, and sex are being made, sometimes with lifelong consequences. Preventative actions to diminish risk-taking behaviour in all adolescents, and to reach those who are truly dysfunctional, need innovative strategies. In southern Africa, such services are virtually underdeveloped and because of limitations in the health budget, new ideas will have to be not only practical, utilizing and sharing available resources, but also accessible to the majority of adolescents. In a heterogeneous society such as ours, cultural differences, opportunities, and pressures are important considerations, and health promotion and health services should therefore be tailored to the values, resources, and sociocultural patterns of all our young people.

As our region undergoes economic development and rapid migration of large populations to the major urban centres, diseases associated with the adoption of a Western lifestyle – obesity, hypertension, diabetes – become more common and are affecting younger age groups. Programmes that prevent risk factors may have to be put in place to control the expected emerging epidemic of diabetes and cardiovascular disease (CVD) in the adult population. They are both feasible and affordable for the developing world. However, implementation of these approaches in young people is hampered by a lack of awareness of cost-effective CVD control options and the concern that involvement in diabetes and CVD prevention will detract from efforts to control communicable diseases and improve perinatal and nutritional disorders.

The second decade of life is considered to be one in which most people enjoy very good health. However, the demands of physical and emotional maturing, coupled with an unprecedented rapid societal transformation, are bound to result in specific adolescent health problems encompassing a broad spectrum of conditions. In addition, significant advances in medical science have increased dramatically the number of adolescents with chronic paediatric conditions who survive to adulthood and who therefore need transitional care from child-centred to adult-oriented systems.

144

## New proposals for national health reform

These ought to ensure that health services for adolescents:

- provide health education and preventative health services;
- provide optimal outpatient and inpatient medical and rehabilitative services for adolescents with physical and emotional problems;
- ensure transitional programmes as a link between paediatric, adult specialized, and psychiatric services for adolescents and co-operate with other services and agencies concerned with adolescents;
- provide training for health workers in the field of adolescence; and
- undertake research on different programme models with a view to improving adolescent health and health care.

# Components for health programmes for adolescents

The changes occurring in adolescents have important implications for health risks and health promotion. The multiple forces pulling the adolescent simultaneously in different directions may strain the capacity of some youngsters, leading them to health-compromising behaviours. Pubertal development with the associated increased sexual motivation and attractiveness puts the adolescent, in particular the girls, at greater risk for body image problems and eating disorders. It also increases the health risk of pregnancy for girls and the risk of contracting sexually transmitted diseases for both sexes. However, adolescent changes involving cognitive and emotional maturity may facilitate efforts to promote a healthy lifestyle. The process of becoming a self-reliant, self-governing individual may lead to health-compromising choices such as unprotected sex or drunken driving but may also provide opportunities for the promotion of health. Cognitively mature adolescents are better able to understand health risks and the consequences of their actions.

It may also be possible to capitalize on the adolescent's desire for autonomy by presenting health as a personal responsibility and choice as something the adolescent can control. Youngsters should be given the opportunity to exercise their autonomy by choosing certain behaviour patterns such as a proper diet and individual or team sport. The risk of negative consequences should be minimized by ensuring that adolescents are well informed, by improving their self-confidence, their decision-making and peer-resistance skills, so they are better able to consider alternative perspectives and thus resist antisocial peer influence.

Health services specifically directed at adolescents are virtually non-existent in South Africa. Family practitioners are available for those who can afford private care. Hospital outpatients departments, community health centres, and antenatal clinics deal with the rest as part of their general services. School health services have the potential to reach a large section of the population, but more often than not this is virtually restricted to cursory school health screening examination at very infrequent intervals (see Chapter 29: School health). With a few notable exceptions, there is a particular lack of special facilities for youngsters with chronic disorders requiring ongoing attention. To be effective, the following aspects of adolescent health surveillance should be integrated (Kibel et al., 1992):

## HEALTH PROMOTION

A conceptual model for adolescent health promotion should encompass physical, social, psychological, and spiritual well-being and should target behaviour patterns that promote short- and long-term physical and mental health. More specifically the multiple changes and various phases of adolescent development would suggest the following goals:

- to promote physical health through proper nutrition and exercise;
- to promote a positive body image, healthy sexuality, and a healthy lifestyle;
- to promote cognitive maturity, social-cognitive skills, and autonomous decision-making;
- to promote self-esteem and a positive sense of personal identity including positive future goals, a sense of self-efficacy, and social responsibility;
- to promote supportive relationships with family, peers, and other important adults;
- to promote opportunities for educational and occupational success; and
- to avoid pitfalls that would interfere with the positive developmental outcomes outlined above.

These goals reflect a dual emphasis on promoting health-enhancing behaviours and simultaneously decreasing health-compromising behaviours (Percey & Jessor, 1985).

Health promotion programmes may have greater impact if they are tailored to the developmental competences and needs of the adolescents they aim to serve. Early in adolescence they need more concrete methods whereas later they may benefit from more abstract and symbolic approaches. Since adolescent development does not occur in isolation but in a social context defined by family, school, peers, the work place, and the community, health promotion efforts need to target not only individual adolescents but also the social context in which they live.

For the third millennium, a multicomponent approach to health promotion should be considered (Percy et al., 1993). Intervention should be designed for the specific environmental spheres:

- microsystems (families, peers, school);
- mesosystems (interaction of families, peers, school);
- exosystems (mass media, community structures); and
- macrosystems (national culture, subcultures).

Already intervention strategies that have been proposed include family involvement programmes, peer leadership training, school-based life-skills, and social competency curricula. The other major socializers of youth – mass media, community-wide activities, including school and places of worship – should be used to reinforce pro-social values and enhance health.

It is encouraging that a Health Education Radio Initiative will combine the efforts of the Department of Health and the South African Broadcasting Corporation. In addition, a healthy public policy promotion should discourage drug, cigarette, and alcohol use, and encourage safe sex, low-fat eating habits, and balanced exercise. Examples of such ventures are the ambitious national anti-smoking campaign and the 'Love Life' youth sexuality initiative, developed by the Department of Health, National Youth Commission, UNICEF, and other public and private sector bodies.

## PRIMARY AND SECONDARY PREVENTION

Primary preventative care focuses on immunization, dental prophylaxis, contraception and condom availability, accident prevention, high-risk behaviour, and disturbed eating patterns.

Secondary prevention involves case finding and individual screening for age-related prevalent conditions. Physical examination should include blood pressure, growth and sex maturation monitoring, the severity of acne, tests for visual and hearing defects, and the detection of scoliosis. Moreover, an evaluation of normal emotional growth should explore areas such as emancipation from the family, heterosexual development, vocational progress, and ego identity.

## TRANSITIONAL CARE FOR ADOLESCENTS WITH CHRONIC CONDITIONS

In adolescence, severe chronic illness or disability such as asthma, diabetes, epilepsy, or physical handicap may lead to serious maladaptive behaviour, non-adherence, frequent hospital admissions, and poor social integration in adult life. Specific comprehensive programmes providing transitional care from child- to adult-oriented systems have been shown, particularly in diabetes (Kibel et al., 1992; Philotheou, 1991), to help negotiate the adolescent crises and support maturing patients and concerned parents in the process. This successful approach, emphasizing social support networks as well as medical care, could serve as a model for the management of other chronic disorders or disabilities.

## SITING OF FACILITIES

Adolescent health care facilities are preferably placed at community health centres rather than at hospitals. Every high school and higher education institution should have a health co-ordinator capable of providing limited medical assessment and treatment. School-based and school-linked clinics are emerging as a very promising approach and are extensively used and well supported.

## Categories or problems needing specific management

- Problems related to sexual activities, teenage pregnancy, and sexually transmitted diseases including HIV infections.
- Drug problems.
- Alcohol-related problems.
- Sports injuries.
- Mental health, e.g., depression, alienation, violence, anti-social and violent behaviour patterns.
- Physical and sexual abuse, including incest.
- School learning difficulties, which might be due to mild intellectual disability or family dysfunction.
- Chronic conditions: asthma, diabetes, epilepsy, gastrointestinal, renal and cardiovascular disease, physical handicaps.
- Growth and sex maturation problems. The wide range in age at which the height spurt and puberty manifest themselves result in major discrepancies in development and associated stresses in peer groups. Transitory gynaecomastia in boys, asymmetrical breast development and obesity in girls, and acne in both sexes are common causes of concern and distress.
- Gynaecological problems such as dysmenorrhoea (painful menstruation), irregular menstruation, amenorrhoea (the absence of menstruation), and hirsutism (excessive, coarse body hair in girls).

Health transition programmes increase independent behaviour and personal autonomy in adolescents with chronic disorders. They need not entail a change in health professionals, and are far from being limited to the simple referral to a physician caring for adults. They could take the form of *disease-specific* models in which a young patient moves from a paediatric specialist team to a transition team with the expertise of both paediatric and adult specialist units, thereby ensuring continuity of care in all settings. Alternatively, *single-site* models offer a general basic clinical environment and a range of ancillary services but the treating doctor changes as the patient matures.

Ideally, adolescent units should be available for inpatients in large hospitals. They should provide multidisciplinary wards, have an area for socializing where there are games, television, and special facilities for schooling.

## Adolescent and youth health policy guidelines

The Maternal, Child, and Women's Health Directorate of the Department of Health is in the process of compiling the first national policy guidelines for South African adolescents and youths. They will be based on a framework developed by the World Health Organization, and will take account of key legal, policy, and treaty obligations, including the United Nations Convention on the Rights of the Child, the Constitution of the Republic of South Africa, and the National Youth Policy. The guidelines will appear at a time when there is increasing international recognition that dedicating resources to adolescent and youth health is one of the most important cost-effective long-term investments a society can make.

## The adolescent interview

Adolescents may consult any one of the various specialists for specific problems but often remain with their paediatrician, family, or community practitioner for treatment of problems not needing specialized services.

Good medical care depends less on the location or speciality of the provider than on the sensitivity of the clinician to the enormous physical and psychological changes during the teenage years. The clinician must also have additional knowledge of legal and ethical issues relevant to adolescent care, and be able to obtain a properly focused but comprehensive history, physical examination, and laboratory evaluation.

The adolescent should be seen individually as well as with the parents. If the clinician sees the parents alone, it can seriously affect confidentiality and alienate the young patient. However, parents know more about the family's medical history, and often their perspective of the teenager's problems may differ from that expressed by the youngster.

The first interview, in a sense the most important, should be unhurried and, after putting the teenager at ease, should concentrate on getting to know the patient as a person. Adolescents respond well to direct questioning, if asked gently and with sincerity, whereas they may feel threatened by abstract and non-specific questions. Sensitive subjects like substance abuse or sexual activity may be opened with non-threatening questions such as: 'Many of my patients report using alcohol. Do you and your friends drink?' or 'Are most of your friends sexually active?'

It is worth remembering that many risk behaviours tend to be linked, for example, smoking is associated with much greater risk of alcohol or marihuana use, unprotected sexual activity, violence, and school failure.

Since the adolescent's life involves several distinct spheres, it is vital to obtain information pertaining to each of the following areas for a complete picture:

- medical – past, present history
- home – family structure, family dynamics

- school, vocational choices
- peer relationships (including questions on substance abuse), romance (including questions on sexual activity)
- sport, recreation, hobbies
- work.

Although most adolescents are in a constant state of embarrassment, the physical examination need not be a trying experience for either the adolescent or the clinician. A routine physical examination carried out with sensitivity, in a professional manner, should not embarrass the youngster. A gynaecological examination is necessary in any adolescent female who is sexually active. An informal verbal consent of the patient is needed, and having a chaperone in the room makes good medico-legal sense. Some adolescents are happy to have their mothers in the examination room, others prefer the nurse who should, in any event, be present to assist the clinician. It is important to include the adolescent in the examination by explaining what is to be done before it is done.

The issues of consent and confidentiality are of great importance in the adolescent–clinician relationship. At the first visit, the adolescent and the parents should be told that the information exchanged between the adolescent and the clinician is privileged but this information may be shared with the parents and other health professionals with the adolescent's permission.

A successful interview with an adolescent requires a delicate balance between empathy and authority, a non-judgemental approach, candour, good humour, and the maturity and confidential communication that teenagers seek during their emerging adulthood.

For youngsters with chronic disorders such as asthma or diabetes, many obstacles are in the way: socio-cultural characteristics, personal beliefs, the burden of being responsible for one's own treatment, denial, loss of self-esteem, depression, and most of all, a traditional, rigid education system.

We spend more time discussing the disease than trying to help our adolescent patients learn the coping skills required for daily living. We need to learn to listen actively to read body language, to hear facts and feelings, silences and hesitations, and to be sensitive to the non-verbal communication that is a key to a successful rapport between teacher and learner (Burnard, 1992).

## Staffing

As resources grow scarcer, the diversity of programmes and fragmentation of service models may adversely affect the efforts to improve adolescent health. Co-ordinated systems will be necessary in order to consolidate the various activities, and to successfully integrate health, education, and social programmes. Intersectoral co-ordinating councils organized by the communities themselves will go beyond the provision of comprehensive health services to include mental health counselling, case management services, and vocational and recreational opportunities.

A multidisciplinary team with clear co-ordination of efforts will succeed in creating links between various professional disciplines, and will have easy access to sub-specialist care or advice if necessary. Specific training in the field of adolescence for doctors, nurses, psychologists, and social workers will greatly enhance their impact, particularly in the organization of health services.

The disease profile of urbanized black adolescents in South Africa is similar in many respects to that in the United States. Substance abuse, trauma, attempted suicide, and pregnancy-related conditions are major causes of admissions both to Chris Hani Baragwanath Hospital (Rosen, 1985) and to Groote Schuur and Red Cross Children's Hospitals (Philotheou,

1991; Ferreira & Lachman, 1991). Rheumatic heart disease and infections are developing world problems still found in South Africa.

Despite past recommendations, very few services are available specifically for the teenager. Success for implementing an innovative programme will depend on the provision of concrete, practical, and feasible ideas, reflecting the immediate needs of young people in our society. Creativity and considerable dedication will be necessary to achieve true and lasting improvement.

## Acknowledgements

The assistance of Dr John Kulig MD, Director of Adolescent Medicine, New England Medical Center, Boston, USA, is gratefully acknowledged.

## References and further reading

BURNARD P. 1992. *Effective communication skills for health professionals.* London: Chapman & Hall.

FERREIRA M & LACHMAN P. 1991. *Adolescent health care at two teaching hospitals.* Proceedings of the conference on child health priorities. Cape Town.

KIBEL MA, PHILOTHEOU A, and SPRINGER P. 1992. Health services for adolescents: Two models. *CHASA Journal.* 3:241–4.

PERCY CL & JESSOR R. 1985. The concept of health promotion and the prevention of adolescent drug abuse. *Health education quarterly.* 12:169–184.

PERCY CL, KELDER SH, and KOMMO KA. 1993. The social world of the adolescent: Family, peers, schools and the community. In: SG Millolein, AC Petersen, and EO Nightingale (eds.). *Promoting the health of adolescents.* Oxford: Oxford University Press.

PHILOTHEOU A. 1991. Psychosocial factors and metabolic control in adolescent diabetes. *South African Medical Journal of Continuing Medical Education.* 9:220–1.

ROSEN EU. 1985. The disease profile of hospitalised third world urban black adolescents. *Journal of adolescent health care.* 6:448–52.

# PART SEVEN

# Comprehensive health care

Comprehensive or 'holistic' care has long been a basic tenet of the discipline of paediatrics. Children's problems should never be viewed in isolation. Their growth, development, family, and environment always merit consideration. Comprehensive health care makes provision for primary, secondary, and tertiary provision both at individual and community level. The Road to Health Chart is an invaluable tool in this respect, and is one of the important components of global strategies to improve child survival and health. Oral health is an integral part of over well-being, and deserves an equal place in the comprehensive health care.

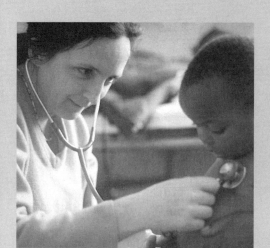

# 19

# Global strategies for child health

ME JACOBS &
LA WAGSTAFF

At the turn of the 21st century, the world's population numbered 6 billion. Of the 130 million babies born in 1999, fewer than 10 per cent will live in relative prosperity, about 30 per cent will be subject to extreme poverty, with approximately 40 per cent being only marginally better off (UNICEF, 1999). Half of the world's poor are children.

Throughout the world, many millions of children are engaged in a daily fight for their survival under conditions of extreme adversity and serious deprivation. Children die from malnutrition and other preventable disorders, and wars, environmental hazards, abuse, neglect and exploitation may threaten those who survive (see Chapter 60: Children in difficult circumstances: An overview).

For decades, there has been broad agreement that global strategies are needed to overcome obstacles to the achievement of a reasonable state of health for all the world's children.

International consensus focuses on a broad approach with two components:
- A framework, which embodies society's responsibilities to children and provides a set of standards for meeting the basic rights of children.

- Within that framework, plans and strategies to meet the needs of children in terms of their survival, development, protection, and participation (see Chapter 1: Introduction).

The Convention on the Rights of the Child, adopted by the UN General Assembly in 1989, provides the societal framework and sets out minimum global standards against which to test the treatment of all children. Based on the Declaration on the Rights of the Child (1959), the Convention was formulated out of many international meetings and consultations, and has now been widely accepted as the foundation for all child-focused global strategies.

Prior to the 1970s, interventions to promote and protect child health concentrated on disease control and treatment. In 1978, the Alma Ata conference on primary health care, sponsored by WHO and UNICEF, challenged this piecemeal approach to health. Through a synthesis of the experiences of nearly all the countries around the world, this landmark gathering issued the Alma Ata Declaration on Primary Health Care – a policy statement on principles and actions to achieve health for all the world's people by the year 2000.

Acceptance of the Primary Health Care philosophy by the international health community signalled a significant shift in approaches to child health and has been pivotal in subsequent global strategies for child health. Primary health care is also the foundation of South Africa's health policy.

## The Declaration of Alma Ata

The Declaration identified the following eight essential elements of primary health care:

- education concerning prevailing health problems and the methods of identifying, preventing, and controlling such health problems;
- promotion of an adequate food supply and proper nutrition;
- an adequate supply of safe water;
- basic sanitation;
- maternal and child health care (including family planning);
- immunization against the major infectious diseases;
- appropriate treatment of common disease and injuries; and
- provision of essential drugs.

These elements rest on multisectoral involvement, community participation, and are contingent on strong political commitment to plan policies for implementing and sustaining primary health care as part of a comprehensive health system, and in pursuit of equity.

The year after the Declaration of Alma Ata, 1979, was designated the International Year of the Child. Great enthusiasm for the well-being of children was generated nationally and internationally and attention was focused on issues affecting the survival, development, and protection of children throughout the world. Discussions and meetings resulted in an analysis of problems related to child health and development, and to the formulation of plans to improve the health of children, especially those in the developing world.

These events set the stage for a new approach to child health, which was given further impetus in 1981, when WHO adopted the global strategy of Health for All by the Year 2000.

Attention was directed at policy formation, economic resources and their distribution, primary health care service components, and improvements in nutrition, literacy, mortality, and income. While all these are associated with good health in general, the approach fell short on listing explicit ways in which the health of children could be improved. The prevailing deteriorating economic situation, together with the millions of child deaths from preventable diseases, called for a creative solution, which would combine effective low-cost health technology with social mobilization.

## GOBI-FF

A 1983 meeting of concerned parties, including UNICEF, WHO, and an international group of specialists in child health, made specific proposals for the attainment of health for all the world's children. These were announced in UNICEF's 1982/3 report, *The state of the world's children*, as a 'children's revolution for survival and development'. The strategies of this 'revolution' were based on concerns about the health of children, and especially about the unacceptably high rates of child deaths from preventable conditions in the developing world. Bearing the acronym 'GOBI-FFF', the elements were **g**rowth monitoring, **o**ral rehydration therapy, promotion of **b**reast-feeding, universal child **i**mmunization, **f**amily planning (birth spacing), and **f**ood supplements, with the later addition of **f**emale education(**F**).

153

The separate components of the GOBI-FFF strategy receive more detailed attention in other chapters in this book.

# Growth monitoring

(See Chapter 4: Physical growth and development; Chapter 20: Child health cards – The Road to Health Chart; and Chapter 15: Infant and child nutrition.)

The child health card, or the Road to Health Chart (RTHC) has long been advocated as being the best method of monitoring growth and can also be a valuable health and growth-promoting tool.

For the health worker, the RTHC is an aid to the identification of growth faltering. It gives the health worker a chance to discuss with parents the child's health, growth, and nutrition.

For parents and caregivers, the RTHC is a very visible record of the child's development. Parents can be shown how to plot weight on the chart, and how to recognize problem growth patterns. The chart therefore provides an opportunity for them to participate in the monitoring of their child's nutrition.

For children, it shows whether steady weight gain is taking place, and when nutritional intervention is needed.

However, the Road to Health Chart has limited application, and will be an ineffectual tool in situations of extreme deprivation, and where resources and infrastructural support are inadequate.

# Oral rehydration therapy

(See Chapter 38: Diarrhoeal disease.)

Oral rehydration therapy (ORT) programmes have been implemented in many countries in an effort to reduce child mortality from diarrhoea and dehydration.

Programmes differ in scope and approach, with some using packets of powder for making up oral rehydration solution (ORS), some cereal-based solutions, others distributing spoons for measuring household sugar and salt, and yet others using measuring tools such as finger pinches or bottle tops. The basic principle of ORT is to give parents the knowledge and confidence to be able to use simple ingredients available in every household for the prevention of dehydration.

# Breast-feeding

(See Chapter 15: Infant and child nutrition.)

Promotion of the scientific facts about the advantages of breast-feeding, together with practical and logistical support for potential and actual breast-feeding mothers, has been one of the major impacts on the health and well-being of young children. In 1981 the World Health Assembly adopted an 'International code for the marketing of breast-milk substitutes' which set out practices conducive to breast-feeding. A similar code applies in South Africa. The promotion of baby-friendly hospitals is a further structured strategy to encourage breast-feeding.

# Immunization

(See Chapter 25: Immunization; and Chapter 24: Vaccine-preventable infectious diseases)

Immunization is one of the easiest and most cost-effective health services. An immunization service is also easy to evaluate. To achieve adequate and appropriate implementation internationally, WHO established the 'Expanded Programme on Immunization (EPI)' in 1974. The goal was to provide universal child immunization (UCI) by the year 1990.

It was also intended to strengthen primary health care through immunization delivery as part of other maternal and child health services. The successes of the strategy have been encouraging, and the lessons learnt through evaluation have proved invaluable. For this reason, immunization will be discussed here in greater detail as an example of the way in which technology and social mobilization have been used as a low-cost, effective health intervention. The importance and value of the EPI has resulted in it remaining a key health service policy.

In the EPI, emphasis was placed not only on vaccine quality control but also on staff development and health service support. Through EPI, WHO encouraged the development of national programme monitoring and evaluation through the use of standardized data systems and review processes. This also involved the development of epidemiological surveillance and methods of outbreak investigation.

A five-point action programme was formulated in 1982, which called for:

- promotion of EPI in the context of primary health care;
- investment of adequate human resources;
- investment of adequate financial resources;
- ensuring continuous programme evaluation and adaptation to achieve high coverage and maximum reduction in cases and deaths; and
- pursuit of research and development.

Two breakthroughs have facilitated UCI. The first relates to vaccine supply. With the development of heat-stable vaccines, improvements in the cold chain, and training and service support to health workers, the delivery of immunization has been more effective.

A second factor was the demand for immunization by people in the community, which has been facilitated by all forms of social communication. Conventional media, such as television and radio, have been joined by ministers of religion, politicians, and other channels to convey immunization messages, and so motivate parents to demand immunization for their children.

## Strategies for EPI outreach

National programmes have explored various strategies to provide UCI. These include involving members of the community and a range of health workers in carrying out home visits to identify, register, and motivate eligible children and their families. School children have also been involved as motivators, to ensure immunization of younger siblings. There needs to be collaboration between ministries, organizations, and individuals in both public and private sectors.

As programmes achieve greater coverage it is important to set clear targets for the reduction of illness and mortality from these infections.

Recommendations from the EPI Global Advisory Group include:

- a mix of complementary strategies;
- provision of immunization at every contact point;
- reduction in drop-out rates between first and last immunizations; and
- improvement in immunization services to the disadvantaged in urban areas.

Continued efforts are also required to:

- strengthen disease surveillance and outbreak control;
- reinforce training and supervision;
- ensure quality of vaccine production, management, and administration; and
- pursue research and development.

## The Three F's of GOBI-FFF

*Food supplementation, family spacing,* and *female education* have the potential to contribute greatly to reducing the great number of infant deaths and nutritional problems found in the underdeveloped world. In comparison with the simple, inexpensive measures of GOBI, the three F's are more difficult in technical, political, and financial terms, and require a different approach, but they are nevertheless important.

## FOOD SUPPLEMENTATION

(See Chapter 15: Infant and child nutrition; Chapter 11: The low birthweight infant.)
In any community, infants, young children, and pregnant or lactating mothers are the groups most likely to suffer the effects of undernutrition. The major contributing factor to low birthweight, a prime cause of infant death, is the mother's own level of nutrition. Food supplements for at-risk pregnant women have been shown to be effective in the prevention of low birthweight, and therefore in the promotion of child survival.

Because of the complex web of causes of childhood undernutrition, demonstrating the value of supplementary feeding has proved difficult, and the benefit is debatable unless combined with general health care.

## FAMILY SPACING

(See Chapter 23: Family spacing.)
Family planning is often regarded as a political tool used for population control. Yet it has been shown that the spacing, timing, and number of births are crucial determinants of maternal health and child survival. Numerous closely spaced pregnancies lead to maternal nutritional deprivation, low birthweight babies, and greater risks to the health of mother and child and older siblings.

## FEMALE EDUCATION

Many studies have shown a clear link between low levels of infant and child mortality and high levels of female education. Although female literacy is an obvious indicator of general living standards, it is also a powerful independent force in child survival. Empowering women through education has enormous potential for improving maternal and child health.

Discrimination against girls and women, which applies not only to education but also to virtually all facets of life, remains a major challenge. In some societies this persists relentlessly, while in others it is being vigorously tackled.

It was hoped that these simple low-cost interventions would help reduce the vast numbers of childhood deaths associated with malnutrition, diarrhoea, and preventable infectious diseases, and would also strengthen health care infrastructure, especially in the developing world.

The approach was fraught with limitations. While encouraging and enabling family participation empowered caregivers, the limited attention paid to fundamental issues such as dealing with the social and economic causes of diarrhoea, and other causes of childhood deaths, reduced the potential impact of the strategy. A further disadvantage was the development of a number of vertical programmes based on the elements of GOBI-FFF. This diluted the good intentions and efforts, leading to fragmentation at the locus of child health care delivery. Consequently, GOBI strategies have been included in a more comprehensive strategy for the promotion and protection of child health in the early years – the 'Integrated Management of Childhood Illness' (IMCI) (see Chapter 36: Integrated management of childhood illness).

For all children the aim should be to reduce the differences between economic, religious, social, and political groups, and to make affordable child care universally available.

While it is well known that the major problems of developing countries' mothers and children are related to malnutrition, infection, and unregulated fertility, these conditions do not exist in isolation from social, economic, and environmental deprivation. Use of a fragmented and selective approach to child health care leads to inefficient use of scarce resources and sub-optimal use of services. This needs to be countered by interventions that are sustainable and effective. The international response has been the formulation of an integrated strategy that focuses on survival, development, and protection of children, and that places greater emphasis on the mother–child dyad (see Chapter 3: Psychosocial factors in child health; Chapter 5: Neurodevelopment; Chapter 6: Emotional and cognitive development).

This was the basis of the discussions at the World Summit for Children held in 1990, at which more than 150 heads of state and senior government officials committed themselves to improving the survival, development, and protection of children, and set goals and targets for meeting this challenge.

# Goals from the world summit

These goals locate health within the framework of human and economic development, and highlight the symbiotic relationship between health, education, and other sectors that are concerned with children. While addressing the need for the acceleration and elimination of hunger and disease and the elimination of illiteracy, an overall goal has been the attainment of economic growth.

The epidemiology of diseases responsible for most mortality and morbidity, and the relative cost effectiveness of the interventions, will be the basis for determining child health interventions needed to promote child health. At the same time the highest priority must be given to the provision of universal access to safe drinking water, sanitary means of excreta disposal, and basic education for all.

In 1990, member states of the Organization of African Unity drafted their own charter on the rights and welfare of the child. Subsequently over 100 countries, including South Africa, have developed national plans of action (NPA) for children. In some countries these plans have followed the World Summit Goals, while in others, plans have been formulated in accordance with the wider mandate provided by the Convention on the Rights of the Child. South Africa has adopted the latter approach, and has deemed children to have a 'first call' in all spheres, including the country's Constitution. Child-oriented plans that are rights-based are thus aimed at ensuring that any decisions relating to children are in their best interest.

# Global child health in the new millennium

## THE SITUATION

International statistics indicate that millions of lives have been saved by the child survival strategy. Despite considerable successes, the needs of the world's children remain largely unmet. The world's poorest countries are crippled by unsustainable debt burdens with women and children bearing the main brunt of associated poverty and adverse circumstances. Large numbers of children suffer in especially difficult circumstances. These include those separated from their parents or street children, abused children, refugees, children who are victims of war and natural disasters, orphans, disabled children, drug abusers, and children who are commercial sex workers. (See Part 15: Children in difficult circumstances – Chapter 60: Overview, and Chapter 61: Child abuse.)

HIV/AIDS is a major threat to child health, and will have to be attacked with the same zeal that led to the eradication of smallpox (see Chapter 39: HIV infection).

157

UNICEF is spearheading the development of a new 'child risk measure' based on five factors that impact on child well-being. These are under-five mortality, moderate or severe underweight, and primary schooling, as well as the likelihood of risk from armed conflict and from HIV/AIDS. The composite scores range from the highest risk groups (average 61) in sub-Saharan Africa to the lowest risk groups (6) in Europe. South Africa's child risk score is 25, compared to 63 in Mozambique and 6 in Cuba (UNICEF, 1999).

## THE UNFINISHED AGENDA

Many children in industrialized countries also have unmet needs. Increasing environmental hazards such as lead, allergens, and other toxins, and nuclear waste call for flexible strategies in planning and delivery of health services, and intersectoral collaboration in sustainable interventions (see Chapter 2: Environmental influences on child health).

There are two further groups of disorders affecting the global child health community that are worthy of more attention. These are lifestyle-related problems (such as substance and tobacco abuse, and disorders related to sexual practices) and adult diseases arising in childhood (such as atherosclerosis and hypertension).

In an era of epidemiological transition, these newer health problems will have to be addressed together with those that have dominated the spectrum of diseases linked with high child mortality experienced by less developed countries.

Special efforts should also be made to promote positive health behaviour, and to secure the health of the unborn child (see Chapter 7: Inherited disorders and congenital abnormalities, and Chapter 9: Fetal Alcohol Syndrome).

## CHILDREN AND DEVELOPMENT

The link between children's healthy growth and development has been universally acknowledged as the cornerstone of any society. International focus has concentrated resources on interventions aimed at reducing unacceptably high levels of preventable child deaths ('the one out of thirteen who die') with less attention being given to the quality of life of 'the twelve who survive.'

## REACHING ADOLESCENTS

Although the internationally accepted definition of childhood extends to those aged less than 18 years, the needs of adolescents have largely been ignored by global strategies. Adolescents have special health and development needs (see Chapter 17: Growth and pubertal development; Chapter 18: Health care services for adolescents). Initiative, flexibility, and willingness on the part of providers to include adolescents in both the planning and delivery of services will improve their well-being. Services will have to reach those in schools and out of school (see Chapter 18: Health care services for adolescents).

## PLANNED INTERVENTIONS

It is generally accepted that human progress depends on the realization of children's rights. These are now recognized in law rather than being dependent on charity (see Chapter 62: Children and legislation in South Africa).

Partnerships between rich and poor nations are proposed to ensure the rights of children. There is an optimistic belief that intergenerational patterns of poverty, violence, disease, and discrimination can be broken in a single generation (UNICEF, 2000). The tools to achieve this are early childhood care and quality education with participation and development of adolescents.

The eradication of poliomyelitis is in sight. The present thrust to achieve this goal involves widely publicized and intensively implemented national immunization days. Such access opportunities can also be used, when indicated, for administering regular anti-worm medication, and giving necessary micronutrients.

Where vitamin A deficiency is a public health problem or under-five mortality is high, supplementation programmes are indicated. One strategy is to incorporate vitamin A administration into immunization programmes. South Africa is on the brink of introducing such a programme. Ending vitamin A deficiency is considered to be as effective in saving lives as has been immunizing against the six major vaccine-preventable illnesses and the use of ORT (UNICEF, 1999).

A total of 12 million children have been spared from mental retardation caused by iodine deficiency.

## INTERSECTORAL COLLABORATION

The notion of intersectoral collaboration has been proposed as a key component of plans to overcome many of the world's problems, as well as to promote child health. Initiatives such as the child-to-child approach with children partners in their own health promotion and care have been cited as examples of intersectoral collaboration worthy of replication on a wider scale. Other strategies include mass media and partnerships with sectors ranging from sport and recreation through to environment, welfare, and the legal system.

In September 2001, the United Nations General Assembly will convene a special session on children. This will aim to review progress in the well-being of children, with special reference to the Convention on the Rights of the Child, and to plans made by the World Summit for Children more than a decade before. At this meeting world leaders, practitioners, and child advocates will have an opportunity to renew their commitments to children, and to consider future action, including practical solutions to the problems facing them. For the health sector, it offers a chance to review our progress, to examine our current practices against the tenets of the Convention, and to affirm our belief that health is a basic right for all the world's children.

The late Doctor James P Grant, Director of UNICEF, enunciated as a fundamental principle 'that the lives and normal development of children should have first call on society's concerns and capacities, and that children should be able to depend upon that commitment in good times and bad, in normal times and in times of emergency, in times of peace and in times of war, in times of prosperity and in times of recession.'

## References and further reading

GRANT JP. 1985–94. *State of the world's children.* New York: UNICEF.

INITIAL COUNTRY REPORT. 1997. South Africa – Convention on the Rights of the Child, November, 1997. Government of National Unity South Africa.

UNICEF. 1984. *Assignment children, 65/68.* New York: UNICEF.

UNICEF. 1989. *Strategies for children in the 1990s* (UNICEF Policy Review). New York: UNICEF.

UNICEF. 1999. *Progress of nations.* New York: Oxford University Press.

UNICEF. 2000. *State of the world's children.* New York: Oxford University Press.

# 20    Child health cards – The Road to Health Chart

LA WAGSTAFF

A variety of home-based personal child health records are used in different parts of the world. Their common purpose is to promote comprehensive child health through the complementing actions of the mother or caregiver and all involved health care personnel. Child health cards have application in virtually all societies. There are examples in booklet form from the United Kingdom, with records of growth and immunization, together with checklists on developmental milestones and behavioural issues during the pre-school years, and advice on general care, including dental health, accident prevention, and management of minor ailments and emergencies.

There are also family-held health cards for school-age children.

The original 'Road to Health Chart' and later 'Teaching Aids at Low Cost' (TALC) were developed by David Morley, using the concept of simple visual records for continuing comprehensive health care. Variations of this chart have been widely used in developing counties for decades.

Recently, after country-wide consultation, the Department of Health in South Africa has produced an updated and improved national 'Road to Health Chart' based on the TALC chart and incorporating beneficial features of other charts. The format of the chart is meant to be uniform throughout the country to accommodate children moving from one area to another, and to facilitate training and ongoing support.

## The benefits of the chart

Phenomenal growth and development, which are the hallmarks of healthy infancy and early childhood, make growth monitoring an extremely valuable health measure. An accurate home-based record of a child's health and development has the potential to allow sharing of information and to promote good relationships and interactions between health workers and the parent/caregiver/family of the child. Children at risk or needing extra care can be identified. The cards are also valuable diagnostic and educational tools and have wider applications for community studies.

Figures 20.1, 20.2, and 20.3 illustrate the areas for recording on the chart. These deserve detailed study to appreciate the amount of useful data recorded, the details of which will not be repeated here. Particular

160

**Figure 20.1** A Road to Health Chart (courtesy of Department of Health)

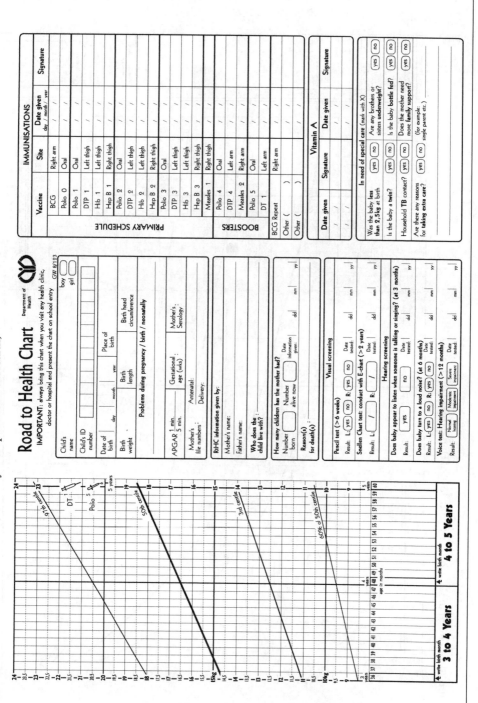

**Figure 20.2** A Road to Health Chart (courtesy of Department of Health)

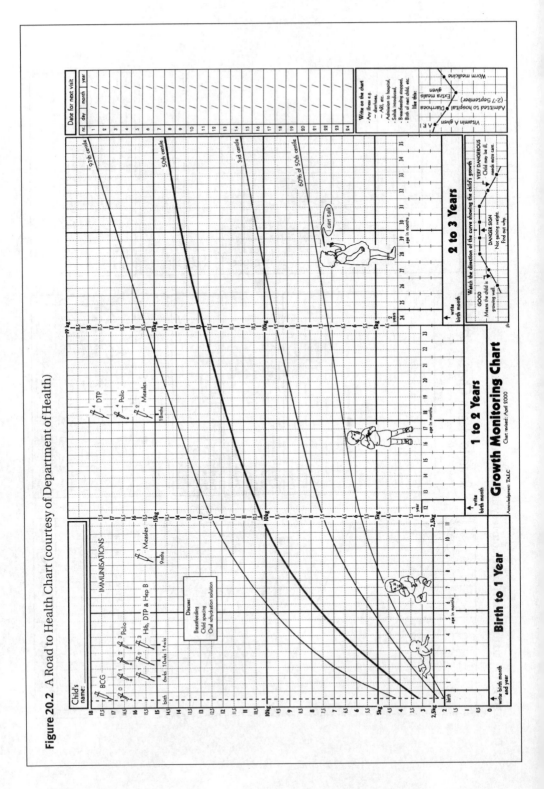

**Figure 20.3** A Road to Health Chart (courtesy of Department of Health)

# Road to Health Chart (RtHC)

## HEALTH WORKER CONSULTATION

Child's name : _____

Date of birth : | dd | mm | yy |

| Date | Clinical notes, diagnosis & treatment  (and signature)<br>( use key words, write legibly - 2 to 8 lines per visit ) |
|------|---------------------------------------------------------|
|      | ① |
|      |   |
|      |   |
|      |   |
|      |   |
|      |   |
|      |   |
|      |   |
|      |   |
|      |   |
|      |   |
|      |   |
|      |   |
|      |   |
|      |   |
|      |   |
|      |   |
|      |   |
|      |   |
|      |   |
|      |   |
|      |   |
|      |   |
|      |   |
|      |   |
|      |   |
|      |   |
|      | continue in column 2 |

attention is drawn to correct use of the calendar system on the weight-for-age chart. Accurate charting is made easier by entering the month of birth in the first heavy block along the horizontal axis, and subsequent months in the blocks along this line. It is easy to show and explain to the mother and avoids having to calculate the child's age at each visit.

This family-owned record is designed to be durable, waterproof, and 'user friendly'. It is also noteworthy that the vertical weight axis has one kilogram intervals (solid lines) exactly one centimetre apart, allowing the cards to be used with hanging scales designed by TALC – a strategy facilitating parent and lay worker involvement and understanding. The weight curves used are derived from the National Centre for Health Sciences (NCHS), currently the most frequently used reference standards. Weight-for-age measures are discussed in Chapters 4: Physical growth and development and 16: Malnutrition. The rate or trend of growth and weight gain is more important and informative than any single plot on the chart.

The Road to Health Chart should be issued at birth by the health service concerned, or as soon as possible thereafter. The National Health Department provides bulk packs of cards together with guidelines on their use, and recognizes that ongoing training and support are essential. Use of the Road to Health Chart implies acceptance of the positive objective of *promoting* adequate growth rather than only detecting malnutrition or other health problems. It is nevertheless true that growth faltering or failure allows important early detection of protein-energy deficiencies, and/or that these may be indicators of poor physical and emotional health and adverse personal and community circumstances.

This most informative and 'mobile' health data bank is for the benefit of the child, health workers, and the mother. The mother is a vital partner in the health care of her child, and

## Features of the Road to Health Chart

These include:

- immunization records and reminders;
- time ranges for selected key milestones;
- spaces for recording appointment dates and any hospital admissions;
- additional data sheets for noting health worker consultations, using brief five- to eight-line summaries; and
- records for the child's height and head circumference (on some charts).

she should never be treated as a mere messenger, carrying the card because she has been instructed to do so!

Growth monitoring is meant to be promotive, preventive, and pre-emptive, allowing early recognition of growth failure, and appropriate action before there is overt malnutrition. Plotting growth enables mothers as well as health workers to envisage progress and to react accordingly, and can thus serve as an educational, intervention, and evaluation tool.

### HEALTH CHARTS AS EPIDEMIOLOGICAL TOOLS

Community studies using collective data from the cards can provide valuable information, for example, on the number of malnourished children or on vaccination coverage. These sequential or area-based studies may influence health and nutrition policies and planning.

# Problems with the chart

Despite the many positive aspects and the great potential of this now widely practised strategy, it has to variable extents fallen into disrepute.

A number of studies have noted pitfalls and problems associated with growth monitoring, making it an expensive exercise in terms of time and effort when measured against the benefits. It has been suggested that resources could be better used in other immediate and direct interventions.

A satisfactory rate of growth implies sufficient protein and energy intake, but may not reveal an inadequacy of vitamins (e.g., vitamin D deficiency rickets in a rapidly growing infant) or trace elements (e.g., iron deficiency because of excessively prolonged and exclusive intake of milk and porridge).

Another major problem encountered is failure of health professionals – including doctors – to use the card properly, thus detracting from its perceived value as well as limiting their own holistic functioning.

## Conclusion

Health cards provide the opportunity for early and therefore less costly action when growth faltering is recognized before there is overt ill health.

In summary it seems fair to say that the strategy is an excellent one, but its proper implementation is crucial. Involvement and participation of caregivers and the community is considered mandatory.

If used correctly, child health cards are multi-purposed and of great value.

### References and further reading

ANON. 1985. Growth monitoring: Intermediate technology or expensive luxury? (Editorial). *Lancet.* II:1337–8.

DIXON RA. 1991. Monitoring the growth of the world's children. *Annals of Tropical Paediatics.* 11:3–9.

### Pre-requisites for 'success' of the Road to Health Chart

These include:
- technical issues – sufficient, properly functioning equipment;
- health workers must be able to weigh and plot correctly. Otherwise, this can become a meaningless ritual;
- necessary knowledge and understanding for the health worker to assess and interpret the findings;
- ability to identify the probable cause of any growth faltering, whether this be related to infections, due to insufficient food intake, or other emotional and social factors;
- access to resources both human and, when necessary, material to react appropriately and effectively. Actions taken may range from complimenting and reinforcing 'good progress' to instituting or arranging for essential health care; and
- emergency food supplements or access to further clinical care have to be available or accessible when needed.

CHOPRA M & SANDERS D. 1997. Growth monitoring – is it a task worth doing in South Africa? *South African Medical Journal.* Jul 87:7:875–8.

DEPARTMENT OF HEALTH – RSA. *Road to health chart guidelines for health workers.* April 2000.

GARNER P, PANPANICH R, and LOGAN S. 2000. Is routine growth monitoring effective? A systematic review of trials. *Archives of Disease in Childhood.* 82:197–201.

MORLEY D. 1979. *See how they grow.* London: Macmillan Press.

MORLEY D. 1979. *Paediatric priorities in the developing world.* London: Butterworth.

# 21     Health surveillance

MA KIBEL &
PI LACHMAN

All children have the right to the benefits of preventive health care. The integration of preventive measures with curative treatment has long been established in paediatric care, but among medical professionals there is still too much emphasis on treatment and too little on prevention. The allure of treating acute medical conditions often overshadows the long-term gains to be derived from prevention programmes.

Perhaps this is because of the paradox that the better prevention works, the less conscious people are that it is working – and so its value is likely to be underrated (Forfar, 1988).

## Prevention

From a public health perspective, prevention of ill health can be divided into three categories, though the distinction is not finite.

*Primary prevention* involves taking effective steps to prevent a condition occurring at all. This is the most complete form of prevention, but is unfortunately not possible for very many conditions. Some examples of primary prevention are:

- immunization prevents many infectious diseases including measles, rubella, and polio;
- penicillin prophylaxis prevents recurrences of rheumatic fever;
- chemoprophylaxis prevents malaria, TB (in contacts);
- fluoridation of water prevents dental caries;
- genetic counselling prevents inherited defects;
- amniocentesis (with the abortion of affected fetus) prevents many congenital disorders including chromosomal disorders such as Down syndrome, spina bifida, and many inborn errors of metabolism;
- good obstetrics prevents perinatal asphyxia and hence many cases of cerebral palsy and intellectual disability;
- fostering and adoption prevent child neglect and abuse; and
- the provision of clean water prevents faecal–oral transmission of diseases such as cholera, typhoid, and gastroenteritis.

*Secondary prevention* involves taking steps to deal with a condition in its earliest stages so as to minimize its impact. In general terms the provision of simple curative services near to where children and their families live will allow problems to be dealt with at an early stage, and so prevent further hospitalization, morbidity, and mortality. Curative services of this type are an essential feature of primary care. Specific examples of secondary prevention are:

- oral rehydration, which prevents severe dehydration and hence morbidity and mortality in gastroenteritis; and
- treatment of a TB primary complex, which prevents progression and adult reactivation.

Early detection to enable pre-symptomatic intervention includes:

- metabolic screening, which permits early treatment of hypothyroidism and phenylketonuria; and
- Ortolani test, which allows early effective treatment of congenital dislocation of hip.

*Tertiary prevention* involves continuing supportive or rehabilitative therapy for a chronic condition in order to maintain the child at his or her optimal level of functioning.

Examples are:

- asthma therapy, which maintains respiratory function as near normal as possible;
- diabetic therapy, which maintains a normal lifestyle and prevents many long term complications;
- physiotherapy for cerebral palsy, which avoids contractures and promotes optimal motor development;
- day training for intellectual disability, which promotes optimal socialization, thus limiting the impact of the problem on the family; and
- changing the environment of a person with a physical disability, which ensures wheelchair accessibility, etc.

# Delivery of holistic child health care

In general terms the provision of a package of health care to all children and their families will include a number of factors: health promotion, health services, and child health surveillance.

## HEALTH PROMOTION

Health promotion includes the following aspects:

- health promotion prior to the birth of the child;
- parental education to allow for optimum involvement in health surveillance programmes; and
- education of teenagers on child health, positive living, and child rearing (rather than concentrating only on high-risk behaviour such as the effects of smoking, alcohol, and drugs, and teenage pregnancy).

## Health services

Health services should provide the following:

- services designed to promote good health and prevent disease, e.g., monitoring of growth and development, and immunization;
- simple curative services near to where children and their families live to allow problems to be dealt with at an early stage, and so prevent further hospitalization, morbidity, and mortality (curative services of this type are an essential feature of primary care); and
- good secondary and tertiary services for the minority of children who may need them.

## CHILD HEALTH SURVEILLANCE

Child health surveillance programmes should be offered to *all* infants and children to:
- prevent ill health by immunization and education;
- promote optimal growth and development; and
- allow early detection of disorders by screening and then referral for assessment.

A health programme should contain general provisions applicable to all children, involve parents, and aim to reach all children. Specific interventions should be designed for those individual children who have special needs.

A framework for child health surveillance is given in Figure 21.1. The intention is to provide a continuum of health care covering all aspects of the child's well-being. Principles and basic elements of child health are universal, though each society will adapt these to the individual needs of the children in the area, and may focus on different priorities. The move over the past decade has been to develop a programme that can be delivered within the available resources, and that reaches all children. In essence child health surveillance has become more focused, more parent centred, and more appropriate. Much of the traditional surveillance carried out in the past is now regarded as unnecessary. The emphasis is on the effectiveness of the surveillance rather than the frequency.

Although the components of a *Health Surveillance* programme are interwoven, a number of individual elements can be defined.
- *Parental involvement* in the growth and physical and mental development of their children is the foundation on which all

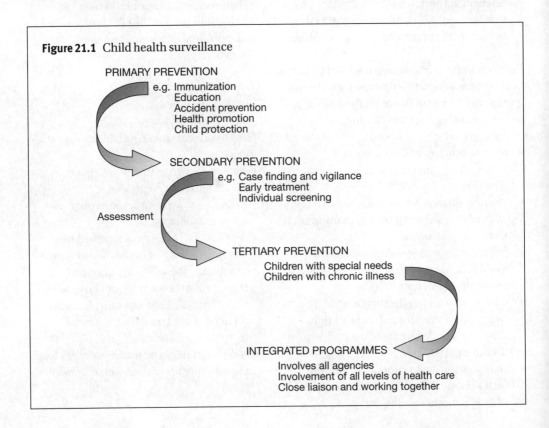

**Figure 21.1** Child health surveillance

PRIMARY PREVENTION

e.g. Immunization
Education
Accident prevention
Health promotion
Child protection

SECONDARY PREVENTION

e.g. Case finding and vigilance
Early treatment
Individual screening

Assessment

TERTIARY PREVENTION

Children with special needs
Children with chronic illness

INTEGRATED PROGRAMMES

Involves all agencies
Involvement of all levels of health care
Close liaison and working together

health surveillance programmes are based. Parents have the opportunity to detect deviations from the norm if they are empowered to do so.

- *Screening* is aimed at the detection of specific conditions in seemingly healthy children in the asymptomatic or early stage (secondary prevention). Tests must be readily applicable and socially acceptable, specific for the condition to be detected, and able to be carried out rapidly and cost-effectively. A screening test is not intended to be diagnostic. After identifying the abnormality it must be confirmed by more detailed investigations.

    Screening may be applied in different settings. Large populations may be tested in community-wide programmes – referred to as 'mass screening' – or groups of children may be selected as being especially at risk (e.g., certain ethnic groups for genetic disorders, or communities at risk for exposure to lead toxicity) – referred to as 'group screening'.

- *Case finding* refers to opportunistic screening on an age-appropriate basis whenever there is a contact between the child and a health professional. It requires ongoing awareness of child health and development.

- *Non-specific vigilance* means that the professional is constantly on the look-out for social, cultural, environmental, or family factors that may place the child at risk for deviations from the normal in the child's development, and for potential problems in parent–child relationships.

All health professionals, teachers, and voluntary sector workers should take every opportunity for case finding and non-specific vigilance. In the ideal situation there will be continuity of care by a family doctor or primary health care nurse whose knowledge of the family and the child's history will place him or her in a position to recognize problems.

## The principles of screening

The WHO criteria for justifying the introduction of a screening test, as outlined by Wilson and Jungner in 1968, remain relevant. They are:

- the condition should be important in terms of the needs of the society and the public perception;
- there should be a suitable test or examination;
- there should be a form of treatment acceptable to the clinician and to the parents and child;
- facilities for diagnosis and treatment should be available, and referral patterns should be established;
- the natural history of the condition should be understood by the health profession. Hypertension, obesity, and vascular disease are believed to have their origins in childhood and to be potentially controllable. However, there is no evidence that modification of risk factors such as weight, blood pressure, and blood lipids reduces harmful effects in adult life;
- there should be an agreed policy on when to treat;
- there should be a latent or asymptomatic phase during which intervention could be initiated;
- the test should be acceptable to the population;
- screening should be a continuing process. Large one-time only screening drives have little long-term benefit except for survey purposes; and
- the cost of case-finding should be realistic in relation to available resources.

- *Assessment* is the evaluation of the problem detected, i.e., the appropriate follow up of the child by a specialist in the field. This therefore implies that, while detection takes place at the primary care level, assessment takes place at the secondary or tertiary care level. The purpose of the assessment is to arrive at a definitive diagnosis and to plan an intervention programme. The provision of assessment facilities is essential to underpin a surveillance programme.

The moral and ethical benefits of a test are often in conflict with the economic reality of the health service. It is essential that these issues be considered with the best interests of the child in mind. For example, as discussed below, prolonged disability and dependency can be avoided if hypothyroidism is diagnosed in the neonatal period, and if it can be effectively treated.

A test should not cause harm and should be accurate. It should clearly distinguish between the normal and the abnormal. It must have a sufficiently high degree of sensitivity (positive when the individual has the condition) and specificity (negative when the individual does not have the condition). There is a great potential for harm in falsely identifying problems that are not confirmed by subsequent tests, just as there is harm in raising false optimism when test results are wrongly reported as negative. Many tests are unsatisfactory for screening purposes because there is a 'grey zone' between those who have a problem and those who do not. Examples of these are tests for anaemia, albumin and blood in urine, hypertension, lead toxicity, and hyperlipidaemia.

## Important screening procedures

There are a number of ways in which a child can be screened for an abnormality:

- History taking is the foundation of all screening and involves a detailed family history and the past history of the child;
- Physical examination builds on the history taken and may be general or specific. Certain conditions are detected on physical examination alone, e.g., congenital dislocation of the hip, congenital heart disease, and genital abnormalities. When performed as part of a comprehensive health care visit, many aspects of the physical examination are both sensitive and specific It is important that conditions that are not pathological are recognized, e.g., functional heart murmurs, as children and parents may suffer psychological harm from unwarranted concern;
- Laboratory tests to detect some conditions that may be latent prior to presentation with the secondary effects of the disease, e.g., metabolic screens at birth for congenital hypothyroidism, phenylketonuria;
- Screening of the special senses are a major part of all programmes, e.g., looking for cataracts, squint, problems with vision, and hearing disabilities;
- Growth monitoring, i.e., weight, height, and head circumference;
- Developmental screening provides a composite view of the progress of the child, (see below);
- Screening for behavioural and psychological problems are aspects often neglected, particularly in settings where life-threatening illness is more common .

## Monitoring growth

Weight is the most important measurement of growth and nutrition and the single most important screening procedure in children. A more composite picture can be obtained from weight, length, and head circumference and these should be recorded regularly on a growth chart. There is a need for care and reasonable precision in measurement of length and height (see Chapter 4: Physical growth and development).

The Road to Health Chart is the key instrument for child health surveillance in southern Africa (see Chapter 20: Child health cards – the Road to Health Chart). Parents, given adequate explanation, can see evidence of their child's progress, and become active partners in surveillance. More elaborate home-based records are used effectively in many countries. These incorporate written material on prevention of ill health and accidents, immunization, normal development, and health promotion.

## Monitoring development

The holistic developmental examination should be part of the standard examination of the child (Hall, 1998; Dworkin, 1989). This involves the ongoing observation of mental and physical development, with a focus on hearing, vision, speech, and language.

The aim of the screening is early detection of impairments that would result in permanent disability, e.g., cerebral palsy, learning difficulties, and other neurological disorders.

All health professionals should have a clear understanding of the normal growth and development of the child, and basic milestones and warning signs for referral must be known. Tests include an assessment of locomotion and posture, of vision and manipulation, of hearing and speech, and of social and emotional development (see Chapter 5: Neurodevelopment).

Developmental assessment cannot stand on its own and must take into account the family and environment, as well as the child. Tests lack sensitivity, so many children who prove subsequently to have problems may be missed by the tests. They are also relatively non-specific, and most children who fail one or other test turn out to be normal. Failure to have an open mind on each child will lead to over- or underdetection of problems. There is a wide range of normality. As the majority of problems detected in these screening programmes have already been recognized by the parents or caregivers, the best approach is to work together with them.

Dynamic surveillance of the child over time, with special attention when possible risk factors are present, and parental education on what to look out for, are the preferred methods. In a society where the basic health needs are barely met, it is important to adapt the surveillance programme to the priorities set by the needs of the children.

## Talking with parents

Education of parents is the positive way forward. The parents should always be asked before, during, or after an examination whether they have any specific queries concerning their child's development, health, and behaviour, such as sleep problems, feeding, temper tantrums. This may form the guide for subsequent surveillance.

## Basic screening

Table 21.1 is an overview of the surveillance programme at each possible age. Although health surveillance is an ongoing continuum, there are five specific opportunities for child health screening, associated with planned contact with health professionals. These are opportunities to detect problems early and to plan for intervention. Screening questionnaires may be a useful tool to help detect children who need a more detailed evaluation.

**Table 21.1** Summary of surveillance programme (a UK model)

| Test | Neonate | 6–8 weeks if possible | 9–10 months | 18 months | 48–60 months | Who |
|---|---|---|---|---|---|---|
| Bonding and relationship to child | ✓ | ✓ | ✓ | ✓ | ✓ | Doctor/nurse Family member |
| Feeding and nutrition | ✓ | ✓ | ✓ | ✓ | ✓ | Nurse/doctor |
| Weight | ✓ | ✓ | ✓ | ✓ | ✓ | Nurse |
| Length or height | ✓ | ✓ | ✓ | ✓ | ✓ | Nurse |
| Head circ. | ✓ | ✓ | ✓ | | | Nurse |
| Appearance | ✓ | ✓ | ✓ | | | Nurse/doctor |
| Hips | ✓ | ✓ | | | | Doctor/nurse |
| Heart | ✓ | ✓ | | | ✓ | Doctor |
| Skin | ✓ | ✓ | | | | Nurse/doctor |
| Tone | ✓ | ✓ | | | | Nurse/doctor |
| Genitalia and testes | ✓ | ✓ | ✓ | | ✓ | Nurse/doctor |
| Gross motor development | | | ✓ | ✓ | ✓ | Nurse, parent |
| Fine motor development | | | ✓ | ✓ | ✓ | Nurse, parent |
| Vision | | ✓ | ✓ | ✓ | | Nurse, parent |
| Language | | | ✓ | ✓ | ✓ | Nurse, parent |
| Hearing | | ✓ | ✓ | | | Nurse, parent |

# The newborn period

## PHYSICAL EXAMINATION

The routine physical examination is really a series of screening procedures that fulfil most of the criteria already outlined. The immediate examination after birth assesses the physiological state of the infant, and detects any gross abnormalities. The rating system developed by Virginia Apgar (Apgar, 1953) is now used universally, and is a quick and reliable measure of the infant's immediate condition. A clinical examination should follow in the next few hours or days to assess maturity and nutrition and to detect abnormalities which may not be overtly apparent. Weight, length, and head circumference are recorded. Of special importance are examination of the eyes, heart, hips (see Figure 21.2), and genitalia.

# Metabolic disorders

Of the several hundred metabolic disorders in which the responsible molecular defect has been elucidated, an effective treatment is only available for a few, and then only if these are begun before symptoms appear. Technology has been employed to develop cheap and reliable tests to detect such affected newborns.

By far the most important of these disorders is *hypothyroidism*, which occurs in all ethnic groups and if properly managed can be totally corrected by a cheap and effective treatment (oral thyroid hormone). Mass screening for hypothyroidism has already been introduced in some urban areas of South Africa. The financial implications and logistical difficulties of introducing this screening test on a wider scale would be enormous, and at present there are far greater health priorities.

Examples of conditions that may require a more focused approach include:

- *phenylketonuria,* which occurs in about one in 10 000 births among infants of Caucasian origin, but is said to be rarer than this in South Africa;
- *cystic fibrosis,* which occurs in about one in 2 500 infants of Caucasian origin and less commonly in other ethnic groups; and
- *galactosaemia* and *maple syrup urine disease,* the widespread screening of which is desirable but the benefits need to be considered.

Early detection of many of these disorders can be beneficial to parents and the affected child.

# Infancy and pre-school period

The surveillance of children before school age is linked to the administration of immunization. The three key ages are:

- *Four to six weeks after birth:* Not only can physical progress be assessed and the infant rechecked for hip dislocation and other abnormalities that may have been missed, but the maternal–infant interaction can also be gauged, and infants at possible risk can be marked out for special surveillance. This should be combined with maternal care for the post-partum period and the mother can be screened for post-partum depression.
- *Eight to ten months:* This is another important period, especially for the detection of hearing and vision defects and other developmental problems.
- The period from *18 months* (when the immunization programme is completed) to school entry: This period is one of particular vulnerability, as children are not brought to clinics on a regular basis – hence the importance of using every opportunity for screening, case finding, and general vigilance.

# School entry

Surveillance at school entry is a selective process. Children are selected for surveillance on the basis of parental concern, concern of health professionals from previous screening, and concern of teachers. This decreases the unnecessary surveillance of healthy children.

For those children who are selected, a focused examination and screening will be indicated, based on the reason for the selection. Screening procedures at school entry may include a physical examination, monitoring of growth, dental screening, testing for visual acuity and colour vision, hearing and school readiness. Examination of children in the first year of school must be directed at specific areas, such as vision and hearing testing. School readiness is the domain of the education authorities, though health professionals may be involved if there are concerns about the child's development.

Table 21.2 indicates when it is appropriate to refer children for assessment.

**Table 21.2** When to refer common problems

| | |
|---|---|
| Late sitting | 9 months |
| Late walking | 18 months |
| Late talking | 24 months (but check hearing) |
| Inguinal hernia | As soon as possible |
| Umbilical hernia | Referral generally unnecessary |
| Squint | On diagnosis |
| Undescended testes | When detected |
| Abnormal cardiac murmur | When detected |

# Specific screening tests and methods

## CHECKING FOR CONGENITAL DISLOCATION OF THE HIP (CDH)

Although congenital dislocation of the hip is rare in black children, consider predisposing factors known to be associated with an increased incidence of CDH. These include:

- family history of CDH;
- female sex;
- first-born child;
- history of oligohydramnios;
- breech delivery or late version;
- Caesarean section; and
- presence of a foot deformity such as talipes equinovarus or calcaneovalgus.

For details on how to conduct the examination see Box 1.

## HEART EXAMINATION

The examination of the heart should be undertaken at birth, if possible at 6 to 8 weeks of age and then at the pre-school age. A prac-tical approach is given in Box 2.

## EXAMINATION OF THE GENITALIA

Boys should be screened for undescended testes (see Box 3) as correction in the second year of life will prevent long term sequelae. The genitalia of girls are often not examined and should be part of any routine examination of children.

## HEARING SCREENING OF PRE-SCHOOL CHILDREN

At all ages ask for family history of hearing loss, antenatal infections, perinatal problems such as hypoxia and jaundice, response to sound, language development and history of

---

BOX 1

## Examination for dislocation of the hip

The baby must be naked and lying on a flat surface. The hips are flexed to 90 degrees with the knees bent. Take the thighs in both hands so that the bent knees are in the palms and the thumbs high up in the middle of the inner aspect of the thighs. Each leg is tested separately. The tested hip and leg is moved inwards (adducted) pressing out-wards at the same time with the thumb, with gentle downwards pressure from the palm along the line of the thigh. If the hip is dislo-catable, the head of the femur under the thumb is moved outwards onto the posterior aspect of the acetabulum. The hip and leg are now moved outwards (abducted) until nearly flat on the surface, and at the same time pressure is exerted inwards (medially) with the middle finger. As the head of the femur returns to the acetabulum (if the hip has been dislocated) a definite jerk or click is detectable. If this is elicited the child should be referred for ultrasound examination or to an orthopaedic surgeon (see Figure 21.2).

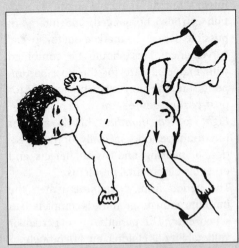

**Figure 21.2** Examination for dislocation of the hip

ear infections, meningitis or head injury. Parental concern is important.

The hearing distraction test – see Box 4 – is the screen performed at nine months of age, but can be performed at subsequent checks. The discrimination test as shown in Box 5 can be used at an older age. (See also Chapter 35: Speech pathology and audiology.)

BOX 2:

## Listening for heart murmurs

Six in every thousand children are born with congenital heart disease. However, an *innocent* or *functional* murmur is present in about 50 per cent of children and adolescents. It is therefore important that those involved in making such assessments should be able to distinguish between significant heart disease and innocent murmurs. Murmurs that are not significant are of four types.

1 **Innocent or functional cardiac murmurs**
   These murmurs:
   - are systolic with no diastolic component;
   - are soft, and always graded as less than 3/6;
   - are short ejection murmurs;
   - are well localized, usually at the second left interspace at the sternal border, but sometimes present at the apex or in the pulmonary area;
   - may disappear on deep inspiration;
   - are never associated with symptoms of heart disease (such as cyanosis, breathlessness, abnormal pulses, etc.)
   - change with posture, being louder when the child is supine and softer when the child is erect;
   - are accentuated in the presence of pyrexia;
   - have normal heart sounds, especially the splitting of the second sound; and
   - are associated with normal electrocardiograms or chest x-rays.

2 **Murmurs due to mild congenital heart disease**
   These murmurs, due to conditions such as small ventricular septal defects, or mild pulmonary stenosis, have no significant effects on life expectancy but do require bacterial endocarditis prophylaxis. These occur in about four children per thousand.

3 **Carotid bruit**
   These usually occur unilaterally, more frequently on the right than on the left, and if innocent are never associated with a palpable thrill.

4 **Jugular venous hums**
   These disappear when the child is horizontal and the legs raised. They also vary in intensity when the head is turned.

   Significant heart disease should be diagnosed if one of the major signs or two of the minor signs listed below are present:

   *Major signs*
   - systolic murmur 3/6 or louder;
   - diastolic murmur;
   - congestive heart failure; and
   - cyanosis.

   *Minor signs*
   - systolic murmur softer than 3/6;
   - abnormal pulmonary second sound;
   - abnormal blood pressure;
   - abnormal electrocardiogram; and
   - abnormal x-ray.

   *Always feel the femoral pulses to exclude coarctation!*

BOX 3

## Checking for undescended testes

It is important to check as early as possible that both testes are descended because this is extremely easy to do in a baby, but subsequently becomes more difficult, both because of the behaviour of boys and also because the testes may become retractile at a later age. If the testes are present in the scrotum at birth there is never any need to worry at a later stage, even if the testes are not easily palpable at a subsequent examination.

If there is doubt about undescended testes, the examination should be repeated. If only one testis is felt, note should be made of whether left or right as the other may be obvious on some future occasion. Warmth, squatting, and milking down the inguinal canal may render the testes palpable. Orchidopexy (if necessary) is recommended at 18 to 24 months.

BOX 4

## Distraction test for hearing loss

Tester calls the baby's name in a quiet voice, then makes five sounds on right and left.
1  'Oo oo' – quietest voice – not a whisper
2  Two wooden bricks tapped together
3  Spoon scraped on cup edge
4  'ss' 'ss'
5  High-tone Manchester rattle *gently* agitated.

Baby *must* locate sound and *turn head*. Thus, both hearing and head control are tested.

Care must be taken that the infant is responding to sound and not to a visual stimulus. The tester must be outside the field of vision, but not directly behind the head as the sound cannot then be localized. Retest babies who fail in one month and refer for assessment if the baby fails the test again.

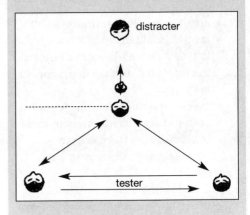

BOX 5

## Discrimination test for hearing loss

First identify seven toys with tester at child's side (speech can be observed here).

Use ball, doll, plane, car, ship, stick, or brick.

Tester uses quietest voice, without whispering, and covers mouth (no face pattern) at three metres from right to left.

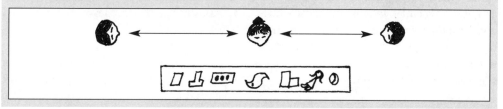

BOX 6

## The heel-to-ear test

The heel-to-ear test is an easy and effective test for tone in the seven to nine month old child. It is performed with the child lying flat on his back with his legs held in extension at the knee. Both legs are then flexed at the hip in an attempt to gently bring the heels as close to the child's ears as possible. Failure to achieve more than 90 degrees should raise the possibility of significantly increased tone in the child's legs.

The legs should be kept in gentle extension throughout the manoeuvre. Make sure that clothing does not limit movements at the hip.

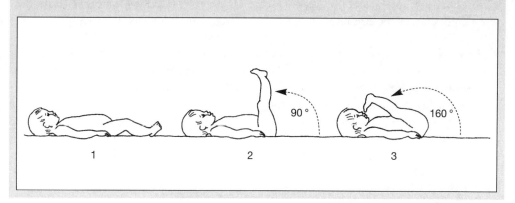

Above the age of four or five *sweep audiometry* is the commonly used screening method for testing large numbers of children. The child is tested with a range of sounds of fixed intensity (usually 25 decibels) and frequencies of 2 000, 4 000, 8 000, and then 250, 500 and 1 000 Herz. If one of these is failed, a full *audiometric test* is performed. All pure tones are presented at varying intervals and intensities. *Free field testing* using instruments such as pitch pipes, xylophone, or tuning fork can be used in younger children or in the developmentally retarded.

## SCHEDULE FOR VISION SCREENING OF PRE-SCHOOL CHILDREN

Special attention should be paid to infants who are at risk for visual problems. These include infants who were preterm and/or in intensive care, growth retarded infants, and those with a positive family history of eye problems such as squint, genetic blindness, cataracts, retinoblastoma, or glaucoma. Specific indicators of possible visual problems include:

- lack of fixing on the mother's face when feeding;
- drifting of the eye from one side to another when awake and placid;
- a white spot in the pupil (a cataract);
- the child holding an object very close to the face to observe it; and
- a squint that persists beyond six months of age.

In terms of developmental sequence, screening tests should encompass eye pathology, near vision, squint, distant vision and colour vision (see Boxes 7 and 8).

---

BOX 7

# Squint detection

## Equipment
Equipment required is a pen torch or other similar light source and fixation targets with detail, such as pictures stuck on spatulae.

## Position
Ensure child is seated so that the eyes are on a level with those of the examiner.

### Light reflex
## Method
This is carried out by shining a light on the eyes from a distance of about 1 metre. In the normal eyes the corneal light reflex should be seen on the centres of the cornea. When a squint is present the light reflex will be off centre in the affected eye. The presence of large epicanthal folds often gives the erroneous impression of a squint. In such children the corneal light reflex will be seen to be normal.

### Cover/uncover test
This is to detect a manifest squint (18 months of age and older).

## Method
Watch the uncovered eye.
- Hold the fixation target, preferably a picture, *at one-third metre from the child* on a level with the child's eyes. Cover each eye in turn with the palm of the hand or a card, allowing the child to fix with both eyes open before covering the second eye. If the uncovered eye moves to fixate the target a manifest squint is present.
- Repeat the test, asking the child to fixate an object at approximately *six metres*.

Note: some squints are only present at one or the other distance.

Squints associated with over-accommodation (focusing) may be missed if only a light and not a detailed target is used.

Alternative cover test to detect latent squints examines the movement of the covered eye. This test is not essential in this age group unless the child complains of symptoms, which may be ocular in origin.

Note: If the child objects to one eye being covered but not the other, suspect amblyopia. Searching fixation is also an indication of this condition.

BOX 8

## Schedule for screening of vision

### 1 Six to eight weeks

The infant's eyes should be checked with a bright light for pupil reactions, cataracts, for wandering eye movements, and for the beginnings of focusing on coloured objects. Pupil reaction to light is normal with cortical blindness, but there is generally ample other evidence of severe defect. Blinking is a normal reaction to bright light. The reflex is checked to exclude cataract, retinoblastoma, etc. Following and focusing develops at this age and can be ascertained from the parent. Obvious squint or different reaction to covering either eye can be detected. Roving eye movements may suggest a blind child.

### 2 Nine months

At this age the more important test is to exclude a squint (Cover test for squint: see Box 7). There is still no accurate test suitable for screening visual acuity at this age.

### 3 Eighteen months

Vision testing at this age is difficult. However, if a 'fine pincer grip' is checked with small objects it can be a rough guide to acuity. Near vision is assessed by the child's ability to fix on small objects such as a raisin or small sweet. Ideally the eyes should be examined with an ophthalmoscope for the normal red reflex in order to exclude cataract and retinoblastoma.

### 4 Older children

Sheridan's letter type test or E charts in pre-schoolers assess the child's ability to read small letters up to N5 or 6/6 for *near vision*, while the ability to see *distant letters*, preferably held at six metres is tested by key cards placed in front of the child (Sheridan Gardiner test).

*Colour vision deficiency* is common in boys. Partial deficiency in red–green colour vision is by far the most common form and has implications regarding future career and employment. Colour vision can be assessed using the Ishihara plates, though this should not be part of a routine screening programme.

# Conclusion

The surveillance of the growth and development of children is the foundation of all health programmes. In the short term it may not appear to be a cost-effective process. Yet if it is focused, responsive to the realities of the society, and carried out in full partnership with empowered and educated parents, it can be a positive process.

The question of whether surveillance is economically worthwhile is difficult to resolve and depends on the resources required to conduct each individual programme and the cost benefit of the programme. This needs to be calculated for each situation and must be balanced against the cost of treatment if early diagnosis is not achieved. A regular programme may increase the use of preventive services; foster a relationship between parents and health services, and promote regular preventive programmes, e.g., immunization.

Surveillance should not be done simply because it has always been done. It is a process that will deliver dividends if it is flexible, appropriate, and relevant. Constant audit of the programme is required to ensure its effectiveness.

## References and further reading

APGAR V. 1953. A proposal for a new method of evaluation of the new-born infant. *Anesthesia Analgesia.* 32:260–7.

BUTLER J. 1989. *Child health surveillance in primary care – A critical review.* London: Her Majesty's Stationery Office.

DWORKIN PH. 1989. American and British recommendations for developmental monitoring: The role of surveillance. *Pediatrics.* 84(6):1000–10.

FORFAR JO (ed.). 1988. *Child health in a changing society.* Oxford: Oxford University Press.

HALL DMB (ed.). 1998. *Health for all children – A programme for child health surveillance,* 3rd ed. Oxford: Oxford University Press.

LAST JM. 1983. *A dictionary of epidemiology.* Oxford: Oxford University Press.

LINGHAM S & HARVEY DR. 1988. *Manual of child development.* Edinburgh: Churchill Livingstone.

POLNAY L. 1997. *Manual of community paediatrics,* 2nd ed. Edinburgh: Churchill Livingstone.

POLNAY L & HULL D. 1993. *Community paediatrics.* Edinburgh: Churchill Livingstone.

WILSON JMG & JUNGNER G. 1968. *Principles and practice of screening for disease.* Public Health Papers. No. 34. Geneva: World Health Organization.

# 22    Oral health

MJ RUDOLPH &
HA LEWIS

Dental caries (tooth decay) is the world's most prevalent disease, affecting up to 80 per cent of the population. Some African countries have reported dramatic increases, which is a cause for great concern. In South Africa, this rise is occurring in rural and poor urban communities, while in higher socio-economic groups dental caries has declined. Reasons given for the decline are a more sensible approach to sugar consumption, increased use of fluorides, and improved oral hygiene.

Dental caries is a very significant health, social, and economic problem with huge cost implications. It is the major cause of tooth loss in South Africa. The peak of caries activity occurs during childhood, with up to 60 per cent of six-year-olds in South Africa being affected. It causes progressive destruction of the crowns of the teeth, often accompanied by severe pain and infection. From an early age various aspects of health may be affected including speech, nutrition, and school performance. Extraction is the predominant form of treatment for dental caries in public dental clinics.

## Promoting oral health

The importance of prevention and control of oral disease and of promotion of good oral health is indisputable. The challenge is how best to apply known preventive measures and to find those cohorts within a population who are at high risk so that these may be targeted for appropriate interventions. The huge backlog of untreated dental disease can and must be reduced so that limited dental public health resources can be used most effectively.

Dentists, dental therapists, and oral hygienists are the main providers of oral health care, but very few of them work where the oral health needs are greatest. Many primary health care clinics do not have an oral health professional available, so it is very important that all primary health care workers have a working knowledge of the mouth, the main oral diseases, and their prevention. All health care providers, who have contact with client groups, can make a major contribution to promoting oral health by encouraging and supporting successful oral health self-care.

The focus has shifted from treatment to prevention and health promotion. Local community involvement in the development and implementation of preventive methods and materials is increasingly sought. Medical, nursing, and pharmaceutical professionals, teachers, community leaders, parents, pupils, patients and the press should be encouraged to participate and become active in facilitating, enabling, and supporting oral health programmes. Oral health knowledge is expanding rapidly and disease patterns are changing. It is important that all health care professionals provide consistent, accurate, up to date advice.

# The oral cavity

## PRIMARY TEETH

Children have 20 primary teeth (deciduous or 'milk' teeth), which erupt into the mouth from the age of six months to three years of age (see Figure 22.1 for approximate eruption dates). These dates are variable and neither early nor late eruptions are likely to be a problem. Very occasionally children are born with teeth; these should not be removed unless they are so loose that there is a possibility of the child inhaling a shed tooth. Other reasons for removal include discomfort during breast-feeding or trauma to the child's tongue.

## PERMANENT TEETH

The permanent or secondary teeth appear in the mouth from the age of six years and, with the exception of the third molars, or 'wisdom teeth', the permanent dentition is complete by the age of 12 to 14 years (see Figure 22.1). At this stage there should be 28 teeth, seven in each quadrant. The first permanent teeth to appear are usually the lower central incisors and the first molars. The appearance of the second molars at age 12 may often go unnoticed by parents or the child and consequently they may not be adequately cleaned. These teeth are at high risk of tooth decay, which

may progress without detection and result in extraction.

# Oral diseases

While dental caries and periodontal disease are the two major oral diseases causing pain, infection, and tooth loss, dental trauma from domestic or criminal violence and road traffic accidents affects a significant number of people. The oral manifestations of HIV/AIDS are of increasing importance because hundreds of thousands of children are affected.

## DENTAL CARIES

Dental caries affects the tooth itself and its consequences can be severe. The process begins with a small patch of demineralized (softened) enamel anywhere on the tooth surface, often hidden from sight in fissures, grooves, or pits or between the teeth. The destruction spreads into the dentine, which is the softer more sensitive part of the tooth lying under the enamel. The weakened enamel then collapses to form a hole or cavity and the tooth, if untreated, is progressively destroyed.

## CAUSES OF DENTAL CARIES

The important local factors that interact to influence the severity of a caries attack are dietary sugars, plaque, saliva, and fluoride. Dental caries is caused by the action of organic acids on the enamel of the tooth surface. The acid is produced from certain components of the diet and by bacteria living in plaque that adheres to the teeth. If not adequately cleaned, plaque builds up and ensures the retention of carbohydrates and micro-organisms on the enamel surface. These carbohydrates are principally sugars, of which sucrose and glucose are the most important. They may be consumed as table sugar, added to hot drinks, sprinkled over food such as cereals, or in processed foods and drinks that have added sugar. Sugars promote the growth of plaque and within minutes produce acid as a by-product, causing a small outflow of minerals (calcium and phosphate) from the enamel. This process is called *demineralization*, which is the earliest stage of dental caries.

## Host/tooth resistance

Within forty minutes to two hours of demineralization, the acid dissipates and the lost minerals may be slowly replaced by minerals from saliva, a process known as *remineraliza-*

*tion.* Dental caries occurs when this delicate balance between de- and remineralization is tipped towards increased demineralization or when the outflow of minerals from the enamel surface is greater than the repair from saliva or other foods and liquids that might dilute or neutralize the acid. If this imbalance persists, for instance, when sugar intake is high and frequent, gradual loss of minerals from the enamel will eventually lead to the formation of a cavity.

The mouth has its own defence mechanisms, of which saliva is the most important. This bathes the plaque, helps to neutralize the acids, and cleanses the mouth of sugars and bacteria. The salivary benefits are enhanced if

**Figure 22.1** The tooth timetable, showing average ages at which the teeth appear and are shed (reproduced from *A guide to oral health and dental ABC, level one* with the permission of the Department of Community Dentistry, University of the Witwatersrand)

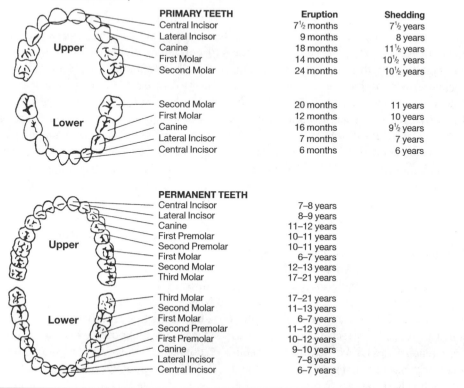

| PRIMARY TEETH | Eruption | Shedding |
|---|---|---|
| **Upper** | | |
| Central Incisor | 7½ months | 7½ years |
| Lateral Incisor | 9 months | 8 years |
| Canine | 18 months | 11½ years |
| First Molar | 14 months | 10½ years |
| Second Molar | 24 months | 10½ years |
| **Lower** | | |
| Second Molar | 20 months | 11 years |
| First Molar | 12 months | 10 years |
| Canine | 16 months | 9½ years |
| Lateral Incisor | 7 months | 7 years |
| Central Incisor | 6 months | 6 years |

| PERMANENT TEETH | |
|---|---|
| **Upper** | |
| Central Incisor | 7–8 years |
| Lateral Incisor | 8–9 years |
| Canine | 11–12 years |
| First Premolar | 10–11 years |
| Second Premolar | 10–11 years |
| First Molar | 6–7 years |
| Second Molar | 12–13 years |
| Third Molar | 17–21 years |
| **Lower** | |
| Third Molar | 17–21 years |
| Second Molar | 11–13 years |
| First Molar | 6–7 years |
| Second Premolar | 11–12 years |
| First Premolar | 10–12 years |
| Canine | 9–10 years |
| Lateral Incisor | 7–8 years |
| Central Incisor | 6–7 years |

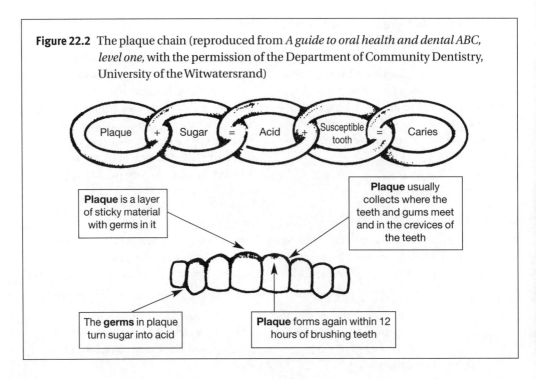

**Figure 22.2** The plaque chain (reproduced from *A guide to oral health and dental ABC, level one,* with the permission of the Department of Community Dentistry, University of the Witwatersrand)

salivary flow is stimulated by fibrous foods, fruit, vegetables, cheese or sugar-free, fluoride-enriched chewing gum. Saliva 'heals' the demineralized tooth surface by depositing calcium and phosphate, and together with fluoride, accelerates remineralization. Thus the early stages of dental caries can be described as a contest over the tooth surface between the acids that cause demineralization and saliva and fluorides that promote remineralization.

## Signs of dental caries

The first signs of dental caries are chalky white patches of demineralized enamel, which may be near the gum margin. These white patches could also be developmental defects and will require an oral health professional to make a correct diagnosis. At this stage dental caries is reversible, the use of fluoride tooth pastes and regular tooth brushing will enable these patches to remineralize and

not progress to a cavity. Pain when eating, especially hot and cold foods and drinks, can be another early sign. More persistent pain is usually a sign that caries has affected the nerve centre of the tooth. A dull or acute pain on biting or pressure may suggest the beginning of an infection. A final stage is the appearance of a large facial swelling, a clear sign of a dental abscess resulting from the spread of bacterial infection from the nerve and blood supply at the centre of the tooth into the surrounding alveolar bone.

## Dental caries in children

Some parents say their child's teeth 'came through rotten' and while it may appear this way, it is more likely that feeding practices such as the frequent use of drinks containing sugar in baby bottles are the main problem. Toothache is a very unpleasant experience, which no parent would wish a child to suffer. Badly decayed teeth need to be extracted,

**Figure 22.3** The events of demineralization–remineralization, adapted from Harris and Garcia-Godoy, 1999. Above the dotted line, demineralization is occurring. Below the dotted line, remineralization is occurring (adapted from Harris and Garcia-Godoy, 1999)

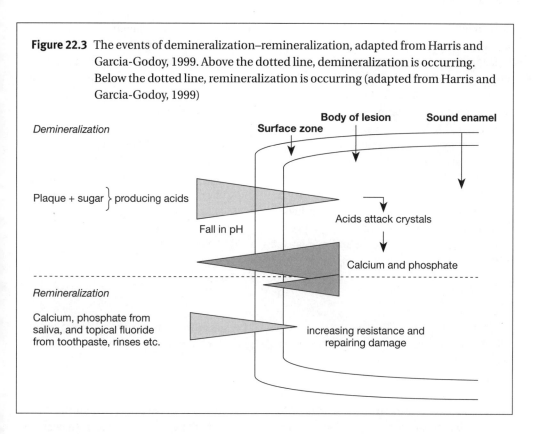

often under general anaesthesia and this can be traumatic for both the child and parents. Early loss of primary teeth may cause the permanent teeth to drift because they use the primary teeth to track into place. This may result in crooked or misaligned teeth and the need for expensive orthodontic treatment.

## Periodontal diseases

Periodontal diseases are a group of related conditions that begin as inflammation of the gum (gingivitis) during childhood. Most populations have gingivitis (the earliest or mildest form) and some periodontitis (a more severe form of destructive loss of bone, loss of attachment and tooth mobility). However, progression of the disease is usually slow, with moderate levels of bleeding or calculus in some communities, and a high prevalence but low severity in others, such as the young black population in South Africa.

Periodontal disease can be seen in children and young adults as childhood gingivitis, puberty gingivitis, and acute necrotizing ulcerative gingivitis. It may be localized or generalized with plaque as the main aetiological factor. However, periodontal disease is no longer considered to be a single entity caused mainly by accumulated plaque. Current classifications tend to be based on clinical phenomena, in particular age at onset, distribution of affected teeth or tissues, and rate of progression. Both gingivitis and periodontitis in children can be associated with systemic diseases such as leukaemia, malnutrition, HIV/AIDS, and other immunosuppressive states.

Gingivitis and periodontitis are often asymptomatic, but can result in halitosis

185

(bad breath), bad taste, and bleeding after brushing or eating.

Dental caries and periodontal diseases are not inevitable. Both can be prevented by changes in personal behaviour. However, knowledge and motivation are prerequisites to changing behaviour, which in turn are influenced by social and economic pressures on individuals and communities. These factors may account, in part, for rising levels of dental caries in economically depressed communities compared to more affluent areas where caries levels, which were previously high, are now declining and appear to be controlled at much lower levels.

# Dental fluorosis

Because of the importance of fluorosis in South Africa, a more detailed background of various aspects of fluoride is presented here. Dental fluorosis is a specific disturbance of tooth formation caused by excessive intake of fluoride during the formation of the dentition. The manifestation of this form of chronic fluoride intoxication depends upon the amount ingested, the duration of exposure, and the age of the subject.

### SIGNS OF FLUOROSIS

The first signs of fluorosis are fine, horizontal white lines distributed evenly over the enamel surface. The lines can become broader, occasionally merging to form irregular paper white areas. With increasing severity, more extensive areas are affected. Pitting, sometimes with brown staining, can occur either as minute depressions or as single or multiple circular holes indicating a loss of the outermost surface enamel. Fluorosis occurs symmetrically within the dental arches. The premolars are the worst affected followed by the second molar and maxillary incisor. Both

the primary and permanent dentition may be affected. The primary dentition appears to be less affected because the placenta modifies fluoride transfer to the fetus, and there is a shorter period of enamel formation.

# Prevention of oral diseases

There are a variety of ways of preventing or controlling dental caries. These include:
- the use of fluorides that promote remineralization;
- dietary control;
- plaque control;
- dental education; and
- dental visits.

The last three interventions also apply to periodontal diseases.

### FLUORIDATION

Fluoride is the one factor that has been shown, beyond doubt, to decrease susceptibility to tooth decay. The most important effect of fluoride is that its direct contact with the tooth after eruption increases the resistance of the enamel of the teeth to attack by acid. There is some benefit to ingesting fluoride but there is no doubt that the topical effect is by far the most beneficial.

## Sources of fluoride

The principal source of fluoride is water. Food is a small contributor to the total daily fluoride intake with an estimated maximum of 0,27 ppm (parts per million = mg/litre) fluoride per day. Fish, particularly tinned fish has high fluoride levels. Tea and green leafy vegetables have varying concentrations of fluoride that can contribute to dietary intake. Fluoride is available in toothpastes, mouth rinses, gels, and tablets.

## Action of fluorides on the teeth

Children who are exposed to fluoride during the two-year pre-eruptive stage of permanent teeth benefit from the fluoride intake. After eruption, and throughout the maturation stage of the teeth, fluoride is absorbed from water, food, and saliva. The absorption is rapid on the enamel surface immediately after eruption.

## Community water fluoridation

Community water fluoridation is the process of adjusting the amount of fluoride that is present naturally in a community's water to the best level for protection against dental caries. It is the most cost-effective public health measure for preventing dental caries. The link between the presence of fluoride in public water supplies and reduced dental caries is supported by more than 30 surveys in over 20 countries.

## Fluoride concentration

Until recently, 1,0 ppm was considered the most appropriate concentration of fluoride in drinking water. 'Most appropriate', meant the concentration at which maximum caries reduction could be achieved while limiting dental fluorosis to acceptable levels of prevalence and severity. By the early 1990s, it became clear that these standards were not appropriate for all parts of the world. The recommended range for South Africa is 0,5–0,8 ppm, taking into consideration variations in conditions like climate, age, dietary habits, and the availability of dental-related products.

## Safety, cost, and general benefits

The safety of water fluoridation is well documented. Numerous studies on both natural and artificially fluoridated water have failed to show any adverse effects on general health at these concentrations. Water fluoridation is cheap; the cost of adjusting the fluoride concentration in the water supply is less than R1,00 per person per year. It is 18 times cheaper than toothpaste and 61 times cheaper than filling a tooth. Analyses of dental treatment needs have shown considerable savings in personnel and resources and a large decrease in the numbers of extractions and general anaesthetics administered to children. The preventive benefits of fluorides save many days that might otherwise be lost from work and school. Water fluoridation benefits everyone with natural teeth and the greatest benefit goes to those least able to help themselves, namely children. Children from impoverished communities benefit most. For most people in South Africa the cost of a toothbrush and toothpaste is often too high. Water fluoridation transcends class and race barriers and eventually will level out oral health differences and contribute to greater equity in oral health status between communities.

There are many areas in South Africa where the fluoride content of the natural water exceeds that recommended for dental caries reduction. Long-term intake of fluoride at high levels can cause mottling of children's teeth. Where fluoride levels exceed the recommended level, it needs to be adjusted downwards.

### DIETARY CONTROL

Sugars in the diet are the main cause of dental caries. While any simple sugars can be metabolized by plaque bacteria to generate acid, those most implicated are the non-milk extrinsic sugars (NMES). These include mainly sucrose and glucose, which are consumed directly or added to a wide range of foods by manufacturers during food preparation and processing, and by consumers during food preparation.

They also include sugars in baby drinks, fruit juice, and honey. Many paediatric medicines still contain sucrose or glucose. NMES do not include lactose in milk and other dairy products, or the fructose in fruit and vegetables (intrinsic sugars). Starch in products such as bread is only slowly degraded in the mouth to sugars and together with fruit, vegetables, and dairy products is *not* strongly linked to caries.

Food labels may refer to sugars as glucose, glucose syrup, fructose, lactose, invert sugar, dextrose, concentrated fruit juice, and other names. All of these sugars have the potential to cause dental caries.

The frequency of sugar consumption determines the severity of the caries attack. With every sugar intake, no matter how small, acid is generated in the plaque and for a period of between 40 minutes and 2 hours the enamel undergoes demineralization. If sugar intakes are repeated at such intervals,

the enamel surface is continually demineralizing with little chance of remineralization and repair from the minerals in saliva. This is illustrated in Figure 22.4. It shows the effect of frequent sugar intake on the pH level in plaque on the tooth surface.

The most important advice for parents is to avoid sugar-sweetened drinks from the beginning, and never put any sugar-sweetened drink into a feeding bottle for the infant to hold. Nor should comforters be dipped in anything sweet. These habits can result in prolonged contact between the newly erupted teeth and the sugar solution causing rapid decay of the front teeth, known as early childhood caries (previously known as 'nursing bottle caries'). A cup should be introduced from six months, and from one year a feeding bottle should be actively discouraged.

Parents need to be advised of the dangers to primary teeth of adding sugar to hot drinks

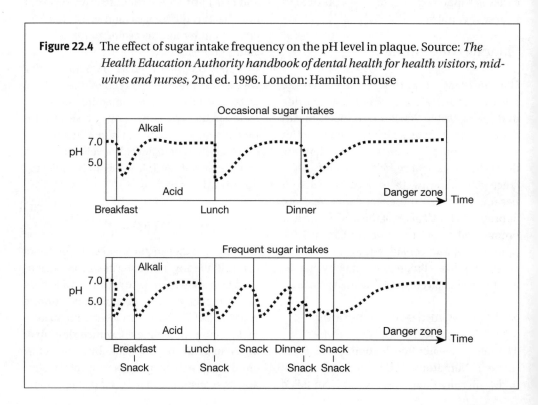

**Figure 22.4** The effect of sugar intake frequency on the pH level in plaque. Source: *The Health Education Authority handbook of dental health for health visitors, midwives and nurses*, 2nd ed. 1996. London: Hamilton House

and concentrated fruit juices that often contain large amounts of sugars or are very acidic even though they are promoted as 'natural' products. Many parents give their children these drinks throughout the day in the mistaken belief that they are benefiting their health. The worst time to give any sugary drinks to a child is at bedtime. The salivary glands 'close down' for the night, their natural neutralization effect is lost, and the acid generated from the sugar persists on the teeth for hours. Cooled boiled water is the best drink for extra fluid. Sugary drinks should also be avoided between meals.

Once children become used to having sweetened drinks it can be traumatic and very difficult to get them to change. Diluting drinks a little and increasing the dilution as the child becomes accustomed to it until it is just water coloured by the syrup or juice is a useful tip. From six to nine months, finger foods such as small pieces of fruit, carrots, or cheese are suitable for snacks. Infant medication needs to be sugar free especially where long-term use and frequent doses are involved. If a sugar-based medicine has to be taken at bedtime then teeth should be brushed with a fluoride toothpaste immediately afterwards.

## PLAQUE CONTROL

## Tooth brushing and flossing

### The objectives of tooth brushing

These are:
- to remove plaque and disturb reformation;
- to clean teeth of food debris and stain;
- to stimulate the gingival tissue; and
- to apply fluoridated toothpaste.

A *routine brushing* pattern should be established to avoid exclusion of any area. Brushing twice a day with fluoride toothpaste gives major benefit. Fluoride toothpastes were introduced in South Africa among the economically advantaged in the early 1970s and they have proved to be widely effective in controlling dental caries. Their use is the single most effective personal means of improving oral health.

Use of dental floss removes plaque and debris in between the teeth but requires good co-ordination and dexterity, and patients should be assisted to achieve proficiency.

The use of a toothbrush and dental floss to remove plaque is also the most important strategy for the prevention of periodontal disease. Chemical anti-plaque mouth rinses can be used to supplement tooth brushing in special cases. Clinicians are also responsible for removing plaque and calculus when it is necessary.

## Plaque control for children

As soon as the first teeth appear in the mouth they need to be brushed. If the child resists brushing, a finger wrapped with a clean piece of gauze with a tiny spot of fluoride toothpaste rubbed over the teeth is sufficient. At two years, twice-daily brushing using an infant brush and a small pea-sized amount of toothpaste should be routine. Special infant toothpaste with a *low* fluoride content is available, but it might not be the best choice for children with dental caries already present. An oral health professional is the best person to give advice in such cases.

Young children often love to brush their own teeth and should be encouraged to do so under supervision as the child may lack the co-ordination and dexterity needed to clean teeth thoroughly. Brushing is best done with an adult or older sibling standing just behind the child with the child's head tilted backwards. Most authorities recommend a brush with a small head with soft to medium bristles. Just a small pea-sized amount of fluoride toothpaste should be used and the child should spit out the excess toothpaste but not rinse with water. Rinsing has been shown to reduce the benefit of fluoride toothpaste.

Plaque disclosing agents (tablets or solutions) dye plaque to make it visible and can be an effective way of improving and monitoring the thoroughness of cleaning the teeth.

## ORAL HEALTH EDUCATION

Health education must be an integral part of any individual or group preventative programme. Health education is used to inform, educate and reinforce health messages. Health education alone is not an adequate preventive method and many health education programmes have not shown the degree of success anticipated. Nevertheless, accurate information consistent with current scientific knowledge is important because it enables individuals, groups, or agencies to make informed decisions about oral health. Education materials should be appropriately designed for specific ages, levels of literacy, and cultural groups.

## ORAL HEALTH CHECK-UPS

One of the most valuable things a health professional can do is advise everyone –irrespective of age or condition – to have regular oral health check-ups. The period must be flexible and based on professional assessment of the risk of oral disease. The maximum period between check-ups should be one year. Children might need to be seen more frequently to have their whole mouths monitored, for appropriate oral health advice, and for early treatment.

Parents need to be encouraged to take their young children to primary health care clinics or dental facilities to get oral health advice before or shortly after the first tooth appears, i.e., before two to three years of age. Children can be introduced to dentistry in an unthreatening manner, thereby winning their trust and confidence.

# Dental care

## PIT AND FISSURE SEALANTS

Prior to cavitating, a non-invasive preventive method, namely pit and fissure sealant, can be applied. Approximately 90 per cent of all carious lesions in the mouth occur on the occlusal surfaces of the posterior teeth, which are approximately eight times as vulnerable as all the other smooth surfaces. Pit and fissure sealants have been effective in reducing this problem. With their use, a thin layer of an epoxy plastic is flowed into the deep pits and fissures of teeth, effectively isolating those areas from the oral environment. No pain or discomfort accompanies sealant placement.

## ATRAUMATIC RESTORATIVE TECHNIQUE (ART)

Once cavitation has occurred, ideally the tooth should be restored. However, many teeth with minimal caries are extracted, particularly in the public service.

In the ART approach, caries is removed by hand instruments only. The cavity is cleaned with a weak acid and a filling material that bonds chemically to tooth tissue is applied to the cavity and the pits and fissure. In this approach a restoration and sealant are obtained in one procedure. The filling material also contains fluoride, which reduces the solubility of the tooth. The idea of ART ensures maximal prevention and minimal invasiveness. ART has already demonstrated that it can be applied to very young children, anxious and fearful patients, and many people who do not have access to traditional dental care.

## COSMETIC DENTISTRY

Chipped, fractured, or stained teeth can be easily corrected today through effective techniques called 'bonding or bleaching'. The bonding techniques improve the appearance of teeth, or rebuilds, reshapes, restores, and covers tooth defects through the use of tooth-coloured plastic materials. The tooth whiteners or bleaching agents improve the discolouration on teeth. The application of these materials should be discussed with an oral health clinician.

## ORAL HEALTH AND PREGNANCY

The oral health of a mother has been shown to be the best predictor of the dental health of her children. Before the child is born, or even conceived, the mother should be advised by a midwife or other health worker of the importance of regular and thorough plaque control and regular oral health check-ups. Establishing effective tooth brushing before pregnancy is

### What to do in an emergency

If a child has a tooth knocked out, it should be washed (not scrubbed) and re-implanted within 24 hours. Get the child to an oral health professional as quickly as possible, carrying the tooth in water or milk, or have the child tuck it in the side of their cheek next to the gum. When playing contact sports, it is important for children to wear a mouth protector or gum guard as these reduce the risk of trauma to front teeth.

important. The hormonal changes in the mother during pregnancy cause an inflammatory response of the gum margin and plaque will accumulate. Bleeding gums are therefore a common problem during pregnancy and usually indicate a pre-existing problem. The important advice here is *not* to stop tooth brushing, but to brush effectively and to see an oral health professional for advice. Reinforcement of the tooth brushing habit at this time may well benefit the child indirectly, because healthy routines will become part of everyday life and children will copy them.

## Oral health messages in summary

- Encourage parents to get early preventive oral health advice.
- Advise an annual oral health check-up once the child's first tooth appears at about two to three years of age.
- Warn against putting any sugar-sweetened drink into an infant's feeding bottle, especially at bedtime. Encourage the use of a cup from six months.
- Encourage the use of sugar-free medicines.
- Use a small soft-bristled toothbrush with fluoride toothpaste as soon as the first teeth appear.
- For pre-school children, advise against excessive consumption of sugar-sweetened drinks, sweets, and biscuits between meals and especially at bedtime.
- An adult or older sibling should assist children up to six to eight years of age to brush twice daily using a small pea-sized amount of fluoride toothpaste.

Good healthy teeth and gums are important for general health and help children to look attractive, feel confident, enjoy food, speak clearly, and have freedom from pain and discomfort.

## References and further reading

BLINKHORN AS & DAVIES RM. 1996. Caries prevention: A continued worldwide study. *International Dental Journal.* 46:119–25.

CLEATON-JONES PE. 1997. Dental caries, sugars, plaque and fluoride. *The Journal for the General Dental Practitioner of South Africa.* 10(4):20–4.

ENWONWU CO. 1981. Review of oral disease in Africa and the influence of socio-economic factors. *International dental journal.* 31:29–38.

FEJERSKOV O. 1997. Concepts of dental caries and their consequences for understanding the disease. *Community Dentistry and Oral Epidemiology.* 25:5–12.

GLASS RL. 1996. Fluoride dentifrice: The basis for the decline in caries prevalence. *Journal of Social Medical Sciences.* 79:15–19.

HARRIS NO & GARCIA-GODOY F. 1999. *Primary preventive dentistry,* 5th ed. Standford and Connecticut: Appleton and Lange

HOLM AK. 1990. Caries in the preschool child: International trends. *Journal of Paediatric Dentistry.* 18:291–5.

HUME R. 1998. Restorative dentistry : Current status and future directions. *Journal of Dental education.* 62:781–90.

JEBODA SO & OGUNBODEDE EO. 1994. Dental caries in Africa. *Nigeria Quarterly Journal of Hospital Medicine.* 5:57–64.

RUDOLPH MJ & CLEATON-JONES P. 1984. The oral health of black and white pregnant women. *Journal of the Dental Association of South Africa.* 39(3):173–6.

# 23    Family spacing

HA VAN COEVERDEN DE GROOT

Family spacing is far more than just birth control. It is a way of life, the major objective of which is to improve the quality of life for everybody. Those caring for children should recognize the interdependence of maternal and infant health and well-being. Increasing the birth interval has benefit for both the mother and children. The physiological and nutritional demands of closely spaced pregnancies and intervening lactation are added to the mother's burden of already having to care for two or more young infants. A multi-country study has found that the infant mortality among those born after a birth interval of less than two years was 80 per cent higher than where the birth interval was two to four years. Furthermore a child was 40 per cent more likely to die before the age of two if its sibling was born within 18 months than if the birth interval was longer than this.

Babies born after a birth interval of 24 months or less develop significantly poorer verbal and perceptive abilities than do their toddler siblings. By contrast, the nutritional deprivation of the displaced *older* sibling, when breast-feeding was interrupted by a further pregnancy, was described in the classic study of Cecily Williams. She also drew attention to the fact that when the quality of life improves, a reduction in family size follows (Williams, 1933).

It is essential to remember that family spacing is an integral part of primary health care.

## Features of family spacing

Family spacing has many facets. Some of the more important are:

- promoting a caring and responsible attitude to sexual matters;
- obtaining prior community acceptance of and promoting community participation in any family spacing programme planned for that community;
- ensuring that every child is a wanted one;
- encouraging the planning and spacing of the number of children, bearing in mind the family's socio-economic potential;
- providing the highest quality maternal and child health care;
- creating awareness, particularly among young people, of the disastrous effects on the environment of unchecked population growth; and
- remembering that problems of infertility are also worthy of attention.

193

# Motivating a person to accept family spacing

A good way to motivate people to accept family spacing is to discuss with them – preferably with couples – what effects another child (or further children) would have on the health and socio-economic circumstances of the families concerned.

It is generally futile to try and promote family spacing by itself. To gain community credibility family spacing must be seen as being part of total primary health care. A high perinatal or infant mortality rate in a community is not conducive to its acceptance of family spacing.

# Counselling a woman about family spacing

A number of points should be discussed when a person asks (or has been motivated to ask) for advice on family spacing. These include the woman's reproductive career, appropriate methods of contraception, side effects of contraception, and the health benefits of contraception.

## THE WOMAN'S REPRODUCTIVE CAREER

A woman must be encouraged to consider her reproductive career as early as possible in her life, just as she would consider her professional career. Unfortunately, this hardly ever happens in practice and, if it does, it is often when the woman is already pregnant.

When considering her reproductive career, the woman (or where appropriate the couple) should decide on:
- the number of children desired;
- the length of the intervals between pregnancies. This will influence the method of

contraception used in the intervals; and
- the contraceptive method of choice when the family is complete. The logical method would be female or male sterilization.

## THE APPROPRIATE METHODS OF CONTRACEPTION

This aspect is best discussed by considering the appropriate methods of contraception for a number of categories of people. In this way nearly all people likely to be encountered will be included. The most appropriate contraceptive methods for maximum efficacy in each category are listed in Table 23.1. Some women want a method with few or no systemic side effects, and then one of the less effective methods may have to be selected. It must, however, not be forgotten that the use of even a relatively ineffective method of contraception, such as barrier contraception, is much better than no contraception at all.

Regardless of the method of contraception chosen the woman must also be counselled about the vital importance of:
- *regular check-ups*, which may include blood pressure checks, breast and pelvic examinations, and Papanicolaou smears;
- timeous *return visits*, e.g., for repeat contraceptive injections;
- adopting an effective *alternative method of contraception* if she discontinues a method because of some problem associated with it;
- *ignoring 'advice'* to stop a hormonal method periodically to 'give the body a rest'. There is no medical justification for such advice;
- taking additional contraceptive precautions in all circumstances where *contraceptive efficacy may be impaired*, e.g., starting or changing a method, diarrhoea, or taking certain drugs (amoxycillin, cotrimoxazole, phenytoin, rifampicin, tetracyclines); and

- seeking *specialist family planning* help if the local family planning clinic is unable to deal satisfactorily with the woman's problems.

It cannot be overstressed that if a woman's family spacing problems are not properly catered for, she will become most antagonistic to that method, or even to the whole concept of family spacing. Worse, she will often demotivate other women about family spacing.

The contraceptive methods listed in Table 23.1 are appropriate for *healthy* women. For contra-indications to the various methods and further details, a standard text (e.g., Guillebaud, 1993) should be consulted.

instances, however, side effects are transient or become less marked in time. It is therefore very important to counsel women carefully about the important side effects of the various contraceptive methods, and to ascertain whether they would find any of them unacceptable. At the same time they can be reassured that some side effects will most likely diminish or disappear after a few months' use. In this way the side effects will be put into their proper perspective, thus allowing the woman to make an intelligent decision on the eventual contraceptive method to be adopted. Table 23.2 lists the major side effects of the various contraceptive methods.

## THE SIDE EFFECTS OF THE VARIOUS CONTRACEPTIVE METHODS

Virtually every contraceptive method has its specific side effects. Some side effects are unacceptable to the woman and cause her to discontinue a particular method. In many

## THE HEALTH BENEFITS OF CONTRACEPTIVES

The main objective of all contraceptive methods is to prevent pregnancy. In developing countries, pregnancy is a major cause of mortality and morbidity in women. The prevention of pregnancy is therefore a very important

**Table 23.1** Appropriate contraceptive methods for various categories

| Category | Appropriate contraceptive methods |
| --- | --- |
| Lactating woman | Injectables/Minipill – for three months, thereafter a combined oral contraceptive pill<br>Intra-uterine contraceptive device |
| Woman spacing her family | Combined oral contraceptive pill<br>Minipill<br>Intra-uterine contraceptive device<br>Injectable – not within one or two years of a planned pregnancy |
| Woman whose family is complete | Tubal occlusion or vasectomy<br>Injectable<br>Combined oral contraceptive pill – no age restriction, provided the woman has no risk factors for cardiovascular disease and does not smoke |
| Adolescents | Injectable – best for compliance, efficacy and safety<br>Combined oral contraceptive pill – requires daily compliance. Condom in addition unless monogamous |

**Table 23.2** The major side effects of the various contraceptive methods

| Contraceptive method | Side effects |
| --- | --- |
| Sterilization | Regret : 3–5 per cent of women<br>N.B. Menstrual abnormalities are NOT a problem |
| Injectables (Progesterone) | Menstrual abnormalities<br>Weight gain<br>Decreased libido<br>Headaches<br>Delayed return to fertility |
| Combined oral contraceptives (Oestrogen & Progesterone) | Menstrual abnormalities<br>Nausea and vomiting<br>Fluid retention<br>Breast tenderness<br>Loss of libido<br>Dry vagina or mucorrhoea<br>Acne<br>Chloasma<br>Headaches<br>Migraine<br>Depression |
| Minipill (Progesterone) | Menstrual abnormalities<br>Loss of libido<br>Headaches<br>Weight gain |
| Intra-uterine contraceptive devices (Copper wire) | Expulsion in 5–15 per cent of women<br>Pain: at insertion; dysmenorrhoea<br>Menorrhagia or spotting<br>Vaginal discharge<br>Increase in pelvic inflammatory disease, which is, however, more likely to be a reflection of the woman's sexual lifestyle – in monogamous unions this increase is short lived<br>Perforation of the uterus is uncommon<br>Ectopic pregnancy : the risk is 0,12/100 women-years |
| Emergency contraception | *Hormonal* (High dose Oestrogen & Progesterone)<br>Nausea in 50–60 per cent of women<br>Vomiting in 20–30 per cent of women<br>Menstrual abnormalities<br>*Intra-uterine contraceptive devices*<br>Vaso-vagal attack<br>As for intra-uterine contraceptive devices given above |
| Diaphragm | 'Messy'<br>Recurrent urinary tract infection |
| Condom | Decreased sensation for both partners<br>Aggravation of erectile or ejaculatory problems |
| Spermicides | 'Messy'<br>Penile 'burning'<br>Decreased sensation for either partner<br>May cause vaginal irritation and increased risk of HIV transmission<br>Increased risk of vaginal candidiasis |
| Coitus interruptus | Sexual dysfunction in either partner |
| Safe period | Marital stress |

health benefit of all contraceptives. Some methods have a number of other health benefits as well. Although these additional health benefits are often very substantial, they are not generally understood by women or by health care workers. Table 23.3 lists the important additional health benefits of the various contraceptive methods.

Most people in developing countries have little or no knowledge of family spacing.

Because of this, all health care workers must develop the counselling skills and empathy necessary for promoting family spacing as an essential part of primary health care. Only then will each woman be able to make an informed and appropriate choice of the method to achieve family spacing.

**Table 23.3** The additional health benefits of the various methods of contraception

| Contraceptive method | Health benefits |
|---|---|
| Sterilization | This has no long-term adverse effects on health |
| Injectables | Decrease in |
| | • Dysmenorrhoea |
| | • Premenstrual tension |
| | • Iron-deficiency anaemia |
| | No effect on lactation |
| Combined oral contraceptives | Decrease in |
| | • Dysmenorrhoea |
| | • Pelvic inflammatory disease |
| | • Ectopic pregnancy |
| | • Iron-deficiency anaemia |
| | • Menorrhagia |
| | • Premenstrual tension |
| | • Functional ovarian cysts |
| | • Benign breast disease |
| | • Endometrial carcinoma |
| | • Ovarian carcinoma |
| Minipill | No effect on lactation |
| Diaphragm | Decrease in |
| | • Pelvic inflammatory disease |
| | • Cervical intra-epithelial neoplasia |
| | • Sexually transmitted diseases caused by chlamydia and gonorrhoea |
| Condom | Decrease in |
| | • Pelvic inflammatory disease |
| | • Cervical intra-epithelial neoplasia |
| | • Human papilloma virus infection |
| | • All sexually transmitted diseases, i.e., including syphilis and AIDS |
| Spermicides | Decrease in |
| | • Sexually transmitted diseases, possibly including AIDS, but see Table 23.2 |

## References and further reading

GUILLEBAUD. 1993. *Contraception – Your questions answered,* 2nd ed. London: Churchill Livingstone.

MARTIN EC. 1979. A study of the effect of birth intervals on the development of 9 year old school children in Singapore. *Journal of Tropical Paediatrics.* 25(2–3):46–76 (monograph).

ROYSTON E & ARMSTRONG S. 1989. *Preventing maternal deaths.* Geneva: World Health Organization: 214.

WILLIAMS CD. 1933. A nutritional disease of children associated with a maize diet. *Archives of Disease in Childhood.* 8:423.

# PART EIGHT

# Immunization

Immunization must rank as the greatest success story in preventive medicine. One infection, smallpox, has already been eradicated as a result of successful immunization campaigns. Poliomyelitis is no longer seen in many countries, measles is far less common, and diphtheria rare, thanks to the Expanded Programme on Immunization (EPI). Because of rapid developments and changing policies in this field, the subject is discussed here in some depth.

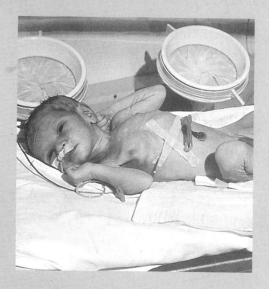

# 24 Vaccine-preventable infectious diseases

## PM JEENA & HM COOVADIA

## Vaccine-preventable diseases

Infectious diseases cause considerable morbidity and mortality at both global and national levels. In recent decades, five million children were estimated to have died every year from measles, tuberculosis, poliomyelitis, tetanus, whooping cough, and diphtheria, while another five million would be crippled, blinded, or mentally damaged.

Infectious diseases account for roughly 11 per cent of all disability world-wide, disability being defined as difficulty in seeing, speaking, hearing, writing, walking, conceptualizing, or performing any other function within the normal range. About 70 per cent of all disabilities in the developing world are caused by only four factors: infectious diseases, malnutrition, perinatal problems, and injury.

Diarrhoea, respiratory diseases, tuberculosis, and HIV disease are the four major infections causing illness and death in South African children. Diarrhoea, tuberculosis, and measles together account for most deaths due to infectious diseases, while the contribution made by whooping cough is uncertain because of unreliable reporting. This morbidity and mortality can be considerably reduced by the implementation of existing interventions. Routine available vaccines include those for measles, tuberculosis, poliomyelitis, diphtheria, whooping cough, tetanus, Haemophilus influenzae type B, and hepatitis B. Diseases caused by pneumococci and meningococci have high mortality rates and are potentially vaccine preventable.

Vaccination must be seen as one part of a broad policy of development for poor people. Campaigns for vaccination can mobilize large numbers of people and release untapped social energies, which can facilitate broader upliftment. Interventions, which have an immediate bearing on health, and can improve living standards, are the provision of food, clean water, sanitation, and housing. In 1977, The United Nations estimated that at existing prices, it would cost nine billion dollars annually to provide community water supplies and sanitation for all by 1990.

Immunization is a far more effective intervention in preventing death than attempted behaviour modification, for example, for ischaemic heart disease.

Since the early 1990s, vaccination coverage in South Africa has increased substantially to current levels of 97 per cent for BCG, 85 per cent for measles, 82 per cent for poliomyelitis, and 81 per cent for DPT. This high coverage has resulted in substantial falls, nationally and regionally, in the numbers of all vaccine-targeted diseases, except tuberculosis (see Table 24.1). The tuberculosis epidemic is in part being fuelled by the HIV epidemic (see Chapter 41: Tuberculosis; and Chapter 39: HIV infection).

Predicted global trends in the ten commonest diseases are shown in Table 24.2. It is shown that infectious diseases are likely to play a smaller role in the overall burden of disease if appropriate interventions are enforced.

Vaccine-preventable diseases are viewed here in the context of child health and detailed clinical descriptions are not included.

# Viral diseases

## MEASLES

### Extent of the problem

Widespread use of live attenuated vaccine over the past two decades has resulted in significant decreases in the incidence of measles in the industrialized world. For example, it is uncommon in the United States, and outbreaks occur only in non-immunized or inadequately immunized adults. The inclusion of measles as one of the diseases targeted by the Expanded Programme on Immunization (EPI) indicates the prime importance of this disease as a cause of sickness and death in developing countries. In the mid 1980s, it was estimated that about 2,1 million children under the age of five years were dying each year

**Table 24.1** Changes in some vaccine-preventable diseases in Durban (1985–1999)

|  | 1985 |  | 1999 | % Reduction | % Reduction in ICU Admissions |
|---|---|---|---|---|---|
| Measles | 2 171 | → | 1 | 99,6 | 100% |
| Varicella | 592 | → | 151 | 74,5 | - |
| Pertussis (whooping cough) | 203 | → | 4 | 98,0 | N/A |
| Typhoid | 237 | → | 21 | 91,2 | N/A |
| Neonatal Tetanus | 41 | → | 6 | 85,4 | 85,4% |
| Mumps | 25 | → | 2 | 92 | - |
| Poliomyelitis | 14 | → | 0 | 100 | 100% |
| Diphtheria | 18 | → | 0 | 100 | 100% |
| Cholera | 248 | → | 0 | 100 | - |
| Overall | 3 549 | → | 179 | 95 | - |

*Mortality changes (%)(1985–1999)*

|  | 1985 |  | 1999 |
|---|---|---|---|
| Measles | 11,9 | → | 0 |
| Varicella | 0,3 | → | 1,3 |
| Pertussis | 0,9 | → | 0 |
| Typhoid | 0,4 | → | 0 |
| Neonatal tetanus | 24 | → | 33 |
| Poliomyelitis | 0 | → | 0 |

**Table 24.2** Predicted global trends in the ten
commonest causes of ill health
(1990–2020) (%) Deaths

|  | 1990 | 2020 |
|---|---|---|
| Lower Respiratory Infection | 9,0 | 3,4 |
| Diarrhoea | 8,1 | 3,0 |
| Perinatal disorders | 7,3 | 2,7 |
| Depression | 3,4 | 5,6 |
| Tuberculosis | 3,1 | 3,5 |
| Measles | 3,0 | 1,3 |
| Malaria | 2,6 | 1,3 |
| Ischaemic heart disease | 2,5 | 5,2 |
| Road accidents | 2,2 | 5,2 |
| Ulcers | 2,2 | 2,7 |

from measles, accounting for roughly 15 per cent of deaths from all causes in this age group. In 1988 the number of preventable deaths from measles in under five-year-olds was 1,9 million; in 1991 this figure was 0,9 million. With the progress of EPI, 77 per cent of the developing world's infants had been immunized against measles by 1991. The programme prevented about 1,6 million deaths from this disease. However, measles still accounted for 50 per cent of the deaths occurring from the common vaccine-preventable diseases of infancy in poor countries in 1991.

Notification data in South Africa for measles give an annual average of 10 to 20 cases per 100 000 of the population. A measles campaign between 1989 and 1991 produced a dramatic drop in the yearly totals. Recent outbreaks (1992–1996) have occurred mainly in school-going children and adolescents, because younger infants have been reached and protected by vaccine. Revaccination at older ages has resulted in further decreases in the number of cases. The incidence of measles in under one-year-olds was 337,8 per 100 000 in 1989 and had decreased to 37,1 per 100 000 by 1994. There is a consistent excess of notified cases from some rural areas. The case

fatality rate when measles is endemic ranges from 1,28 per cent to 3,43 per cent. In epidemics this rate rises to about 13 per cent. Most recent deaths have occurred in HIV-infected individuals with a case fatality rate of 40 per cent. HIV infection increases the risk of acquiring measles by 3,8 times in infants less than nine months of age. The measles mortality rate in HIV-infected individuals is decreased by vaccination.

The main reasons for measles outbreaks are inadequate coverage by the vaccine (urban 85 per cent vs. rural 75 per cent), overcrowding in urban ghettos or within cramped homes, and the wide prevalence of protein energy malnutrition. Overcrowding probably works through a number of mechanisms, chief of which is the transmission of a higher load of virus. Furthermore, overcrowding encourages early transmission of the virus so that younger children get the disease, which is universally more severe in infancy.

A very important method of the spread of measles is through clinics and hospitals where susceptibles come into contact with infectious cases.

## Threat to health

Although measles in South Africa is now uncommon, until eliminated it remains a threat to health. The clinical presentation of measles is quite characteristic and has been reliably recognized by communities in Asia, Africa, and Central America. The features, which allow this recognition, are given in Figure 24.1.

The major organ system to be affected is the respiratory system, and much of the serious damage takes place during the post-measles period through secondary infection. A mild catarrhal inflammation of the respiratory tract gives way in severe cases to pneumonia resulting from the measles virus itself, other organisms, or both. Laryngotracheobronchitis, often due to herpes simplex infection, is less common but can be particularly distressing; marked obstruction of the upper airways is a potentially fatal emergency. Herpes simplex oral ulcers are a frequent feature, leading to fever, salivation, and a refusal to eat. Pneumomediastinum and subcutaneous emphysema are frightening to children and parents alike, although these often resolve spontaneously.

Infection of the middle ear is common. Conjunctivitis is usually associated with photophobia, but permanent damage to the eyes only results if there is severe vitamin A deficiency, or if toxic home remedies have been applied. Diarrhoea is frequent, especially in infants, causing dehydration and metabolic changes. Encephalitis complicates one case of measles in a thousand, causing neurological abnormalities; the course is variable but

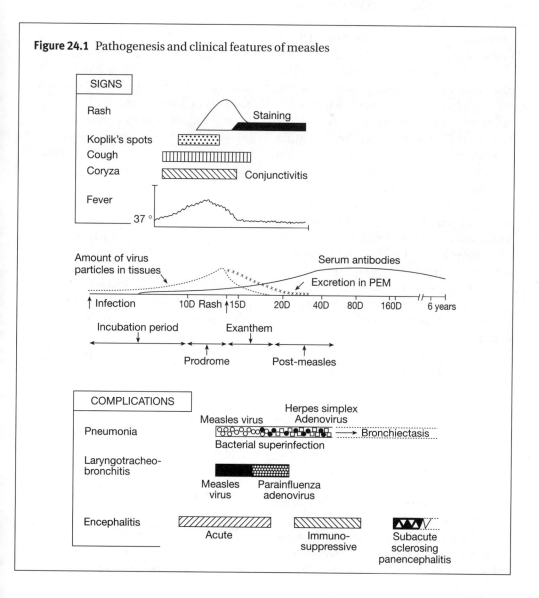

**Figure 24.1** Pathogenesis and clinical features of measles

roughly 60 per cent recover, 25 per cent have neurological sequelae, and the remainder die.

The post-measles state is characterized by a failure to recover and deterioration into chronic illness. Pneumonia does not completely resolve in a few patients, and leads to bronchiectasis in a small minority (see Figure 24.1). Diarrhoea causes growth retardation; it is more common in those under two years of age and most marked in the first two months. Recovery may take four months or longer. Prolonged diarrhoea precipitates marasmus or kwashiorkor and increases the risk of dying in the subsequent months. Tuberculosis may be exacerbated by measles-induced depression of cell-mediated immunity, and must be considered when there is unsatisfactory catch-up growth during convalescence. It is important to recall that false negative tuberculin tests are found in these circumstances. Oral herpes may on rare occasions disseminate to the lungs, liver, and brain with great risk to life. Corneal ulcers and associated vitamin A deficiency can lead to scarring and blindness within three months of acute measles. Late onset encephalopathies (e.g., subacute sclerosing panencephalitis) cause profound neurological impairment and are often fatal.

Uncommon complications are gangrene of fingers and toes, cancrum oris, and septicaemia.

## Protecting health

Use of live attenuated vaccine has produced impressive reductions in the incidence of measles. However, difficulties have arisen with the use of this vaccine in developing countries for the reasons given below. Heat-stable vaccines are now available.

Protection usually occurs three weeks after vaccination.

The main difficulty in South Africa has been inadequate coverage. Extremely high coverage (about 95 per cent) is required for

### Reasons for failure of measles vaccination programmes in developing countries

These include:
- lack of sustained financial support;
- faulty refrigeration of vaccine (breaks in the cold chain); and
- ineffective immunization of those aged less than eight months.

herd immunity. Under moderate levels of immunization there will be pockets of non-immunized children. The integrity of the cold chain needs to be maintained. In urban ghettos and squatter settlements the provisions by WHO for 'special populations' should probably be applied, e.g., additional measles vaccination at six months.

It may be possible not only to prevent measles, but also to reduce its severity if it occurs. After measles, monitoring of growth, and intervening as necessary, is essential. The general health of children should be improved by better nutrition, by encouraging breast-feeding, increasing child spacing, and by the provision of adequate housing. Primary health care services need to be strengthened. Large doses of vitamin A can be given at the time of measles immunization, and vitamin A 200 000 IU orally or 100 000 IU IM should be given on diagnosis to prevent ocular and other complications.

Children with chronic lung and neurological sequelae need the multidisciplinary care alluded to in other chapters.

## POLIOMYELITIS

### Extent of the problem

The natural history of poliomyelitis has been profoundly influenced by sanitation and by the age of the person infected. The disease was endemic in industrialized countries until the end of the nineteenth century. The appalling sanitary conditions of the period led to a rapid spread of the virus among young children, but in this age group the infection was mostly unapparent and only occasionally paralytic. With improved living conditions, especially sanitation, spread of infection was delayed to a later age among children. The virus, which survived the intervention of hygienic measures, seemed to be more virulent and appeared in epidemics. Accordingly, the disease in older children and young adults was more often associated with paralysis. The point at which sanitation was sufficiently improved to reduce the infant mortality rate (IMR) to 80 per 1 000 live births was the level at which endemic poliomyelitis changed to the epidemic form. The subsequent introduction of polio vaccine was followed in about ten years (in the United States) by reduction of the incidence virtually to zero. In developing countries, poor sanitation encourages the rapid spread of the virus, but if immunization coverage is extensive, children are protected and the infection is not a serious problem. However, if immunization coverage is inadequate, then spread is delayed until infection attacks a large pool of susceptibles with a high paralysis rate.

Immunization coverage with three vaccine doses against poliomyelitis has increased globally. In South Africa an additional neonatal dose is given.

Since 1993 the Western Hemisphere has been declared polio free, while in South Africa the last two cases of poliomyeltis were seen in 1991 (one in the Transkei – now renamed Eastern Cape – and one in Lebowa). Prior to this, the polio incidence followed a cyclical pattern with peaks occurring every three years.

Oral polio vaccine has been in use since 1960. With improved vaccination coverage, poliomyelitis in southern Africa may soon be eradicated.

## Threat to health

The greatest threat to well-being posed by polio is paralysis. Fortunately the overwhelming majority of infected children have no obvious disease or have a mild influenza-like illness (see Figure 24.2).

Some get signs of meningism with pains in the neck, back, and legs. A small minority develop full-blown paralysis of skeletal or cranial muscles or the 'bulbar' form with circulation and respiration affected.

Combined forms may also occur. There is considerable wasting of muscles but improvement occurs within three months from onset. The 'encephalitic' type results in irritability, disorientation, drowsiness, and tremors. Occasionally there is heart failure from myocarditis, and the formation of kidney stones from long immobilization.

Complications depend on the degree and site of paralysis and often include pneumonia, suffocation, bed sores, etc.

## Protecting health

Poliomyelitis can be eradicated. The World Health Assembly (WHA) of the United Nations aimed to do this globally by the year 2000, by raising and sustaining immunization rates of infants to 80 per cent by improving surveillance, strengthening laboratory capabilities for diagnosis, increasing public awareness to sustain political and financial commitment, improving rehabilitation services (especially through community-based programmes), and promoting appropriate research. In 1988, WHA launched a programme aimed at global eradication. Since then there has been a greater than 90 per cent reduction in the global number of cases of poliomyelitis with only 3 512 cases reported in 1996. During this time, over half the world's children numbering 600 million in 90 countries have received polio vaccination through a process of national

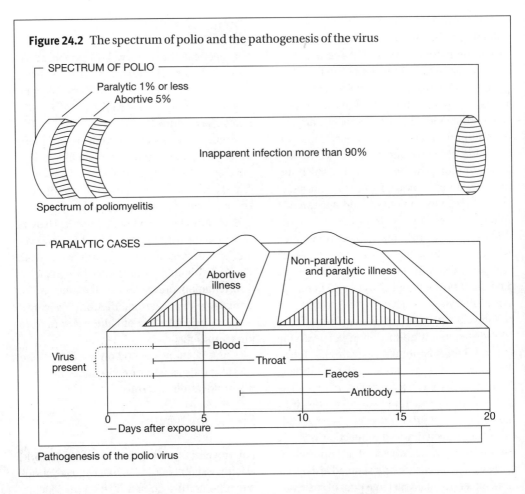

**Figure 24.2** The spectrum of polio and the pathogenesis of the virus

SPECTRUM OF POLIO

Paralytic 1% or less
Abortive 5%

Inapparent infection more than 90%

Spectrum of poliomyelitis

PARALYTIC CASES

Non-paralytic
and paralytic illness

Abortive
illness

Virus
present

Blood

Throat

Faeces

Antibody

0        5                    10              15            20
Days after exposure

Pathogenesis of the polio virus

days of immunization and mopping up campaigns.

It is estimated that global eradication could be achieved by the year 2005. The cost of such an exercise (US$140 million) over ten years is negligible when compared to the expected benefit (a saving of between US$1,5 billion and US$1,7 billion annually) once eradication is achieved. For certification as a polio-free country, the WHO laid down criteria stating that greater than 80 per cent of cases of acute flaccid paralysis (AFP) in children under 15 over the last three years have to be investigated and found not to be poliomyelitis, and an immunization coverage of more than 80 per cent must be recorded.

In South Africa, only 34 of 144 expected cases of AFP have been notified, with no confirmed case of polio detected. The greatest threats to eradication are wars and civil strife. For example, in Afghanistan less than 20 per cent of children are immunized and a recent outbreak of 361 cases resulted in 26 deaths. Similarly, war-torn Angola remains endemic for polio with a recent epidemic in 1999.

Acute flaccid paralysis has been made notifiable for surveillance purposes (see Notifiable Medical Conditions). The definition is as follows: All cases with acute onset of paralysis in persons less than 15 years of age, for any reason other than severe trauma, *or* paralytic illness in a person of any age in which polio is suspected.

Any such case must be notified immediately, and if possible two stool samples taken 24 to 48 hours apart sent for virology.

The programme also includes immunization campaigns, house-to-house immunization in high-risk areas, outbreak immunization around suspect cases, and a better regional laboratory network.

During the acute paralytic phase, it is necessary to protect painful muscles and to prevent contractures and aspiration pneumonia. Ventilatory support may be needed if respiratory effort fails. During the recovery phase, active physiotherapy, the use of splints (to hold joints in optimal position), and the use of callipers (to support flailing limbs) is necessary. Orthopaedic and surgical interventions may be required during the phase of residual paralysis.

Appropriate health workers such as village or community health workers should undertake rehabilitation in underserved communities. Children can become participants in child-to-child health programmes. Appropriate technology can provide crutches, casts, and low wooden trolleys made from simple materials. It is important to reduce dependency by encouraging those affected to achieve their maximum potential through personal effort. Even where trained therapists are available it is advisable to encourage the disabled to make demands on themselves.

## HEPATITIS B VIRUS

## Extent of the problem

This is a major cause of disease world-wide. Over 200 million persons are said to be carriers and the virus is believed to be responsible for the majority of primary liver cancers which are the main type of malignancy in adult African males. The virus is prevalent throughout South Africa and carrier rates of between 13 and 14 per cent have been detected in adult black males in some areas. There were about 1,5 million carriers in the country as a whole in 1993. A community-based study in KwaZulu-Natal showed that the carrier rate of hepatitis B was 10 per cent in urban black children. The rates are much higher in rural and institutionalized children. The infection is not transmitted from mother to baby, and the carrier rates in the very young are therefore low (2,5 per cent in those below six years of age) but peak between six and eight years (14,4 per cent). The prevalence rates in adults are lower, and it would therefore appear that some children clear the hepatitis B antigen. Multiple mechanisms are involved in horizontal transmission of the virus; some identified in KwaZulu-Natal are scarification, ear piercing, intra-familial spread, and probably mosquito bites. The carrier rates for hepatitis B are much higher in South Africa than in industrialized countries where they are usually less than one per cent. Notifications of acute hepatitis B number several hundred every year, and about 40 per cent of these cases occur in those under 18 years of age. The case fatality rate is roughly four per cent.

## Threat to health

Asymptomatic carriers of hepatitis B, who are the reservoir for this virus, may develop membranous nephrotic syndrome, and are at long-term risk for cancer of the liver. Children may develop acute hepatitis, which usually resolves but in rare cases may go on to chronic active or chronic persistent hepatitis. Cirrhosis may develop in some of these chronic cases. A minority of patients with the acute disease develop fulminant hepatic failure in which the mortality rate exceeds 80 per cent.

## Protecting health

Since 1995, the South African Department of Health have implemented the routine use of hepatitis B vaccine for infants in the first year of life. Despite over 80 per cent immunization coverage, this strategy has failed to produce tangible benefits as the disease rarely presents in the newborn or early childhood periods but rather occurs in the pre-school and primary-school children. In order to assess this issue and accelerate observed benefits, an immunization policy change was instituted in 1998 in KwaZulu-Natal. This involved the additional use of the vaccine in the pre-school period in conjunction with DT.

Hepatitis B antigen vaccine can be used for children in endemic areas, for those with high-risk health occupations and for others at risk. A number of other procedures (not discussed here) can limit the spread of hepatitis B. These include screening of blood and blood products for hepatitis B, using disposable needles, and taking protective measures when taking blood, and so on.

## RABIES

## Extent of the problem

India has the highest incidence of deaths from rabies (50 per million of the population), while Ethiopia (12,6 per million), Sri Lanka (10,3 per million), and Thailand (7,6 per million) all report high incidences.

Between 1924 and 1988 the number of human cases in South Africa ranged between one and nine every year except for peaks in 1937 (31 cases), 1938 (25 cases), 1941 (50 cases), 1961 (10 cases), and 1984 (14 cases). Of the 76 human rabies cases seen in South Africa between 1990 and 1993, 71 occurred in KwaZulu-Natal. The disease is endemic among a number of different wild animals, and these probably constitute the main reservoir. The yellow mongoose is the main culprit, but civet cats, foxes, and jackals are also involved. Rabies is also endemic among domestic animals, with dogs and cattle accounting for 87 per cent of these. Stray animals, especially dogs, may be the link in the transmission between wild and domestic animals. Rabies is a winter disease among animals. The proportion of rabies in domestic and wild animals varies from province to province. In most parts of the world the dog is the main vector. Humans are infected from these animal sources.

## Threat to health

Rabies is a neurological disease. In 'furious rabies' there is hyperactivity, bizarre aggressive behaviour, hydrophobia (fear of water), and aerophobia. Ascending symmetrical paralysis supervenes, leading to respiratory muscle paralysis, arrhythmias, and coma. 'Paralytic rabies' is characterized by ascending paralysis only. The disease is uniformly fatal in non-immunized cases even with mechanical ventilation.

## Protecting health

Measures can be taken to limit the growth of the mongoose population and to keep domestic animals vaccinated with live attenuated virus vaccine. Stray animals should be eliminated during epidemics, domestic animals revaccinated and restricted, the movement of animals between rabies and non-rabies areas cut down, and high-risk humans (veterinarians, health inspectors, etc.) vaccinated. Following exposure, wounds should be cleansed with soap, water, and a viricidal solution, and the subject treated with Rabies Immune Globulin and Rabies Vaccine (see Viral vaccines).

## GERMAN MEASLES (RUBELLA)

Rubella is endemic in many communities throughout the world and epidemics occur every six to eight years in non-immunized populations. About 65 per cent of infections are asymptomatic. There are no reliable data on the disease in South Africa. The rarity of congenital rubella in blacks suggests that there is immunity among women of child-bearing age as a result of early exposure in childhood or young adulthood.

Rubella causes low-grade fever, a measles-like rash, tender lymph nodes in the neck (posterior cervical), and conjunctivitis. Arthritis develops in some young adults. Rubella virus is teratogenic and produces a recognizable syndrome of multiple abnormalities in infected babies, particularly if the rubella occurs in the first trimester. Rubella vaccine is discussed in Chapter 25: Immunization. Coverage in South Africa is patchy because rubella immunization is not seen as being a high priority. The diagnosis is confirmed during pregnancy by a single measurement of specific IgM antibody to rubella or by a rise in titre of paired samples of sera taken two weeks apart. Inadvertent immunization of a pregnant woman is not an indication for termination of pregnancy.

## CHICKEN POX (VARICELLA)

Chicken pox is attended infrequently by a number of complications, some of which are severe. Encephalitis, transverse myelitis, and Reye's syndrome are a few examples. In order to prevent severe disease, immunodeficient children (those with primary immunodeficiencies, neoplasms, or those on cytotoxics) should receive Varicella Zoster Immunoglobulin (VZIG), 0,15 ml/kg/IMI, within three days of exposure to chicken pox or zoster. Newborns whose mothers get varicella in the period between seven days before and 30 days after delivery should also receive VZIG. Acyclovir (10 mg/kg/dose), given IVI slowly over one hour for three doses in 24 hours, is given for treatment of severe varicella or herpes zoster. Oral acyclovir (40–80 mg/kg/day) may

be used for less severe cases. A live attenuated vaccine can prevent fulminating disease in children with haematological malignancies. Vaccinated leukaemic children develop milder disease if breakthrough infection occurs. There is also greater protection against the development of zoster and the disease is less contagious. Varicella infection often occurs more than once in HIV-infected individuals. Most varicella deaths currently occur in HIV co-infected patients. (see Table 24.3). Wider use of the vaccine is being suggested in order to reduce the likelihood of complications developing, and to cut down on loss of school days occasioned by the disease.

## MUMPS

The main area of concern is the development of epididymo-orchitis, encephalomyelitis, and deafness. The live attenuated vaccine is given to children in the second year of life and may be offered to susceptible post-pubertal males to avoid orchitis.

## INFLUENZA

### Extent of the problem

The annual attack rate of influenza is 10 to 20 per cent. It is higher in winter and in children with chronic respiratory and heart disease. Influenza disease in HIV-infected children is more prolonged and more severe. Regular antigenic variations are responsible for new epidemics.

### Protecting health

(See Chapter 25: Immunization.) The benefits of vaccination include reduction in hospitalization by 30 to 70 per cent, and in deaths by 80 per cent. In those infected with HIV, there is a transient post-vaccination rise in HIV

**Table 24.3** Impact of HIV on vaccine-preventable diseases in the Durban Functional Region (1994–1999)

| | N | % of those Tested & adm HIV infected | % of total HIV infected | Overall % MR | % of deaths with HIV infection | MR for HIV infected |
|---|---|---|---|---|---|---|
| Measles | 1 073 | 13,0% | 1,3% | 0,9 | 60% | 42,9% |
| Varicella | 1177 | 67,9% | 26,5% | 1,4 | 81,3% | 6,1% |
| Pertussis | 74 | 33,3% | 2,7% | 2,7 | 100% | 100% |
| Typhoid | 141 | 13,3% | 1,4% | 0 | 0 | 0 |
| NNT | 60 | 23,5% | 6,67% | 11,7% | 42,8% | 17,6% |
| Mumps | 49 | 100% | 2,0% | 0 | 0 | 0 |
| Overall | 2 574 | 51,2% | 9,1% | 1,36%(n=35) | 68,6% | 14,9% |

MR = Mortality rate
NNT = Neonatal tetanus
Adm = Admissions

replication but this is not yet proven to have long-term ill effects. There is reduced response to vaccination in these patients.

Other protective measures against influenza include chemoprophylactic agents such as amantidine hydrochloride. This agent provides 70 to 90 per cent protection against Influenza A if given within 48 hours. The vaccine may exacerbate an asthmatic attack and rarely causes Guillain-Barré syndrome.

# Gastrointestinal infections

## GASTROENTERITIS, TYPHOID FEVER, AND CHOLERA

The main thrust of programmes against these diseases should be the improvement of sanitation, provision of clean water, encouragement of breast-feeding, promotion of oral rehydration, better food supplies, and establishment of an extensive network of primary health care centres. Diarrhoeal diseases are a major cause of morbidity and mortality among children in South Africa (see Chapter 38: Diarrhoeal disease). Deaths due to diarrhoea account for half the total mortality from all infectious diseases and this condition contributes substantially to the IMR in black children. Roughly 15 per cent of cases of gastroenteritis in South African children are due to *rotavirus*, for which heterologous vaccines are available. Rotavirus vaccines using human and animal derived *rotaviruses* have shown efficacy; evaluation of adverse events is still incomplete. The judicious use of such vaccines may play a small part in the reduction in morbidity and mortality from gastroenteritis.

*Typhoid* is endemic in South Africa. The incidence in South Africa has decreased substantially from 17,0 per 100 000 in 1985 to 2,1 per 100 000 in 1994; with the greatest decrease in Africans. The incidence rate is highest in the five- to nine-year age group with roughly 50 per cent of cases being under 15 years of age. It is mainly a disease of blacks in the rural areas and peri-urban squatter settlements. The annual case fatality rates are usually under two per cent although in epidemics they may be as high as 5,8 per cent.

Although oral vaccines are available and partially effective (see Chapter 25: Immunization), improvement in primary health care and clean water supply in high-risk areas such as Mpumalanga provides most benefit.

Yearly epidemics of *cholera* have re-emerged from the beginning of the 1990s. Current outbreaks in KwaZulu-Natal, Rwanda, Zimbabwe, and Mozambique make vigilance for this disease essential on account of migratory patterns. An oral vaccine is available and is being evaluated (see Chapter 38: Diarrhoeal disease).

# Bacterial infections

## WHOOPING COUGH (PERTUSSIS)

### Extent of the problem

Pertussis accounts for significant mortality and morbidity among children at a global level. It was one of three infections (the other two were measles and tetanus) that together caused more than 1,7 million childhood deaths in 1991. This figure is probably conservative, as the importance of pertussis has always been underestimated, especially in the developing world. Difficulties in accurate diagnosis caused by unreliable laboratory techniques and atypical presentation in very young babies are responsible for the lack of precision of such data. The problem is further compounded by the fact that other organisms such as *Bordetella parapertussis, B. bronchiseptica, adenovirus,* and *influenza virus* all produce illnesses that resemble whooping cough. The prime reason for such wastage of young lives is inadequate coverage by vaccine, although this coverage had reached 78 per cent for developing countries by 1991. A minimum effective coverage is about 80 per cent; which recently appeared to have been attained in South Africa.

The disease is notifiable in South Africa, but there is no accurate information on incidence or disease characteristics. Pertussis is, however, widespread throughout the country, as is indicated by hospital and anecdotal data. It is largely a neglected disease with all cases being diagnosed on clinical grounds alone; laboratory confirmation is virtually non-existent. It follows that most patients with pertussis are in fact 'suspected cases'. The description given under 'Threat to health' is based on an analysis of 1 525 cases admitted to six major infectious diseases hospitals in the country.

### Threat to health

It would appear that this disease poses a greater danger to the health of children in Africa than in industrialized countries, and this in part parallels the experience of the developed world at the turn of the century. The median age of occurrence of whooping cough in Africa is between two and three years whereas it is between four and five years in the wealthier countries. In South Africa, about a third of hospitalized cases were under a year of age and 7,2 per cent under two months. This feature has serious overtones as deaths occur more frequently in the younger age group. In parts of Africa, more than 60 per cent of all pertussis deaths are in infancy. The comparable figure in South Africa is 53 per cent, with 10 per cent of deaths being in those under two months of age. For unexplained reasons, the death rate is higher in females. The overall mortality for South African children is 3,3 per cent and is greatest for blacks and coloureds. It may account for part of the ill-defined causes of infant mortality.

Pertussis seriously affects the well-being of the child and causes considerable distress because of the protracted course it runs – the Chinese knew it as the '100-day cough'. The condition can be recognized clinically on the basis of the features listed in Table 24. 4.

**Table 24.4** Helpful features for diagnosis of pertussis

• *In children*

| | |
|---|---|
| Cough | spasmodic, choking, stringy sputum, ends with vomiting/whoop, lasts more than 21 days |
| Oedema of eyelids | |
| Bleeding | epistaxis, subconjunctival, haemoptysis |
| Contact | with another person with similar problems |
| Lymphocytosis | only in two-thirds of cases |

• *In young infants*:

Apnoea

Cyanosis

Convulsions

Cough – later onset, no whoop

Sudden death

In general, the children are well between attacks of coughing, extremely anxious just prior to a bout of coughing, and they have a clinically clear chest.

The main threat to health is posed by lung complications, of which bronchopneumonia is the most important. Sudden severe rises in intrathoracic pressure may lead to mediastinal emphysema, pneumothorax, and the escape of air to subcutaneous tissue. Encephalopathy is less frequent but more dangerous because of the possibility of neurological sequelae.

Weight loss occurs in about half the children and, although less profound than in measles, it may lead to marasmus in the younger child, or kwashiorkor in older children. This wasting appears to be primarily on account of decreased calorie intake. To regain weight may take as long as 12 weeks in a sixth of the patients. As with other infectious diseases, dormant tuberculosis may be reactivated. The neurological deficits, which include mental retardation and motor deficits, are permanent and lead to disability and handicap. Severe lung damage can lead relentlessly to bronchiectasis.

## Protecting health

Immunization is the main measure to protect children against the destructive effects of whooping cough. It has been estimated that if a full course of triple vaccine were to be administered universally, it would prevent 0,6 million annual global deaths. The momentum gained by the EPI increased vaccine coverage to 78 per cent in poor countries by 1991. Among the children with pertussis in this country, 27 per cent had been given three doses of DPT, 26 per cent were non-immunized and 47 per cent partly immunized. Transmission is maximal within four weeks of the onset of disease; therefore cases should be isolated from susceptibles. Even partial immunization is better than none, as it is believed to protect against severe disease (see Chapter 25: Immunization). The care of children with long-term sequelae such as bronchiectasis and neurological deficits requires team effort by many disciplines if rehabilitation is to be achieved.

There is some evidence to suggest that better nutrition may lessen the severity of the disease. In any respiratory disorder, overcrowding and clustering around closed areas where bio-fuels are being burnt are to be avoided. Proper housing is therefore a requisite for good health.

## TETANUS

## Extent of the problem

Given the effectiveness of the currently available vaccine and the knowledge about the best means of delivery, it is reasonable to expect that tetanus can not only be prevented but also eliminated. In the 1980s, tetanus, measles, and whooping cough were responsible for the deaths of 25 million young children, which is more than all the children under five years of age in western Europe or the United States. In 1996, 450 000 infants died from neonatal tetanus world-wide. Immunization of women can protect newborns by passive transfer of maternal antibody. A total of 28 per cent of pregnant women in developing countries, but only 20 per cent in Africa, received tetanus toxoid.

In South Africa the incidence of neonatal tetanus has decreased from 356 per 100 000 in 1981 to one per 100 000 in 1998. The case fatality rate has also decreased from 50 per cent to 8 per cent over the same period. The coverage by three doses of DPT vaccine is 79 per cent, though pockets of low coverage are found. The World Health Assembly's aim to eliminate neonatal tetanus by the year 2000 has progressed successfully with up to 60 per cent of developing countries reaching the target of less than one case per 1 000 births, and 58 countries progressing towards elimination. Over 90 per cent of all global cases of neonatal tetanus that occur currently are found in 26 countries, 16 of which are in Africa. In South Africa, 50 districts have reported neonatal tetanus as a problem between 1995 and 2000. A major threat to elimination is the lack of an appropriate surveillance system including the lack of a proper notification system. WHO estimates that less than five per cent of cases are reported annually and therefore refer to the disease as a silent killer.

## Threat to health

Tetanus is a dreaded disease, mainly because many die and the patient remains conscious and aware during the most violent convulsions. Respiratory complications are the most frequent cause of death. Painful and uncomfortable hypertonia of muscles in mild cases leads to focal signs or extension of the neck and spine. Pronounced arching of the back with clamping of the jaws occurs during recurrent muscle spasms. Drooling of saliva appears when the muscles of the pharynx go into spasm; inhalation of saliva predisposes to pneumonia. Impaired breathing, apnoea, cyanosis and sweating are due to laryngospasm and spasms of chest wall muscles and diaphragm. Muscles may be torn from their attachments, and the spine affected by compression fractures of vertebrae. Lockjaw and trismus are prominent features in the neonate. Untreated severe cases survive for about three days; if the patient survives more than ten days, recovery usually occurs. In the absence of special care facilities, the mortality rate in neonatal tetanus is 90 per cent and in older children 50 per cent; at King Edward VIII Hospital, Durban, where 40 paediatric tetanus patients are admitted annually, the mortality in neonates is 20 to 30 per cent.

## Protecting against tetanus

Three strategies are utilized in protection: immunization, clean deliveries, and surveillance. There are two approaches to immunization: one is to immunize women of childbearing age to prevent neonatal tetanus, and the other is to provide adequate coverage by triple vaccine in infancy and childhood to secure against tetanus at an older age. The recommendations made to achieve this are:

- to have a trained person attend each birth
- to conduct births in safe conditions;
- to immunize all women of childbearing age (especially pregnant women) against tetanus;
- to immunize all women who attend health services for immunization of their children, or for any other reason; and
- to identify high-risk groups and develop strategies for immunization and safe

delivery in such groups. Monitoring all cases of neonatal tetanus can facilitate identification.

All children should receive a full course of initial and booster doses of the triple vaccine. Moreover, appropriate therapy of wounded patients with surgical debridement, toxoid, and human anti-tetanus immunoglobulin can prevent the disease.

Intensive care facilities are absolutely necessary for severe tetanus. This is needed for most neonatal cases. Rehabilitation of patients with neurological damage, continuing chest problems, or with complications arising from ventilatory support need, a multidisciplinary approach. Clean deliveries should be facilitated by neonatal and delivery kits. Surveillance should be regarded as 'good' if 80 per cent of confirmed cases are reported within seven days and 80 per cent of suspected cases are investigated by a district medical officer of health within 48 hours by a home visit and

## Tetanus immunization doses for pregnant women

In a non-immunized pregnant woman, two doses of tetanus toxoid should be given with an interval of at least four weeks between them, and the second dose given at least two weeks before expected delivery. One booster dose for a previously vaccinated pregnant woman is sufficient. In order to cover the childbearing period, five doses of toxoid are necessary; a four-week interval is required between the first and second doses, six months between the second and third doses, one year between the third and fourth doses, and at least a year between the fourth and fifth doses.

given supplemental immunization. This should be followed by a community-based strategy of immunization because prenatal immunization has failed.

## DIPHTHERIA

## Extent of the problem

Diphtheria is one of the six diseases targeted for control or elimination by the EPI. The disease still occurs in poorer communities, but the marked decline in incidence of this disease in South Africa is illustrated in Figure 24.3. The annual number of cases notified is fairly small and the case fatality rate is about seven per cent. Localized outbreaks may occur. Local surveillance and mass immunization campaigns have been successfully employed in controlling outbreaks.

## Threat to health

The main dangers posed by diphtheria are severe upper airway obstruction produced by a membrane in the oropharynx and a 'bull-neck', myocarditis in the first or second week of the disease, and nerve inflammation resulting in paralysis of muscles. Bleeding and kidney failure are seen in severe cases.

## Protection of health

Even though the last cases of diphtheria occurred in 1992 in South Africa, continued stimulation of memory cells by vaccination is essential. Vaccination by initial and booster doses of DPT provides adequate protection. Disease surveillance and high immunization rates are essential to prevent epidemics. The acute case has to be treated with antibiotics, diphtheritic anti-toxin, and bed rest. Endotracheal intubation and mechanical ventilation are indicated for specific complications.

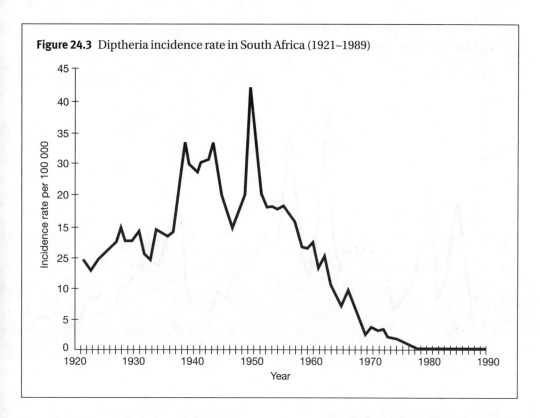

**Figure 24.3** Diptheria incidence rate in South Africa (1921–1989)

## MENINGOCOCCAL INFECTION

### Extent of the problem

The disease occurs in winter epidemics that last for about three to five years and which occur at irregular intervals of about 11 years. The epidemiological features of this infection have been gradually changing with time. Whereas the disease used to afflict young black males between the ages of 15 and 30 years who often were mineworkers in the Transvaal (renamed Gauteng), meningococcal infection is now primarily a problem of pre-school coloured children in the Western, Eastern, and Northern Cape. Both sexes are equally affected.

There is an overall decrease in incidence of meningococcal disease, the mortality being 11,2 per cent.

In 1989, coloureds from Western Cape had an incidence of 13,2 per 100 000 and this had decreased to 6,1 per 100 000 by 1994. Similarly the incidence in infants less than one year of age has decreased from 16,6 per 100 000 to 6,9 per 100 000 in the same period.

### Threat to health

Meningococci (along with *Haemophilus influenzae* and *Streptococcus pneumoniae*) account for the overwhelming majority of cases of acute bacterial meningitis in children. Septicaemia presents with purpura, arthritis, and (rarely) circulatory collapse. The disease carries an excellent prognosis in most cases, provided there is prompt therapy.

### Protecting health

Intravenous penicillin is recommended for the established case, but local drug sensitivities must be remembered. Complications should

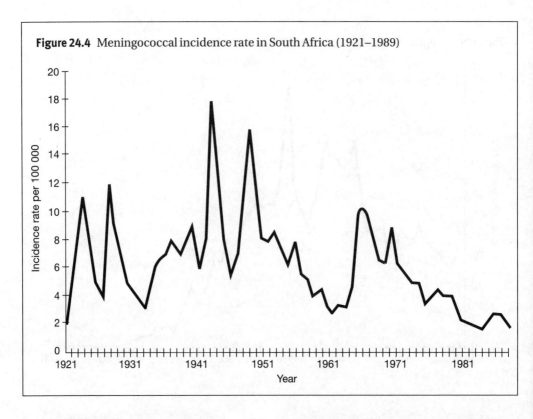

**Figure 24.4** Meningococcal incidence rate in South Africa (1921–1989)

be prevented or treated and general care provided for those with impaired consciousness. Close family and household contacts are treated with rifampicin. Sulphonamides are no longer recommended for prophylaxis because of high levels of resistance. During epidemics it is necessary to suggest that large social gatherings be avoided. Vaccine is indicated as a means of controlling outbreaks of meningococcal disease, for travellers to epidemic areas, and as prophylaxis for household contacts of cases. Immunity lasts for about three years (see Chapter 25: Immunization).

### HAEMOPHILUS INFLUENZAE TYPE B

### Extent of the problem

World-wide, *Haemophilus influenzae* type B

(HiB) is responsible for 20 per cent of cases of severe respiratory infections and over 200 000 cases of meningitis per year with an overall case fatality rate (CFR) of 30 per cent. In South Africa, an estimated 5 000 cases are seen annually; 70 per cent with pneumonia, 24,5 per cent with meningitis, and 5,9 per cent with septicaemia. The CFRs for each of these diseases are 15 per cent, 5 per cent, and 40 per cent respectively with 20 per cent of survivors of meningitis having permanent brain damage. The annual risk of death in children less than one year of age is 169 per 100 000.

### Protecting health

Prior to the initiation of routine HiB vaccine in July 1999 in South Africa, the burden of haemophilus influenza disease had already decreased between 1995 and 1999 (see Chapter 25: Immunization).

## Threats to health

Recent data of 110 HI type B isolates from King Edward VIII Hospital, Durban, have shown resistance to ampicillin and chloramphenicol at 9 per cent and 5,5 per cent respectively. In 1994, HIB disease became notifiable in South Africa. To counteract failures in the surveillance systems, an active laboratory surveillance system has been instituted. All blood and CSF HI isolates are sent to central reference laboratories together with clinical data. Sero-typing and sensitivities are also performed. The surveillance system aims to monitor the impact of the vaccination policy especially in HIV-infected individuals.

## PNEUMOCOCCAL DISEASE

### Extent of the problem

Over 150 million cases of pneumococcal disease are seen annually world-wide, and occur most commonly in young children and the elderly. The CFR for pneumococcal bacteraemia is 15 to 20 per cent, being higher in meningitis and bacteraemic pneumonia than non-bacteraemic pneumonia. The annual incidence in South Africa is 50 per 100 000 in children under five. An overall CFR of 13,5 per cent has been recorded. HIV seropositivity increases the risk of acquisition of pneumococcus by 36,9 times in children and 8,2 times in adults. Pneumococcal meningitis is the most common type of childhood meningitis at Chris Hani Baragwanath Hospital. Pneumococcal otitis media occurs commonly in children less than two years of age, and currently available vaccines are not protective against this.

### Protecting health

There are over 90 serotypes of the bacteria with the current capsular polyvalent polysaccaride vaccine containing 23 serotypes. These represent 85 per cent of common serotypes causing invasive disease and are also the serotypes affecting HIV-infected individuals. The vaccine is not effective in children under the age of two years (see Chapter 25: Immunization). Efficacy studies of the polysaccharide vaccine has been confirmed at 80 to 90 per cent for low-risk bacteraemic pneumonias, 56 to 81 per cent for invasive pneumococcal disease and 56 per cent for non bacteraemic pneumonia. Vaccine efficacy in HIV-infected individuals has not been proven, but if used it should be given early as immunization is more beneficial with higher CD4 counts. A transient increase in HIV replication after vaccination has raised concerns. The vaccine is otherwise recommended in children post splenectomy, other immune deficiencies, malignancies, chronic heart, and lung diseases (e.g., bronchopulmonary dysplasia) and those with CSF leaks.

### Threats to health

Resistance of pneumococci to penicillin was first described in 1967 from Australia, New Guinea, and South Africa. For penicillin-resistant pneumococcal pneumonia, high doses of penicillin are adequate in effecting cure, but in meningitis and otitis media an alternative agent should be used. The cost effectiveness of routine administration of the vaccine to children in developing countries is still under review.

### LEPROSY

The incidence of this disease has declined steadily in South Africa since 1912. About 120 to 130 cases are seen annually, almost exclusively in blacks. With a prevalence of 0,37 per 10 000 population it is no longer a public health problem and is not a disease of childhood. BCG has been found to be effective in preventing leprosy in some countries.

## MALARIA

### Extent of the problem

Malaria continues to ravage children and adults in areas adjacent to our borders, namely Mozambique, Zimbabwe, and Rwanda. As such it provides a major threat to health services in the northern provinces, Mpumalanga, and Northern Kwazulu-Natal. In 1996, 20 000 cases and 124 deaths related to malaria were seen in these areas with 38 per cent of these cases originating from neighbouring countries. The incidence of malaria in KwaZulu-Natal increased from 48,6 per 100 000 in 1989 to 63,8 per 100 000 in 1994. Major outbreaks have occurred in 1999 in KwaZulu-Natal and two-thirds of the recorded deaths occurred there. The sources of these outbreaks are migrants from Mozambique who are chronic carriers and spread the disease.

### Protecting health

The mainstay of management for malaria is prevention. The use of appropriately impregnated mosquito-repellent nets is most beneficial. The use of DDT remains controversial. Reducing mosquito infestation is also an important strategy. The use of chemoprophylaxis for visitors entering malarial areas is essential. Those with malaria need effective therapy. Resistance to anti-malarials is a major problem (see Chapter 42: Malaria). Malaria vaccines are still undergoing evaluation.

## Legislation or regulations relating to infectious diseases

Government departments of health may promulgate that:

- vaccination against certain diseases be mandatory or compulsory;
- certain diseases must be notified to the local health authority; or that
- quarantine periods be observed and that, where the disease constitutes a risk to others, treatment be enforced.

### COMPULSORY VACCINATION

In South Africa, BCG and polio immunization was made mandatory by the Department of Health, but this was rescinded in 1988. The reason for so doing was that the regulations were unenforceable, and compulsion was considered ethically unacceptable and ineffective. There is no planned or intended reduction in the free availability of the vaccines.

A difficulty now experienced by some health workers is that, when informed consent is sought, there may be undue delay while rural mothers consult distant migrant-worker fathers.

Objectors to vaccination, for whatever reason, pose a difficult problem as the parent can overrule the right of the child to be thus protected against disease.

Travellers to or from high-risk areas may be obliged to produce the required vaccination certificates when crossing borders.

Other forms of compulsion are requirements such as that a valid vaccination record or doctor's report of a prior disease be an essential prerequisite for acceptance at a crèche/nursery school, for school entry, or for participation in health care services.

Such practices are widely enforced in the United States and are variously applied in South Africa. Medical and nursing personnel should ensure that they can neither contract nor spread conditions such as hepatitis B or rubella.

**Table 24.5** Quarantine/isolation of communicable diseases, showing when patient and contacts may return to teaching institutions

**Acquired immunodeficiency syndrome (AIDS)**
No exclusion apart from that dictated by severity of illness or as certified by a health professional. It is advisable for immuno-compromised individuals to avoid exposure to infectious diseases.

**Chicken pox**
*Patient:* until rash has dry crusts/scabs – usually seven to ten days
*Contact:* immediately

**Cholera**
*Patient:* on submission of a medical certificate
*Contact:* according to quarantine measures

**Diphtheria**
*Patient:* on submission of a medical certificate, and after two nose and two throat swabs at appropriate intervals have proved negative
*Non-immune contacts:* eight days after removal from source of infection
*Immune contacts:* immediately

**Epidemic typhus**
*Patient:* on submission of a medical certificate
*Contact:* immediately

**German measles (rubella)**
*Patient:* seven days after appearance of a rash
*Contact:* immediately

**Haemorrhagic fever diseases of Africa**
*Patient:* on submission of a medical certificate
*Contact:* according to quarantine measures

**Haemorrhagic viral conjunctivitis**
*Patient:* seven days after beginning of symptoms
*Contact:* immediately

**Hepatitis A**
*Patient:* seven days after appearance of jaundice or on submission of a medical certificate
*Contact:* immediately

**Other hepatitis**
*Patient:* on production of a medical certificate
*Contact:* immediately

**Leprosy**
*Patient:* on submission of a medical certificate
*Contact:* immediately

**Louse infection**
*Patient:* after complete cleansing and delousing and removal of nits from head, body, and clothing
*Contact:* immediately, but must be kept under surveillance

**Measles**
*Patient:* seven days after appearance of rash
*Contact:* immediately

**Meningococcaemia**
*Patient:* on submission of a medical certificate
*Contact:* immediately, provided the necessary prophylactic medicine is taken

**Mumps**
*Patient:* nine days after appearance of swelling
*Contact:* immediately

**Plague**
*Patient:* on submission of a medical certificate
*Contact:* according to quarantine measures

**Poliomyelitis**
*Patient:* on submission of a medical certificate
*Contact:* immediately

**Scabies**
*Patient:* no exclusion but should receive proper treatment
*Contact:* immediately

**Tuberculosis of the lungs**
*Patient:* on submission of a medical certificate. If on treatment, exclusion only depends on severity of illness
*Contact:* immediately

**Typhoid fever**
*Patient:* on submission of a medical certificate
After three negative stool tests done at appropriate intervals (at least 48 hours) and not less than 72 hours after cessation of antibiotic policy
*Contact:* immediately

**Whooping cough**
*Patient:* 21 days after beginning of paroxysms or on submission of a medical certificate
*Contact:* immediately

## Notifiable diseases

The purpose of notification is to:
- establish the incidence and mortality of potentially preventable diseases;
- identify high-risk areas and situations to enable intervention for control;
- monitor the success of immunization programmes; and
- alert the health authority and thus mobilize their expertise and resources.

Notification is frequently incomplete for many reasons, a major one being poorly motivated health care personnel. If potential 'notifiers'were to fully appreciate the benefits of notification, they may well prove more compliant. This calls for improved communication and feedback from the health authority to doctors and other health workers.

Not all 'cases' may present at a health care service. Not surprisingly, the youngest and sickest patients are most likely to reach clinics and hospitals where notification is generally better practised, and this may have given a biased view of the age-specific incidence of infectious diseases such as measles. Older children with less severe illness may be managed at home, particularly in communities accustomed to the condition.

## Quarantine periods

Schools and other institutions may need quarantine guidelines, and these are given in Table 24.5.

Compulsory treatment is indicated in conditions such as typhoid, and if necessary, such patients can be kept in hospital by court retention orders.

## References and further reading

ANON. *Epidemiological Comments*. Pretoria: Department of Health. (Numerous issues referred to in preparation of this text.)

DE QUADROS CA, HERSH BS, OLIVE T, et al. 1997. Eradication of Wild Poliovirus from the Americas: Acute flaccid paralysis surveillance, 1988–1995. *Journal of Infectious Diseases*. 175(supp):S37–42.

JEENA PM, WESLEY AG, and COOVADIA HM. 1998. Infectious diseases at Clairwood Hospital, Durban. Trends in admission and mortality rates and the early impact of HIV infection. *South African Medical Journal*. 1:81–6.

OKWO-BELE J, LOBANOV A, BIELLIK RJ, et al. 1997. Overview of poliomyelitis in the African region and current regional plan of action. *Journal of Infectious Diseases*. 175(Suppl):S10–5.

# Notifiable medical conditions

| Code (ICD10) | Name |
|---|---|
| AFP- | Acute flaccid paralysis |
| A22 | Anthrax |
| A23 | Brucellosis |
| A00 | Cholera |
| A50 | Congenital syphilis |
| A98 | Crimean-Congo haemorrhagic fever Other haemorrhagic fevers of Africa |
| A36 | Diphtheria |
| A02&A05 | Food poisoning |
| HiB | *Haemophilus influenzae* type B |
| T56 | Lead poisoning |
| A48 | Legionellosis |
| A30 | Leprosy |
| B54 | Malaria |
| B05 | Measles* |
| A39 | Meningococcal infection |
| A01 | Paratyphoid fever |
| A20 | Plague |
| T57&T60 | Poisoning from any agricultural or stock remedies |
| A80 | Poliomyelitis (acute)* |
| A82 | Rabies |
| 100 | Rheumatic fever |
| A35 | Tetanus |
| A33 | Tetanus neonatorum |
| A71 | Trachoma |
| A16.7 | Tuberculosis primary |
| A16.5 | Tuberculosis pulmonary |
| A16.9 | Tuberculosis of other respiratory organs |
| A17.0&G01 | Tuberculosis of meninges |
| A18.3 | Tuberculosis of intestines, peritoneum |
| A18.0 | Tuberculosis of bones and joints |
| A18.1 | Tuberculosis of genito-urinary system |
| A18.8 | Tuberculosis of other organs |
| A18.9 | Tuberculosis miliary |
| 010-8(ICD09) | Tuberculosis total |
| A01 | Typhoid fever (ICD 10: Typhoid fever and other) |
| A75.0 | Typhus fever (lice-borne) |
| A75.2 | Typhus fever (ratflea-borne) |
| B15.9 | Viral hepatitis type A (ICD10: Acute hepatitis A) |
| B16.9 | Viral hepatitis type B (ICD10: Acute hepatitis B) |
| B17.8 | Viral hepatitis non-A non-B (ICD10: Other V H) |
| B19 | Viral hepatitis unspecified |
| 0701-9 (ICD09) | Viral hepatitis total |
| A37 | Whooping cough |
| A95 | Yellow fever |

* Cases investigated by provincial EPI teams. (As at April 2000 – changes may be made periodically)

Source: Department of Health, Republic of South Africa.

As published in *Epidemiological Comments*

# 25 Immunization

**BD SCHOUB &
KP KLUGMAN**

*'I am hard-hearted enough to let the sick die if you can tell me how to prevent others from falling sick'*

Mahatma Gandhi

The two most effective means of preventing morbidity and mortality from infectious diseases are sanitation and immunization. Global strategies are now aimed not just at controlling but at eliminating and eventually eradicating vaccine-preventable conditions. A notable success has been achieved with smallpox, and there are very significant declining incidence rates of other infections as immunization coverage increases (see Chapter 19: Global strategies for child health; and Chapter 24: Vaccine-preventable infectious diseases).

The safety and efficacy of currently available vaccines place a great responsibility on health care personnel to ensure that all children are duly immunized and that no possible opportunity is missed.

There are few valid contra-indications to immunization and it is a serious decision to withhold a vaccine. Health workers who administer vaccines need and deserve to be well informed and to be guided and supported. They should not feel left uncertain of their decisions and afraid of criticism.

Six major vaccine-preventable diseases (measles, poliomyelitis, diphtheria, whooping cough, tetanus, and tuberculosis) were targeted for control by the World Health Organization Expanded Programme on Immunization (EPI) launched in 1974 with the goal of Universal Child Immunization (UCI) by the year 2000.

South African government health services have also concentrated on these six infectious diseases. Since 1995, hepatitis B, and more recently *Haemophilus influenzae* B, have been added to the routine schedule.

In this chapter the general principles underlying vaccination will be discussed, the eight major vaccines will be dealt with in some depth, and other available viral and bacterial vaccines will be described.

## Definitions

### VACCINATION VS. IMMUNIZATION

The words 'vaccine' and 'vaccination' were originally derived from the Latin word for 'cow', *vacca*, which referred to the first human

**Table 25.1** Immunization schedules

Recommendations from the Department of Health (South Africa), United Nations Children's Fund, and World Health Organization (1994)

Infants and Children

| AGE | VACCINE |
| --- | --- |
| Birth | BCG (*Bacillus Calmette- Guerin* – Mycobacterium bovis – attenuated tubercle organism) TOPV (Trivalent Oral Polio Vaccine) |
| 6 Weeks | DPT1 (Diphtheria, Pertussis, Tetanus) TOPV1 HBV1 (Hepatitis B Vaccine)* HiB1 (*Haemophilus influenza* B)~ |
| 10 Weeks | DPT2 TOPV2 HBV2 HiB2 |
| 14 Weeks | DPT3 TOPV3 HBV3 HiB3 |
| 9 Months | Measles Vaccine 1 |
| 18 Months | Measles Vaccine 2 DPT4 TOPV4 |
| 5 Years | DT (Diphtheria, Tetanus) TOPV5 |

- HBV * – Provided by the State from 1995
- HiB ~ – Provided by the State from 1999
- Rubella vaccine – depends on arrangements by local authorities, generally reserved for pre-pubescent girls
- Tetanus vaccine for women – given in high-risk areas to protect newborn infants against neonatal tetanus

vaccine – Edward Jenner's cowpox virus vaccine introduced in 1798. Immunization, strictly speaking, refers to the production of an immune response in the host after introduction of a foreign antigen. However, the terms 'vaccination' and 'immunization' tend to be used interchangeably.

## Passive vs. active immunity

*Passive immunity* denotes immediate but temporary protection provided by antibodies formed outside the child. This applies to:
- the transplacental passage of antibodies (against measles, for example) from mother to fetus. This is natural passive immunity;
- the administration of pooled globulin preparations precipitated from the blood plasma of about a thousand random donors, and administered by intramuscular injection;
- the specific 'hyperimmune' globulins. These are made from plasma derived from donors who are recovering from or who have recently been immunized against the particular infection. These are examples of artificial passive immunity.

'Antitoxins' such as those used in the treatment of diphtheria, tetanus, snake-bite, scorpion, and spider bites are derived from horse serum. Prior testing for sensitivity must precede administration.

'Active immunity' refers to the stimulation of the host's immune system in order to develop resistance to disease after the introduction of vaccines or as a result of natural infections.

'Herd immunity' refers to the situation where the level of immunity in a population is sufficient to result in the interruption of transmission of a pathogen, the survival of which is dependent on susceptible human hosts. A higher level of herd immunity is needed when the infecting load is great, as occurs with measles virus in crowded disadvantaged communities.

## Vaccines

These may consist of *attenuated live pathogens*, which may be viral (such as measles, mumps, rubella, poliomyelitis – Sabin oral vaccine, or yellow fever) or bacterial (such as BCG).

*Purified antigen extracts* used in first generation hepatitis B vaccine and soluble capsular material, such as pneumococcal polysaccharide.

*Toxoids* are bacterial toxins rendered non-toxic, but remaining antigenic, and able to stimulate the formation of protective antitoxins, such as diphtheria toxoid and tetanus toxoid.

Another vaccine type comprises *killed pathogens,* such as bacteria (pertussis) and viruses (poliomyelitis Salk vaccine, rabies, and influenza).

*Conjugate vaccines* – purified capsular carbohydrate is chemically linked to a protein, e.g., tetanus or diphtheria toxoid to make the carbohydrate immunogenic in children (e.g., *Haemophilus influenzae* conjugate vaccines).

*Recombinant vaccines* – see Hepatitis B.

## The immune response to immunization

The administration of live attenuated vaccines results in the multiplication of the organism in the vaccinee with stimulation of production of antigen until the intended specific immune response arises. In this way the vaccine induces an immunological response more like that resulting from a natural infection. Inactivated vaccines rarely give rise to lifelong immunity so boosters are necessary if high levels of protective antibody are to be maintained.

On first exposure to a vaccine antigen, the primary immune response takes several days to occur. These antigens are processed by T-cells and cause B-cell stimulation with the appearance first of IgM antibodies, and then sustained high levels of IgG antibodies. These IgG antibodies fix complement, and opsonize, or neutralize, or precipitate their stimulating antigens.

Following a second (booster) exposure to the same vaccine antigen, heightened T-cell and B-cell responses are elicited with earlier appearance of specific antibodies. This secondary response reflects the induction of immunological memory by the primary vaccination. Immunological memory reflects an ongoing defence system, which allows speedy reaction when dealing with subsequent exposures to micro-organisms.

Despite a fall over time in the measurable titre of antibodies to some vaccines, a typical secondary response consisting of IgG with or without IgM is usually observed upon rechallenge, denoting persistence of immunological memory. Thus the absence of measurable antibody doesn't necessarily mean that immunity is absent. In contrast, for some vaccines the mere presence of antibodies is insufficient to ensure adequate protection, but rather a minimum titre of antibodies is needed (e.g., more than 0,01 IU/ml of tetanus antitoxin).

Immunity to polysaccharide vaccines is not directly dependent on T-cells (polysaccharides stimulate a T-cell-independent response by directly stimulating B-cells to produce antibody). The IgG molecules produced in this way may not, however, be of all IgG sub-classes, complement may not be bound, and opsonization may be defective. This is a particular problem with the first generation *Haemophilus influenzae* type B vaccine, because young children do not make these T-cell independent antibodies. T-cell-independent immunity does not generate memory T-cells, and therefore there is no booster response.

# Routes of administration

The administration of attenuated live viral vaccine, such as *oral Polio* (Sabin), by the same portal of entry as is used by the natural infection leads to identical immunity (see Table 25.2).

Live virus entry by an unnatural route, such as parenteral (IMI or subcut) administration of measles, mumps, and/or rubella vaccines, results in replication of the virus throughout the body with good systemic but relatively little epithelial immunity and no spread to contacts. Thus, a child who develops vaccine measles (a mild measles-like illness eight to ten days after measles vaccination) is not infectious and need not be isolated.

In the case of measles vaccine, systemic administration has the advantage of a shorter incubation period, thus allowing post-exposure prophylaxis.

The following viral vaccines are administered by subcutaneous injection, which should be given into the deltoid region of the arm – measles, mumps, rubella, rabies, Trivalent inactivated polio vaccine (TIPV). Depot antigens, e.g., diphtheria toxoid (formalinized toxin adsorbed with alum), should be given by deep intramuscular injection. More superficial injections may result in cyst formation.

Intramuscular inoculation should be carried out on the antero-lateral part of the thigh in infants, and into the deltoid muscle in older children. The buttocks are not suitable for intramuscular injection because of the possibility of inoculation into fatty tissue. Immunogenicity via this route has been shown to be sub-optimal. Influenza and hepatitis B are administered intramuscularly. It has been suggested recently that *all* parenteral vaccines be given intramuscularly rather than subcutaneously as absorption is better (Zukerman, 2001).

# Measles

### MEASLES VACCINES

The measles vaccine presently in major use throughout the world is derived from the Schwarz strain of measles virus, which is attenuated by the multiple passage of wild-type virus through both fertilized chicken eggs and chick embryo fibroblast culture. Another attenuated strain of measles vaccine is derived from the Edmonston-Zagreb (EZ) strain of vaccine virus, which is attenuated by passage through human diploid fibroblast cell culture.

### ADMINISTRATION

Both vaccines are administered by subcutaneous injection, and both produce a greater than 95 per cent rate of seroconversion when administered at the optimal age of 15 months as recommended for developed countries.

## Know your vaccines

Knowledge and understanding of the type of vaccine being used has *practical implications*. For example, *live viral vaccines*:
- may be destroyed by improper handling;
  - unsatisfactory cold chain (see EPI in Chapter 19:Global strategies for child health),
  - poor administration techniques (destruction by cleansing spirits),
  - excessively prolonged storage (check expiry dates);
- are potentially hazardous
  - during fetal development (contra-indicated in pregnancy), and
  - when there is significant immune deficiency.
- Antibodies in gammaglobulin or plasma/blood transfusions are likely to destroy live viral vaccines if given within four weeks.

The health worker armed with this information can comply with immunization directives more intelligently.

Immunity thereafter is long lasting. In developed countries, measles infection is rare before 18 months, and delaying immunization until 15 months to take full advantage of its efficacy at that age is therefore quite safe. However, in developing countries, measles has been a major cause of infant death and morbidity. It occurs frequently below one year of age and significantly even below nine months of age. Earlier immunization is therefore a practical necessity. The WHO recommended age of measles immunization for developing countries is nine months. Using the Schwarz strain of vaccine, an 80 per cent rate of seroconversion can be expected at that age, because of some interference by residual maternal immunity. It would be desirable to be able to immunize at an even earlier age (say six months), but maternal antibody interference reduces the efficiency of the Schwarz strain to a prohibitively low level of about 60 per cent. Nevertheless, early immunization of such young infants may still be the preferred option when there is considerable risk on account of exposure to wild measles virus. In these circumstances the measles vaccine must be repeated at or after the age of nine months. Previous concern that measles vaccination at a very young age might impair long-term immunity is now considered unfounded. The immune response, although altered, is probably not deficient.

In South Africa the official recommendation is for a two-dose schedule – at nine months and at 18 months of age. Children admitted to hospital or facilities where others may have measles should be routinely immunized if over the age of six months.

Measles vaccine can be used for post-contact prophylaxis provided it is administered within 72 hours of exposure.

### STORAGE

Measles vaccine should be protected from light, and should always be stored in a refrigerator (4–10 °C). Freezing will not harm the vaccine. In the field the vaccine must be carried in a suitable 'cold-box'. Measles vaccine is very susceptible to heat, and should always be kept cold. The reconstituted vaccine should be used immediately, *and certainly within one hour unless stated otherwise* by the manufacturer, for it rapidly loses its potency. Measles vaccine is killed by ether, alcohol, and detergents, and these agents should not be used for sterilizing syringes prior to immunization. Before giving the injection, wait for the skin to dry after swabbing. The shelf life of measles vaccine is limited to 12 months from the time of manufacture, and the vaccine should not be administered after the expiry date printed on each vial.

## SIDE EFFECTS

Mild pyrexia about seven days after measles immunization is not uncommon, but of little concern. In some ten to 20 per cent of cases a mild measles-like illness, sometimes with morbilliform rash, may complicate immunization. Vaccine measles is not contagious.

## CONTRA-INDICATIONS

There are essentially two contra-indications to measles immunization – egg hypersensitivity and immunosuppression. The attenuation of the Schwarz strain of vaccine in fertilized chicken eggs and chick embryo cell culture results in minute traces of egg protein being present in the vaccine, despite purification, which can cause hypersensitivity reactions in children allergic to eggs (this does not apply to the EZ vaccine). In practice, however, very few such reactions have been reported, and then only in children with histories of severe hypersensitivity, e.g., anaphylaxis following ingestion of eggs.

Anaphylaxis manifests with generalized urticaria, swelling of the mouth and throat, difficulty with breathing, hypotension, or shock. Such cases are rare. An anaphylactic reaction to neomycin is another extremely rare occurrence, and would be a contra-indication to measles vaccine.

It is only in these situations that measles vaccine is contra-indicated. Mild or even moderate egg allergy should not be used as a reason to deprive a child of the benefits of a vaccine which gives such effective and safe protection from a potentially lethal infection.

The immunodeficiency disorders again represent only relative contra-indications. It is especially this group of children who need to be protected from the ravages of measles infection. Thus, children with severe immunosuppression, such as those with the congenital immunodeficiency syndromes, should *not*

receive live measles vaccine. Immunodeficiency of a lesser degree, such as children with underlying tuberculosis, children on steroid therapy, malnourished children, and asymptomatically as well as symptomatically HIV-infected children, should all be immunized with measles vaccine.

During acute febrile illnesses it may be preferable to postpone measles vaccination. However, children admitted to large hospitals or attending clinics where there is an immediate danger of measles contact should, regardless of their illness, be given measles vaccine unless this is specifically contra-indicated. This policy has been adopted by several South African paediatric departments, and is applied to all health service attenders between the ages of six months and five years unless they have available documented evidence (Road to Health Charts) of prior measles immunization. If the illness may become life threatening because of complications caused by measles or measles vaccine, use can be made of measles hyperimmune globulin. Thereafter measles vaccination should be given after three months if the child is well. Ensure that a delayed vaccine does not in fact become a missed vaccine.

## MEASLES VACCINES ADMINISTERED TOGETHER WITH OTHER VACCINES

There is no contra-indication to giving measles vaccine simultaneously with any other live or killed viral or bacterial vaccine (including BCG). However, if not given simultaneously, at least a month should lapse after administration of any live vaccine before giving another live vaccine.

Tuberculin testing on the same day as measles immunization is acceptable, but a few days to a few weeks thereafter may give a false negative result because of depressed immune responses.

## Non-contra-indications

The following are *not* contra-indications to measles vaccination:

- a previous seizure or idiopathic epilepsy in a parent or sibling. Advise parents to watch out for fever a week after the vaccination, and to administer paracetamol at the first sign of fever;
- hay fever, asthma, eczema, or food allergies other than anaphylaxis to egg protein;
- previous exposure (or absence of exposure) to egg protein;
- antibiotics or other medications including topical or low-dose oral steroids;
- chronic illness. Vaccination is especially important here;
- failure to thrive or low weight, marasmus, and kwashiorkor;
- prematurity;
- child of breast-feeding or pregnant mother; and
- uncertainty about previous measles vaccination. If in any doubt as to previous vaccination or a history of natural measles it is far safer to vaccinate.

There is seldom a need to immunize pregnant women with measles vaccine, and this is generally not recommended. However, no teratogenic effects of the vaccine have been recorded.

# Poliomyelitis

Two kinds of polio vaccine incorporating the three types of poliovirus are used for routine immunization. An inactivated vaccine given by injection, and named after Salk – trivalent inactivated polio vaccine (TIPV) – and a live attenuated oral vaccine named after Sabin – trivalent oral polio vaccine (TOPV). The comparative characteristics, advantages, and disadvantages are listed in Table 25.2.

In some developed countries, such as Scandinavia and Holland, where excellent health care services have provided exceptionally high levels of immunization cover, polio has been eliminated by routine immunization with TIPV. However, in most parts of the world, routine immunization is carried out using TOPV. An increasing number of developed countries, such as France, Canada, and the USA have recently switched to using TIPV.

## DOSAGE SCHEDULE OF TOPV

Routine administration of TOPV is carried out in South Africa at six, ten, and 14 weeks, and booster doses are given at 18 months and on school entry.

## NEONATAL IMMUNIZATION

The World Health Organization has recommended that a further supplementary dose of TOPV be given at birth because of the accessibility of newborns for immunization, as well as the lack of interference at that age.

## BREAST-FEEDING AND POLIO IMMUNIZATION

There is no scientific evidence that breast-feeding in any way interferes with polio immunization, and there is no contra-indication to breast-feeding either before or after receiving polio vaccine. The same would apply to formula feeding or any other feeding.

## INTERCURRENT GASTROENTERITIS

Viral interference with polio immunization as a result of infection of the gut with enteric viruses is far more likely in the presence of gastroenteritis, and rotavirus is known to

**Table 25.2** Comparative characteristics of TIPV and TOPV

| | TIPV (Salk) | TOPV (Sabin) |
|---|---|---|
| Preparation | 1  Growth of wild- type virus in monkey kidney cell culture<br>2  Inactivation by formaldehyde | 1  Multiple passages in monkey kidney cell culture to produce live attenuated strain |
| Route of administration | 0,5 ml subcutaneous injection in single or multi-dose vials<br>–  vaccine may be combined in same injection with DPT | Orally – three drops onto tongue in 20-dose vials |
| Type of immunity | Serum and pharyngeal (transudation from serum) | Serum, pharyngeal, and gut |
| Type of protection | 1  Protection against paralytic polio<br>2  Protection against respiratory spread poliovirus infection | 1  Protection against paralytic polio<br>2  Protection against gut infection, faecal-oral, as well as respiratory spread virus |
| Herd immunity | Reasonably good herd immunity for respiratory spread polio (in developed countries). Poor herd immunity for faecal-oral spread polio (in developing countries) | Good herd immunity for faecal–oral and respiratory spread polio. Vaccine virus spread to the unvaccinated via same routes as wild-type polio. Lower percentage of cover required to achieve herd immunity |
| Interference | Nil | Problem in developing countries – interference with 'take' of vaccine virus by endogenous viruses in the gastrointestinal tract |
| Safety | Very safe – side effects of sensitivity very rare and usually mild | Danger of back-mutation to virulent polio virus, especially type 3 in about one in five million vaccine recipients and can cause paralysis<br>Danger not only to vaccine recipients but also to susceptible contacts. Potential danger of contaminating virus in cell culture, e.g., SV40 |
| Cost | Relatively expensive | Cheap |

interfere with oral polio immunization. One may therefore delay immunization until after recovery from the intestinal infection if there is reasonable certainty that the child will not be lost to immunization. An often safer alternative is to give the vaccine, and note the need for an additional precautionary dose when opportunity presents. Should vomiting occur soon after receiving TOPV, a repeat dose should be given. No harm results from extra dosing with TOPV.

## POLIO IMMUNIZATION AND IMMUNODEFICIENCY

Recovery from infection with polio virus is mediated by the humoral arm of the immune system. Individuals with deficiency of humoral immunity, such as hypogammaglobulinaemia, agammaglobulinaemia, or severe combined immunodeficiency, are particularly liable to the paralytic complications of polio virus infection even with the attenuated vaccine strain. In these subjects, TOPV is absolutely contra-indicated, and TIPV should be administered because it is safe, although the efficiency of protection, because of humoral immunosuppression, is considerably lowered (such subjects should have their immune response checked serologically after immunization). Children with other immunodeficiencies (e.g., those on steroid therapy and children with asymptomatic or symptomatic HIV infection) should receive TOPV. The WHO recommendations, which are followed by developing countries and South Africa, recommend TOPV for *all* HIV-infected children.

## POLIO VACCINE IN PREGNANCY

There is no evidence that TOPV is teratogenic, and during an outbreak non-immune pregnant women should be protected with TOPV. If possible, however, pregnant women should preferably not receive TOPV during the first trimester.

# Tuberculosis

## BCG VACCINE

BCG is widely used in many developing countries to prevent disseminated tuberculosis. The vaccine consists of a freeze-dried live attenuated strain of *Mycobacterium bovis* known as the *Bacillus Calmette-Guerin*. A number of different strains of BCG are used around the world. All are derived from the original strain produced in Paris by Calmette and Guerin but they now differ widely in potency and probably also in their protective properties. The method used in South Africa for many years has been percutaneous, using a nine-pronged vaccination tool. This is currently being changed to the intradermal method because of doubts as to the efficacy of the percutaneous method. The vaccine should be given in the days immediately after birth, and is no longer repeated.

A normal reaction to intradermal BCG is a raised papule at the site of vaccination, reaching a maximum at four to six weeks, and then fading to leave a faint scar. Scars remain visible in only about 40 per cent of vaccinees. Prolonged ulceration at the site, with lymphadenitis may occur in one to ten per cent of cases. A rare complication is BCG osteomyelitis. In an estimated one in a million vaccinees, disseminated BCG disease may occur. This rare complication usually results from underlying immunosuppressive illness.

BCG vaccination stimulates the cellular immune response to *Mycobacterium tuberculosis*, and thus induces skin reactivity to tuberculin. Tuberculin test reactions of 5–9 mm induration are usual, but a number of children will show reactions of 10–15 mm, i.e., *positive* tests. However when a child shows a reaction greater than 15 mm, or Tine Test of 3+ or 4+, it can be assumed that natural (tuberculous) infection has occurred. The reactivity is maximal for six months after vaccination, and fades after about two years.

## GENERAL GUIDELINES

BCG can be given to HIV-infected asymptomatic infants. It is contra-indicated in AIDS cases because of the risk of dissemination of the BCG bacillus. BCG should only be administered 24 hours after discontinuation of INH or other anti-TB therapy when this is given prophylactically. BCG can be given to premature infants when they are ready for discharge. Eczema is *not* a contra-indication but injecting into an eczematous or other abnormal areas should be avoided.

## STORAGE OF VACCINE

Refrigeration or cold box at 2–10 °C (*not frozen*). Once reconstituted, the vaccine will remain active for 8 hours but it is destroyed by direct sunlight.

## Diluent

Store in a cold cupboard.

## VACCINE EFFICACY

The degree of protection conferred by BCG against tuberculosis in infants and young children remains controversial. A meta-analysis of fourteen prospective trials and twelve case-control studies concluded that BCG conferred 50 per cent protection against active disease. In seven trials using tuberculosis death as an end point, protection was 71 per cent, and the five studies on TB meningitis gave a protective efficacy of 64 per cent. It should be noted that the majority of the studies used the intradermal and not the percutaneous method. Serious and extensive tuberculosis may occur despite previous BCG vaccination, and the clinician should not be lulled into a false sense of security by the presence of a BCG scar. BCG must thus be combined with active case-finding strategies and treatment of persons with open tuberculosis for optimal efficacy.

# Diphtheria–pertussis–tetanus

## DIPHTHERIA TOXOID

Diphtheria toxoid is highly effective in inducing antibodies that will neutralize diphtheria toxin, thus protecting against disease. It may not, however, protect against acquisition or carriage of *Corynebacterium diphtheriae*. Two preparations are available: an adsorbed, more immunogenic, higher-dose vaccine intended for use in children up to the age of seven years; and a lower-dose formula intended for use in persons over this age. For children under the age of two years, diphtheria toxoid is usually administered together with tetanus toxoid and pertussis vaccine (DPT). A formulation without pertussis (DT) is given to older children.

Immunization with DPT consists of three doses, four weeks apart, which may be given from the age of six weeks, and a fourth dose given six to 12 months later. Booster doses of diphtheria toxoid may be given every ten years.

Local pain and tenderness are frequently encountered after diphtheria immunization. Rarely, there may be fever. The only known contra-indication is in those extremely rare individuals who have previously had severe hypersensitivity or neurological reactions after the administration of diphtheria toxoid.

## TETANUS TOXOID

Tetanus toxoid is an inactivated, yet highly antigenic, preparation of tetanus toxin. It is usually adsorbed to alum to render it more immunogenic, and administered as a course of four injections as part of the DPT vaccination schedule. Protective antibodies develop in over 95 per cent of vaccinees. Older children who were not vaccinated in infancy should receive a primary course of two injections four to eight weeks apart, followed by a third injection six to 12 months later. In this situation, tetanus toxoid should be combined with diphtheria toxoid (DT) to ensure protection against both toxin-mediated diseases. Since the risk of pertussis is substantially lower in older children, and since adverse reactions to this vaccine appear to increase with age, DPT is not given to children over the age of two years in South Africa. Not all countries practise this age restriction for pertussis vaccine.

In areas where neonatal tetanus is common, routine vaccination of pregnant women in pregnancy or during the childbearing years may provide excellent protection for the newborn, because maternal tetanus antibodies cross the placenta efficiently and at high levels.

The only known contra-indication to tetanus vaccination is in those rare individuals who have shown severe hypersensitivity or neurological reactions to prior tetanus immunization.

## PERTUSSIS VACCINE

The conventional vaccine against whooping cough consists of a suspension of killed *Bordetella pertussis* organisms. It is usually given in conjunction with diphtheria and tetanus toxoids as the DPT vaccine. The primary immunization starts as early as six weeks of age, and consists of three injections given four weeks apart, with a fourth dose administered about one year later.

Vaccine efficacy is high, in the region of 80 per cent, but immunity may wane in young adults.

As there is no neonatal protection against pertussis, infectious cases in the community may have serious consequences.

Pertussis vaccine has been associated with a higher incidence of adverse events than other vaccines in general use. About 60 per cent of vaccinees experience pain at the injection site and fever. Prolonged crying is estimated to occur in about five per cent of recipients, and a high-pitched, abnormal cry in one in one thousand doses. Convulsions and hyporesponsive collapse are rare complications that have not been definitely associated with long-term ill effects.

Contra-indications to pertussis vaccination include a history of severe reaction to a previous dose including a fever greater than 40,5 °C, collapse, convulsions, prolonged or abnormal screaming, or encephalopathy. A personal history of convulsions should lead to deferment from vaccination. In the United Kingdom, a family history of convulsions or a family history of adverse reaction to pertussis vaccination is also considered a contra-indication to immunization.

Because of the fear of irreversible acute encephalopathy associated with pertussis vaccination in the United Kingdom and elsewhere, despite the fact that a causal role in this association remains unproven, the numbers of children vaccinated dropped markedly in the mid-1970s. The result was two major epidemics of pertussis in the late 1970s and early 1980s in Britain, with considerable morbidity and mortality. This experience indicated the need for ongoing vaccination against pertussis while research into improved vaccines continues. New pertussis vaccines (acellular vaccines) have recently been developed consisting of various components of the organism, including the filamentous haemagglutinin, pertussis toxoid, surface agglutinogens, and outer membrane proteins. These vaccines are immunogenic in experimental animals, and studies on protective efficacy in humans are the subject of ongoing randomized double-blinded clinical trials. Because these preparations lack endotoxin, they may be less likely to cause serious adverse reactions.

## Storage

- In refrigerator or cold box at 2–10 °C. *Must not freeze* as this causes irreversible clumping of antigen, and leads to irregular dosage and cyst formation.
- Avoid *direct sunlight*.

## Contra-indications to combined diphtheria, pertussis, and tetanus

- A severe local reaction. The definition of a severe local reaction is as follows: an extensive area of redness and swelling that becomes indurated and affects a large part of the surface of the limb. This is usually seen in people who have been immunized more frequently than is necessary.

- A severe general reaction. This may take several forms:
  - a fever of over 40,5 °C within 48 hours of immunization;
  - convulsions, prolonged unresponsiveness, or prolonged inconsolable screaming occurring within 72 hours of immunization;
  - anaphylaxis, bronchospasm, laryngeal oedema, or generalized collapse.

The first two reactions mentioned here constitute absolute contra-indications to giving pertussis immunization again. Only diphtheria and tetanus toxoids should be given in future immunizations. In the case of the third reaction, all three should be omitted. If tetanus toxoid is subsequently required, it should only be administered under careful supervision.

- Acute illnesses. Postpone immunization if the child is febrile (T > 38,5 °C). However, a slight cough or cold, diarrhoea, or mild skin rashes are not contra-indications to immunization.
- A history of convulsions or a progressive neurological disorder.

## Preventing febrile reactions

Paracetamol can be given immediately after DPT immunization, and repeated in four hours, to reduce chances of febrile reactions and/or seizures in susceptible infants.

## HAEMOPHILUS INFLUENZAE TYPE B VACCINE

Vaccination of children under two years of age is now possible with the use of conjugate *Haemophilus influenzae* vaccines. The use of

## Non-contra-indications

The following are not contra-indications to DPT immunization:
- mild local or mild general symptoms, which are to be expected six to eight hours after immunization;
- convulsions in siblings or close relatives;
- a history of asthma, eczema, hay fever, migraine, or food allergy;
- antibiotic or any other medication;
- developmental delay or stable neurological conditions (such as established cerebral palsy);
- failure to thrive, marasmus, or kwashiorkor;
- prematurity;
- previous history of pertussis; and
- HIV seropositivity or AIDS.

these vaccines in developed countries has resulted in a dramatic reduction in the incidence of invasive Haemophilus disease. The impact of vaccination has been greater than that predicted by consideration only of the number of children vaccinated in these countries. The reason for this increased impact is that there is evidence that conjugate *Haemophilus influenzae* vaccine prevents colonization of the nasopharynx with this pathogen. This impact on colonization interrupts the spread of organisms in the community so that vaccinated children may protect unvaccinated children from disease by interrupting the transmission of the organism to susceptible children.

## CONJUGATE HAEMOPHILUS INFLUENZAE TYPE B VACCINE (HIB)

There are four vaccines currently available world-wide. However, only two of these (HbOC and PRP-T (polyribosyl phosphate-T) are available in South Africa at the present time. The selection of these was based on field trials where conditions were comparable to those found locally including socio-economic circumstances and average age at which children were likely to experience their first infection.

HbOC vaccine and the PRP-T vaccine elicit similar immunogenicity. The HbOC vaccine consists of PRP conjugated to CRM (cross-reacting molecule). This is a mutant form of diphtheria toxin. The PRP-T conjugate is tetanus toxoid. The HbOC vaccine was shown to be efficacious in children in California when given at two, four, and six months of age. The protective efficacy in that trial was 100 per cent. The trial was conducted in a health maintenance organization with a patient demography representing a more affluent population than those at highest risk in South Africa. The organization did include some children of lower economic status. Preliminary data from immunogenicity studies on African children suggest that the vaccine is immunogenic, but slightly less so than that found in Californian children. The PRP-T vaccine gives similar immunogenicity to the HbOC vaccine. Immunogenicity data as well as the results of a prospective double blind clinical trial carried out in the Gambia will be available within the next few years. Although both of these vaccines are immunogenic in young children, the maximal immune response is found following only the third dose of the vaccine, suggesting that full immunity to disease is conferred only at about two weeks following the third dose. These data do raise some concern as to the efficacy of these vaccines in Africa where poor socio-economic status and overcrowding results in a high density of transmission with severe disease occurring commonly before the sixth month of life.

The final vaccine formulation available abroad is PRP-OMP. This vaccine uses the outer membrane proteins of the meningococcus as the conjugate. The vaccine was found to be 93 per cent to 100 per cent effective in preventing invasive disease in Navajo children when given at two and four months of age. The immune response to this vaccine is different from that of the HbOC and PRP-T vaccines in that there is good immunity after the first dose of the vaccine, but no subsequent significant booster response. This is the reason that the vaccine can be given in two doses. The early immunogenicity of this vaccine is attractive for use in Africa, but its production and standardization are complex. No clinical trials of this vaccine have been carried out to date in Africa.

## Recommendations for the use of *Haemophilus influenzae* vaccine

The new conjugate vaccines have been shown to be highly immunogenic and effective in the reduction of invasive *Haemophilus influenzae* disease in developed countries. They are protective against *Haemophilus influenzae* meningitis, pneumonia, epiglottitis, and osteomyelitis, but *not* against otitis media. The latter is often caused by infecting organisms that are non encapsulated (i.e., not Group B). Vaccination is now given free of charge to all children in South Africa at six, ten, and 14 weeks combined with DPT. There is a surveillance programme in place, and all children in South Africa who have HiB isolated from blood or CSF should be notified to the surveillance team to investigate whether the child has been vaccinated. It is possible that the vaccine may be less effective in HIV-infected children.

# Hepatitis B

Infection with hepatitis B virus (HBV) is one of the most important causes of chronic morbidity and mortality from cirrhosis, chronic liver failure, and primary liver cell cancer in sub-Saharan Africa and the Far East. In South Africa, up to 15 per cent of rural blacks have been shown to be HBV carriers. Transmission occurs horizontally in the first one or two years of life, and can be prevented by prior HBV immunization. Routine infant immunization has been recommended for such parts of the world by many agencies including WHO. Infants born to carrier mothers should receive HBV vaccine as a matter of urgency together with hyperimmune hepatitis B globulin.

The first generation of HBV vaccines were prepared by very extensive purification of HBsAg particles from blood units of donors who were carriers of the virus.

A second generation of vaccines produced by recombinant technology has been developed – the only human vaccines in current use produced by such means. Recombinant vaccines are prepared from yeast cultures where the viral gene coding for HBsAg protein is spliced into the DNA of the yeast cells. In this way, large amounts of particularly pure protein are produced. Both first- and second-generation vaccines are amongst the safest human vaccines known, and no contraindications exist.

The vaccine is routinely administered to all infants by intramuscular inoculation at

## Administering vaccines

### Simultaneous administration of vaccines

All vaccines may be administered simultaneously. MMR is a mix of three viral vaccines. When other viral vaccines, either live or attenuated, are administered at the same time as other immunizing agents, separate sites should be used. It is not necessary to restart an interrupted series of immunizations.

### Staggered administration of vaccines

If live attenuated viral vaccines are not given simultaneously, a succeeding live viral vaccine should not be given before a lapse of at least a month because of inactivation by induced interferon or other antiviral factors. This does not apply to inactivated vaccines, which can be staggered.

### Staggered administration of vaccines and globulins

Following the administration of hyperimmune globulin the corresponding vaccine should generally not be given until at least six weeks, but preferably three months, have elapsed. A blood or plasma transfusion may also inactivate a live virus vaccine given within the succeeding four to six weeks.

A period of at least four weeks is advisable between the commencement of any infectious disease and any immunization procedure.

### Economic and logistic factors

Immunization programmes are inevitably dependent on available resources. The distribution and accessibility of health care facilities determine whether immunization is integrated into comprehensive health care, provided by mobile outreach services, or delivered through intermittent mass campaigns. The latter may also be a crisis response to epidemic outbreaks.

It is noteworthy that the EPI programme takes cognizance not only of the provision of satisfactory vaccines, but also staff development, middle management, and community involvement.

the dosage schedule of six, ten, and fourteen weeks to fit in with routine EPI immunization protocols (Schoub et al., 1991).

# Other currently used viral vaccines

## MUMPS

Mumps vaccine is seldom administered on its own, but usually together with measles and rubella vaccines as a combined measles–mumps–rubella vaccine given by subcutaneous injection at 15 months of age. The vaccine is a live, attenuated vaccine, grown in fertilized chicken eggs and egg embryo cell culture. It is thus also contra-indicated in children with a history of severe egg hypersensitivity, and should also not be given to children with severe immunosuppression. Like measles, it is not known to be teratogenic.

## RUBELLA

Rubella vaccine is also a live, attenuated vaccine, but is grown in human diploid fibroblasts so that there are no contra-indications with respect to egg hypersensitivity. Being a live vaccine, however, it should, as with mumps and measles vaccine, not be given to individuals who are severely immunosuppressed.

Rubella vaccine is administered routinely, either combined with measles and mumps vaccine to all infants at 15 months of age, or as a single vaccine to the target population of schoolgirls just before they reach the reproductive age group. In developing countries selective immunization programmes of schoolgirls should be aimed for, as universal immunization of 15-month-old infants with MMR may be more detrimental if it is incomplete as the main age of infection could be shifted to an older age, i.e., the childbearing age when rubella is most problematic.

Rubella vaccine is absolutely contra-indicated during pregnancy, but no cases of teratogenicity were observed in some 2 000 cases of accidental immunization investigated and monitored by the Center for Disease Control. Inadvertent rubella immunization is therefore *not* a ground for termination of pregnancy. As with measles and mumps, administration of rubella vaccine by an unnatural route, subcutaneous inoculation means that vaccine-related illness is not contagious. In outbreak situations, immunization of children living in the same home as a susceptible pregnant mother is often recommended to prevent the infection from reaching her.

## INFLUENZA

Influenza vaccine in current use is prepared annually from circulating strains of virus as recommended by WHO. The vaccine consists of three strains, one from each of the influenza subtypes (WHO, 1999), H3N, H1N1, and influenza B, respectively. Influenza vaccine is prepared by inactivating by formaldehyde, virus strains grown in fertilized chicken eggs. The vaccine should therefore not be given to children with a history of severe hypersensitivity to eggs, but it is not otherwise contra-indicated.

Recommended indications for influenza immunization in paediatric practice include children who have been hospitalized and are receiving regular medical care for asthma, fibrocystic disease of the lungs, chronic heart disease with heart failure, children on immunosuppressive therapy, children symptomatically affected with HIV, and children on long-term aspirin therapy (because of the danger of Reye syndrome).

Influenza vaccine should be given by intramuscular injection as the immunogenicity is somewhat better and the side-effects somewhat less than with subcutaneous injection.

Side-effects with influenza vaccine occur more frequently in children. A split-product vaccine (prepared in the same way as the inactivated whole virus vaccine, but further purified by digesting off the lipid membrane from the surface haemagglutinin and neuraminidase proteins) or purified subunit vaccine are the preferred vaccines in paediatric practice. Children less than nine years of age who have never previously been vaccinated should receive two full doses of vaccine separated by one month, and those less than three years of age, half the adult dose on two occasions separated by a month.

## YELLOW FEVER VACCINE

This vaccine should be used for travellers journeying to countries where yellow fever is endemic, such as tropical Africa and tropical south and central America. The vaccine is a live, attenuated vaccine made in fertilized chicken eggs, and is consequently contraindicated in children hypersensitive to egg protein. It is also contra-indicated in infants less than six months of age as the majority of encephalitis complications from the vaccine have been observed in children of this age. Immunosuppressed children must also not receive yellow fever vaccine. It is administered as a single subcutaneous inoculation at least two weeks before leaving for travel. Immunity is of some ten years' duration.

## RABIES VACCINE

The rabies vaccine is an inactivated viral vaccine made from virus grown in human diploid cell culture, and then inactivated with B-proprionolactone. The vaccine is consequently safe, and no contra-indications exist. It is administered by subcutaneous injection (although for pre-exposure prophylaxis the intradermal route has been used to save costs). Children exposed to rabies from the bite of an infected animal or an animal suspected to be rabid should receive post-

exposure prophylaxis. Injections of vaccine should be carried out at days 0, 3, 7, 14, and 30. Unless the wound is superficial or the exposure is only via mucous membranes, the first dose should be supplemented with hyperimmune rabies globulin, and a further vaccine dose given at 90 days.

## HEPATITIS A

Passive immunization is available for protection against hepatitis A. It can be used for:
* pre-exposure, e.g., susceptible travellers in high-risk situations – immunity lasts for up to three months;
* post-contact – early administration may abort the infection. If given later but within 10 to 14 days (and preferably as early as possible) of contact the disease may be attenuated;
* the control of outbreaks and protection of susceptible contacts.

The following general guidelines are useful in selecting individuals for immunoprophylaxis:
* family members or other persons living in the same house as an index case with hepatitis A;
* children or adults living in the same boarding school, institution, barracks, etc. as an index case of hepatitis A, and who share sleeping quarters and who eat together.

It is worth noting that because a larger proportion of adults in South Africa (50 per cent) have hepatitis A antibodies, locally prepared pooled globulin is probably more effective against hepatitis A than is the European product.

An inactivated hepatitis A vaccine has recently become available, and is administered by intramuscular injection as two doses separated by six months.

## CHOLERA VACCINE

The routinely used cholera vaccine consists of killed *vibrio cholerae* organisms and can be administered intramuscularly or subcutaneously to infants six months of age or older. The efficacy of the vaccine is poor, and immunity is short lived. It is administered only to comply with travel requirements for certain countries. Optimal protection against cholera consists of avoiding food and water that might be contaminated.

The most common adverse reactions are local tenderness, malaise, and fever.

# Other currently used or available bacterial vaccines

## MENINGOCOCCAL POLYSACCHARIDE VACCINE

Vaccines are now available for protection against meningococcal types A, C, Y, and W135. There is no vaccine against type B, which remains common in many areas, thus limiting the efficacy of routine immunization. Vaccination is indicated for protection of individuals at high risk of infection, e.g., during epidemics in closed institutions.

A single intramuscular injection stimulates high antibody levels in individuals over the age of two years. Booster doses are not recommended. Adverse reactions, including local pain, are rare, and there are no known contra-indications to the use of this vaccine.

## PNEUMOCOCCAL VACCINE

This vaccine initially contained 14 different capsular types of *Streptococcus pneumoniae*, but an improved 23-valent vaccine has since become available. The types contained in the vaccine represent the majority of those that cause bacteraemic pneumococcal infection in the community. The vaccine is quite immunogenic, giving rise to detectable antibody levels in over 80 per cent of vaccinees. Clinical efficacy has been shown by the marked reduction of pneumococcal disease among vaccinated South African gold miners. The efficacy of the vaccine in the general population not considered to be particularly at risk for pneumococcal infection has been less well documented. Only a few of the 23 antigens are immunogenic in children, and the major childhood invasive serotypes 6A, 6B, 9V, 14, 19A, and 23F are not immunogenic in young children. Conjugate vaccines similar to those licensed for *Haemophilus influenzae* are under investigation for use in children.

Paediatric indication for the existing 23-valent pneumococcal vaccine is primarily in individuals with functional or anatomical asplenia. While efficacy is greatest when administered prior to splenectomy, protective levels of antibody are induced when the vaccine is administered after removal of the spleen. A single dose is given by intramuscular injection, and boosters should be given to children at risk within five years.

## TYPHOID FEVER VACCINE

The routinely available typhoid fever vaccine consists of killed *Salmonella typhi* bacilli. It is administered as two subcutaneous injections, two weeks to one month apart. The protection afforded by the vaccine is in the region of 60 to 70 per cent and lasts for up to three years only. Typhoid vaccination is occasionally recommended for travellers to endemic areas or for household contacts of typhoid carriers. For travellers, avoidance of potentially contaminated food and water is probably more efficacious in preventing typhoid fever than is vaccination. For household contacts, newer, more immunogenic vaccines may be of great benefit for the protection of individuals in communities where typhoid fever is endemic.

Local reactions and fever occur commonly after typhoid vaccination. There are no known contra-indications to its use.

Several new candidate typhoid vaccines have emerged, offering potentially greater protection without significant adverse reactions. These include the attenuated *S. typhi* strain used as a live, oral vaccine (TY21a) and a purified subunit parenteral vaccine consisting of the Vi polysaccharide antigen of virulent *S. typhi*. The TY21a must be given in four doses, maintenance of the cold chain is essential, and it should not be given together with mefloquine prophylaxis for malaria, because the mefloquine may inactivate the vaccine. The currently available formulation in an enteric-coated capsule has shown variable protective efficacy, and has not been proven to be effective in highly endemic areas. A formulation in which a live suspension of organisms is given may be more effective, but it is not yet commercially available.

The Vi capsular polysaccharide vaccine was first documented to be efficacious in a large clinical trial in South Africa. It is given as a single intramuscular dose. Typhoid vaccines only give short-lasting and incomplete protection against typhoid fever, as, unlike most viral diseases and many vaccine-preventable bacterial diseases, the natural disease of typhoid itself does not confer long-lasting immunity, and a sufficiently large infective dose will cause reinfection. These vaccines should therefore be restricted to travellers, outbreak situations, and in rural areas where there are high levels of endemic disease without the prospect of improved sanitation and water supplies. The control of typhoid rests on these latter engineering provisions, and not on a typhoid vaccine.

# Future vaccines

Rotavirus vaccines are currently being evaluated (see Chapter 24: Vaccine-preventable infectious diseases). The use of synthetic peptides for a malaria vaccine has shown promise in a number of South American countries and is under investigation in the Gambia.

No significantly effective HIV vaccine has been documented to date.

A large number of childhood infections are theoretically amenable to prevention by vaccination, including Group A and Group B streptococcal disease, as well as the remaining important bacterial and viral pathogens causing pneumonia and diarrhoeal disease. The development of these vaccines will be one of the challenges of the next few decades.

# Conclusion

It is repeatedly emphasized that vaccination is the single most cost-effective strategy in medicine and public health. It would seem to be axiomatic that universal provision of vaccines that protect against diseases of the greatest severity would be seen as the highest priority of every health ministry, and that community-based immunization programmes would be standard practice in every country in the world. This still remains an unattainable goal, particularly in developing countries. Various global programmes such as EPI are addressing these issues, but every child health worker must accept the responsibility for the promotion of universal immunization (see Chapter 19: Global strategies for child health).

# References and further reading

ANON.1988. Report of the Committee on Infectious Disease, 21st ed. Evanston: American Academy of Pediatrics.

BLACK SB, SHINEFIELD HR, HIATT RA, et al. 1991. Efficacy in infancy of oligosaccharide conjugate *Haemophilus influenzae* type B (HbOC vaccine) in a United States population of 61,080 children. *Pediatric Infectious Disease Journal*. 10:97.

COLDITZ GA, BREWER TF, BERKEY CS, et al. 1994. Efficacy of BCG vaccine in the prevention of tuberculosis. *Journal of the American Medical Association*. 271:698–702.

HINMAN AR, BART KJ, and ORENSTEIN WA. 1985. Immunisation. In: *Principles and practice of infectious disease*. London: John Wiley.

KLUGMAN KP, GILBERTSON IT, KOORNHOF HJ, et al. 1987. Protective efficacy of Vi capsular polysaccharide against typhoid fever. *Lancet.*: 1165–69.

NICHOLL A, ELLIMAN D, and BEGG NT. 1989. Immunisation: Causes of failure and strategies and tactics for success. *British Medical Journal*. 299:808–12.

SCHOUB BD, JOHNSON S, MCANERNEY JM, BLACKBURN NK, KEW MC, MCCUTCHEON JP, and CARLIER ND. 1991. Integration of hepatitis B vaccination into rural African primary health care programmes. *British Medical Journal*. 302:313–16.

WORLD HEALTH ORGANIZATION. 1999. *Weekly epidemiological record*. 74:321–8.

ZUCKERMAN JA. 2001. *British Medical Journal*. 321:1237–8.

# PART NINE

# Measuring and monitoring

All child health professionals should have a basic understanding of the skills required to monitor the health of the child population they serve, and the quality of their service. Knowing the extent and size of anything that is to be studied or assessed enables planning of interventions and evaluation of outcomes. Strategies to achieve this and to determine the validity of findings are incorporated in the following chapters.

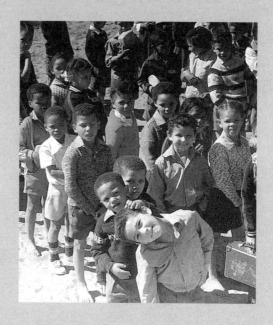

# 26    Epidemiology

D YACH, D BRADSHAW
& J IRLAM

Epidemiology is defined as the study of the distribution and determinants of disease in human populations. The word is derived from the Greek words 'epi' (upon) and 'demos' (people). It is concerned with the health of populations rather than individuals, and is used to study relationships between people, their diseases, and the agents that cause or prevent or cure these diseases in the environment. Research is a systematic plan used to discover facts or principles, and the central focus of epidemiology is on the use of research methods. Clinical epidemiology incorporates the principles and techniques of epidemiology in patient care (Sackett et al., 1988).

The purpose of epidemiological research in child health is to improve the quality of health care for children and to determine which interventions are necessary to achieve their maximum health potential. Epidemiological methods are of use to all health professionals involved in child care, whether they work in private practice, in a hospital/clinic setting, or are public health professionals mainly interested in community health.

This chapter serves as a guide for the child health practitioner who is interested in epi-

demiological research. An understanding of epidemiology will also provide practising doctors with a valuable tool for evaluating their own work and that of others.

## Epidemiological methods

Epidemiological methods are used to describe, investigate, or evaluate:
- the extent of health problems in the community and identifying inequalities;
- the availability and use of health services;
- the causes of disease and their ways of transmission;
- the natural history of disease;
- the basis for prevention programmes; and
- the effectiveness of preventive, therapeutic, or overall health service interventions.

## General epidemiological concepts

Epidemiology involves the use of *qualitative* and *quantitative* methods.

242

*Qualitative methods* such as participant observation, in-depth and semi-structured interviews are methods derived from the disciplines of anthropology and sociology, which are used to formulate precise research questions. These methods should precede any quantitative approach. This chapter will deal only with quantitative approaches and should be read in conjunction with Chapter 27: Some statistical concepts.

Central to the notion of quantification is the need to have a clear method of defining what is being measured.

# Categories of information used in epidemiology

There are three major categories of information: outcomes, exposures, and confounders. This information is collected either as *categorical* data (such as gender or social class) or *continuous* data (e.g., age, weight). Continuous data can assume a potentially infinite number of values along a continuum.

Information relating to the *outcome* may include mortality data (deaths), morbidity data (disease, including notifiable diseases), nutritional status, psychological status, and dental health status.

*Exposure* information includes risk factors for disease such as quality of housing, water supply or sanitation, as well as factors beneficial to health such as immunization and breast-feeding.

A *confounding factor* is associated with both the exposure and the disease. Depending on the strength and direction of these associations, a confounding factor may either spuriously strengthen or dilute an association. For example, when studying the relationship between indoor air pollution from wood fires and acute respiratory infections, it is necessary to take into account the role of tobacco smoking. Parental smoking would be the con-

founder or nuisance variable that must be controlled (see below) in order to obtain an undistorted estimate of the effect of air pollution.

# Measurement error

All three categories of information are subject to error. There are two broad types of possible measurement error.

Systematic measurement error (or *bias*) occurs when an observer or instrument measures an attribute repeatedly higher or lower than the real value. *Random error* occurs when measurements are sometimes higher and sometimes lower than the true value being estimated and results in imprecise or unreliable summary measures of effect. Random measurement error refers to the concordance reached in repeated measurements, irrespective of how close they are to the true value.

*Inter-observer reliability* refers to the concordance between two (or more) observers if they use the same instrument to measure an attribute in the same individual under the same conditions.

Systematic error affects the *validity* (or truth) of the estimated effects, and random error affects the *precision* of estimated effects (Sackett et al., 1988).

In all research projects it is essential to identify potential sources of both systematic and random measurement error and to take steps when planning to minimize important sources of error. Training observers, excluding sloppy observers, calibrating measurement tools, and standardizing the measurement techniques are all important in this regard.

# The case definition

An adequate definition is needed to determine which patients qualify as cases for the purpose of epidemiological studies. Case definitions

243

may be rigorous or loose, but ideally incorporate as many of the true cases, while excluding as many of the false cases, as possible.

Rigorous case definitions have the advantage of excluding nearly all the non-cases but may exclude cases that supply important clues to the cause of the condition. On the other hand, a loose case definition will tend to dilute the association between exposure and risk of disease by including many non-cases. For these reasons, epidemiological and clinical case criteria are rarely identical. The clinician must identify all true cases and avoid treating non-cases, while comparability and reliability are important considerations in epidemiological research.

## Sensitivity and specificity

*Sensitivity* is a measure of the ability of a test to correctly identify all true cases, while *specificity* is a measure of the ability of a test to correctly identify non-cases. Sensitivity is syn-onymous with the true positive rate (i.e., true positives as a percentage of all positive test results) and specificity is synonymous with the true negative rate (i.e., true negatives as a percentage of all negative test results). *Positive predictive value* refers to the ability of the test to correctly identify true positives (i.e., the percentage of positive test results that are true positives), while the *negative predictive value* refers to the percentage of negative test results that are true negatives.

In practice, the predictive values of the test are more important to the clinician than sensitivity and specificity but they are strongly influenced by the prevalence of the disease being studied.

In general, the ability of a screening or diagnostic test to correctly identify positive and negative cases is less in the community than in the clinical setting.

In Table 26.1 the trade-off between having a highly sensitive test (1) or a highly specific test (4) is illustrated. For epidemiological purposes the definition of a cough as lasting for

**Table 26.1** Sensitivity, specificity, and predictive values of clinical definitions for pertussis (compared with culture results)**

|  | CULTURE RESULTS | | |
|---|---|---|---|
|  | + | − | Sensitivity=A/(A+C) |
| Clinical symptom + | A (true positive) | B (false positive) | Specificity=D/(B+D) <br> Positive predictive value (PPV) = A/(A+B) |
| − | C (false negative) | D (true negative) | Negative predictive value (NPV)=D/(C+D) <br> Accuracy+(A+D)/(A+B+C+D) |

| SYMPTOMS USED | A | B | C | D | SENS* | SPEC* | PPV | NPV |
|---|---|---|---|---|---|---|---|---|
| 1 Any symptom or sign of acute respiratory illness | 118 | 115 | 0 | 0 | 100% | 0% | 51% | n/a |
| 2 Acute cough | 116 | 83 | 2 | 32 | 98% | 28% | 58% | 94% |
| 3 Cough – more than 14 days | 99 | 43 | 19 | 72 | 84% | 63% | 70% | 79% |
| 4 Sleep disturbance, fever | 16 | 4 | 102 | 111 | 14% | 97% | 80% | 52% |

\*   Values derived from 2×2 table above
\*\*  Patriarca et al., 1988

at least 14 days (3) provides reasonable sensitivity and specificity, and very adequate predictive values (Patriarca et al., 1988).

## Incidence and prevalence

Two measures of disease frequency are incidence and prevalence.

The incidence reflects the rate of new cases and the prevalence reflects the current cases (old and new).

Prevalence constitutes a balance sheet between incidence (new cases) on the inlet side and death/recovery on the outlet side (see Figure 26.1).

Under stable conditions, prevalence reflects the incidence and the duration of the condition studied.

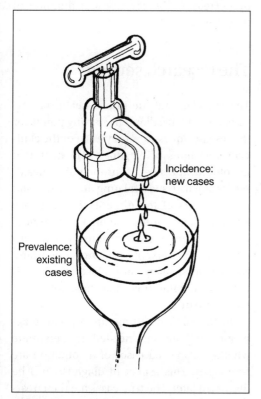

**Figure 26.1** Incidence vs. prevalence

From this we can deduce that prevalence serves as a measure for chronic diseases or the burden of chronic illness in the community, but it may be quite misleading as a measure for acute diseases or acute episodes of chronic illness.

More formally, incidence refers to the number of new cases reported during a specified follow-up period in a defined population. The source of this information can either be specially designed follow-up studies or routine public health surveillance. For example, the notifications of infectious disease and the registration of deaths are both examples of the measure of incidence. Incidence is therefore a useful measure for evaluating the effect of preventive measures on the occurrence of new cases.

Prevalence and incidence do not necessarily measure the same trend. If, for instance, a new and effective therapy is introduced, prevalence may well increase as a result of increased survival despite incidence remaining unchanged or even decreasing.

Incidence is a dynamic measure, whereas prevalence is a static measure. The prevalence of disease refers to the number of people who have a particular condition during a specific period, usually a single point in time. Several *prevalence measures* are commonly used in child health as indicators of the burden of chronic illness in communities (see Table 26.5). These include disability and nutritional deficiency rates. Whereas the source for incidence data is usually routinely available records or follow-up studies, information for prevalence studies must generally be obtained from community-based surveys. Registers maintained by a variety of organizations dedicated to specific disorders (e.g., cerebral palsy, intellectual disability) are also useful sources of prevalence data.

Both incident and prevalent cases form the numerator for calculating rates, a rate being the expression of the frequency with

The image labels read:

Incidence: new cases

Prevalence: existing cases

which an event occurs in a defined population. The use of rates rather than raw numbers (the numerators) is essential for the comparison of populations at different times, in different places, or among different classes of people (Last, 1988).

*Rate* = number of events in a specified period/average population during the period $\times 10^n$ per time period.

The *incidence rate* most often used in public health practice is calculated by the formula: number of new events in a specified period/number of persons exposed to risk during this period $\times 10^n$ per time period.

In a dynamic population, the denominator is the average size of the population, while in a follow-up study (e.g., a birth cohort study) the initial size of the cohort of persons being followed makes up the denominator.

Incidence rates can be calculated using hospital/clinic data or (preferably) community-based data. The number of first-time visits to a specific hospital in a specified time period divided by the total number of children at risk for that condition in the drainage or referral area of that hospital would be an example of an incidence rate derived from hospital data.

This rate will probably reflect the most severe cases of disease. Further, it will probably represent those cases with the best access to health care. To have a more complete picture of incidence, it is necessary to add to this total all first-time visits to GPs and clinics of children from the same drainage or referral area of the hospital, within the same period. To determine the total incidence it will be necessary to obtain the total number of new cases arising in the same community who do not seek care during the period of interest (see Follow-up studies below).

Death or *mortality rates* are the purest forms of incidence rates. The numerator can only occur once! Table 26.2 gives the formulae for commonly used infant and child mortality rates. The most important ones for child health include the infant mortality rate (IMR) which is made up of a neonatal (NMR) and a post-neonatal mortality (PNMR) component. The IMR is an overall indicator of child health and of the health of the population. Distinguishing between the NMR and PNMR can determine whether environmental/social factors or perinatal/delivery factors are the more important contributors to the IMR. The second most commonly used incidence rates are those for notifiable diseases. In South Africa these are predominantly infectious diseases such as tuberculosis, measles, and hepatitis.

Incidence and prevalence are influenced by different intervention strategies. Primordial and primary prevention aim to reduce the incidence of disease in a community. Secondary prevention reduces the prevalence of disease by decreasing the severity and duration of that disease.

# The research setting

The clinician and the public health professional often have different starting points for the research questions they ask. For the clinician, questions of diagnosis and treatment are of critical concern. For the public health professional, issues relating to causes and determinants of the disease, the incidence and prevalence of disease on a community-wide basis, and the effectiveness of community-based interventions are important. Nevertheless, there are close similarities between community- and hospital/clinic-based research.

In the clinical setting, appropriate diagnostic methods are needed to determine whether suspected cases of a condition are true cases. This aspect of diagnosis will be discussed later. The true cases are then treated, and it is important to determine the

**Table 26.2** Selected measures or indicators of infant and child mortality

| | | |
|---|---|---|
| Infant mortality rate = (IMR) | $\dfrac{\text{Number of deaths in a year of children under one year of age}}{\text{number of live births in the same year}} \times 1000$ | This index not only reflects the health status of children under one year of age, but it also reflects the overall environmental and health service inputs in a community. It is a key indicator for comparing the health status of countries or regions. |
| Neonatal mortality rate = (NMR) | $\dfrac{\text{Number of deaths of infants under 28 days of age in a year}}{\text{number of live births in the same year}} \times 1000$ | This reflects the effectiveness of maternity/child services at the time of delivery. It reflects the quality of antenatal care and access to ICU. |
| Postneonatal mortality rate = (PNMR) | $\dfrac{\text{Number of deaths of infants between 28 days and one year of age in a year}}{\text{number of live births in the same year}} \times 1000$ | This reflects the quality of the physical environment (water, sanitation, fuel), the social environment (quality of care), immunization status, and nutrition (breast-feeding). |
| Perinatal mortality rate* = | $\dfrac{\text{Stillbirths over 500 g plus deaths in first week of life}}{\text{total number of stillbirths and live births in the same year}} \times 1000$ | This reflects the effectiveness of maternity/child services at the time of delivery. It reflects the quality of antenatal care and access to ICU. |
| Child death rate = | $\dfrac{\text{Number of deaths of children aged between one and four years in a given year}}{\text{number of children in this age group}} \times 1000$ | Similar to PNMR with even more emphasis on the physical environment. |
| Under-five mortality rate = | Probability of a newborn dying before the age of five. $\dfrac{\text{Number of deaths of children aged 0–4 years in a given year}}{\text{number of children in this age group.}} \times 1000$ | This is a general child health status indicator that also reflects the overall environmental and health service inputs in a community. It is increasingly becoming important for comparing regions and countries. |
| Cause-specific mortality rate = | $\dfrac{\text{Number of deaths from cause A in a given year}}{\text{number of children in the appropriate age group}} \times 1000$ | This rate indicates the extent of mortality due to a particular cause. |
| Case fatality rate ** = (percentage) | $\dfrac{\text{Number of children dying during specified period after disease B onset or diagnosis}}{\text{number of children with disease B}} \times 1000$ | This reflects the proportion of children with a particular disease who die from that disease. |

\* Several definitions are used. The World Health Organization definition is used here
\*\* Actually a ratio (not a rate)

efficacy (whether the treatment works when given under ideal circumstances) and the effectiveness (if it works when given under field conditions). Randomized controlled trials are used in this context.

In reality, the number of cases of disease seen by clinicians reflects only a small proportion of the true cases that may arise in a community over a period of time. Furthermore, it is possible that a larger proportion of cases from higher social classes attend the clinic/hospital. To determine the true burden of disease, it is therefore not sufficient to use clinic/hospital data alone, but information on the prevalence and incidence in the community must also be available.

The setting has a bearing both on the type of epidemiological research carried out and on the inferences that can be drawn from it. For example, a clinician in a hospital or private practice is able to describe the characteristics of his or her patients seen during a certain time period. This constitutes a case series. A summary of these patients may be useful in drawing inferences about the quality of clinical care provided and enable the clinician to set priorities within that setting. However, a major drawback to clinically based research is that the attendance pattern is unclear – the likelihood of individuals in the community presenting to a specific clinical practice is not known. This limits the possibilities of drawing inferences beyond the specific clinical setting.

Since the quality of follow-up, particularly in specialist clinics, is likely to be very high, long-term studies to examine the natural history of a disease are well suited to such settings.

In contrast, public health professionals need to make inferences regarding health service provision at a community or population level. In this chapter, epidemiological concepts and methods useful for all child health professionals are discussed.

# Types of studies

In epidemiology three broad categories of study are used: descriptive studies quantify the extent of a problem; analytic studies aim to identify risk factors amenable to intervention; and intervention studies broadly assess the effectiveness of interventions.

## DESCRIPTIVE STUDIES

## Use of information collected routinely

Descriptive studies are used to quantify the extent of health problems applying to people, places, and times, as well as the availability of health services and their use in a population. The place to start when conducting a descriptive study is by exploring the availability and quality of data routinely collected and its transformation into information.

Table 26.3 summarizes the source and quality of child health data routinely available in South Africa.

As can be seen from Table 26.3, each source of information has certain problems with respect to quality. By and large, black mortality suffers particularly from severe under-registration and misclassification of the causes (Botha & Bradshaw, 1985). The latter refers particularly to the high proportion of deaths that are categorized as ill-defined.

With respect to notifications (see Table 26.4), diagnostic inaccuracies, incomplete identification of cases, and failures of the recording systems all contribute to errors in identifying cases accurately and completely.

It can be seen from Table 26.4 that in the general population there has been a dramatic increase in the incidence of malaria, a significant decrease in measles and typhoid and a swing from a decrease to an increase in TB. The extent of under-reporting with respect to notifications and the under-registration of mortali-

**Table 26.3** Child health statistics routinely available in South Africa

*Mortality* – *national*
Source – Central Statistical Services (tables), CERSA, MRC (computer tape)
Quality – (a) under-registration, mainly of African deaths
(b) misclassification of the cause of death with a high percentage of ill-defined causes.
*Mortality* – *local*
Source – Local authorities (MOH reports)
Quality – (a) misclassification of the cause of death with a high percentage of ill-defined causes.
(b) not complete due to lack of exchange between authorities.
*Morbidity: notifiable conditions – national*
Source – Department of Health (Epi Comments)
Quality – (a) under-reporting
(b) variation in diagnostic reporting practices by geographical area
*Morbidity: notifiable conditions – local*
Source – Local authorities (MOH reports)
Quality – (a) under-reporting
(b) variation in diagnostic reporting practices by geographical area
*Births* – *national*
Source – Central Statistical Services, birth registration and censuses (1980, 1985, 1991, and 1996)
Quality – (a) birth registration – extensive under-registration
(b) national census – incomplete as the deaths are omitted
*Births* – *local*
Source – local authorities (MOH reports)
Quality – under-reporting among blacks

ty has not been adequately assessed. There may therefore be large errors in the comparison of areas and population groups. Despite this, errors are likely to be smaller when assessing trends over time within the same area.

A common problem relating to morbidity and mortality data is that the population at risk (the denominator) is often underestimated or unknown. However, the Human Sciences Research Council produces population figures corrected for the undercount and extrapolations between the censuses. Births, which form the denominator for several of the rates in Table 26.2, are particularly poorly documented for blacks in rural areas. There is a need in most countries for correlation between birth and death certification that would allow, for example, ongoing national surveillance of birthweight-

**Table 26.4** Notifications of selected infectious diseases in South Africa, 1998

| Disease | Total | Incidence Rate per 100 000 Population (All Race Groups) | | | |
|---|---|---|---|---|---|
| | | 1970* | 1980* | 1990* | 1998+ |
| Malaria | 26 388 | 0,6 | 10,7 | 18,3 | 65,0 |
| Measles | 1 058 | – | 65,8 | 28,6 | 2,6 |
| TB | | | | | |
| – Meninges | 470 | – | – | – | |
| – Pulmonary | 73 928 | – | – | – | – |
| Total | 87 090 | 274,4 | 189,6 | 216,2 | 214,5 |
| Typhoid | 419 | 19,1 | 15,0 | 5,8 | 1,0 |

*Epidemiological Comments, March 1994
+Epidemiological Comments, September 1999

specific mortality trends, and changes in the causes of death (Arden-Miller et al., 1989).

Annual reports published by the Medical Officers of Health in the larger local authorities usually include data on child health in the area served. This information is often neglected.

With increasing computerization of hospital and clinic records, it is likely that hospitals will become a useful source for child health statistics. However, for the foreseeable future, the variable reporting formats and definitions used for disease, the difficulty of defining who constitutes an admission or what the appropriate denominator should be, and the variable referral patterns between hospitals imply that hospital data are unreliable for epidemiological purposes. This also applies to several other child health indicators such as birthweight and iron deficiency anaemia.

Health service information is difficult to compare and interpret because of discrepancies in data collection.

Despite several problems with routinely available data, it still constitutes an essential body of information that has been underused. Greater use of available sources by child health professionals would, in all likelihood, result in improvements in the quality and coverage of data collection.

Until national data are available, the emphasis should be on sentinel, regional or district level child health groups collecting only the key indicators of child health. Selected aspects of health (or its indicators) can be used to show progress, and to measure change. Indicators often consist of measurements and are expressed in numbers, such as percentages, rates, and ratios. Table 26.5 compares key child health indicators from the United States (Arden-Miller et al., 1989) and the United Kingdom (Allsop et al., 1989) with those developed by the Department of Health (September 1997) for evaluating its goals and objectives for maternal, women's, and child health by the year 2000. It can be seen that in the United

## Sources of measurement error: birthweight

Birthweight is the most universally reliable indicator of fetal maturity. It is subject to several sources of measurement error.

**Subject variation**
This includes:
- the amount of placental blood infused (which may vary according to the local policy about when to clamp the cord); and
- when the child is weighed (may vary from immediately after birth to two or three days later).

**Observer variation**
This includes:
- the presence of inaccurate or poorly calibrated scales;
- inaccurate reading of the scales;
- rounding up or down of readings; and
- end-digit preference (with a high proportion of weights in clinics being recorded exactly on the 2 500 g point. This is particularly problematic as 2 500 g is the point below which children are defined as being of low birthweight).

States, age-specific indicators are used, while several broad areas relate to the aims of child health services in the United Kingdom.

The Year 2000 Indicators are based on the health objectives contained in the draft White Paper for the Transformation of the Health System in South Africa. The definitions of these indicators arise from internationally accepted definitions, and from the National and Provincial Departments of Health. A copy of the Year 2000 Indicators can be accessed via the website: www.hst.org.za/pubs/year 2000.htm.

Indicators appropriate to southern Africa are needed, and could be adapted from these

**Table 26.5** Child health indicators in the United States, United Kingdom, and South Africa

*United States of America (1989)*
(all 12 indicators shown)
1   Newborn, infants
  – inadequate antenatal care
  – low birthweight
  – IMR, NMR, PNMR
2   Children
  – inadequate immunization
  – population-based growth stunting
  – elevated blood lead level
  – non-motor vehicle traumatic deaths
3   Adolescents, young adults
  – births to school-age mothers
  – suicide
  – motor vehicle accident deaths
4   All ages
  – iron deficiency anaemia
  – child abuse

*United Kingdom (1989)*
• Death
  – IMR, NMR, PNMR, CMR, deaths from accidents, diarrhoea, pneumonia
• Immunization coverage
• Acute illness
  – notifications for measles, rubella, pertussis
  – admission to hospital for fractures, asthma
• Chronic illness
  – severe disability
• Psychological and behavioural disturbances
  – rates of marital breakdown
  – school failure and drop-out
• Health promotion
  – alcohol, smoking, drug use
  – teenage pregnancies

• Optimal child development
  – changes over age in height, weight
  – birthweight
• Social and geographical equity
  – variation in birthweight, immunization coverage
  – smoking rates by area and social class

*Year 2000 Health Goals, Objectives, and Indicators for South Africa* (September 1997)
1   Child health
  – immunization status at one year
  – proportion of low birthweight infants
  – nutritional status
  – growth monitoring
  – breastfeeding rates at 4–6 and 12 months
  – cause-specific mortality rates (neonatal, infant, under 5)
  – incidence of acute flaccid paralysis and neonatal tetanus
• Maternal, reproductive, and women's health
  – proportion of deliveries in institutions attended by trained personnel
  – proportion of pregnant women who receive antenatal care
  – contraceptive prevalence rate
  – proportion of pregnant women immunized against tetanus
• Adolescent health
  – prevalence of substance abuse (smoking, alcohol, drugs)
  – suicide rate
  – proportion of teenage births
  – STD prevalence
  – HIV prevalence

lists. The indicators should be selected to demonstrate the extent to which social policies in general and health services in particular have been effectively directed to meet child health needs. They should include specific reference to assault among young adults, substance abuse, and HIV infection. More specifically they should:
• reflect important health concerns;
• be understandable to policy makers;
• use data easily obtained; and
• relate to conditions that could be prevented or greatly reduced by using available interventions.

251

## Community-based surveys

After determining that information required is not available from routine sources or, if available, that the information is of dubious quality, a survey may be carried out, and this should be carefully planned.

The cross-sectional or descriptive study is a useful means of obtaining estimates of a number of key indicators of child health. These may relate to outcome, such as infant mortality or nutritional status, to health service process measures such as immunization coverage, knowledge of mothers and caregivers about sugar/salt solution preparation, or to the extent of growth monitoring in an area. All of these questions require careful attention to the sampling strategy as well as to measurement issues discussed earlier.

It is rarely feasible or desirable to include all the children of a given area (i.e., the population) in a study. Rather, a selected subset of the population (i.e., a sample) is chosen so that results are representative of the whole population.

Random sampling ensures that all individuals in a population have a known chance of being selected. This means that the results of a random (or probability) sample can be reliably used to make inferences about larger populations.

Such samples are either simple random, stratified random, systematic, cluster, or a mixture of these. In any sampling scheme, the key concept is always to ensure that the resulting sampling is representative (qualitatively) of the target population. Sampling is discussed further in the section on statistics.

## Selection bias

Selection bias is a reflection of failed sampling. In conducting a study there will almost always be some omissions (in cross-sectional studies) or drop-outs (in follow-up studies). It is important to try to limit the number of missed individuals, since they may have some special characteristics that could bias the results of the study. For example, when conducting a nutritional study of pre-school children, a high proportion of children may not be at home at the time of the survey, but at a crèche. If children in the crèche are better (or worse) nourished than those present in the community, the results would be biased.

In community surveys, several visits late in the afternoon may be required to ensure that all potential respondents are included.

## Reporting bias

Problems with reporting constitute a common measurement bias. In most epidemiological studies that involve children, information is required that necessitates the mother or caregiver being present at the time of the study. Studies conducted in the South African setting indicate that anywhere between 20 and 40 per cent of mothers may be absent at the time of the interview, so that the interviewer is dependent on information obtained from the caregiver. Since the quality of information regarding knowledge and attitudes of the mother is often not reliably obtainable from a caregiver, this information should be coded separately, so that separate analyses can be conducted according to the identity of the respondent.

Wherever possible, verifiable sources should be used to obtain information. For example, immunization status should be obtained from a clinic or Road to Health Chart.

## ANALYTIC STUDIES

Analytic studies are conducted to try to determine the causes of disease. In general epidemiological texts, emphasis is placed on the infectious, chemical, and physical agents, and on the host and environmental factors modified by health service interventions, which influence disease incidence.

This model, however, is not particularly useful for paediatric epidemiology as it generally neglects the socio-economic determinants for child survival. An alternative framework, developed by Moseley and Chen (1984), uses the concept of proximate determinants (Figure 26.2). These are intermediate variables and mechanisms that may be used interchangeably.

Maternal factors (age, parity, birth interval) exert an independent influence on pregnancy outcome and infant survival. Environmental contamination refers to the transmission of agents to children (and mothers). Nutrition and nutrient deficiency relates to the intake of three major classes of nutrients; calories, proteins, and the micronutrients (which would include vitamins). A critical point is that the

survival of children is influenced by nutrients available not only to the child, but also to the mother.

Injury includes physical injury, burns, and poisoning. Personal illness control refers to measures taken to avoid disease. These may include traditional behaviours as well as modern practices such as immunization. An important inclusion here is the practice and quality of care during pregnancy and child birth.

The second component, medical treatment, relates to those measures taken to cure diseases after they have become manifest (i.e., secondary prevention).

Proximate determinants influence the rate at which healthy individuals become sick. Ultimately, there is either complete recovery, increasing degrees of permanent growth faltering or other disability among the survivors, and/or death.

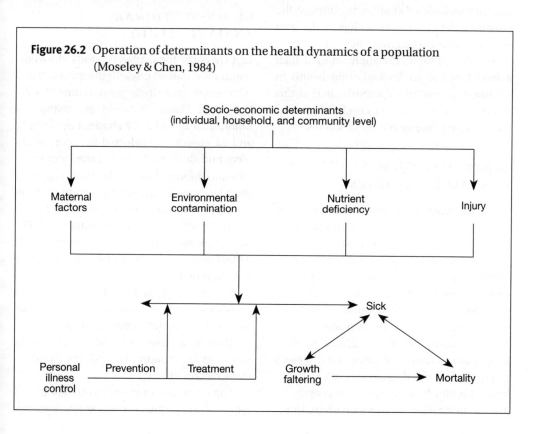

**Figure 26.2** Operation of determinants on the health dynamics of a population (Moseley & Chen, 1984)

An important aspect of the model is the definition of a specific disease state as being a result of the operation of proximate determinants rather than a single cause of illness or death. The aim of the model is to emphasize the social as well as the medical roots of ill-health.

This approach to child survival parallels methods used in the epidemiology of chronic diseases. It is recognized that chronic diseases have multi-factorial causes, may have long latencies between disease exposure and manifestation, and are powerfully influenced by lifestyle and socio-economic circumstances. There is ample evidence in the medical literature to show that child mortality also possesses these attributes, especially in developing countries. The implications of this model for epidemiological research are that there is a need to ensure that socio-economic determinants are considered as operating through the proximate determinants to influence the level of growth faltering and mortality.

Figure 26.3 shows the application of such a model to the analysis of child health in Mamre. A community diagnosis such as this should be a first step in conducting area-based analytic and intervention studies.

## GENERAL APPROACH TO ANALYTIC STUDIES

Figure 26.4 presents a simplified approach to the design, analysis, and interpretation of epidemiological studies. Exposure variables can either be risk factors for disease or protective factors beneficial for health. A represents the number of individuals with both the exposure and the outcome present. B represents the number with the exposure present but the outcome absent, etc. However, when looking at causes or risk factors for disease, a single risk factor acting alone is rarely identifiable. Certain factors may be necessary for disease to develop (e.g., tuberculous infec-

tion), but other factors are required before the disease progresses (in the case of TB these may relate to nutrition or to the immunological state of the child).

In a clinic setting, data are usually only obtainable with respect to A and C. The total number of children with the disease disorder (A + C) are identified, and the proportion having a particular risk factor A/A+C can be determined.

It is, however, impossible to decide whether the proportion represents an increase or decrease on what is expected since there is no control group of non-diseased children.

For example, if A + C represents all measles cases seen at a clinic, and A/A+C the proportion of those cases immunized, then insufficient information is available to comment on measles immunization efficacy.

## CROSS-SECTIONAL ANALYTIC STUDY

In a cross-sectional analytic study, the information is obtained on both the exposure and the outcome at a single point in time (A + B + C + D in Figure 26.4). As an example, a random sample of 2 000 children between 12 and 23 months are selected in a peri-urban area, and their mothers or caregivers interviewed. Information is obtained regarding their histories of measles and immunization status, as recorded on the Road to Health Chart. All four cells could be completed. The rate of measles among those immunized is A/A+B, and the rate of measles among those not immunized is C/C+D.

Vaccine efficacy is defined as: incidence rate (non-vaccinated) − incidence rate/incidence rate (non-vaccinated) (Orenstein et al., 1958).

Thus, in a cross-sectional analytic study, sufficient information is available to determine vaccine efficacy.

There are, however, shortcomings to this approach. In a cross-sectional study, one relies

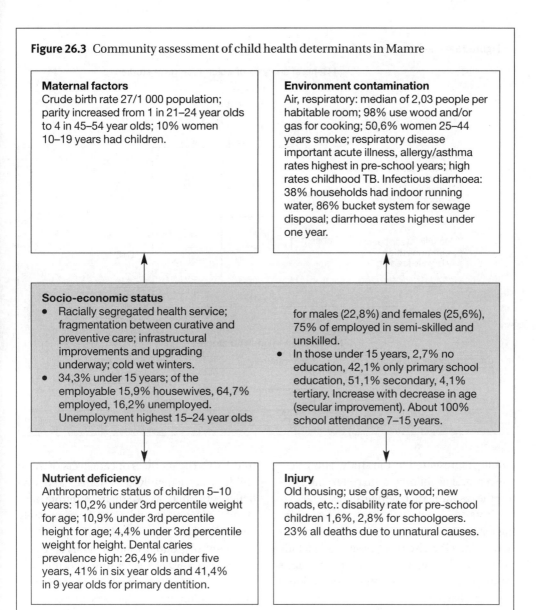

**Figure 26.3** Community assessment of child health determinants in Mamre

**Maternal factors**
Crude birth rate 27/1 000 population; parity increased from 1 in 21–24 year olds to 4 in 45–54 year olds; 10% women 10–19 years had children.

**Environment contamination**
Air, respiratory: median of 2,03 people per habitable room; 98% use wood and/or gas for cooking; 50,6% women 25–44 years smoke; respiratory disease important acute illness, allergy/asthma rates highest in pre-school years; high rates childhood TB. Infectious diarrhoea: 38% households had indoor running water, 86% bucket system for sewage disposal; diarrhoea rates highest under one year.

**Socio-economic status**
- Racially segregated health service; fragmentation between curative and preventive care; infrastructural improvements and upgrading underway; cold wet winters.
- 34,3% under 15 years; of the employable 15,9% housewives, 64,7% employed, 16,2% unemployed. Unemployment highest 15–24 year olds

for males (22,8%) and females (25,6%), 75% of employed in semi-skilled and unskilled.
- In those under 15 years, 2,7% no education, 42,1% only primary school education, 51,1% secondary, 4,1% tertiary. Increase with decrease in age (secular improvement). About 100% school attendance 7–15 years.

**Nutrient deficiency**
Anthropometric status of children 5–10 years: 10,2% under 3rd percentile weight for age; 10,9% under 3rd percentile height for age; 4,4% under 3rd percentile weight for height. Dental caries prevalence high: 26,4% in under five years, 41% in six year olds and 41,4% in 9 year olds for primary dentition.

**Injury**
Old housing; use of gas, wood; new roads, etc.: disability rate for pre-school children 1,6%, 2,8% for schoolgoers. 23% all deaths due to unnatural causes.

on those present at the time of the interview (i.e., survivors) as well as on the quality and availability of information with regard to both exposure and outcome.

In deciding whether selection bias has occurred, one needs to consider whether any of the four cells present in Figure 26.4 are likely to be under- or over-represented in comparison with any other cell. In the example just given, the children most at risk would be those recently arrived from the rural areas. These mothers might have a poor understanding of what measles is, and little information about the child's immunization history. This group would also be subject to the highest death rates for measles, and thus not

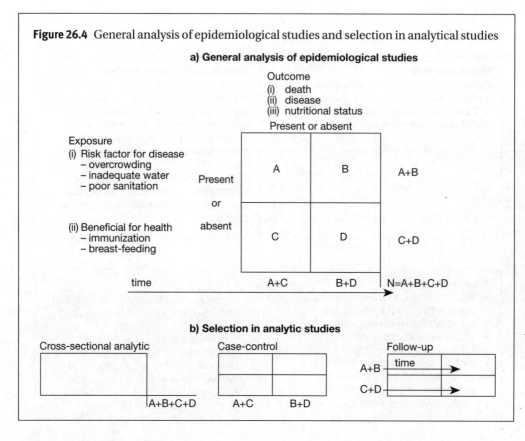

**Figure 26.4** General analysis of epidemiological studies and selection in analytical studies

**a) General analysis of epidemiological studies**

Outcome
(i) death
(ii) disease
(iii) nutritional status
Present or absent

Exposure
(i) Risk factor for disease
   – overcrowding
   – inadequate water
   – poor sanitation

(ii) Beneficial for health
   – immunization
   – breast-feeding

Present or absent

|       | Present or absent | |       |
|-------|---|---|-------|
|       | A | B | A+B |
|       | C | D | C+D |
| time  | A+C | B+D | N=A+B+C+D |

**b) Selection in analytic studies**

Cross-sectional analytic     Case-control     Follow-up

A+B+C+D     A+C   B+D     A+B   time    C+D

be fully represented in the study. This selective removal of children from cell B could distort the resulting vaccine efficacy.

Cross-sectional analytic studies examining risk factors for comparatively rare events such as specific diseases (these even include measles and tuberculosis) require very large samples to accumulate sufficient children who have had disease.

## CASE-CONTROL STUDY

An alternative analytic design is the case-control study. To illustrate this, the example of immunization status and measles will again be used. Cases of measles are interviewed at a clinic or hospital, care being taken to ensure that only cases occurring during a specified time period are included. They would consti-

tute A + C. The mothers or caregivers of these children are carefully questioned, and evidence obtained as to their immunization status, allowing A and C to be separately determined (see Figure 26.4).

A control group without measles is selected in such a way as to ensure that they are similar to the cases in all respects except immunization status. One way of achieving such control selection is to use neighbourhood controls. They are comparable in terms of socio-economic status and prior residential history. By the latter is meant that, in general, one would expect people living near each other to have an equal chance of having come from a rural area where immunization would be poorer. This generalization, however, may not apply in rapidly growing townships. The information obtained from the mothers and caregivers of controls allows one to compare the proportion of the cases who were exposed (A/A+C) with the proportion of the controls who were exposed (B/B+D).

An example of the use of a case-control study to determine measles vaccine efficacy is shown in Table 26.6. The age-stratified analysis in this example demonstrates that vaccine efficacy in the six- to eight-month group is much lower than in the nine- to fifteen-month group.

## FOLLOW-UP STUDY

Follow-up studies (also called prospective or cohort studies) are particularly useful methods of determining the natural history of a disease, evaluating the role of risk factors in causation or association, and evaluating the role of interventions in preventing disease. In Figure 26.4, a possible follow-up study would involve selecting two groups of children, A + B, who live in overcrowded conditions, and C + D, who live in less crowded conditions. At the start of the study, the children would be

tested to ensure that they are equal as far as their immunization status and their past histories of measles are concerned.

Over a five-year period, children would be visited regularly and surveillance would be equal among the overcrowded and less crowded children. The incidence rate of measles among the overcrowded children A/A+B divided by the incidence rate among the less crowded children C/C+D produces a relative risk as an estimate of the effect of overcrowding on measles incidence.

In this study care has to be taken to ensure that the difference does not result from differences in immunization status or the age distribution of children. Such factors would be confounders of the relationship between overcrowding and measles.

The group to be followed up is often referred to as a cohort. In general, a cohort is a group who share a common experience (e.g., they may be born within a similar time period or be of the same sex). In paediatric epidemiology, birth cohorts have played an important role in the identification of several risk factors and determinants of growth and development in children in both developed and developing countries.

## INTERVENTION STUDIES

### Randomized clinical trials

The randomized control trial (RCT) is regarded as the best method for assessing whether or not an intervention produces a beneficial result under ideal conditions (i.e., determines the efficacy of an intervention). The key components of a randomized control trial are that the intervention and allocation of individuals to groups is under the control of the investigator, and that allocation is determined by the study goals and not by the patients' needs or characteristics. For ethical reasons, ran-

**Table 26.6** Theoretical example of a case-control study to determine measles vaccine efficacy

Pooled results (six to 15 months)

|  | Measles cases | Controls |
| --- | --- | --- |
| Vaccinated | 20 | 60 |
| Unvaccinated | 80 | 40 |

Odds ratio (OR) = $[20 \times 40]/[60 \times 80] = 0{,}167$
Vaccine efficacy (VE) = $[1 - OR] \times 100\% = 83{,}3\%$

Stratified by age

|  | Six to eight months | | Nine to 15 months | |
| --- | --- | --- | --- | --- |
|  | Measles | Controls | Measles | Controls |
| Vaccinated | 15 | 30 | 5 | 30 |
| Unvaccinated | 40 | 20 | 40 | 20 |
|  | OR = 0,25 | | OR = 0,083 | |
|  | VE = 75% | | VE = 91,7% | |

domized control trials are not appropriate for the study of most risk factors, and are difficult to use to evaluate the outcome of community-based interventions. They are best known for assessing drug and vaccine efficacy.

Using Figure 26.4 again, if a study were to determine the true vaccine efficacy for measles, children at the start of a study would be randomly selected to receive the new vaccine, A + B, or not receive the vaccine, C + D. The groups, A + B and C + D, are followed over time, using equal surveillance and diagnostic methods to determine what proportion of vaccinated A/A+B as opposed to unvaccinated C/C+D children contracted measles.

Vaccine efficacy = [(C/C+D)]-[(A/A+B)] divided by (C/C+D).

In this study design, unlike that of a case-control or follow-up study, the effect of confounding has been reduced. Randomization of the two groups ensures that these groups are alike with respect to both known and, more importantly, unknown risk factors.

It is critical that, after the intervention has been applied, equal follow-up occurs in both groups and that those following the groups are unaware of which groups seek intervention. Similarly, the person(s) observing the outcome should (where possible) be blinded to the intervention. Blinding ensures that neither the patient nor the investigator can be biased by knowledge of the treatment received.

Finally, the prevention of contamination (the control group erroneously receiving the new therapy) and co-intervention (one of the groups receiving an intervention that could influence the result) needs to be carefully avoided.

## Randomized field trials

Field trials and community trials may be better suited for looking at the impact of interventions under service conditions (i.e., measure effectiveness) than randomized con-

trol trials. An example is given of a study conducted in the Ciskei to determine whether or not village health workers were able to teach mothers how to prepare sugar/salt solutions safely (see Table 26.7) (Yach et al., 1989). At baseline, experimental and control villages were similar with respect to the availability of the key ingredients needed, environmental risk factors, and the incidence of diarrhoea. Experimental and control villages were randomly selected from villages in the community. Verification of the fact that visits really did occur (validating the intervention) was achieved by determining the availability of forms in the control and experimental villages.

The high proportion of these forms in the control villages (not visited by village health workers) was due to their being made available in the surrounding clinics during the course of the study since it was felt that withholding information was unethical. This is an example of contamination, i.e., the control group received the experimental intervention.

The experimental villages had a lower proportion of diarrhoeal cases treated with home remedies and enemas, and a higher proportion treated with the correct sugar/salt solution.

Such a study used process measures of outcome. To be sure that the intervention really works, it may be necessary to demonstrate in larger studies that a decline in the death rate from diarrhoeal disease has occurred.

## Health service evaluation

It is necessary to have a means of evaluating entire child health services that does not require the complexities of a randomized design. A major restraint to health service evaluation is that services frequently do not have stated goals or objectives. Where this is the case, general goals relating to equity (a useful social goal that involves determining the distribution of resources, their use and availability by group), efficacy, effectiveness, and efficiency (which has economic aspects, and includes the extent to which resources are used to provide a specific service) should be used.

Before and after follow-up studies are useful for health service evaluation provided that one takes account of secular changes outside the health sector (e.g., education, income, or food availability), which could explain differences in health status that occur in communities over time. Ideally, the researcher should ensure that if a community-based intervention is applied, at least a baseline should be conducted in a neighbouring community with a subsequent post-evaluation cross-sectional study conducted in both communities to ensure that the control community had not similarly improved.

It is likely that rapid changes in health status in a community would be due to services and service inputs or to severe natural or civil disasters. Often, it is less important to identify the specific intervention than to know whether an entire primary health care package worked.

Health service evaluation was pioneered by Kark in South Africa in the 1950s (Kark & Cassel, 1952). Table 26.8 gives a local example of the results of the evaluation of a child health service (Bac, 1986). A number of key measures of outcome were used in the study

**Table 26.7**  Randomized field study to determine if village health workers are able to teach mothers to safely prepare sugar/salt solutions (SSS)

| | Experimental Villages (N=11) | Control Villages (N=11) |
|---|---|---|
| **Baseline characteristics** | | |
| (i)  children under five years | 556 | 584 |
| (ii)  availability of water, salt, sugar, litre bottles | equal | |
| (iii)  water/sanitation services | all villages 'traditional' with similar services | |
| (iv)  diarrhoea incidence (14-day recall period) | 13,8% | 15,6% |
| **Intervention** | | |
| (i)  definition | village health worker visits to all homes, teach mothers re SSS, leave information card | issue information card in clinic |
| (ii)  validation of coverage: percentage with card after six weeks | 81,5% | 29,7% |
| **Results** | | |
| (i)  treatment received for diarrhoea (percentage): | | |
| – home remedies | 7,8% | 28,6% |
| – enema | 2,6% | 12,1% |
| – sugar/salt solution | 76,6% | 50,5% |
| (ii)  percentage prepared correct SSS | 81,0% | 48,0% |
| (iii)  percentage solutions with sodium less than 100 mmol/l | 7,0% | 36,0% |

including the mortality rate in the ward, the under-five mortality rate measured in a community survey, and the nutritional status of children. These results occurred during a period of increasing drought and economic recession, and are a useful indication of the overall impact (primarily measuring effectiveness) of a primary health care package, but they do not allow the identification of the specific components that resulted in the improvements, nor do they allow comment on changes in equity (i.e., whether or not the gap in health status between the poorest and richest sectors decreased).

## Evidence-based medicine (EBM)

EBM refers to the principle that all clinical and managerial decisions in health care should be based on epidemiological evidence of effectiveness of those decisions. The recent

**Table 26.8** Evaluation of child health services in Gelukspan Community Hospital area**

| | 1978 | 1983 | Percentage change 1978–1983 |
|---|---|---|---|
| Number of children 0–4 years* | 9 658 | 11 307 | +17,1% |
| Outpatient visits* | 13 843 | 21 570 | +55,8% |
| Clinic visits* | 25 344 | 96 283 | +280,0% |
| Ward mortality rate (%) * | 5,5% | 3,7% | -32,7% |
| Mortality rate 0–5 years in community (%)* | 9,5% | 1,8% | -81,1% |
| Weight for age less than 80% of Harvard mean (%) | 5,1% | 3,1% | -39,2% |
| | (1980) | (1984) | |

* Community-based survey
** Bac M, 1986. Three year average 1978–80; 1983–5

growth of EBM can be attributed to international collaborative efforts to systematically review all intervention studies (both published and unpublished) in a broad range of specialities, using strict criteria for quality assessment.

An example is the Cochrane Collaboration, which disseminates the results of these reviews in frequently updated databases to its subscribers. Abstracts of systematic reviews can be accessed free of charge, however, from the websites of the Cochrane Collaboration and many others (see the list of EBM websites at the end of this chapter for details).

# Application of epidemiological concepts

Several concepts discussed earlier in this chapter will now be applied to the analysis of South African paediatric mortality data. *Race is presented here as a distinguishing personal characteristic of childhood mortality. This reflects the close relationship between several social, economic, and health service factors, and race resulting from apartheid policy, levels of urbanization, and development.*

Table 26.9 indicates that there is a clear difference in the profile of causes of diseases between the different race groups. For blacks and coloureds: infections, nutritional deficiency, and ill-defined conditions are particularly important, while congenital abnormalities, accidents, and poisoning are the most important causes for whites. Non-natural causes become more significant as causes of death in children over the age of five years.

## TEMPORAL AND SPATIAL VARIATIONS IN THE INFANT MORTALITY RATE (IMR)

The IMR is regarded as a key indicator of the general health of the population, and is used

**Table 26.9(a)** Age-cause-specific mortality rates (per 100 000 children) and proportional mortality rates (per cent) by race for South African children, 1990

| Under 1 Year | Asian | | White | | Coloured | | African |
|---|---|---|---|---|---|---|---|
| Cause of Death (ICD) | MR* | PM** | MR | PM | MR | PM | PM |
| Gastroenteritis (001–009) | 71,3 | 5,8 | 6,3 | 0,7 | 706,0 | 15,9 | 17,4 |
| Congenital (740–759) | 160,4 | 13,1 | 185,1 | 21,3 | 258,2 | 5,8 | 3,2 |
| Perinatal (760–779) | 718,8 | 58,7 | 494,3 | 57,0 | 2 198,8 | 49,6 | 47,8 |
| Ill-defined (780–799) | 53,5 | 4,4 | 15,7 | 1,8 | 185,1 | 4,2 | 10,5 |
| Nutritional (240–279) | 23,8 | 1,9 | 6,3 | 0,7 | 103,0 | 2,3 | 3,8 |
| Respiratory (460–519) | 41,6 | 3,4 | 33,0 | 3,8 | 476,2 | 10,7 | 8,2 |
| Non-natural (800–999) | 35,6 | 2,9 | 18,8 | 2,2 | 43,3 | 1,0 | 1,4 |
| Measles (55) | 5,9 | 0,5 | 1,6 | 0,2 | 11,9 | 0,3 | 1,3 |
| All other (remaining codes) | 112,9 | 9,2 | 106,7 | 12,3 | 452,3 | 10,2 | 6,5 |
| Total deaths | 206 | | 553 | | 2 971 | | 11 746 |

*MR = Mortality rate
**PM = Proportional mortality rate

**Table 26.9(b)**

| 1–4 Years | Asian | | White | | Coloured | | African |
|---|---|---|---|---|---|---|---|
| Cause of Death (ICD) | MR* | PM** | MR | PM | MR | PM | PM |
| Gastroenteritis (001–009) | 7,4 | 13,3 | 2,8 | 5,0 | 44,2 | 22,1 | 23,1 |
| Congenital (740–759) | 8,6 | 15,6 | 2,1 | 3,8 | 4,9 | 2,5 | 0,9 |
| Perinatal (760–779) | 0 | 0 | 0,4 | 0,6 | 1,0 | 0,5 | 0,2 |
| Ill-defined (780–799) | 4,9 | 8,9 | 4,2 | 7,5 | 12,5 | 6,3 | 21,6 |
| Nutritional (240–279) | 1,2 | 2,2 | 2,1 | 3,8 | 26,4 | 13,2 | 16,7 |
| Respiratory (460–519) | 4,9 | 8,9 | 6,7 | 11,9 | 30,7 | 15,3 | 13,7 |
| Non-natural (800–999) | 18,4 | 33,3 | 22,5 | 40,3 | 30,3 | 15,2 | 7,8 |
| Measles (55) | 1,2 | 2,2 | 0,4 | 0,6 | 0,7 | 0,3 | 4,1 |
| All other (remaining codes) | 8,6 | 15,6 | 14,8 | 26,4 | 49,4 | 24,7 | 12,8 |
| Total deaths | 45 | | 159 | | 607 | | 3 225 |

*MR = Mortality rate
**PM = Proportional mortality rate

**Table 26.9(c)**

| 5–14 Years | Asian | | White | | Coloured | | African |
|---|---|---|---|---|---|---|---|
| Cause of death (ICD) | MR* | PM** | MR | PM | MR | PM | PM |
| Gastroenteritis (001–009) | 0 | 13,3 | 0,3 | 5,0 | 0,7 | 22,1 | 4,2 |
| Congenital (740–759) | 1,5 | 15,6 | 0,6 | 3,8 | 1,0 | 2,5 | 0,8 |
| Perinatal (760–779) | 0 | 0 | 0 | 0,6 | 0 | 0,5 | 0,1 |
| Ill-defined (780–799) | 1,5 | 8,9 | 0,5 | 7,5 | 2,2 | 6,3 | 25,6 |
| Nutritional (240–279) | 0,5 | 2,2 | 0,6 | 3,8 | 0,5 | 13,2 | 3,2 |
| Respiratory (460–519) | 2,0 | 8,9 | 1,9 | 11,9 | 2,9 | 15,3 | 8,2 |
| Non-natural (800–999) | 11,8 | 33,3 | 7,1 | 40,3 | 14,8 | 15,2 | 25,0 |
| Measles (55) | 0 | 2,2 | 0,1 | 0,6 | 0 | 0,3 | 0,7 |
| All other (remaining codes) | 7,4 | 15,6 | 7,3 | 26,4 | 12,8 | 24,7 | 32,2 |
| Total deaths | 50 | | 144 | | 254 | | 1 555 |

*MR = Mortality rate
**PM = Proportional mortality rate

by the World Health Organization as one of the indicators being monitored in the process of moving towards health for all by the year 2000. Temporal and spatial variations in the IMR will be discussed.

Figure 26.5 indicates changes in trends of the neonatal (NMR), post-neonatal (PNMR), and infant (IMR) mortality rates for whites and coloureds over time (Rip et al., 1988). For both population groups there have been substantial declines in the IMR. A major reason for the decline has been the decrease in diarrhoea mortality rates over this period (Yach et al., 1989). The decline in the white IMR is particularly due to a decline in the PNMR. While this has also occurred with respect to coloureds, the rates are still substantially higher.

The current IMR for whites is comparable to that in England and Wales, suggesting that socio-economic conditions and the availability of good health care are similar. In contrast, the IMR for coloureds is much higher, sug-

gesting poor standards of living and inadequate health care, especially before 1970.

Temporal trends need to be supplemented by an examination of spatial trends. The box plots presented in Figure 26.6 and discussed further in the section on statistics show that the overall IMR in the country is higher among coloureds and, more importantly, that the variability of the IMR across the country at any point in time is considerably higher in coloureds than in whites (Rip et al., 1988).

Table 26.9 presents age-cause-specific information by race for 1990. The quality of available data needs to be first interpreted. For whites, coloureds, and Asians, less than five per cent of deaths were ill-defined. For blacks the proportion is higher, and greater uncertainty exists as to the real denominator. For these reasons, rates are not calculated for blacks, but rather the proportion of deaths due to certain causes is given.

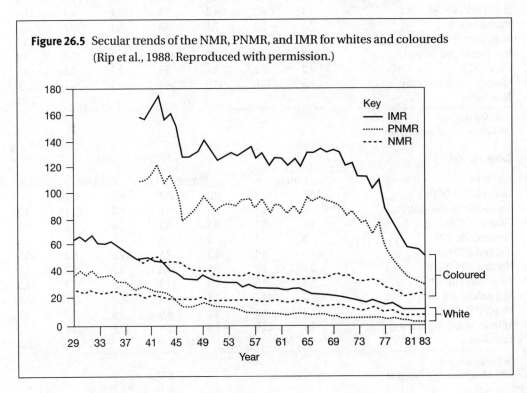

**Figure 26.5** Secular trends of the NMR, PNMR, and IMR for whites and coloureds (Rip et al., 1988. Reproduced with permission.)

Under one year, perinatal causes are major contributors to death in all races. Gastroenteritis, however, is a key preventable cause of death in coloureds and blacks. Non-natural causes (injury, trauma) are the major causes of death in whites and Asians aged between one and 14 years. In contrast, gastroenteritis is the major cause in coloureds and blacks until four years.

Table 26.10 shows that the IMR varies markedly according to socio-economic status regardless of race. This is an example of an ecological or correlational study where information was available at a grouped level with respect to both the outcome (the IMR) and the exposure (socio-economic status derived from the census). Analytical studies involving individuals are needed in order to obtain more personal characteristics with respect to the IMR.

Certain calculations can be carried out to further interpret Table 26.9. It is clear that mor-

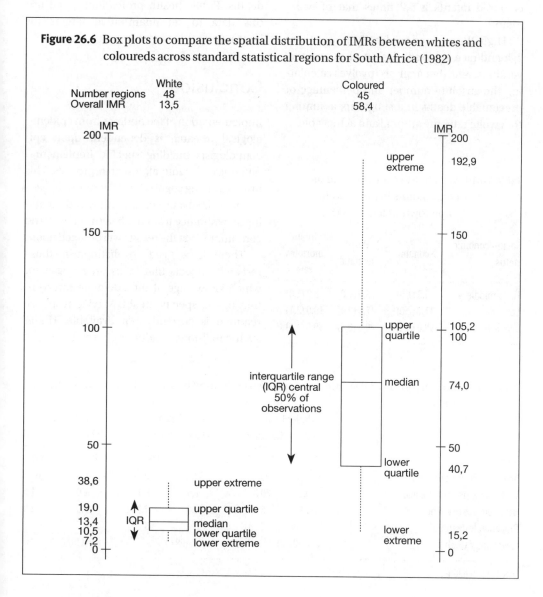

**Figure 26.6** Box plots to compare the spatial distribution of IMRs between whites and coloureds across standard statistical regions for South Africa (1982)

tality rates are age and race related. The overall mortality rate falls with age in all race groups.

Use of the risk ratio (RR): age-specific rate under one year/age-specific rate five to 14 years summarizes the relative effect of age within race. Table 26.11 shows that, within races, the risk ratio for whites under one year compared to five- to 14-year-olds is 30,2.

Similarly, if the white RR is set at one for all ages, it can be seen that the mortality rate in coloured infants is 5,2 times that of white infants.

High RRs are used to identify groups (here age and race are examples) in need of interventions. A further analysis involves calculating the absolute number and percentage of preventable deaths in a subgroup, assuming that white rates are optimal and achievable.

The number of preventable deaths in coloured infants is calculated by first determining the attributable risk or rate difference for this group (5 205 – 996 = 4 209 deaths per 100 000 infants) (see Table 26.11).

This is multiplied by the number of coloured infants (66 144) to give the result that 2 784 deaths were preventable if conditions that led to white rates were to have been applied, i.e., 80,9 per cent of actual observed deaths. Public health professionals can use this data to set quantitative targets for improvements in the future.

# Conclusion

Implementation of the findings from epidemiological research is dependent upon epidemiologists building specific implementation objectives into all research projects. This involves taking cognizance of community perceptions in advance of any study, and obtaining an assurance from the health services and community that the results will be acted upon.

There is a need to distinguish those research projects that focus on diseases for which knowledge of the adequate intervention or the specific health service response required is currently not available. Under such conditions conducting research on the

**Table 26.10** Variability of the IMR and its components in metropolitan Cape Town (relative risk)

| Socio-economic status | Neonatal | Post-neonatal | Infant mortality rate |
|---|---|---|---|
| High-middle | 5,9 (1,0) | 3,0 (1,0) | 8,9 (1,0) |
| Low | 11,7 (2,0) | 7,3 (2,4) | 19,0 (2,1) |
| Very low | 19,0 (3,2) | 20,5 (6,8) | 39,5 (4,4) |

**Table 26.11** Interpretation and summary of selected childhood mortality data for South Africa, 1985

| | Under 1 Year | | 1–4 Years | | 5–14 Years | |
|---|---|---|---|---|---|---|
| | White | Coloured | White | Coloured | White | Coloured |
| All deaths | 758 | 3 443 | 259 | 1 090 | 274 | 443 |
| Age-specific mortality rate* | 996 | 5 205 | 82 | 399 | 33 | 65 |
| Within race risk ratio for age | 30,2 | 80,0 | 2,5 | 6,1 | 1,0 | 1,0 |
| Between race risk ratio | 1,0 | 5,2 | 1,0 | 4,9 | 1,0 | 2,0 |
| Preventable deaths | 0 | 2 784 | 0 | 753 | 0 | 217 |
| (percentage total) | (80,9) | | (69,0) | | (49,0) | |

*per 100 000 children

disease would be justified even if it occurred at a low rate, but was expected to increase over time. AIDS and smoking in township children are two examples.

Finally, epidemiological research needs to look at why known effective interventions are not being applied. Such research would of necessity involve an analysis, not only of health service factors, but also of social, economic, and political impediments to the optimal delivery of health services.

Many of the studies described reflect the impact of fragmented health services along racial, curative, preventive, and geographical boundaries. The current restructuring of the health services is based on the needs identified by such research, and future progress should be monitored using epidemiological methods.

## References and further reading

AFRICAN NATIONAL CONGRESS. 1994. *The Reconstruction and Development Programme: A policy framework.* Johannesburg: Umanyano Publications.

ALLSOP M, COLVER A, and MCKINLEY I. 1989. Measurement of child health. Report of the working party of the Executive Committee of the Community Paediatric Group (associated with the British Paediatric Association), April 1989.

ARDEN-MILLER C, FINE A, and ADAMS-TAYLOR S. 1989. *Monitoring child health: Key indicators.* Washington DC: American Public Health Association.

BOTHA JL & BRADSHAW D. 1985. African vital statistics – A black hole? *South African Medical Journal.* 67:977–81.

KARK SL & KASSEL J. 1952. The Pholela Health Centre – A progress report. *South African Medical Journal.* 26:101–4; 131–7.

KATZENELLENBOGEN JM, JOUBERT G, and ABDOOL KARIM SS (eds.). 1997. *Epidemiology – A manual for South Africa.*

Cape Town: Oxford University Press Southern Africa.

MATHEWS C, YACH D, and BUCH D. 1989. *An overview of issues relating to the evaluation of primary health care projects.* Centre for Epidemiological Research in Southern Africa, Medical Research Council.

PATRIARCA PA, BIELLIK RJ, SANDEN G, BURSTYN DG, MITCHELL PD, SILVERMAN PR, DAVIS JP, and MANCLARK CR. 1988. Sensitivity and specificity of clinical case definitions for pertussis. *American Journal of Public Health.* 78:833–6.

RIP MR, BOURNE DE, and WOODS DL. 1988. Characteristics of infant mortality in the RSA, 1929–1983 – Part I: Components of the white and coloured infant mortality rate. *South African Medical Journal.* 73:227–9.

SACKETT DL, HAYNES RB, and TUGWELL P. 1988. *Clinical epidemiology – A basic science for clinical medicine.* Boston, Toronto: Little Brown and Company.

YACH D & JOUBERT G. 1988. Determinants and consequences of alcohol abuse and cigarette consumption in Mamre. *South African Medical Journal.* 74:348–51.

YACH D, STREBEL PM, and JOUBERT G. 1989. The impact of diarrhoeal disease on childhood deaths in the RSA, 1968–1985. *South African Medical Journal.* 76:472–5.

## Websites on evidence-based medicine (EBM)

COCHRANE COLLABORATION HOMEPAGE: *http://update.cochrane.co.uk/info/*

NETTING THE EVIDENCE: A directory of EBM resources on the Internet: *http://www.shef.ac.uk/~scharr/ir/netting.html*

TURNING RESEARCH INTO PRACTICE (TRIP): Using evidence for primary care in a GP group practice (UK): *http://www.gwent.nhs.gov.uk/trip/*

# 27 Some statistical concepts

G JOUBERT, R SCHALL
& J IRLAM

The best advice to give to medical researchers who need a statistical analysis of data is, where possible, to consult a professional statistician to plan the study before data collection. It is in fact here, in the planning stage, that a statistician can often make the greatest contribution to a research project. Only if an appropriate research design has been used will the results of a study be reliable. Once the data is collected and ready to be analysed, the statistician knows which statistics to compute and which analyses to perform.

In this chapter, the researcher will be familiarized with some statistical concepts, so as to make the interaction between the researcher and a statistician more fruitful for both.

After some details of sampling, the first steps of the data analysis are described, focusing on data quality and data summaries.

This is followed by a brief outline of some important concepts in statistics, namely the normal distribution, confidence intervals, hypothesis testing, and parametric and non-parametric tests.

## Sampling

As outlined in Chapter 26: Epidemiology, a researcher interested in a certain characteristic of the members of a population need not study the entire population. Usually it is sufficient to study a *representative* sample, which ensures that the results can be generalized to the population without bias.

*Random sampling* ensures that a sample is representative of the population under study. But random does not imply haphazard! In *simple random sampling* each individual in the population has an equal chance of being selected into the sample. If, for example, a researcher wishes to investigate certain characteristics of the population of children in a school, it is easy to obtain a full list of children (N) from school records and then draw a simple random sample (n) of children. The sample can be selected by drawing n random numbers from a random number table or by drawing n numbers from a hat containing the total (N) numbers.

If, however, there is some evidence that subgroups/strata of the population differ with regards to the measurement being made, the population should be divided into these strata and individuals selected randomly from each stratum. This is called *stratified random sampling*. Typical strata are age groups, sex, or social class. Strata should be selected so that the variation of the characteristic under study between strata is maximized, and variation within strata minimized. The precision of the estimate of the characteristic is thus improved. It is still necessary to have a full list of the individuals in each stratum.

In *cluster sampling*, certain groups (clusters), and not individuals, are selected at random. Typical clusters are schools, villages, or street blocks. Once a cluster is selected, all individuals, or a random sample of the individuals in the cluster, are included in the sample. In rural research, villages are often treated as clusters. A full list of villages is drawn up, a sample of villages drawn at random, and then individuals within these selected villages included in the sample. In this way less time and money are spent on travelling between villages. However, cluster sampling produces results with less precision than a simple random sample of equal size. Including more clusters in the sample will reduce the risk of bias.

One of the most commonly used forms of sampling is *stratified cluster sampling*. For example, in a Ciskei rural study (Yach et al, 1987) strata were defined according to village type: urban, traditional (rural), resettled, and re-resettled. In an initial field visit all villages in the area were classified into one of the strata. Villages or parts of villages constituted clusters.

In *systematic sampling*, individuals are selected systematically from some ordering, such as a queue of patients. This sampling technique is useful when selecting a random sample of records in clinics or hospitals, or of admissions to a hospital. Using a random starting point, each 10th admission, for example, is selected into the sample. To ensure the representativeness of the sample, the ordering must not be arranged according to a cyclical pattern. If hospital admissions are selected into the sample on every seventh day and the random starting point is Monday, then the sample is only representative of Monday admissions, not of all admissions.

## Sample size

When deciding on the size of the sample the researcher must consider the likely prevalence (or level) and variability of the characteristic of interest in the population under study. This information can be obtained from a pilot study or from published results that can be generalized to the study population. The larger the variability of the characteristic the larger the sample size needed.

One must also decide how precise the sample estimate should be. In general, the more precise the estimate needed, the larger the required sample size. Time and cost constraints often limit the sample size to what is practically feasible. The decision must then be made as to whether the study is worth doing, if a limited sample size results in little precision.

Formulae for calculating minimal sample size are given in standard texts (Ebrahim & Sullivan, 1995; Lwanga & Lemeshow, 1991), or else a variety of computer software packages can be used (e.g., EpiInfo, SAS, Statistica). It is always advisable to consult a statistician, however, to ensure that your assumptions and choice of formulae are correct.

## Data quality

Data, whether gathered by means of interviews or through examinations or measurements, can be flawed. To gauge the *quality* of the data the reliability and validity of the information obtained must be investigated. Data that are *reliable* are sound and consistent in quality, and they are *valid* when their correctness can be confirmed. If data are gathered through interviews a sample of the interviews should be repeated to see whether the information is reliable. Repeated measurements of biological features, such as blood pressure, enable the researcher to assess and adjust for biological variation. Information should be validated by means of documentation wherever possible, for example, age by means of birth certificates. If several observers are used in a study (e.g., to read blood pressure), the observers should be trained and standardized before the study. By repeating measurements on a subsample of the study sample, the variation between and within observers can be evaluated. Various statistical techniques exist to evaluate the agreement between data gathered on two or more occasions (Fleiss, 1981).

Errors can occur in the process of transcribing data from an interview or hospital records onto a coding sheet or into the computer, and these should be detected and corrected before the data is analysed. Some errors can be detected through data summaries, as described here. A more detailed description of steps that should be taken to detect and correct errors in research data is given by Jooste, Jordaan, and Van Eck (1988).

# Summarizing the data

Summary statistics, also known as descriptive statistics, are used to summarize and describe the data in a concise form. Whether one has conducted a descriptive study where the primary interest is the magnitude or distribution of a characteristic within a population, or an analytic study in which associations between characteristics are of interest, the first step of the statistical analysis remains the basic summary of the data. By summarizing the information first, one can also immediately see whether all aspects of the analytic study will be meaningful to explore. If, for example, only two children out of a sample of 100 have a certain characteristic, there is little point in exploring the association of that characteristic with other factors. More basically, by summarizing the data in a meaningful way, the researcher will be able to detect errors in the data that may have occurred during data collection or transfer.

The type of summary statistic used depends on the type of variable. In the case of categorical variables, such as sex, one presents the percentage of the study subjects that are classified into a given category. For continuous variables such as age, however, one needs to indicate where the central location of the data lies, as well as the spread of the data, i.e., how variable the data is.

The most commonly used *measure of the central location* of the data is the *mean*. This is calculated by adding all individual values together and dividing the sum of these by the number of individuals in the group.

The *standard deviation* is the most commonly used *measure of variation*, and is a summary of how widely dispersed the values are around the centre. It is calculated by taking the square root of the variance, which is defined as the sum of the squares of deviations from the mean, divided by the number in the group minus one.

An alternative measure of central location is the *median*. The median (or 50th percentile) is that value which divides the series of values, ordered from small to large, in half. A total of 50 per cent of the sample lie below this value, and 50 per cent above. If the sample size is odd, the middle value in the ordered series is the median. So, for example, if the group has nine values the fifth ordered value will be the median. If the sample size is even, the median is the average of the two middle values. If the group has 10 values the median will be the average of the 5th and the 6th values.

The lower (25th) and upper (75th) quartiles divide the halves of the data set into quarters. The distance between the two quartiles is called the *interquartile range* and can be used as a measure of spread. The median and interquartile range are *robust* alternatives to the mean and standard deviation, i.e., they are not as sensitive to outliers or asymmetry in the distribution of the data.

To decide which measures of location and spread are appropriate to use for one's data, the distribution of the data values should be examined. If the distribution is asymmetric or there are outliers, the robust summary statistics should be used.

Stem-and-leaf plots and box plots (Chambers et al., 1983) enable the researcher to evaluate the distribution of variables. In the *stem-and-leaf plot* each observation is plotted. All possible leading digits form the stem, and each data value is represented by writing its trailing digit in the appropriate row next to the stem, in this way forming the leaves. From the stem-and-leaf plot it is easy to determine whether the distribution is symmetric, and outlying values can be identified for investigation as possible data errors. The digits used for the leaves can also be checked for rounding error, e.g., weight of babies rounded to the nearest 100 g. These leaves should be ordered as in Figure 27.1.

A second graphical technique is the *box plot* (see Figure 27.2). Not all data points are plotted in a box plot, only the following summary values: the quartiles are displayed by the top and bottom of the rectangle that contains the central 50 per cent of the data, and

**Figure 27.1** The stem-and-leaf plot

```
Group A                                              Group B
(n=24)                                               (n=25)
                                   14   8
                                   13
                                   12
                                   11
                                   10   4
                           4        9   3
                      7    1        8   0   4   5
                9  5  4    1        7   1   4   6
       9  9  5  4  3  3    2        6   0   0   1
          9  7  5  2  2    0        5   2   2   4    4   8
                      6    6        4   1   1   1    1   6   6   6   8
                      8    3
```

| | | | |
|---|---|---|---|
| median | = 63,5 | median | = 58 |
| 25th centile | = 52,75 | 25th centile | = 46 |
| 75th centile | = 73,25 | 75th centile | = 76 |
| interquartile range | = 20,5 | interquartile range | = 30 |
| mean | = 64,3 | mean | = 64,6 |
| standard deviation | = 13,6 | standard deviation | = 24,8 |

the median is the horizontal line within the rectangle. The quartiles are connected by lines to the largest and smallest value in the sample. If the distance from the lower quartile to the median approximately equals that of the upper quartile to the median, the distribution is symmetric.

In the following example two groups of children were scored on psychological tests. The scores were (in order):

| Group 1 (n = 24) | | | | | Group 2 (n = 25) | | | | |
|---|---|---|---|---|---|---|---|---|---|
| 38 | 46 | 46 | 50 | 52 | 41 | 41 | 41 | 41 | 46 |
| 52 | 55 | 57 | 59 | 62 | 46 | 46 | 48 | 52 | 52 |
| 63 | 63 | 64 | 65 | 69 | 54 | 54 | 58 | 60 | 60 |
| 69 | 71 | 71 | 74 | 75 | 61 | 71 | 74 | 76 | 80 |
| 79 | 81 | 87 | 94 | | 84 | 85 | 93 | 104 | 148 |

From the back-to-back stem-and-leaf plot in Figure 27.1 it is clear that the values in group 1 follow a symmetric distribution and there are no outlying values (i.e., points far from the bulk of the data). In group 2, the value 148 seems suspect and should be checked. The values in group 2 do not have a symmetric distribution: most of the values are low.

From the box plot in Figure 27.2, the symmetry of group 1 is clear since the median lies approximately halfway between the two quartiles. Group 2 is asymmetric as can be seen from the fact that the median is much closer to the lower quartile than to the upper quartile.

For a distribution such as in group 1, the mean and standard deviation are appropriate summary statistics, since the distribution is symmetric and resembles the normal distribution (see below). The median value (63,5) is close to the mean value (64,25), and it is a feature of symmetric distributions that the mean and median values are very similar. In group 2, however, the median and interquartile range are appropriate summary measures

of location and spread respectively. The influence of the one large extreme value on the mean is clearly seen, whereas the median is robust against the outlying value.

When comparing two groups, one must of course use the same summary statistics for both groups. If the one group does not have a symmetric distribution or has an extreme case (which in a small sample can have a large influence on the sample mean), both groups should be summarized by medians and quartiles.

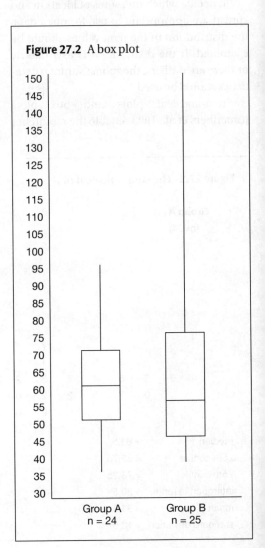

**Figure 27.2** A box plot

150
145
140
135
130
125
120
115
110
105
100
95
90
85
80
75
70
65
60
55
50
45
40
35
30

Group A
n = 24

Group B
n = 25

In the medical literature certain parameters, e.g., the number of decayed, missing, or filled teeth (DMF score) per child, are usually summarized by means and standard deviations. If this conventional summary is not appropriate for the distribution in one's sample, more appropriate summaries should be provided, along with the conventional summaries.

## The normal distribution

(ROSNER, 1990; ALTMAN, 1992)

Most commonly used methods of estimation (e.g., means) and hypothesis testing (e.g., t-tests) are based on the assumption that the continuous variables under investigation follow the normal (Gaussian, bell-shaped) distribution. Indeed, experience shows that some biological variables, for example birthweight, are approximately normally distributed. Furthermore, if the sample size is large, the sample mean will be normally distributed, even if the underlying distribution is not normal. However, in small samples with skew distributions one cannot make these assumptions. The normal distribution is a theoretical distribution characterized by its mean and standard deviation. For example, if a variable follows a normal distribution 95 per cent of the values will lie within two standard deviations either side of the mean.

## Hypothesis (significance) testing

Researchers are often interested in whether groups differ *significantly*, or whether factors are significantly associated with each other. To answer these questions they make the proposition that the groups do *not* differ and the factors are *not* associated. This is termed a 'null hypothesis'. Under this null hypothesis

is a *test statistic*, calculated on the basis of the sample. A *p-value* associated with this test statistic is then computed: the p-value is the probability, under the null hypothesis, of observing the test statistic or a more extreme result. A small p-value (e.g., p = 0,01) can be taken as evidence that there is indeed a significant difference or association, whereas a large p-value (e.g., p = 0,78) indicates that the difference/association is not significant. Often an arbitrary cut-off point of the p-value is chosen, namely 0,05, and p-values are dichotomized into 'significant' (if p is less than 0,05) or 'non-significant' (if p equals or is more than 0,05). However, this habit is now strongly discouraged in the medical literature (Gardner & Altman, 1989). Clearly a p-value of 0,06 should be interpreted rather differently from a p-value of 0,60, and these two values should not both be classified simply as 'non-significant' as often happens in journals. Instead, exact p-values should always be quoted in papers, and the readers can then decide whether or not they agree with the researcher on the 'significance' of a finding.

It must be noted that hypothesis testing determines the *statistical significance* of a result, which may have no relevance to *clinical significance*. If two large samples are compared the observed small difference between the groups may be statistically significant, although clinically unimportant. The clinician must therefore decide whether observed differences/associations are clinically important, and must not be guided purely by statistical significance.

## Confidence intervals

In contrast to hypothesis testing where the researcher is interested in testing some specific hypothesis (e.g., the means of two groups do not differ, or two factors are not associated), the researcher may wish to estimate a population parameter (e.g., what is the size of the difference between the means of two groups, or what is the strength of association between two factors). The sample estimate is the best estimate the researcher has of the population parameter but, because of sampling variation, the estimate could be imprecise. To obtain a range of values that are considered plausible for the population parameter, one can calculate a confidence interval.

A confidence interval is calculated using the sample estimate, the variability of the estimate, and the degree of certainty one wishes to associate with the confidence interval (usually 95 or 99 per cent). If one calculates a 95 per cent confidence interval, one can say that in a series of identical studies on different samples from the same population, 95 per cent of the confidence intervals will cover the true population value. The main purpose of confidence intervals is to indicate the precision of the sample estimates as population values. The more precise the sample estimate, the narrower the confidence interval. Enlarging the sample size leads to more precise estimates. If the sample estimate is not precise the confidence interval is very wide. Formulae for the calculation of confidence intervals for most medical applications are given by Gardner and Altman (1989).

# Parametric and non-parametric methods

(ROSNER, 1990)

If one assumes that one's data comes from a specified distribution such as the normal, one can use tests and confidence intervals based on the assumptions of the underlying distribution. These methods are called *parametric*. However, if these assumptions cannot be made, one must use *non-parametric* methods. These methods are also called distribution-free as they make no, or only weak,

assumptions about the underlying distribution. They are often *ranking* techniques that focus on the order or ranking of sample values, and not on their numerical values. If one wants, for example, to compare two groups on a continuous measurement that can be assumed to be normally distributed, one can perform a *t-test* (a parametric test). If one cannot, or does not want to make any assumptions about the form of the underlying distribution, one could, however, perform the non-parametric Mann-Whitney U-test. Similarly, parametric or non-parametric confidence intervals can be calculated.

The type of analysis that can be applied to one's data depends on the type of variable one is investigating. Looking at the data of the psychological test scores of the two groups of children, we have clearly determined that the scores in group 2 are not normally distributed. A t-test would therefore not be an appropriate test to compare the scores of the two groups. The Mann-Whitney U-test, which uses the ranks of the scores, would be a suitable test to do. This results in a p-value of 0,44, i.e., we conclude that the two groups do not differ significantly.

However, what if we were only interested in knowing if the two groups differed with respect to the proportion of children who scored below 70 points? The data can then be categorized into the following 2 x 2 table (2 rows, 2 columns):

| | Scored less than 70 | Scored more than 70 | Total |
|---|---|---|---|
| Group A | 16 (67%) | 8 (33%) | 24 (100%) |
| Group B | 16 (64%) | 9 (36%) | 25 (100%) |

Whereas before we were comparing two groups with respect to a continuous variable, we are now comparing two groups on a categorical variable. The appropriate test to do is a *chi-square test*. The chi-square test can be used to test the association between two categorical variables, and makes use of the discrepancies between the observed frequencies and the frequencies expected under the hypothesis that the factors are not associated. In the above example the chi-square test results in a p-value of 0,85, i.e., the groups do not differ significantly. As described in the previous chapter, a *relative risk* (risk ratio) or *odds ratio*, with a 95 per cent confidence interval, can also be calculated for this $2 \times 2$ table to determine the strength of association between the two dichotomous variables.

## References and further reading

ALTMAN DG. 1992. *Practical statistics for medical research.* London: Chapman & Hall.

CHAMBERS JM, CLEVELAND WS, KLEINER B, and TUKEY PA. 1983. *Graphical methods for data analysis.* Boston: Duxbury Press.

COHEN J. 1969. *Statistical power analysis for the behavioural sciences.* New York: Academic Press.

EBRAHIM GJ & SULLIVAN KR. 1995. *Mother and child health research methods.* London: Book-Aid.

FLEISS JL. 1981. *Statistical methods for rates and proportions.* New York: John Wiley.

GARDNER MJ & ALTMAN DG (eds.). 1989. Statistics with confidence. Confidence intervals and statistical guidelines. *British Medical Journal.*

JOOSTE PL, JORDAAN E, and VAN ECK M. 1988. Error detection and correction for improving the quality of epidemiological research data: Experience gained from a cardiovascular community study. *South African Journal of Epidemiology and Infection.* 3:12–16.

LWANGA SK & LEMESHOW S. 1991. *Sample size determination in health studies.* World Health Organization.

ROSNER B. 1990. *Fundamentals of biostatistics,* 3rd ed. Boston: Duxbury Press.

YACH D, KATZENELLENBOGEN J, and CONRADIE H. 1987. Ciskei infant mortality study: Hewu district. *South African Journal of Science.* 83:416–21.

# PART TEN

# Health services for children

The overview of health services as described in this part must be seen in the context of rapid structural adjustments presently in progress in South Africa.

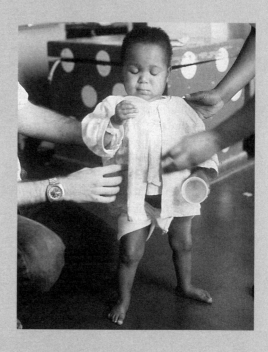

# 28

# Levels of health care with special reference to children

## DJ POWER & MA KIBEL

Every child, regardless of social position, needs access to an adequate service at the primary, secondary, and tertiary levels of care. In reality, the socio-economic and political position of the child largely determines the nature of the service he or she will receive. This should not be so, and health care equality must be a goal of all paediatric services.

## Primary level care

This term is used to indicate the level of health care closest to the patient. It may refer to a GP's consulting room practice, a well-developed group practice, a primary health care nurse in a clinic setting or, on a larger scale, a comprehensive community development programme with health issues as its focus. In any event primary level care has three main elements: the health service aspect, the staff, and the community aspect.

### THE HEALTH SERVICE

This is first contact health care and in its best form is truly comprehensive, meaning that it will provide a full range of the services needed

by the people. It will provide both curative and preventive services, it must serve the whole family (a children-only primary care service is not comprehensive), it will be within an affordable travelling distance of all the people, its hours will be convenient to everyone, and it will provide emergency after-hours cover if no other cover is reasonably available. The specific features, which are discussed in greater detail in various other chapters, include:

- obstetric and neonatal care: antenatal care, facilities for low-risk deliveries, very simple neonatal care including oxygen, resuscitation masks, blood glucose stix, and reflective foil for keeping babies warm during transport;
- family planning, immunization, and provision for oral rehydration as basic preventive measures;
- a simple curative service for all ages with adequate medicines and legal cover for their prescription by non-medical personnel as necessary;
- continuing care of chronic disorders, especially in childhood TB, asthma, epilepsy, and disabilities; and
- emergencies (both medical and traumatic). Examples of paediatric emergencies for which facilities must be available are

severe dehydration, seizures, acute asthma attacks, croup, poisoning, and conditions needing oxygen;
• communication with the associated hospital by telephone and/or radio; and
• transport in order to transfer referred patients to hospital on a 24-hour basis.

## STAFF

The staffing of primary care services will vary from a few individuals in a small community to a large team in a big centre, in which case some specialization of function usually occurs but should be kept to a minimum. It is best if all members of the team are able to carry out most tasks. The categories of staff will include medical, nursing, therapists, domestics, and lay workers. It is essential that all such groups are trained specifically for their work in primary level care and that their knowledge is regularly updated. Enthusiastic leadership is essential to motivate them and to inspire their work.

## Lay health workers

Lay health workers, who are responsible and respected members of the community, can be recruited and given a brief training in simple health and curative measures. They have been shown to have a big impact on the health of disadvantaged communities. Such workers are made responsible for a number of families living in the immediate vicinity of their houses. They know their people, visit their homes regularly, advise on health-related matters, and encourage the use of clinic services such as antenatal care and immunization. They also act as a link between the more formal health services and the people.

## Community rehabilitation workers

It is recognized that disability in children is more prevalent in disadvantaged communi-

ties than it is in more affluent ones, but that the community facilities to deal with the problems are mostly absent. Furthermore the present rate of training of physio-, occupational, and speech therapists is such that the needs of these doubly disadvantaged children will not be met in the foreseeable future.

Community rehabilitation workers form a new category of health worker that is in the process of being formally structured and recognized. They operate in the home of a person with a disability rather than in a hospital or clinic, and aim both to adapt the person's home environment and to provide active therapy so that the effect of the disability is minimized. The training is relatively short, and they work under the general supervision of trained physio-, occupational, or speech therapists who may be hospital based.

## THE COMMUNITY ASPECT

The programme is involved in the promotion of health and the prevention of ill health by involvement with the community in most aspects of its life. Not only must the community be consulted on such issues, but it must be a full partner in the process. The specific items vary with the socio-economic status of the community, but include the following:

## The care of children away from their homes

This involves educare centres, schools, and children's homes. The grouping of children in these situations provides an environment conducive to cross-infection (with, for example, lice, scabies, and viral infections). This situation needs constant monitoring and intervention as necessary. It offers opportunities for preventive and promotive health care such as immunization, health education, nutritional support, detection of silent defects (particularly of vision and hearing), and screening for occult disease such as TB (see Chapter 29: School health).

## Community facilities for children with disabilities

Whether these are residential units or day centres, the children and the staff need simple but regular health service support. These children have a high incidence of problems that need ongoing attention, such as anti-epileptic treatment, physiotherapy, and bowel and bladder care. Community-based physio- and occupational therapists are ideally placed to take care of many of these needs either at primary level centres, or at home when this is indicated.

## At- risk children

In any community it is possible to pick out children at risk because of health-related problems. These may be children on the border of malnutrition, children living in very unfavourable socio-economic situations, children looked after by unsuitable caregivers (alcoholic parents, elderly grandparents, etc.), children who have been abused, children with profound disabilities cared for at home, and so on. These children need to be monitored by regular visits to their homes by the primary level services so that early action can be taken as necessary.

## Education of the community

This involves key health issues appropriate for the community involved, such as alerting parents to drug abuse in teenagers, the avoidance of unwanted pregnancy, oral rehydration for gastroenteritis, the use of recently erected toilets in a rural area, or the need for regular weighing and immunization of babies.

## Relief work

In very poor communities it may be necessary to develop a network of relief centres for the destitute, mainly to provide nutritional support. In many cases, if this is not done, large numbers of children will be admitted to hospital with severe malnutrition. The same is true of the elderly who are often left to look after the children with no means of support.

## Community development

In very disadvantaged communities, the root cause of ill health in children is poverty, and, if that problem is not addressed, little progress can be made. The despair and powerlessness of the very poor needs to be dealt with directly. By encouraging participation in the creation of income-generating schemes, the primary care service helps to foster in people the idea that they can rise up and take charge of their future and that of their children, despite their predicament. This empowerment may spill over at a later stage into activities such as the development of community centres for educare or sports facilities and participation in community service such as lay health work.

## Environmental hygiene

This includes water supply, food handling, solid and liquid waste disposal, the control of domestic animals such as pigs infested with cysticercosis, etc.

## PRIMARY LEVEL HEALTH SERVICES IN SOUTH AFRICA

Because the care provided for children varies so greatly, the ideal service will first be discussed, and then this will be related to the existing position in South Africa.

An excellent Western industrialized society working model of primary level care is that which applies in the United Kingdom. The basic unit is a group of general practitioners providing care to a limited number of families making up their panel. Members of each family are known personally to members of the practice holding their medical records. Usually one member of the practice has a special interest and training in paediatrics and all have had vocational training in general practice. The practice has one or more health visitors who do home visits, social investigations, and supervise home treatment. There is easy access to simple X-rays, laboratory tests, physio- and occupational therapy. There is close liaison with the local community services, which include community-based paediatricians and social workers who are especially relevant for child care and child abuse problems. There is a range of social benefits to support truly indigent and disadvantaged families. Where necessary the social workers will co-ordinate the placing of children in foster or children's homes. There is a range of locally available services for those with disabilities, such as day care centres, institutional care, and community-based physio- and occupational therapists.

The service is based on the philosophy of prevention at all levels. The central activities are the careful supervision of pregnancy and delivery followed by the monitoring of growth and development, and the provision of primary preventive measures such as immunization. The management of episodic illness and chronic disorders, such as asthma and epilepsy, are systematically catered for, as is the active management of disabilities. The general practitioner model is seen as ideal because it maximizes the relationship between the doctor and the family, and allows him or her to see the child developing within the family and the surrounding society.

This sort of model is expensive because it relies on medical personnel, a high doctor–patient ratio, expensive buildings and equipment, as well as on properly trained ancillary staff and community services. It presupposes a well-developed social welfare service with financial support by the State for the indigent and seriously disadvantaged. In those parts of the world where this type of model operates there is practically no distinction between rural and urban communities except for transport factors.

A less expensive model based on family care by specifically trained doctors applies in Cuba. Despite relatively poor socio-economic circumstances they have achieved remarkably low infant mortality rates, and other impressive health indicator outcomes.

## SOUTH AFRICAN PRIVATE GENERAL PRACTICE

In the South African setting, the private general practice resembles the British model but has a number of important flaws. Firstly, the provision and delivery of preventive services such as immunization remain the responsibility of public health bodies and function as a separate service. Secondly, very few practices have attached health visitors or other allied medical professionals. As a result, liaison with community services tends not to be close. For many sectors of the population, community services and social welfare benefits are very scanty indeed. Thirdly, private practice reaches only those who can afford it. On the other hand, there is a growing tendency for new general practitioners to undergo specific vocational training, and therefore their knowledge and skills in the child health field is much greater.

## SINGLE-HANDED PRACTICE

For much of the world's population, the private general practice is out of reach, but many people will seek a personalized service from the single-handed doctor running a high volume dispensing practice on a fee for consultation basis. Such doctors provide a service that responds to the needs and wants of the patient who pays for it directly. As a result, the service is provided at convenient times and locations, and to some extent the type of treatment is tailored to patient expectations. The disadvantage of this type of service is that, because of large numbers, there is very little time available for each patient. This precludes the doctor from dealing with problems that require lengthy discussion or explanation, and rather leads to a concentration on straightforward medication. Preventive measures are rarely provided and links with community or welfare services are tenuous. As a result, community-service-related problems tend to be inappropriately referred to hospital.

## COMMUNITY HEALTH CENTRES

In much of the developing world, primary level care services provided by the State, welfare bodies or relief agencies are in the form of a comprehensive community health centre. Such a clinic is situated within easy reach of most of the community, be it rural or urban. The size of the unit will be determined by the surrounding population density. In an urban situation, a large clinic will cater for a population of about 50 000, whereas in rural areas, the population served will often be far less and the size of the clinic correspondingly smaller. The cardinal factor when determining siting and size is access, as the clinic will be the focus of primary level care in the area, providing, or being linked to, every facet of primary care. These include preventive services, facilities for emergencies, a maternity service, and a basic curative service linked by good communication and transport to the associated hospital. The staff will be a team of health workers – a variable mix of medical practitioners, registered nurses, community

health nurses, domestics, and lay health workers. They will have access to an adequate range of medications and facilities for managing emergencies, and preventive and curative services will be provided at the same time and place. An important guiding principle should be that a curative visit is always used as an opportunity for preventive interventions.

The well-run rural or urban community health centre provides many of the services of the ideal group practice in that it combines preventive and curative services, provides antenatal and delivery facilities, may have simple X-ray and laboratory facilities, has an attached body of community health nurses to do domiciliary work, and may even have an associated social worker. On the other hand, it does not match the ideal in a number of respects. There is usually a high patient turnover with short consultation times and resultant problems similar to those described for the single-handed doctor. Shifting staff and low caregiver–patient ratios mean that health workers do not usually know their patients personally, which leads to problems of understanding and communication. The level of expertise of the health workers in such clinics possibly may not match that of the vocationally trained general practitioner, although the trained registered nurse is capable of providing a very high standard of care.

Historically, health services in South Africa emulated the British model, which separated preventive and curative services, and divided them variously between the provinces, local authorities, and the central government. This resulted in progressive fragmentation of the health services. At the present time extensive planning is underway to restructure the services, but the situation today remains largely unaltered. The separation persists and is a major stumbling block to the logical provision of primary level services in the public sector. Local authorities may provide clinics that offer antenatal care but will not carry out deliveries. They might give immunizations and treat tuberculosis and sexually transmitted diseases, but not other acute ailments. The current restructuring process is addressing this fragmentation and is proposing the adoption of a district-based system under which a single authority would render all public sector primary level services up to and including the non-specialist district hospital, within a defined geographical area. The size of the population covered by a district would vary from about 300 000 in a city to about 70 000 in a widely dispersed rural community.

There are a number of other problems facing the concept of the community health centre in South Africa. While very many clinics have been established around the country over the last 20 years, the number remains inadequate, especially in the rural areas. The nursing staff in these clinics are often not specifically trained for the work, and are posted there armed only with their traditional hospital-based training. They are thus compelled to learn the work through their own mistakes. Although a great deal of excellent primary level training for clinic nurses is being done in various centres and through IMCI courses (see Chapter 36: Integrated management of childhood illness), the quantity and distribution of the training remains very uneven. There is also a considerable lack of uniformity as to syllabuses and certifying authorities, and very little recognition in the form of extra pay or promotion for nurses who have undergone extra training in primary level care. Another limiting factor is that both nurses and doctors may be reluctant to work and live in rural areas.

The lack of adequate transport to clinics is one of the great obstructions to the provision of primary level care in this country. This is especially so in the rural areas. The delivery of staff and supplies to clinics is a key factor, as is the transportation of patients to hospital.

## SOUTH AFRICAN PRIVATE PAEDIATRIC PRACTICE

At present about half of all registered paediatricians practise on a fee-for-service basis. They serve primarily the minority of the child population covered by medical insurance or whose parents have the means to pay for the service. Many provide primary level care, but this is surely a policy that wastes scarce expertise. On the other hand, a considerable number of private paediatricians are paid by the State to carry out service or teaching sessions in government-run hospital wards and outpatient departments. This deserves to be greatly extended. A large fund of knowledge and experience would then be available to the population as a whole. Private paediatricians could be especially effective in the 'community paediatrician' model described below.

# Secondary level care

Secondary care is the next level of care for both inpatients and outpatients who have been referred by the primary level services for more sophisticated management. Patients seen 'off the street' in hospitals are really primary level patients being seen in a secondary care setting. There are two classes of secondary care hospitals – 'district' and 'regional'. In each region there should be several district hospitals, run by general practitioners/medical officers with part-time specialist supervision, falling under a single regional hospital with full-time specialist services.

## DISTRICT HOSPITALS (LEVEL 1)

District hospitals are staffed by general practitioners and/or medical officers and provide care for most of the common conditions that need hospital management. A district hospital will serve a small town and its surrounding rural area. In a city there will be several district hospitals depending on population size. Children's wards tend to be mixed medical and surgical. The neonatal facilities (level 1) are able to deal with normal preterm infants, to give oxygen therapy, to administer phototherapy for neonatal jaundice, and to treat sepsis. Transport incubators and other equipment for the transfer of neonates to the regional (level 2) hospital must be adequate. Facilities for ventilation are not usually available (see Chapter 12: Perinatal services).

The laboratory and X-ray facilities will be basic and may not be available on a 24-hour basis.

From a paediatric point of view these hospitals should be under the regular supervision of a specialist general paediatrician from the regional hospital. This involves a weekly or monthly visit by the paediatrician to see problem patients but more importantly to establish and monitor medical and nursing regimens. Unfortunately, the uneven distribution of paediatricians in the subcontinent precludes this vital supervision that is essential for the maintenance of adequate standards in the face of the inevitable frequent changes of both medical and nursing staff.

At district hospital level, the key medical and nursing staff need to have had post-basic training in paediatric care. Senior nursing staff should have a Diploma in Paediatric Nursing and the medical staff should ideally at least have the Diploma in Child Health. Children's beds, neonatal facilities, and appropriate equipment for the various health care functions are required. Adequate communication and transport to both primary and subspecialist, level 3 centres are very important.

There are a number of problems experienced in district hospitals in this country that are similar to those experienced overseas. There is inadequate provision for newborn infants, both in physical space and in basic equipment such as incubators, oxygen head-

boxes, oximetry, bilirubinometry, and phototherapy. In some hospitals, there is no continuous medical cover for the paediatric ward, and nursing staff are expected to deal with all contingencies between daily or even weekly visits by medical staff. Overcrowded wards and avoidable hospital deaths are the hallmarks of this situation. Lack of structured contact with the public primary level services leads to poor continuity of care and little transfer of paediatric knowledge to the primary care level. Transport is very often a major problem that can prevent timely referral to the next level of care. Both medical and nursing staff at this level frequently have inadequate training in paediatrics. Compounding this, one finds that there is often a lack of specialist supervision in the form of regular visits, teaching, or consultation by the regional paediatrician – because there is no such person.

## REGIONAL HOSPITALS AND REGIONAL PAEDIATRIC SERVICES (LEVEL 2)

The regional hospital usually caters for two groups of patients – those referred from the region who need specialist attention, and those patients who use the regional hospital as their local district hospital. This duality of function is almost inevitable and must be catered for when bed numbers at regional hospitals are being allocated.

At this level there should be at least two resident specialist general paediatricians. About 95 per cent of all patients presenting could be managed without needing to be referred for more specialized care at the associated subspecialist, level 3 centre.

The X-ray facilities should include ultrasound and CT scanning as well as the usual special radiological investigations. The laboratory service should be available 24 hours a day and cover all investigations, except the most highly specialized.

There will be intensive care facilities with the capacity, for example, for ventilatory support for children, and for peritoneal dialysis.

The neonatal care will be at level 2. This implies facilities for ventilation, for performing exchange blood transfusions and for basic neonatal surgery.

## Teaching of primary level staff

Training in primary level care may well become concentrated at the regional hospital for a number of reasons. It is usually economical to teach reasonably large classes and the associated district hospital may not be able to release large numbers of staff for training at one time. Further, the medical staff in the district hospitals are usually few in number and have time constraints that preclude prolonged teaching sessions.

There will be close liaison with the subspecialist level 3 centre for referred patients.

The problems encountered are varied at the regional level. There are many regions where no hospital has been designated and upgraded as the regional centre, and therefore facilities at this level are not available. Patients are then referred directly from district hospitals to distant level 3 centres at great expense to patient and state, when a well-equipped regional centre could have coped with the problems. The lack of a regional centre means that there is no post for a regional paediatrician with regional responsibilities. The lack of a regional paediatrician and paediatric service leads to the familiar situation in which child health services in the region remain poorly developed, thus placing an inappropriate burden on distant level 3 centres. The development of strong regional centres is the key to a sound network of child health services. The regional centre is the powerhouse of the region as it is the focal point of service development for both the district hospitals and the primary level services. At the same time it is in a position to benefit directly from the knowledge and advances of the subspecialist level 3 centre and to pass that information, appropriately modified, down to the smallest primary level unit in the region. At present there are only a handful of properly developed regional centres, and most of the rural population have to deal either with a cottage or a faraway teaching hospital.

The practice of child health requires specific knowledge, a set of skills, and a distinctive overall approach to the problems of children. Health and welfare services for children, on the other hand, form part of a larger provision of services for the whole community and, unless particular care is exercised, the special needs of children are easily overlooked. It is important that in each geographical region there is a person or small group of people responsible for monitoring the provision of child health and welfare services. The multiplicity of bodies involved in the provision of services to any one geographical area makes this especially necessary. For example, it would be wasteful for a number of different health authorities in a region to each provide primary health care training for their nursing staff. It would be more practical for one body to do this for all staff, regardless of their employing authority. At the individual level, when a child is discharged from hospital there may be continuing treatment (as in the case of tuberculosis) that has to be carried out by a different authority. A liaison structure is needed to pass care smoothly between authorities. A proposal for a particular community facility for children with disabilities might come, for example, from medical staff in a hospital, while the authority responsible for the provision of the service might be a welfare body with whom the hospital doctors do not normally have contact. A group is needed in every regional centre to provide this type of practical co-ordination.

## THE REGIONAL PAEDIATRICIAN

Every region should have a regional paediatrician with broad responsibilities for child health services. Such a person is ideally placed to lead a co-ordinating group. He or she would be employed by the regional hospital and would have wide-ranging responsibilities.

## Regional hospital duties

These would include the normal neonatal, general, and outpatient work performed by any specialist paediatric service. It is necessary that the paediatrician(s) have an adequate number of medical officers and junior staff to help them cover the workload.

## Supervision of district hospitals

The district hospitals in the region should be visited regularly, and at such visits there should be three main activities. Firstly, the paediatrician will see the inpatients and discuss their care with the local medical officer. Secondly, he or she will observe and discuss the local medical and nursing routines and intervene as necessary with the hospital administration to ensure that these are correct. Thirdly, he or she will see specialist level outpatients who are conveniently followed up nearer to their homes.

## Monitoring of primary level services

In areas where the primary level services are run by the district hospital, it is easy for the paediatrician to maintain contact with the practice of the clinics. He or she will be able to determine policies for both preventive and curative aspects of the work and to monitor how these are implemented.

In other areas, primary care will be provided by several different organizations includ-ing all the local authorities in a region. He or she will need to have an official mandate to make contact with all of these bodies and to be co-operatively involved with them in policy-setting and with monitoring of their child health practice.

## Involvement with community services

In all areas the paediatrician will need to be involved in a practical and advisory way with community services for children – especially the child welfare services, services for children with disabilities, and the school health service.

## Teaching

One of the most important duties of the regional paediatrician is the teaching of all categories of child health workers in the region. The primary level nurses from clinics form a large part of this work, but it also includes the hospital medical officers, general practitioners, physiotherapists, social workers, school health nurses, and those in the disability services. It is usually practical to do most of this teaching for the region at a central point (usually the regional hospital), so as to have adequate group sizes and the necessary teaching equipment and clinical material available.

## Epidemiology

The gathering and analysing of routine data relating to child health will be an important part of his or her work. This will provide ongoing evaluation of the child health work in the region.

## Liaison with the district hospital

The regional paediatrician plays a key role in passing on new information from the academic centre to the most basic health care workers. In this type of transfer it is essential that information be communicated one level at a time in order to avoid widening the conceptual and practical gap between the giver and receiver. For example, a subspecialist from a level 3 centre may try to tell a group of primary level workers in a rural area about a new concept and its practical implications. His or her message may well not be communicated simply because of the subspecialist's understandable lack of awareness of the problems and limitations under which they work.

It is much more productive for the message to be suitably modified and to be passed on by a regional paediatrician to the district level, and then on to the primary care level. By this time the idea will have been put in a form that is relevant to the primary health care or village health worker.

While it is conceded that each of these activities could be carried out by separate non-paediatric persons, it is only the paediatrician who has the ability and vision to pull all the elements together. Thus, the paediatrician is the central figure for the upliftment of child health in his or her region. A paediatrician is first and foremost an advocate for children's health, and so must be prepared to appear in whatever forum is necessary.

In any region, it is ideal to have at least two paediatricians working together in the hospital. This is desirable for mutual support, for cover over holidays and illness, as well as to cope with the volume of work.

## SUBSPECIALIST OR LEVEL 3 PAEDIATRIC SERVICES

The population supporting a level 3 centre is correctly very large, and will involve university teaching facilities. Patients needing level 3 care will be involved with subspecialists in, for example, oncology, cardiology, nephro-

logy, etc. At this level there are specialist paediatricians with subspecialty expertise in areas such as cardiology, oncology/haematology, nephrology, neonatology, etc.

They will deal with the patients who have been referred by the regional centres and they will be the resource people in the regions covered by their level 3 centre.

The X-ray facilities include the most advanced techniques, such as MRI. Radio isotope studies are available. There are facilities for cardiological investigation and cardiac surgery.

Specialized neonatal care is capable of dealing with all neonatal problems including major surgery.

It is essential that the specialist general paediatricians at the regional hospitals receive regular visits from the subspecialists at the level 3 centre in order to keep them up to date and to provide regional centre staff with in-service training. The regional staff are, in turn, responsible for diffusing information down to the district hospital and primary care levels. It is inappropriate for level 3 staff to make educational visits to primary level centres.

It is ironic that it is at this level that the greatest degree of consensus exists as to what service should be provided. There is more than adequate provision of level 3 paediatric services in South Africa, and these need the least further development. It is in the existing level 3 services that the majority of paediatricians in the public service are to be found. It is the recruitment of paediatricians with extended responsibilities at the regional level that is needed to redress the present imbalance. There is the related need for medical faculties to ensure comprehensive child health care teaching and training at all levels of care for both under- and postgraduate students.

In several tertiary centres, the bulk of the workload is not made up of complicated problem patients referred from distant centres, but rather by patients needing district or at most regional level care. The outpatient departments of many level 3 care centres also carry an inappropriate load of primary care patients attending 'off the street' with minor illnesses. These patients are cared for by many high-quality staff at a cost more appropriate for a level 3 centre. The solution to this problem is not to provide more capacity in the level 3 system, but rather to establish in proper proportions, district and regional facilities in the areas from which the patients come. Some parents are forced by poor health service design to travel over 1 000 km to obtain district hospital care for their children at level 3 centres. These tertiary centres are overcrowded and the staff are stressed. The standard and quality of true level 3 care drops.

## THE COMMUNITY PAEDIATRICIAN

In metropolitan areas where there are level 3 hospitals and more sophisticated facilities at all levels, the paediatrician's orientation will be towards the 'new morbidity'. His or her

special expertise will lie in school health, disabilities, child abuse, or neglect. He or she will then function as the leader of the community team of professionals whose brief is the overall health of the entire population of children. A further important function will be to improve standards of primary care. This will be achieved by consulting, advising,, and teaching in the community health settings.

Experience in the United Kingdom has shown that the provision of one community paediatrician per 100 000 of the total population is a cost-effective ratio. Such paediatricians work entirely, or almost entirely, outside the traditional paediatric ward setting, but there is close liaison and ties with the teaching hospital.

# References and further reading

DEPARTMENT OF HEALTH. 1995. *Maternal, child and women's health.*
DEPARTMENT OF HEALTH. 1996. *Towards a national health system.*

# 29

# School health

CM ADNAMS &
LA WAGSTAFF

School-age children and young people are generally identified as being healthy. As a result, provision of services to these groups has historically carried low priority and status in many countries. School-age children have equal rights to health and health services, whatever their age and wherever they live. Ideally, their health needs should be met by a school health system that is specifically dedicated to this task, but which is itself an integral part of primary health care.

## School health services in South Africa

In South Africa, school health has until recently been a relatively neglected field and has taken second place to services for under fives (Adnams & Lachman, 1994). This deficiency is now being addressed, and national school health policy guidelines are being developed. The policy guideline document, which is presently at discussion stage, sets out the vision and objectives for a new approach to school health care services in South Africa. The broad objective is to promote health through the prevention of physical and psy-

## Aims of a school health system

The aim of a school health system should be to provide an appropriate service in order to:
- achieve the best possible level of health (mental, physical, and social well-being, current and future) for children of school age; and to
- enable children to derive full benefit from their education.

Strategies to achieve this include:
- working in collaboration with other professionals, parents, and children to meet the health-related needs of school-age children
- providing access to primary health care for all schoolchildren;
- age-appropriate health screening and health maintenance activities;
- identification and appropriate referral of children with special needs;
- health education and health promotion; and
- decreasing preventable causes of ill-health and disability.

287

chosocial diseases that may hamper the learner's development, through early identification of health deviation and appropriate treatment and referral.

The most efficient and effective school health care model is that of a unitary service provided by the District Health Department in co-operation with the Education Department providing a comprehensive service that covers all relevant aspects of child care. This should involve joint planning, controlling, and funding between health education and other relevant sectors.

In addition to emergent national school health policy, the concept of the health-promoting school has been adopted in South Africa.

The health-promoting school aims at achieving healthy lifestyles for the total school population by developing supportive environments conducive to the promotion of health. It offers opportunities for, and requires commitments to, the provision of a safe and health-enhancing social and physical environment.

The initiative with its co-ordinated and intersectoral approach to health promotion has been recognized as an effective way to improve South African scholars' health and their ability to learn. The South African Health Promoting Schools Policy Guidelines, currently being developed, outline how the health-promoting schools approach can be expanded to and implemented in all schools.

Ideally, child health care should provide for a smooth transition from the prenatal period (antenatal clinic) through to the child health clinic to the school years. For continuity to be achieved, immunization, developmental screening, school health promotion, and curative care need to be delivered by an integrated health service.

An agreed balance between health surveillance/screening, service, and health promotion should be established. The World Health

## The South African Health Promotion Schools initiative

The five tenets of the South African Health Promotion Schools initiative are:
- appropriate services;
- appropriate skills;
- community action;
- healthy policy; and
- a health-conducive environment.

Organization criteria for screening apply (see Chapter 21:Health surveillance).

The school health team should consist of well-trained nurses and doctors supported by other health professionals (including paediatricians), who are knowledgeable about school health issues. School health professionals need managerial and teaching skills and less complex tasks such as weighing and measuring of children could be undertaken by designated teachers. Schoolteachers and other educational professionals such as educational counsellors and school psychologists are now being trained to provide health education and promotion. The health team can provide a link between different services and facilities in the community, for which they need to be familiar with resources for children with special needs.

School health services in South Africa range from government-paid special nurse–doctor teams to no formal provision whatsoever. The poor and disadvantaged, whose need for comprehensive care exceeds that of the better-resourced communities, tend to receive only episodic curative care from clinics and hospitals. Children from low socio-economic communities are especially vulnerable to developmental problems, such as learning and emotional disorders, and to the long-term sequelae of untreated physical problems, such as hearing loss, speech problems, and poor vision (Creswell & Newman, 1988). Referral facilities and resources for children with special needs are often limited or lacking.

However, even with limited resources, it is possible as an interim measure to improve support for the child's learning needs. For example, in poorly resourced areas where special schools, hearing aids, or spectacles may not be easily available, it is still helpful to identify or confirm sensory impairments or learning difficulties. Explanation to the parents and teachers may reduce pressure on the child and unrealistic expectations in the home and school, so that the child will consequently receive greater understanding and support.

Children with barriers to learning may further benefit from sitting in front of the class and not being chastised or punished for being lazy or stupid. Parents and teachers who stop blaming themselves or each other for the child's poor progress are better able to cope with the child's difficulties.

Many schools have no specific space set aside for school health visitors, and basic facilities for treating primary health care problems are inadequate. Designated clinic areas are desirable to provide the privacy and confidentiality necessary for adolescent consultation and examination. This can be achieved by using existing resources and combining school health and community health facilities (see Chapter 18: Health care services for adolescents).

The ideal situation of, for example, a school nurse in every school is unlikely to be achieved in South Africa. In reality we should aim to provide the minimum service that is effective and appropriate to the needs of the school-going population. Readers need to assess their local situations and gain awareness and understanding in order to promote optimal health care for the school-going learners in their area. Health professionals can interact with local schools through appropriate service delivery and skills transfer, and by supporting the schools' health policies and priorities.

# The role of the school health system

Health inspection is by far the major school health activity and is undertaken routinely wherever school health is practised, although the recommendations vary from country to country (Campbell & McIntosh, 1998).

Examination of school entrants should be regarded as the minimum activity. While children are examined immediately before or after admission to school, examination or screening of children in other age-groups is selective. There is no general agreement about the method of selection. Screening procedures that are usually carried out by school nurses include the following:

- *Growth monitoring* (weight/height-for-age)
- *Vision.* Visual acuity should be tested at least once in all primary and secondary schools and in all special schools.
- *Hearing.* All children should have hearing screening (ideally testing) in their first year of life and most children with sensorineural deafness should be identified before they reach school. The most common cause of hearing loss is middle ear infection, which is especially prevalent in early childhood.

Vision and hearing screening are important because they have direct relevance to learning.

- *Screening for other disorders*
  - skin infections;
  - intestinal infection;
  - orthopaedic conditions (scoliosis, limb deformities);
  - dental caries;
  - heart murmurs in areas of high rheumatic heart disease prevalence; and
  - undescended testes

289

Parents are encouraged to attend when their younger children are being examined, or to communicate their concerns about their child's health to the school health team.

## CONTROL OF INFECTIONS AND TRANSMISSIBLE DISEASES

This includes hygiene inspection and targeted surveillance of children who have been exposed to endemic or epidemic infectious diseases. Some local authorities issue guidelines for the exclusion of infected children from school.

The school-going population in South Africa includes many young people in their late teens and early twenties. This age group is the highest risk group in the country for contracting HIV/AIDS. There has been public discussion around encouragement of sexually active learners at schools to determine their HIV staus and to undergo voluntary testing and counselling. In terms of the Schools Act, teachers and schools may make learners aware of available health facilities where such services are rendered.

## IMMUNIZATION

Pre-school immunization is frequently a prerequisite for school entry (see Chapter 25: Immunization). In some countries boosters are administered in the school years. Of particular importance is rubella vaccine for prepubescent girls, whether or not they have received MMR during infancy. Parental consent is required for immunization.

## HEALTH EDUCATION

Here most school doctors and nurses do not have defined responsibilities, and many initiatives depend upon individual enthusiasm and time. Ideally, teachers supported by the health team should undertake health education and promotion. Health and lifestyle education is included in the South African curriculum system and is part of the health-promoting schools initiative. Health education topics should include nutrition, hygiene, sex education, healthy lifestyles, mental health, first aid and accident, and child abuse prevention.

Schools are encouraged to make information available to scholars on health and other services for family planning, pregnancy counselling, and child abuse.

In turn, the service providers should supply information of their facilities to the schools.

## ENVIRONMENTAL HEALTH

The role of the school nurse and/or school inspector may be to monitor and promote acceptable standards of hygiene in the physical environment. This may include:
- toilets and safe sanitation;
- clean drinking water;
- litter disposal; and
- safety of buildings and play areas.

Of note, many schools in rural areas do not yet have electricity or running water.

## CHILDREN WITH CHRONIC DISORDERS

Where there is a need for long-term therapy for conditions such as asthma, diabetes, epilepsy, or tuberculosis, the school staff should be informed and their co-operation sought as needed. The school nurse or local health service provider can enhance essential understanding, promote treatment adherence, and reduce the risk of the children being stigmatized.

The teacher and scholar's classmates should, when necessary, know about acute asthma attacks and seizures, their immediate management, and about possible complications of the scholar's condition.

## DENTAL SERVICES

(See Chapter 22: Oral health.)

As well as dental screening, these may include instruction on oral hygiene and referral for curative and corrective dentistry.

## SPECIAL EDUCATIONAL NEEDS

Special educational needs arise from a child's disabilities or learning difficulties. In some areas, the school health team may be helped by multidisciplinary academic health teams, and psychological and educational services. This facilitates optimal comprehensive assessment and management of children with special needs in the school environment. However, such resources are limited.

It is important to shift the emphasis from provision for special disabilities to the meeting of special educational needs, i.e., focusing on needs rather than disability. The needs will depend on the degree and type of disability, and whether the children attend mainstream or special schools. The trend internationally and in South Africa is towards inclusion and provision for learners' needs, where possible, in mainstream schools.

## CHILD GUIDANCE AND MENTAL HEALTH

Adolescents, especially, need access to counselling and management of age-related problems, including substance abuse, depression, and eating disorders. Behaviour problems, secondary to home/community environment problems and/or learning and primary behaviour difficulties (e.g., learning disorders, attention deficit hyperactivity disorder) generally manifest in the school environment and are a common source of referral to health professionals. The school health team, and health professionals with knowledge of management of behaviour problems can be of great help in supporting staff and learners to manage these difficulties in the classroom.

## CHILDREN WITH SPECIAL SOCIAL NEEDS

School health personnel may contribute greatly to the welfare of children who are socially and environmentally disadvantaged, such as street children and children who are victims of family disruption or violence.

## CHILD ABUSE

All health professionals caring for the school-age population should be aware of the less obvious manifestations of abuse, and should know how to guide teachers accordingly. They may have a role in counselling, support, and referral for specialized management.

The physical and mental health of scholars is not only important for their individual well-being but also for the long-term effect on the quality of society. Appropriate knowledge and skills gained in the school years should translate into healthier lifestyles and practices with a positive effect on future generations. Scholars, parents, schools, and communities are partners in achieving these goals.

## References and further reading

ADNAMS CM & LACHMAN PI. 1994. The school health service. *Pedmed.* 7 (1):3–6.

BRITISH PAEDIATRIC ASSOCIATION. 1993. *Consultation report of the joint working party. Health services for school age children.*

CAMPBELL AGM & MCINTOSH N. 1998. *Forfar and Arneil's textbook of pediatrics,* 5th Ed. New York. Churchill Livingstone.

CRESWELL WH & NEWMAN IM. 1988. *School health practice,* 10th ed. Mosby-Year Book Inc.

DEPARTMENT OF HEALTH. 1999. *School health care services in South Africa, policy guidelines: Discussion document*

DEPARTMENT OF HEALTH. 2000. *Health promoting schools policy guidelines: Draft 2.*

PRIMARY HEALTH CARE GROUP, KINGS FUND CENTRE FOR HEALTH SERVICES DEVELOPMENT, UK. 1988. *Changing health services.*

WAGSTAFF LA, DE VRIES G, and MKHASIBE C. 1988. Whither school health services for lower primary school children in Soweto? *South African Medical Journal.* 73:117–19

# 30 Community support groups

## J HOLLINGSHEAD

'They get this training, but they do not know how you feel' is a quote often heard in reference to social workers, but one that may well apply to all health care professionals. It also explains one of the reasons why people, either individuals or families, with special needs get together to form community support groups. In this short chapter, an attempt will be made to look at what such groups are, why they exist, what they provide, how to find them, and how health professionals can make them an essential part of health service delivery.

## What are community support groups?

'Self-help', 'natural helping', 'community support', and 'mutual aid support systems' are terms given to groups where people with a common experience join together for emotional support, technical expertise, education, information, friendship, refuge from discrimination, and to lobby for a better deal. Much of the literature on child health concentrates on special interest groups for parents of children with disabilities; for those who have lost a child by accident, stillbirth, neonatal, or cot death; and

for those who are considering alternative birth techniques. There are also groups for children with inherited disorders, diabetes, haemophilia, cystic fibrosis, food allergies, and chronic juvenile arthritis. We are familiar with the groups such as DICAG (Disabled Children's Action Group), Down's Syndrome Association, Compassionate Friends, SHARE, Cot Death Society, Breastfeeding Association, La Leche League, Parents of Twins Association, and many others.

In the field of disability in South Africa, statutory and private welfare organizations have done much for their users. Following a move against paternalism and in favour of self-advocacy, groups such as Disabled People of South Africa (DPSA), South African Inherited Disorders Association (SAIDA), and DICAG were established. They consist of people and families dealing with disabilities and act as pressure, support, information-sharing, and self-advocacy groups.

## Why do community support groups exist?

Community support is as old as human history, based on the simple fact that people who share a particular problem may have something to offer each other. A variety of reasons explain their beginnings. A look at the field of intellectual disability alone gives ample evidence of the advocacy role that participating families have played in starting new services, changing terminology, and promoting more positive attitudes. Groups have been set up to deal with the following problems:

- the monopolization of knowledge by professionals. The pursuit of scientific expertise has transferred *power to specialism*, which gives less consideration to the human aspect. The self-help movement is seen as a means of redressing this imbalance of power;
- marginalization of 'others', such as people with intellectual disability, by society. Such people, or their advocates, act together to strengthen each other against the hostility of society. The growth in numbers and popularity of such groups should be seen in the context of international movements that address political and gender liberation, consumer advocacy, human rights, and minority group issues. Private issues have become public. Existential psychiatry has described this as groups and individuals going through a development from *private to public to political activity*;
- the isolation of families of people with problems. A sociological perspective on mutual help is rooted in the role of the family and what it provides to its members. Each time an individual or family member guides, controls, nurtures, supports, or loves another member, this action personally benefits the giver as much if not more than the receiver. There is mutuality and reciprocity in these actions.

It should be remembered that many community support groups meet middle-class needs. People who have their basic needs met can spend time, energy, resources, and money

## What do support groups provide?

A quotation from the Winter 1988 edition of *Ark/Play Matters*, the publication of the Toy Libraries Association in England, illustrates several points about the value of self-help groups:

It was the first time many mothers felt they could meet each other on an equal footing, compare experiences and give one another comfort and advice. Professionals were pleased to find an informal setting where they could 'get on the floor' and play with the children.

Community support groups are helpful in the following ways:

- they provide an accepting social setting;
- they combat isolation by providing a chance to make new friends and to share information about resources and services;
- they provide a sense of belonging to an understanding group of people;
- they produce a place to become involved in constructive action and to learn by doing;
- they provide a place to regain a sense of personal worth;
- they provide a channel for the positive expression of energy and emotion that might otherwise have been spent negatively or destructively; and
- they provide a place for professionals to share their expertise and to learn from parental expertise in a more equal environment.

Membership of self-help groups may be temporary. Diminishing participation in a group could be seen as a healthy sign of growth in learning to live with a particular problem.

attending meetings, writing newsletters, sharing skills, and exploiting contacts for their mutual benefit. Those struggling for survival have other priorities.

# How can health professionals help?

Health professionals can help by doing the following:

- knowing that self-help groups exist. Information can be obtained from the list at the end of this chapter;
- giving that information to families, preferably in writing. Parents may not seek immediate engagement with a group, but should be able to make that choice when they are ready to do so;
- using their status and power in partnership with parents in lobbying for their children's needs. Dumont says that the redistribution of political power is meaningless if the power residing in professionalism is not redistributed as well (Dumont in Caplan & Killilea, 1976). Health professionals may also play an important role in facilitating the start of a self-help group.

'Parents as partners' is a challenging concept to professionals, but one which has potential for great rewards. It is an acknowledgement that management is not the monopoly of any one group, and that each has a role to play in holistic health care. It gives recognition to the efforts that 'lay' experts make in contributing to the specialist knowledge of a particular field. Families with a vested interest may have the motivation and time for these pursuits; health professionals often need to direct their energies elsewhere, but could continue to assist with training, support, and linkage to updated scientific knowledge.

## Child care information centres

Child Care Information Centre
Red Cross Children's Hospital
7700 Rondebosch
Cape Town
Tel: (021) 689 1519 or (021) 685 4103
Fax: (021) 689 5403
E-mail: lizette@rmh.uct.ac.za
Assessment Clinic (Sr Mac)

The Memorial Institute for Child Health and Development
Private Bag X39
2000 Johannesburg
Tel: (011) 481 5194
Fax: (011) 642.6027

Child Information Centre
Department of Paediatrics and Child Health
University of the Orange Free State
P. O. Box 339 (G69) 9300
Bloemfontein.
Tel: (051) 444 1867
Fax: (051) 444 3230
E-mail: gnddcr@med.uovs.ac.za

## References and further reading

CAPLAN G & KILLILEA M (eds.) 1976. *Support systems and mutual help: Multidisciplinary explorations.* New York: Grune & Stratton.

FOX AM. 1974. *They get this training, but they do not know how you feel.* Horsham: The National Foundation for Research into Crippling Diseases.

GOTTLIEB BH et al. 1981. *Social networks and social support.* California: Sage Publications.

ROBINSON D & HENRY S. 1977. *Self-help and health: Mutual aid for modern problems.* London: Martin Robertson & Company Limited.

ROYAL SOCIETY FOR MENTALLY
    HANDICAPPED CHILDREN AND ADULTS
    (MENCAP). 1984. *Day services today and
    tomorrow*. London: MENCAP.
TOY LIBRARIES ASSOCIATION. 1988. *Ark/Play
    Matters*. Winter 1988. London.

# PART ELEVEN

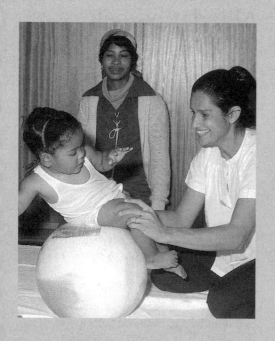

# Allied professions

Optimal health care for children should involve close interaction between professionals in a number of disciplines. This section, which examines the role of allied professions, could well be extended to include education, the judiciary, and other aspects of health care, covering for example, the pyschologist's role and the pharmacist's role. Spatial constraints limit us to the four disciplines most directly allied to clinicians and nurses – occupational therapy, physiotherapy, social work, speech pathology, and audiology. The scope of their work, and their traditional role is described in the following chapters, together with a modern view of their broader scope in southern Africa, where scare resources must be used optimally.

# 31

# Allied medical professionals

## B KATZ & G LLOYD

*'Making the shift to a resource-based approach to meeting child and family needs is possible when we can cease thinking about communities as having limited resources and begin to think of them as having limitless opportunities'.*

(Dunst et al., 1994)

In South Africa, current socio-economic circumstances and diminishing resources are challenging allied medical professionals (AMPs) to find the 'limitless opportunities' of children, their families and communities. Children are our most important capital asset and represent the future productive potential of society. Investing in their education and health is a critical necessity and not a luxury. It is also the goal of a just society.

In the past, early intervention was regarded as the domain of the special educator and the parents' view was either overlooked or considered to be part of the problem. An enlightened approach now acknowledges that parental involvement in early childhood programmes is associated with greater success. With allied medical professionals as facilitators and resource persons, people are assisted and empowered to build on their existing competence and thus maintain a 'sense of control' over circumstances. Inability to promote competence is due to failure to create enabling opportunities.

AMPs are caught in the dilemma of providing a human service that addresses poverty and disadvantage without being paternalistic or encouraging the dependence that was so prevalent under the apartheid regime (Drower & Katz, 1998). Current government policy aims to serve and build a self-reliant nation in partnership with all stakeholders. An integrated social welfare system is envisaged and this should be equitable, sustainable, accessible, people-centred, and developmental. Concepts such as participation, partnership, capacity building, inclusion, and collaboration emerge as focal points for consideration. An understanding of these core issues will enable AMPs to incorporate aspects that are relevant to their individual working environments and to their own needs and values. This does not mean that AMPs should lose their medical identity and frame of reference. There are always instances where the medical model prevails, for example, fitting the appropriate hearing aid. However, what is being suggested is that AMPs broaden their approach in keeping with the South African democratic human rights culture in which children and families now receive care and can participate.

## Participation

The interpretation most suited to the allied medical professions would be 'Participation as empowerment'. This emphasizes the importance of identifying groups with which to work and the use of non-formal education to develop their awareness. Rehabilitative processes, training, the development of programmes and their evaluation would be participatory in nature.

Three obstacles to participation are:

- operational obstacles – where there is too much centralization of power, limited capacity, limited co-ordination, and inappropriate technology;
- culture of poverty – from which people may have difficulty emerging, thus preventing them from contributing meaningfully; and
- lack of structural support – this limits participation.

The AMP emerges from training with all the skills and expertise relevant to that specific field. But it is how that skill and expertise is used that becomes critical when working with families.

From the past, families carry the baggage that may make them insecure about participating in their children's rehabilitative programme. There has always been an emphasis on 'the professional knows best'. Consequently, the AMP cannot expect immediate full parental participation. In the face of this apparent reluctance, the AMP has the mammoth task of empowering the parents, and offering sufficient support to reassure them that their participation and choices will be respected.

The process may take time and may involve the development of not only mutual trust but also of mutual learning between AMPs and parents.

True participation will be evident only when a parent feels sufficiently comfortable to share with an AMP that the home programme suggested is not suitable or could not be carried out. If alternative ideas are initiated, suggested, and tried, participation and the beginnings of empowerment start emerging.

## Empowerment

Swanepoel and De Beer (1996) state that empowerment is a process fed by information, knowledge, and experience. It brings people confidence in their own abilities. This process can help people to emerge from marginalized positions and become creative persons with rights, responsibilities, and strengths. Empowerment of the individual requires assistance from outside communities with regard to skills acquisition and training. The question of control and decision making may necessitate a shift or balancing of power, and this may impact on the AMP. In a developmental approach, structures may be developed from the 'bottom-up' rather than from 'top-down' as occurs in 'health planning'.

The medical model of disability that treats the person with disability as a patient or client with only physical or medical needs is wholly inadequate. Even if 'community-based', a programme is not developmental unless the people play a leading part in its design and implementation.

Professionals may be dubious about 'empowering' non-professionals. This feeling probably arises from the fear of relinquishing their own power and becoming disempowered themselves. Viewed more positively, the AMP can promote the resourcefulness of children and family members by providing opportunities to use and build their own capacity and support networks. With increasing independence, they can then act on their own choices with a sense of responsibility.

Empowerment occurs through positive attitudes, rather than through a type of charity that entrenches negative attitudes and places obstacles in the way of an inclusive society.

## Inclusion

The idea of 'inclusion' has involved a paradigm shift from that of mainstreaming. *Mainstreaming* implies that people with disabilities have problems within themselves and they have to be changed so as to fit in with or be made acceptable to society (Burden, 1995). The term 'mainstreaming' is often used with the same meaning as 'inclusion'. However, 'inclusion' expects society to facilitate the acceptance of those who do not fit in by accepting them just as they are. That is, the programme must fit the child, rather than the child fitting into the programme. The implication is that there is a shift in societal attitudes, which were previously evidenced by the belief that 'handicaps' were absolute characteristics of 'unfortunate' people. The process of 'labelling' a condition, for example 'deafness', provides a description of a condition but may also mean that 'victims' may need rehabilitation to change them rather than seeing them within their societal context.

This gives rise to two truisms stated by McConkey and O'Toole (1995): 'A disability need not be a handicap' and 'Handicaps are in the eye of the beholder'. Inclusion of children with disabilities has been difficult because the 'problem' is located in the child rather than in the often negative or discriminatory attitudes, policies, and institutions of countries.

Solutions that focus on mainstreaming and the prevention and cure of disabilities rather than on changing societal attitudes affect AMPs. Inclusion acknowledges that each family is unique and it accommodates diver-

sity. People do not have to change and become what seems to be normal. Society has to change its mindset and systems so as to accommodate and respond to the needs of all members of a unified, diverse society.

The fallacy about inclusion is to expect that all children, even those with severe disabilities, can be included into the schooling system. If this is not possible, living within a caring community can assist the family in building relationships and accessing resources. The process of inclusive education focuses on the whole system rather than on individual children. It may involve awareness-building, training, and recruitment. Perhaps when there are teachers who reflect the differences in the community, the barriers that exclude children and marginalize families will be broken. AMPs have an important role in promoting and facilitating such mutually beneficial approaches. Inclusion can only be successfully achieved if all stakeholders work collaboratively.

## Collaboration

Three elements of collaboration will be outlined: intersectoral collaboration, the transdisciplinary approach, and parent–professional collaboration.

### INTERSECTORAL COLLABORATION

In order to prevent duplication, view the child holistically, and become more cost effective, government policy promotes the collaboration of different departments, services, civil society, the private sector, and the community. This is particularly important and necessary in the presence of 'rightsizing' because of budget constraints.

A South African conference in 1998, 'Promoting Early Childhood Development – Building

Partnerships', highlighted the need for sharing information about existing resources. Poor communication and networking between non-government organizations (NGOs) and community-based organizations as well as the rivalry between these structures were identified as major barriers to collaborative partnerships. Financial constraints and cutbacks were perceived as a lack of commitment to these human services. The need to respect cultural diversity and develop organizational and marketing skills was emphasized. Teamwork amongst all parties involved in early childhood development (ECD) was also noted as a principal approach in facilitating the process of intersectoral collaboration (Drower & Katz 1998).

## THE TRANS-DISCIPLINARY APPROACH

On a micro level, teamwork gives rise to the trans-disciplinary approach involving the child, the family, therapists, and educators. While the team members may share discipline-specific information and concentrate on functional skills, there is now an emphasis on binding therapy needs into a holistic consolidated programme compatible with the child's natural environment. The ideal is a team of individuals possessing mutually supportive and complementary skills to guide and work in participation with the family in establishing a programme that can satisfy all needs.

If the team members acknowledge each other's expertise without creating barriers and marking territories, acknowledge the terminology of other disciplines, and develop an understanding about the roles, academic preparation and clinical experiences of each member, a solid grounding will be set for building a trans-disciplinary approach beneficial to all. Their values will not only be extended, but also enriched. In turn, this will facilitate some 'role exchanges' between the team members and the parents (Alper et al., 1995).

The ability to role model this approach will give rise to fruitful parent–professional collaboration.

## PARENT–PROFESSIONAL COLLABORATION

Family support is the primary goal of early intervention and families should be able to select services according to their culture, needs, and values, as well as their level of involvement in the decision-making process. Instances where professionals judge parents as being uncooperative or apathetic are often in reality the result of a lack of consensus between the parent and the professional.

Traditionally, parents have had a passive role in the assessment and intervention intended for of their child's disability. They are provided with diagnoses and results and expected to follow recommendations made by the professional, an attitude that affects their perception of their control over life events. The belief that professionals can solve all problems exacerbates their feeling of being disempowered and immobilized. Where AMPs have agreed with this belief, this needs to be reversed.

Helping families determine their own needs and priorities and then respecting their choices will rapidly change service delivery, and will create a new role for the professional with a new set of responsibilities for all participants. Building partnerships between families and service providers and treating these partners as equals were other concerns expressed at the Early Intervention Conference. Communication and counselling skills were identified as vital prerequisites for building such partnerships. Emphasis was placed on the concept of empowerment and involvement of parents in the development and running of community-based services. Central to the creation of barriers in the building of partnerships were factors such as the attitudes, lack of understanding, bureaucratic inefficiency, and rivalry between service providers. Lack of involvement of key community leaders and conflict between the needs of the service providers and those of the families were other obstacles. Priorities include encouraging parents to advocate for their rights, involving fathers, and building on the parents' knowledge and skills.

Collaborative working in a developmental framework on all levels will certainly facilitate the participation of all stakeholders. The more these all actively participate, the more will be the desire to take ownership and responsibility for the children within an inclusive process.

# Conclusion

In terms of Article 23 of the United Nations Convention on the Rights of the Child, the child with disability should be able to enjoy a 'full and decent life in conditions which ensure dignity, promote self reliance and facilitate the child's active participation in the community'.

AMPs have an important role in facilitating this process. They cannot work alone with individuals with disability if they are to participate in a developmental framework. This process may involve changing the stance and attitudes of AMPs and of society, rather than changing the children. With a supportive and inclusive approach, the abilities of children with disability can be emphasized rather than their disabilities or disadvantages. Attention will be directed to their needs and those of their families while also focusing on their 'equalness'. The process may require AMPs to examine and reflect on policies collaboratively so as to ensure there is no danger of reverting back to or perpetuating stigmatization and segregation. Seen more positively, the AMP can influence policy by assisting in monitoring, promoting, and supporting the realization of children's rights.

'Almost every significant breakthrough is the result of a courageous break with traditional ways of thinking', and if AMPs make this break with tradition, and act as role models, they will create limitless opportunities for themselves and others.

## References and further reading

ALPER S, SCHLOSS PJ, ETSCHEIDT, SK, and MACFALANE CA. 1995. *Inclusion – Are we abandoning or helping students?* California: Cronwin Press.

BERNARD VAN LEER FOUNDATION. 1994. *Building on people's strengths: Early childhood in Africa*. The Hague: Bernard van Leer Foundation.

BURDEN A. 1995. Inclusion as an educational approach in assisting people with disabilities. *Educare*. 24; 2:44–57.

DROWER S & KATZ B. 1998. Early childhood development: Promoting intersectoral partnerships through conference participation. *The Social Work Practitioner – Researcher*. II;1:21–39.

DUNST CJ, TIVETTE CM, and DEAL A (eds.). 1994. *Supporting and strengthening families, Vol I: Methods, strategies and practices*. Massachusetts: Brookline Books.

MCCONKEY R & O'TOOLE B. 1995. Towards the new millennium In: B O'Toole and R McConkey (eds.). *Innovations in developing countries for people with disabilities*. Lancashire: Lusieux Hall.

O'TOOLE B. 1989. The relevance of parental involvement programmes in developing countries. *Child Care, Health and Development*. 15:329–41.

SWANEPOEL H & DE BEER F. 1996. *Community capacity building: A guide for field workers and community Leaders*. Johannesburg: International Thompson Publications.

TREURNICHT S. 1997. From modernisation to sustainable development. In: H Swanepoel & F de Beer (eds.). *Introduction to development studies*. Johannesburg: International Thompson Publications.

# 32 Physiotherapy

## M GOODMAN & F SEMPLE

Childhood is characterized by growth and development. Movement, which is the essence of physiotherapy, accelerates this process. An intact neuromusculo-skeletal system is required for normal movement to take place and adequate cardiopulmonary function is also necessary. Physiotherapists thus have a role to play in ensuring that every child is given the opportunity to develop to his or her full potential.

Early diagnosis and treatment of conditions such as Erb's palsy, spina bifida, and club feet can prevent muscle contractures and deformities resulting from a lack of movement. Children with chronic disorders like cerebral palsy, muscular dystrophies, chronic juvenile arthritis, haemophilia, and other genetic and congenital abnormalities need to keep moving. How, when and how often they should move are vital factors influencing long-term outcome.

Efficient oxygen perfusion from the lungs into the circulation and to the tissues depends on adequately functioning lungs and airways. Conditions that interfere with this process, such as asthma and cystic fibrosis, require intervention to ensure that the airways are kept clear and normal breathing patterns are established. Anaesthesia may depress breathing and result in atelectasis requiring post-operative treatment by physiotherapists.

Movement may follow various stimuli. A noxious stimulus such as a pinprick to a limb will lead to its withdrawal. Movement and function are usually initiated by the cognitive and volitional need to move, like reaching for a toy. Children with an intellectual deficit may lack the motivation to move, especially if they are placed in a comfortable position. This may seem unimportant when a child is small and can be carried around, but immobile adults who cannot stand cause enormous nursing problems. Change of position is essential to prevent pressure sores and their serious complications.

Physiotherapists are not simply concerned with movement 'per se' but rather with the important impact that movement has on perception and cognitive growth.

Head control is a pre-requisite for establishing visual fixation on an object and for developing eye–hand co-ordination. Sitting offers the child a new perspective of the world and orientation in space. This, together with the ability to shift weight, balance, and then move around, enables the child to explore the environment. With the acquisition of developmental milestones, the child develops and perfects manipulative skills and the ability to perform functional activities necessary for daily living. The various life skills can be learnt by practice, perseverance, and motivation.

Physiotherapists working in the field of paediatrics will need a thorough knowledge of the development of all the body systems and how this will impact on function in adulthood. Deprivation of the specific and necessary stimulation for this growth and development can have lasting detrimental consequences if early intervention is not timeously instituted.

## Role of the physiotherapist

In the last five years the role of the physiotherapist has changed dramatically.

Treatment initiatives are not only formulated according to the medical model but social and societal needs must also be considered. Health professionals dealing with children can no longer ignore the opinions and needs of the parents, family, and caregiver, or those expressed by their patients. From an early age, children have their own aspirations and their use of an appliance or adherence to an exercise programme will depend on their attitude, motivation, and perseverance as well as the approach of parents and caregivers. Demanding instructions, such as 'You will do as I say', no longer apply.

There will not be enough physiotherapists to meet the needs of all the people. One-on-one treatment situations using expensive electrical equipment are now seldom feasible. Physiotherapists, as scarce expert resources, are called upon to delegate as many tasks as possible to suitably trained but less highly qualified assistants. These include community-based rehabilitation workers and volunteers, who, contrary to the beliefs of many, are

doing mostly excellent work. Carefully planned teaching, training with hands-on experience, as well as continuing education and support are essential. Regular follow-up clinics to correct techniques, handling, and exercises are most important for affirmation and progression of treatments. Associated supervision to discuss the social as well as the medical aspects of their therapy sessions is essential. Ongoing contracting of length and time of treatment is included.

The role of physiotherapists is expanding and changing as more emphasis is placed on primary health care and preventive medicine. The scope of the physiotherapist must necessarily include other dimensions to meet these needs.

## Meeting demands

The 'team approach' is not a new concept, but the emphasis placed on members of the team has changed. Without a doubt, the most important members are the parents and caregivers. As noted above, their understanding, hopes, and expectations are a prime concern. In turn, the objectives of treatment must be explained, negotiated, and agreed upon.

Children are being grouped, whether in primary, secondary, or tertiary care systems, according to their particular and similar needs. All or some of the members of the health team participate in a group. The groups meet regularly to reinforce techniques being taught and to provide support. Advantages of group sessions include increasing the numbers of clients assisted, the sharing and support amongst caregivers and socialization of children. Some such groups have gone on to form the core of a care group and later a nursery school.

Physiotherapists are now taught basic management and organizational skills, teaching and counselling skills, and research principles in order to meet all these needs. They may be movement and exercise specialists but the education, training, and understanding of parents, teachers, and caregivers and the society in which they live are essential. Specialized manual techniques alone are not the key to success.

## References and further reading

ANDERSON G & VENTER A. 1997. Parental experiences of a cerebral palsy clinic in a poor urbanising community. *South African Journal of Physiotherapy.* 53;3:4–8.

FINNIE N. 1974. *Handling the young cerebral palsy child at home,* 2nd ed. Oxford: Heinemann Medical Books.

GOODMAN M & KATZ B. 1998. *Caring and coping.* Johannesburg: Witwatersrand University Press.

LEVITT S. 1994. *Basic abilities.* Souvenir Press.

SHEPHERD R. 1974. *Physiotherapy in paediatrics.* Oxford: Alden Press.

TAUKOBONG NP. 1999. The role of the community based rehabilitation worker within the primary health care service. *South African Journal of Physiotherapy.* 55;1:19–23

# 33 Occupational therapy

## T COETZER

Many children in South Africa experience disabilities or chronic illness that limit their everyday function. A large number of these children will one day be unable to work and earn a living or live independently in their communities because of disabilities, unless they are assisted by rehabilitation professionals to overcome difficulties and maximize their potential.

Occupational therapists (OTs) are part of the team of rehabilitation professionals who provide services and create opportunities for children with a variety of disabilities to achieve independence in their home with their families, at school with their peers, and in their communities within a wider spectrum of people.

Occupational therapy enables children with limited abilities to do the 'day-to-day' activities that are important to them despite impairments, activity limitations, and participation restrictions. The occupational therapist uses goal-directed pursuits that are meaningful to the performer and involve multiple tasks or media.

## Evaluation

The child's functioning is evaluated in collaboration with family, care providers, and relevant others.

The aims of evaluation are to:
- identify performance problems interfering with role fulfilment. These may include difficulties in performing activities of daily living, inability to play with peers, or difficulty with learning and inability to progress at school;
- identify the nature of impairments and the components that interfere with performance potential – these are sensorimotor, cognitive, and psychological or

---

### OT is directed at children who have or are at risk for:

- physical disabilities;
- cognitive disabilities;
- psychosocial dysfunction;
- intellectual disabilities;
- developmental and/or learning disorders;
- maladaptive behaviours;
- co-morbid conditions; and
- chronic illness.

social components of function. Problems are contextualized within biomedical and/or psychosocial realms;

- determine meaningful and purposeful occupations and potential therapeutic activities;
- analyse environmental and social conditions and contexts that may restrict occupational performance;
- determine available environmental resources to facilitate performance; and
- identify intact, retained, or remaining performance component skills that may be effectively used to effect change in performance.

In this evaluation, the influence of age, developmental level, life cycle, health and disability status, culture, and social circumstance are all contextually considered.

Occupational therapists use multiple methods to gather data about occupational performance, not only involving the child but also including input from family members and school or child care personnel. These methods comprise interviews, self assessment questionnaires, checklists, skill rating scales, occupational histories and narratives, standardized tests, skilled formal and informal observation, as well as other non-standardized procedures.

## Intervention

After analysing the results of the evaluation, the occupational therapist collaborates with the child family and care providers such as schoolteachers or child care personnel to establish goals and methods of intervention and the setting where the intervention is to be provided.

Intervention approaches involve remediation and/or restoration, compensation and/or adaptation, disability prevention, and health promotion, or lifestyle restructuring.

This intervention would include:

- developing, improving, sustaining, or restoring skills in activities of daily living (ADL), schoolwork, play and leisure, and preparation for work;
- identifying and facilitating engagement in meaningful and healthy occupations to fulfil life roles appropriate for that individual child;
- developing, remediating, or restoring sensorimotor, cognitive, or psychosocial components of performance. This involves using specific frames of reference, such as sensory integration therapy, neurodevelopmental therapy, perceptual motor training, play facilitation, psychosocial factors or a combination of these approaches (Kramer & Hinojosa, 1993); and
- therapeutic use of purposeful and meaningful occupations. For the child this would primarily mean the skilled use of play because play is the ordinary familiar activity in which the child engages every day. Other media such as music, dance, puppetry, art, craft, and sport are used singly or in combination as therapeutic agents.

Therapeutic occupation, particularly play, is used for a variety of reasons:

- It is used to act as a therapeutic change agent to remediate and restore impaired abilities.
- It facilitates transfer of an acquired performance component (e.g., eye–hand co-ordination) to multiple contexts (e.g., to use a pencil effectively when drawing).
- It enhances motivation and drive for making change.
- It promotes self-expression, exploration, and identification of values and interests.
- It creates opportunities to practise skills.
- It provides the child with feedback that successfully and naturally grades performance.

- The experience of success and mastery in play is the foundation for further achievement of goals.

## Adaptation of environments and processes to enhance performance

This involves changing the task, altering the task methodology, or prescribing adaptive equipment. It may also mean biomechanical adaptation to the living environment.

Adaptive equipment spans the continuum from low-tech devices for ADL, such as grab bars, adapted handles, dressing sticks, and mobility devices to technologically complex equipment, such as a voice-activated computer system that interfaces with a power wheelchair system.

This form of intervention involves choice of design, fabrication, application and training in the use of assistive technology, orthotic appliances, or prosthetic devices.

It is important to educate the child, family, caregiver, or any other relevant persons in carrying out appropriate non-skilled interventions. This will involve home visits, classroom visits, and visits to care facilities or institutions.

It is also important to consult with organizations, projects, groups, or communities to provide community-based services.

## The child within the context of family and community

The child's abilities and disabilities must always be viewed in relation to his or her family and community and all intervention must involve these significant elements. In South Africa this is not always possible as service providers are often inconveniently situated and it is difficult to promote this philos-ophy. Home programmes for parents, collaborative work with resourceful and respected people in the community, and working with families can be useful. The assistance of village health and rehabilitation workers, where they are available, is invaluable in these circumstances because they are familiar with the area, its people, and their resources (Loveday, 1993; Werner, 1988; and DART, 1997).

## Settings for provision of service

Occupational therapists are able to provide services at all health care levels, where such posts exist in the public health sector.

At primary health care level in community settings, non-governmental organizations, educare, and day-care centres, occupational therapists are increasingly acting in an advisory and consultative capacity to community rehabilitation workers, caregivers, and teachers of children with disabilities.

At secondary and tertiary levels, occupational therapists provide services of evaluation and intervention at specialized in- and out-patient clinics and in general hospital ward settings.

In the educational setting, occupational therapists have traditionally been part of the specialist rehabilitation teams at schools for children with special needs (such as cerebral palsy, learning disability, sensory impairments, autism, pervasive developmental disorder etc.) who have not been able to manage with mainstream education. Therapists are increasingly assisting children with special needs who are in the mainstream school setting, in accordance with departmental policy.

In the welfare setting, in children's homes, in places of safety, and in institutions, occupational therapists are increasingly employed in a consulting capacity to advise on developmental and health promotion programmes.

Occupational therapists also work in private practice providing a variety of services to children. The practitioner may choose to see the child and family in the practice setting or at their own home, depending on the model of practice. Most registered medical aid schemes cover the services of occupational therapists registered with the Health Professions Council of South Africa.

Occupational therapists assist the courts and legal profession in medico-legal work by assessing and reporting on the impairments, disabilities, and handicaps that result from personal injury.

# Conclusion

There is a world-wide need for the services of occupational therapists, not only for the rehabilitation of children, but across all age groups and for a variety of disabilities. In South Africa a lack of post structure exists for mid-level health workers in the public sector. In the current plan of inclusive education of children with disabilities in mainstream schools, provision should be made for posts for occupational therapists as a matter of urgency. There is a lack of rehabilitation service provision for people with disabilities in general, but particularly for disadvantaged groups in rural areas.

The contextual management of at-risk children needs to be a priority in South Africa's health, welfare, and educational plans, as it will save on costly rehabilitation once disability is established. Health promotion of adults and lifestyle changes of high-risk families, where infants and children are raised in potentially debilitating circumstances, need urgent attention to ensure child health for all.

## References and further reading

CASE-SMITH J. 1994. Defining the specialization of pediatric occupational therapy. *American Journal of Occupational Therapy.* 48(9):791–802.

CLANCY & CLARK MJ. 1990. *Occupational therapy with children.* Brisbane: Churchill Livingstone.

COSTNER W. 1998. Occupational centred assessment of children. *American Journal of Occupational Therapy.* 52:337–44.

DART. 1997. *Community-based rehabilitation (cbr) database* – A listing of articles, journals, books, and resources. Available from Disability Action Research Team (DART), 12 Millar Street, Howick, KZN, 3290.

KRAMER P & HINOJOSA J. (1993) *Frames of reference for pediatric occupational therapy.* Baltimore: Williams & Wilkins.

LOVEDAY PM. 1993. An evaluation of the SACLA Rehabilitation Worker Project in Cape Town. Unpublished M Phil MCH dissertation.

WERNER D. 1988. *Disabled village children – A guide to community heath workers rehabilitation workers and families,* 2nd ed. Palo Alto: Hesperian Foundation.

# 34 Social work and the child health team

## SJ DROWER

The primary concern of social work is the interaction between people and their environments, i.e. people's social functioning. 'Environment' includes the physical, emotional, interpersonal, and spiritual surround of people. It incorporates intimate groups like the family and the peer group, as well as more distant environments ranging from the school, the local neighbourhood, and the workplace to social, economic, and political systems, through which society's beliefs and values with respect to meeting people's needs are actualized.

To fulfil its functions social work pursues a threefold purpose: first, to strengthen people's abilities to problem-solve, cope, and develop; second, to link people with systems in their environment that provide services, resources, or opportunities to improve their functioning; and third, to promote the effective and humane operation of service, resource and opportunity systems (Pierce, 1989:105).

Facilitating people's empowerment of themselves and promoting mutually beneficial interactions between people and society in order to improve the quality of life for everyone is the nub of all social work activity. Social workers work with individuals, families, small groups, and communities in order to provide direct services. Indirect social work services include colleague and interdisciplinary consultation, programme development, policy formulation, and research.

## Social work intervention and the child health team

There are two distinguishing characteristics of social work that are especially pertinent to the profession's contribution to the child health

### The functions of social work

These include:
- caring;
- protection;
- healing and restoring;
- prevention;
- education;
- resource management;
- social justice and equity;
- policy and programme development;
- professional education/training; and
- practice development.

team. The first is its emphasis on the whole-ness and totality of people and their environ-ments, and the second is the profession's emphasis on the importance of the family as the basic building block of society. While the profession acknowledges the varied and dynamic structure of the family, it also notes the family's importance in moulding and influencing behaviour. Highlighting whole-ness and totality underscores social work's commitment to an interdisciplinary team approach to meeting people's needs. Social workers acknowledge the different dimen-sions of people, including biological, physio-logical, social, psychological, and spiritual aspects. It locates these different dimensions within people's economic, social, and cultur-al contexts in order to 'support, maintain or heal' the whole (Potgieter, 1998:114). The role of the family as 'the basic unit of society' was reaffirmed in the 1997 White Paper for Social Welfare, which noted the need to strengthen family life through family-oriented policies and programmes (Ministry for Social Welfare and Population Development, 1997:20).

The importance of the family rests on its contribution to the stability of society through the socialization of the young, and the provision of protection and nurture for both the young and the vulnerable. The rapidly and constantly changing social, political, and economic con-texts of South Africa have placed enormous strain on the family's ability to make this con-tribution. In addition to the overriding factor of poverty, other aspects of present South African reality have been identified as negative influ-ences on the individual's ability to function optimally. This, in turn, affects the function-ing of the family and the community. These factors include unemployment; malnutri-tion; infant mortality and teenage pregnancy; housing and public health; literacy and educa-tion; alcohol and substance abuse; and vio-lence, abuse, and neglect (Potgieter, 1998). The impact of HIV/AIDS should be added to these.

With much of the present social dislocation in South Africa being attributable to poverty, social work is paying increased attention to interventive approaches that aim to contribute directly towards its eradication. This has neces-sitated a move away from remedial strategies that focus on individual change toward pre-ventive and promotive activities that support the strengths of individuals, families, groups, and communities. This facilitates people's empowerment of themselves. The sharing of information and development of skills are both central to a developmental approach.

In terms of this new paradigm the social work contribution to the child health team may best be illustrated by noting some of the activities of the social worker at the three levels of preventive intervention:

- *Primary prevention:* This refers to early intervention through the timely provision of services to vulnerable persons so that individual and family dysfunction is avoid-ed. Encouraging the immunization of young children, attendance at well-baby clinics and pre- and post-natal care are basic con-cerns of social workers working with fami-lies and young children. In addition, social workers may be involved in the provision of family life education for children and adolescents, and pre-marital and parent education for young adults. Also at the pri-mary level of intervention social workers are active in mobilizing the skills and resources of other team members in the provision of health education programmes, e.g., HIV/AIDS education, family planning, and in ensuring that families are educated about and have access to relevant resources.
- *Secondary prevention:* This 'is aimed at the identification of problems and early inter-vention into the lives of individuals, fami-lies and groups who are at risk of develop-ing social problems before the situation becomes critical' (Ministry for Welfare and Population Development, 1997: 97). Target

311

groups with respect to secondary prevention in child health may include the family with a developmentally delayed child or with a parent who has become mentally ill. When such families find themselves in a precarious socio-economic position, the risk of social dysfunction increases. Encouraging compliance with treatment, attending follow-up appointments at clinics, and mediating between the health care service and the family are important aspects of social work in this regard.

- *Tertiary prevention:* This is concerned with individuals and families who are already experiencing critical problems and dysfunction, and aims to prevent further deterioration. The rehabilitation and support within society of the chronically mentally and physically ill are special foci of social work activities in tertiary prevention. These activities may involve the education and support of family members, for example, addressing the special needs of the adolescent with a parent who is chronically depressed, or those of the young family whose breadwinner has been permanently disabled through a mining accident. Also included are reconstruction services that attempt to reunite parents and children previously separated through statutory provisions enacted to safeguard the interests of minor children.

At all three levels of prevention the social worker encourages consumer responsibility and control by supporting the active involvement of the individual, family, and local community group affected. Likewise, at all three levels of intervention the social worker acts as an important conduit between consumers and other members of the child health team. This latter contribution is especially relevant in the South African context where diversity in culture, religion, and class affects the understanding of health concerns and the use of health services.

# Challenges facing social work

Like other human services in South Africa today, social work is confronted by a situation of considerable need and limited resources. It is challenged to redress the imbalances of its previous services and to identify ways of intervening that are relevant to local conditions. These challenges demand that social workers continually review and evaluate their services with respect to the diverse peoples they serve. Also it requires that people, the recipients of services, are viewed as resources that should be mobilized in addressing health and welfare concerns. This is nowhere more evident than in respect to the HIV/AIDS pandemic. With the looming prospect of an increased number of orphans, an increasing number of HIV-infected babies, and an increased death rate amongst the economically active population, the social worker will be confronted with a family unit that is less likely to be able to serve its function as the cornerstone of society. Addressing this situation will necessitate new and creative responses on the part of social workers and close collaboration between all members of the health care team.

## References and further reading

MINISTRY FOR WELFARE AND POPULATION DEVELOPMENT. 1997. White Paper for Social Welfare: Principles, guidelines, recommendations, proposed policies and programmes for developmental social welfare in South Africa. Pretoria: Department of Welfare.

PIERCE D. 1989. *Social work and society: An introduction.* New York: Longman.

POTGIETER MC. 1998. *The social work process: Development to empower people.* Johannesburg, Prentice-Hall South Africa (Pty) Ltd.

# 35

# Speech pathology and audiology

## G BECKETT

Communication is a highly complex process used by the communicator to express meaning. Learning how to talk or express oneself through sign, which is language acquisition, enables this. Meaning or intent is organized and encoded into language usually through speech or sometimes writing or sign language. The speaker uses voice to produce sound and co-ordinates voice use with breathing and speech articulation. This communication is conveyed through hearing, or, in the case of sign language through sight, to the listener or receiver of the message. This is then decoded in the receiver's brain to convert the symbols of the message back into meaning.

The discipline of speech pathology and audiology is divided into language, voice, speech, and hearing. Students study subjects as diverse as neurology, linguistics, community work, psychology, and educational principles. However, speech pathology, language, and audiology form the backbone of the course. The role of speech and hearing professionals is to diagnose and treat all the disorders that fall within their professional ambit. They need to know when to refer individuals. They need to be able to conduct research into communication difficulties,

and they need to be able to engage in management and various community outreach programmes.

Because communication is such a complex process many aspects of it are vulnerable to breakdown. It is estimated that approximately ten per cent of any population will suffer from communication impairment. This figure is higher in certain sub-groups, particularly among disadvantaged people whose children are at greater risk due to pre-, peri-, and post-natal trauma. They may also have secondary difficulties because of failure to receive adequate treatment.

## Disorders of communication

*Speech problems* may present as inability to articulate or speak clearly, or as an interference with rhythm or fluency of speech production. In mild forms such as the well-known childhood lisp, the child does not produce a clear 's' sound. However, in severe dysfunction, as may occur with cerebral palsy, speech can be apraxic or dysarthric. Such children have difficulty controlling the muscles needed to produce speech sounds and in co-ordinating their breathing. They may not be able to produce any of the speech sounds or they may produce speech that is very difficult to understand. The speech of a child with a cleft lip and/or cleft palate, or with a serious tongue abnormality is also affected. Stuttering is sometimes classified as a speech disorder, but it also may be associated with other language or emotional disorders. The speech of children with hearing loss may be impaired by their inability to hear the sounds they are trying to produce.

*Voice disorders* are due to functional or organic causes. Diagnosis should, whenever possible, be undertaken by a team including both a speech pathologist and an ear, nose, and throat specialist. The help of either or both specialists and co-operation between them is essential for the optimal treatment of the patient.

*Language problems* may be congenital or acquired. Language acquisition is one of the most amazing feats of the human brain and interference with this learning process can result in either delayed or deviant language development. Much of our learning occurs through language. The child with poor language acquisition will have learning problems. High-risk infants and those with Pervasive Developmental Delay are also prone to difficulties or delays in language acquisition.

*Auditory processing disorders* are often linked to language disorders. Children thus affected are able to 'hear' at a peripheral level but at a cognitive level they have difficulty in interpreting auditory signals and therefore in understanding language. Language disorders, untreated during the pre-school years, may manifest as attention deficits or other learning difficulties at school. Such children require specialist help in order to cope with academic demands and in particular with learning to read and write. These kinds of difficulties can have serious social and educational implications.

*Acquired language disorder* implies that the child has developed language and that as a result of some insult such as disease or head injury, aspects of his/her speech and language are interfered with. This can involve both receptive and expressive language.

Early interventionists have identified that the quality of parent–child interaction is crucial in the development of the whole child, and in particular the social, emotional, cognitive, and linguistic aspects.

*Hearing disorders* can be congenital or acquired. The age of onset, degree, and type of hearing loss determine the severity of the disorder. Deaf people fight for the recognition that they can do everything except hear. They are certainly not 'dumb'; they can learn to communicate and there is increasing worldwide acceptance that for deaf people the first language is 'sign'. While some deaf children are also brain injured or intellectually disabled, most deaf people have normal intelligence.

*Hearing loss* is categorized according to its severity, ranging from profound to moderate or mild. Those with some hearing can be assisted to hear at their optimal level. Thorough hearing assessments need to be made over time by an audiologist in order to ascertain the prognosis for the child, and to make the best management decisions about that child. This may involve a hearing aid assessment and auditory training with these aids, as well as speech therapy, language therapy, and lip-reading.

The diagnosis and treatment of *middle-ear infections* in children is very important. Recurring otitis media during the critical pre-school years may interfere with hearing and language-learning resulting in later learning difficulties, or even permanent hearing loss. This is common in economically disadvantaged areas where adequate management may not always be readily accessible. Such children need rehabilitation therapy as well as medical treatment.

In South Africa there is insufficient screening for these disabling conditions. Many children suffering from hearing loss, intellectual disability, cerebral palsy, forms of brain injury, and learning disorders are underserved. There are not enough facilities and professionals to help habilitate them. Children in disadvantaged areas are more likely to have multiple disabilities and their diagnosis and treatment can be both complex and expensive. The importance of early intervention is well recognized internationally, both for humane reasons and because it is cost-effective. In South Africa, the *early childhood development* sector is not yet accepted as an educational priority and the burden therefore falls on non-governmental educational sectors and on health services to identify and assist at-risk pre-school children.

## Speech, language, voice, and hearing professionals

There are two categories of professionals who deal with communication problems. These are speech, language, and hearing therapists (SLHTs) and community speech and hearing workers (CSHWs).

The SLHT holds a four-year university degree and while he/she may engage in some community work, the focus is on individual rehabilitation, including in-depth diagnosis and therapy, as well as research.

CSHWs hold a two-year university diploma. They focus, as the name implies, on outreach primary health care, and work with communities to promote optimal communication and prevent disordered communication. Most CSHWs function in rural areas, sometimes with the more general community rehabilitation workers.

Both categories of worker are registered with the Health Professions Council of South Africa and both may be members of the professional South African Speech, Language, and Hearing Association (SASLHA). They form an integral part of the health care team together with occupational therapists, physiotherapists, doctors, nurses, teachers, social workers, psychologists, and other community workers. There is growing understanding that the medical component alone is insufficient for all rehabilitation therapy and management, and increasing acceptance of equity between the members of the health care team.

## The nature of the work

### PREVENTION

(See Chapter 21: Health surveillance.)
Primary health care takes on a particular meaning within a therapeutic framework.

*Primary prevention* seeks to prevent disability altogether, and in this context, disorders that affect speech and hearing.

*Secondary prevention* refers to early screening and identification of children with disabilities so that timeous intervention can prevent further deterioration and promote optimal outcome possibilities (see Table 35.1). After a full assessment, parents can be advised on how to develop their child's speech and language. They can also be given a home programme together with recommendations for follow up.

A problem still far too common in South Africa is the late identification and referral of disabled children. This is partly because of the poverty and undereducation of the populations concerned, but also because of misguided professionals who advise parents to wait. At-risk and disabled children need to be referred for specialist diagnosis as early as possible. It is neither cost-effective nor humane to leave the parents with the burden of coping alone with a disabled child. Critical periods of learning are often wasted by incorrect advice. The child aged eight years who is brought to hospital seeking admission to a school for the deaf or the cerebral palsied is far more difficult and costly to help than a baby identified and properly managed before six months of age. Disabled children are sometimes hidden away, neglected, or abandoned, again resulting in a lack of, or a delay in treatment. Public and professional education is vital and part of outreach with screening in clinics, pre-schools, and primary schools.

In *tertiary prevention and treatment* the therapist aims to rehabilitate the child who is already suffering in some way, thus helping him/her to reach his/her maximum potential. This does not necessarily mean 'cure' but often includes adjustment and education towards living as full a life as possible together with counselling the parents and teachers, and sometimes managing the child's environment. Therapy can be short or long term and may involve home programmes. There is increasing recognition of the importance of involving parents and teachers in therapy and sharing information with them. Therapy requires a two-way commitment by both patient/parent and therapist. The understanding of the concept of communication is no longer just restricted to speech. Additional devices such as computers are being used increasingly. Children who cannot speak or write normally may be able to express themselves through operating a computer or communication

**Table 35.1** Screening checklist to determine whether a child needs assessment for a speech, language, or hearing problem

| Child's age | Hearing and understanding | Speaking |
|---|---|---|
| Birth | Does child respond to loud noises and to speech? | Does child coo or gurgle ('aagoo')? |
| Three months | Does child respond to speech by stopping crying or by head-turning or by smiling? | Does child babble ('babababa')? |
| Six months | Does child try to find the source of sounds? Does child respond to 'no' or to his/her name? | Has child's babbling increased and become more complex ('badaba', 'lalalam')? |
| Nine months to one year | Is the child beginning to understand some words, e.g. his/her name and some simple questions or statements, e.g. 'Come to Mummy', 'Do you want milk?' Is he/she beginning to listen to your conversations? | Is child beginning to imitate sounds and say one word, e.g. 'Mama, Dada, Baba'? |
| $1\frac{1}{2}$ to two years | Can child follow two instructions, e.g., 'Fetch your shoes and bring them to me?' | Is child's vocabulary increasing and becoming clearer? Is child putting two words together e.g. 'Me up', 'Want milk', 'Where Dada'? |
| $2\frac{1}{2}$ to four years | Does child follow simple conversation? Does child hear quiet speech or when called from · another room? | Is child using 200–300 words? Is he/she putting at least three or four words together, e.g., 'me go dad', 'Where big dog go?' Can you and other people understand most of what child says? |

(adapted from other checklists, including one from SASLHA)

board. Deaf people can read telephone messages. Cochlear implants in infants can, where appropriate, allow them to hear a form of speech they can learn to understand from infancy. Deaf children and their families are encouraged to use sign language from a very early age so that the child's language development is not delayed.

## The range of the work

Working with communication impairment involves working with the individual, his or her family, school, the health care team, and the broader community in which the child lives. Therapy can be aimed at the child, the family, or the group; while education, including promotion and prevention of disorders, is often aimed at the community. 'Community' here includes the geographical as well as the functional community, examples of the latter are the parents of children who are intellectually disabled or a group of adolescents who stutter.

Therefore both CSWHs and SLHTs have to be multi-skilled. They have to be able to screen for communication difficulties and other developmental disorders and refer when necessary to other professionals. They have to be skilled in educating groups, such as child caregivers on topics such as language stimulation, and teachers in handling communication problems in the classroom.

Parents who are coming to terms with loss, either the loss of functioning in the child or the loss of the perfect or normal child, need counselling to assist in the process of grieving or adjustment. The marriage is often strained because of a disabled child, and parent counselling is essential. Helping the adolescent who stutters with his/her image or helping the mother of a newborn baby with a cleft palate with her anxieties and practical difficulties about the feeding of her infant are a vital part of this work.

Diagnostic tools are becoming increasingly sophisticated, particularly as our knowledge of brain function increases. Speech and language assessments form an important part of the overall assessment of a young child. A growing area of interest and concern in this country is the possible effect on the language system(s) experienced by the bilingual or multilingual child. Ethical issues, including the right of the child to essential health care and the role of therapists, are gaining increasing attention. Viewing the child holistically within his/her family, school, and community is important, as decisions about the management of the child's life are taken.

## What to teach parents when there is no professional

The SLHT aims to get the child communicating as early and as fully as possible, an aim shared by the parent/s. The earliest communication with a baby and child would start with playful turn-taking – making sounds, pulling faces, and then incorporating the use of gestures and words into this play. The mother or infant may initiate a communication and the other would respond with mutual enjoyment and an interchange of meaning-making. It is vital for parents of disabled children to understand this and to realize that they should persevere with such interactions. Through this, language develops. If parents mistakenly think they do not need to communicate with a child who is deaf or intellectually disabled, the child will become far more disabled. Despite the child's disability, there may still be capacity to develop language and some form of signalling, and thus the ability to communicate.

Parents should understand that children learn through play and that exploration of their world is essential to their normal early development. This also applies to the child with a disability who needs as full a range as possible of appropriate experiences using all kinds of sensorimotor experiences within their capacity.

Children need caring adults to mediate the world to them, to talk about the world, to point out things to them, to focus on certain things, to explain things to them. Children learn both language and thought through this mediation which is essential to their successful learning.

# Conclusion

It is unfortunate that while there is a huge need in South Africa for the services of both CSHWs and SLHTs, there are insufficient posts. Moreover, remuneration, particularly in relation to their levels of training and the complexity and importance of their work, is inadequate.

More rehabilitation facilities are needed for all groups of disabled people.

It is hoped that in the new South Africa we will express our care as a nation by placing a higher priority on four aspects of development:

- *Pre-school education:* This will lead to better early stimulation of children. More parental education with an increase in their involvement in their children's education and welfare, and early detection and prevention of disabilities;

- *Rehabilitation of disability;*
- *Action at local level:* It is necessary to identify and to follow up those at risk for disability through a thorough and caring health and education system. Resources available to high-risk infants are extremely disparate. Currently, there are far too many at-risk children not being identified for intervention, who start life at risk and who grow up without reaching their full emotional, linguistic, or cognitive potential;
- *the creation of appropriate community-based rehabilitation posts and facilities for child care specialists:* These can treat and possibly prevent communication disabilities and a broad range of mental health disabilities.

South Africa's children need to be seen, heard, and understood!

## References and further reading

FRAIBERG S. 1959. *The Magic Years: Understanding the problems of early childhood.* London: Methuen & Co.

HALLIDAY MAK. 1985. *Spoken and written language.* Oxford: Oxford University Press.

ROSETTI LM. 1996. *Communication intervention: Birth to three.* London: Singular Publishing Company.

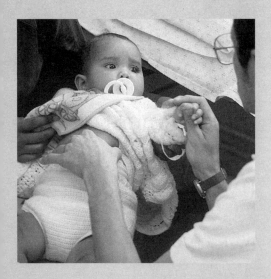

PART TWELVE

# Childhood illness

Gastrointestinal infections, respiratory disorders, bacterial, viral and parasitic infections, injuries, and poisonings account for the bulk of deaths outside the perinatal period. In this section, these major causes of mortality and morbidity will be addressed. There are also short chapters on medications for common ailments, and the management of emergencies.

# 36

# Integrated management of childhood illness (IMCI)

## WEK LOENING

The integrated management of childhood illness, now well known by the acronym IMCI, is a strategy designed by the World Health Organization and UNICEF in the early 1990s. Since then, it has been introduced in many countries throughout the world. The underlying principles are long standing, and are universally applicable to the health care of all children under the age of five years. IMCI has the greatest impact in those countries where mortality of children is well above that of industrialized countries. Nevertheless, it is advocated for impoverished and underserved communities even in developed countries.

Initially, the focus of IMCI was on reducing childhood mortality and morbidity caused by the main killers in that age group, namely, diarrhoeal disease, acute respiratory infection, measles, malaria, and malnutrition. However, it became obvious that the paediatric disease profile varied considerably from one country to another, and even within countries. Moreover, because culture and traditions may influence the care of the sick child, it became necessary for countries to adapt the strategy to their own needs and circumstances. This is best illustrated by the profound effect that AIDS is having on the health of children in most sub-Saharan countries.

Recognizing that the health of children is determined by more than the common pathogenic organisms, IMCI extends well beyond the immediate care of the sick child by addressing essential elements of support within the health sector, as well as practices in the family and community.

Experience has shown that much of what follows below is already accepted practice at health facilities, but unfortunately it is frequently practised inadequately. The strategy does not claim to be new but it does bring all facets of child health together and aims to improve the quality of the care.

## What is integrated? And why?

At the heart of the IMCI strategy is the child and not the disease. Again, although this concept is generally supported in principle, it is seldom put into practice. All health workers will acknowledge that one is inclined to be satisfied with labelling a sick child with a diagnosis, such as pneumonia or gastroenteritis and providing treatment accordingly. How often does one look at the whole child, who might very well have another serious or at least potentially serious problem? For example, is the nutritional state of every under-five-year old that attends our health facilities assessed?

Integration refers to:

- considering more than one problem;
- always checking the immunization and nutritional status; and
- involving the primary caregiver in continuing treatment at home and preventive measures.

This is best illustrated in the case of a child with diarrhoeal disease: immediate assessment of the state of hydration and consideration of other illnesses leads to prompt oral rehydration therapy (ORT) and treatment of all coexisting conditions. Any outstanding immunizations are administered. Counselling of the caregiver includes continuing ORT and the importance of proper nutrition, both during the illness and the recovery phase, as well as good hygiene and sanitation at home.

# Component 1: Case management

The central focus is on the quality of care of the sick child presenting at a first level health facility. The process is delineated in a Chart Booklet in a series of algorithms.

## ASSESSMENT, CLASSIFICATION, AND TREATMENT

There are several unusual features in the clinical approach of IMCI in that it is based on a triage system, which comes into operation as soon as the child is seen. Triage in turn is based on carefully selected and validated symptoms and signs that are clearly defined. The presence of any one of five *Danger Signs*, (i.e., vomiting everything up, unable to take

any feeds, lethargy or unconsciousness, convulsion during this illness, or convulsing at present) signifies pre-referral treatment, rapid assessment, and then immediate referral.

Similarly, determining the severity of the main symptoms is based on a combination of signs. (For instance fast breathing in an infant under the age of 2 months is 60 and over, whereas from the age of 2 months up to 12 months, it is 50 and over, and in the child over the age of one year, it is 40 and over.) Signs of chest indrawing, dehydration, malnutrition, and anaemia, among others, are similarly clearly defined. Accordingly, the problems are classified and well-designed treatment protocols govern further management. No attempt is made at a diagnosis, which at times requires more detailed technical investigation, but often adds nothing of consequence to the management. It is therefore of fundamental importance that the classification is correct to ensure that the severely ill child is referred promptly. On the other hand, unnecessary referrals, which are a burden for the mother and child and on the referral centre, are avoided.

Treatment protocols are consistent with the Essential Drug List and include country- or province-specific antibiotics. Generally, drugs are kept to a bare minimum and do not include placebos, such as cough mixtures. Indications for analgesics/antipyretics are few and the number of doses is limited. Moreover, the mother is carefully counselled, so that there is no doubt that she has understood when and how to give the medication.

## COUNSELLING THE MOTHER

Although it seems obvious, the child's primary caregiver needs to have a good understanding of the child's illness as well as the treatment required. Nevertheless, this is one of the most frequent omissions in primary care practice. Considerable time is devoted to counselling in the 11-day 'Case Management' training programme: not only does it focus on treatment but also includes the importance of follow-up visits and signs that indicate the need for immediate return. The latter then also empowers the mother to make a decision in subsequent illnesses whether there is need for urgent attention or whether care of the child at home is preferable. Needless to say, this avoids unnecessary clinic visits to the advantage of all concerned.

The child's nutritional needs are stressed, both in sickness and during convalescence as well as under healthy circumstances.

## PREVENTIVE AND PROMOTIVE MEASURES

The importance of the child's nutrition cannot be stressed sufficiently. This is dealt with in detail in Chapter 15: Infant and child nutrition. Here, it is only necessary to say that a careful assessment of the nutritional status of every under-five-year old child is imperative at every primary care consultation. On entry into the facility, the child needs to be weighed by a health worker specifically trained for this task and for recording the weight accurately on the Road to Health Chart. If growth faltering was identified on what was meant to be a routine visit to a so-called 'well child' clinic, the child must then be directed for a full Case Management, as described above.

The importance of breast-feeding is reinforced by IMCI practitioners who pay attention to correct positioning of the infant and attachment to the breast during feeding. The issue of breast-feeding by the HIV-positive mother is given careful consideration in the training.

The immunization status of every child is similarly assessed and any outstanding vaccinations given at that visit, whether the child is ill or well. Furthermore, the date for the next vaccination is agreed upon with the mother.

## TRAINING

The three IMCI training courses are meticulously structured:

The 11-day *Case Management course* is based on individual attention to the learner by a facilitator. One-third of the time is spent in a clinical setting, both in a primary care setting and in a paediatric ward to learn to recognize the signs of severe disease. The rest of the time is devoted to a range of classroom activities, which include video exercises. As there is a high ratio of facilitator to learner, the capacity of the latter to practise good quality care of the sick child is readily established. Within four to six weeks of completing the course a follow-up visit is paid to the facility where the learner is practising, in order to ensure that skills are being implemented and that the circumstances at the facility are supportive.

The purpose of the *Facilitators' course* is to ensure that the Case Management course is a facilitative and not a didactic process and to equip the participants with confidence in all the educational modes used in the IMCI strategy.

A *Supervisors' course* is intended to equip senior staff members with the information, skills, and approaches to ensure that a high quality of child management is being practised.

Supervisors' duties are two-fold, namely, to monitor and support IMCI practitioners and to ensure that necessary health system requirements are in place.

Regular follow-up is essential to avoid a gradual downhill slide of the quality of care of children.

The World Health Organization has recognized that in-service training is too costly and will take too long for countries to be adequately provided with IMCI practitioners. Hence there is a move afoot to introduce the Case Management courses into the undergraduate curriculum of nurses and medical students.

# Component 2: The health system

There are certain essential elements in the health system – listed below – that have to function efficiently in order to provide good quality care of children.

## Health system components essential for good quality of primary clinical care

- supply of essential drugs;
- good stock control;
- reliable referral system; and
- effective and efficient health data collection.

Over and above this, it is preferable that there is a line for waiting mothers and children separate from the general waiting queue, as generally children are more vulnerable and more susceptible to cross infection. Furthermore, there are considerable advantages for the child to be seen by the same health worker when coming for a follow-up or repeat visit.

These issues and the presence of a functional ORT corner (amongst others), should be seen to on a supervisory visit.

# Component 3: Family and community practices

It is self-evident that the environment, both immediate within the family setting as well as in the wider community, needs to be child friendly for healthy development. The Convention on the Rights of the Child (see Chapter 19: Global strategies for child health) outlines these in considerable detail. For the purposes of the IMCI strategy some key practices have been selected.

Clearly these practices cannot be implemented in isolation nor can it be imposed upon the community. Hence existing structures and groups – particularly those concerned with improving living conditions – must be consulted and drawn into the process where feasible.

## IMPLEMENTATION OF THE IMCI STRATEGY

As the strategy has the potential for a considerable improvement in childhood mortality and morbidity, it is of fundamental importance that the ultimate decision makers are involved at an early planning stage. If it is intended to be a country-wide process the approval and commitment of top government officials must be obtained. However, the support of every level of government is essential, as management needs to be participating in developing and sustaining the framework that is essential for successful implementation. In this endeavour, it is important to emphasize that existing health workers and management structures will need to take on these tasks. Moreover, in the long run there will be cost saving, particularly in respect of the drug bill, which invariably is an important budget item.

Experience has shown that the identification of a focal person, who can drive the process, has been a key element of successful implementation of the strategy.

## MONITORING, EVALUATION, AND RESEARCH

IMCI provides a rich field for both quantitative and qualitative research:

In order to establish whether the strategy is having the desired impact, it is essential to develop indicators that will determine the

## Key family practices

- Breast-feed infants exclusively for at least four months and, if possible, up to six months. (Mothers found to be HIV positive need counselling about possible alternatives to breast-feeding).
- Starting at about six months of age, feed children freshly prepared energy and nutrient-rich complementary foods, while continuing to breast- feed up to two years or longer.
- Ensure that the children receive adequate amounts of micronutrients (vitamin A and iron, in particular), either in their diet or through supplementation.
- Dispose of faeces, including children's faeces, safely, and wash hands after defaecation, before preparing meals, and before feeding children.
- Take children as scheduled to complete full course of immunizations (BCG, DPT, OPV, measles, HBV, and HiB) before their first birthday.
- Protect children in malaria-endemic areas, by ensuring that they sleep under insecticide-treated bednets.
- Promote mental and social development by responding to a child's need for care, and through talking, playing, and, where possible reading suitable material to the child and providing a stimulating environment.
- Continue to feed and offer more fluids, including breast-milk, to children when they are sick.
- Give sick children appropriate home treatment for infections.
- Recognize when sick children need treatment outside the home and seek care from appropriate providers.
- Follow the health worker's advice about treatment, follow-up and referral.
- Ensure that every pregnant woman has adequate antenatal care. This includes having at least four antenatal visits with an appropriate health care provider, and receiving the recommended doses of the tetanus toxoid vaccination. The mother also needs support from her family and community in seeking care at the time of delivery and during the postpartum and lactation period.

Adapted from the WHO/UNICEF publication 'Improving family and community practices – A component of the IMCI strategy'.

achievement of the set aims and objectives. Although one can base these on experience elsewhere, adaptation to local circumstances may be necessary. Some important management decisions are at times best based on local operational research.

Adaptations of treatment or assessment protocols to the needs of a country or region need to be validated by research.

## Conclusion

The IMCI strategy has unquestionably had a major positive impact on the well-being of children in those countries where it has been successfully implemented. Because the approach to the management of the sick child is not the conventional one used by health professionals, it is necessary to obtain the support of the medical and nursing professions. Once this has been achieved and the commitment of important decision makers has been obtained, one can look forward to successful implementation of the strategy.

# 37

# Acute respiratory infection in the developing world

## MA KIBEL

*'A family is a unit composed not only of children, but of men, women, an occasional animal, and the common cold.'*

Ogden Nash

No child escapes acute respiratory infection (ARI). ARI is more frequent and more severe in children living in disadvantaged settings, where, on average, a toddler in an urban area will experience between five and eight episodes each year (WHO, 1985). Low socioeconomic status, poor nutritional status, crowding, indoor air pollution, and the group care of young children increase the frequency of ARI. Although the great majority of such acute infections are mild and self-limiting, ARI is the world's leading killer of children under five years of age. Of the 12,9 million deaths of children under five that occurred in 1990, some 4,3 million were attributed to ARI (WHO, 1994), and two-thirds of these deaths were in infants. Increased mortality is associated with low birthweight, early weaning, lack of maternal education, and reduced health care access. Figure 37.1 shows the huge contribution made by ARI to overall childhood deaths (WHO, 1994). ARI is the commonest infection in HIV-infected chil-

dren, and often the presenting feature of this disease (see Chapter 39: HIV infection).

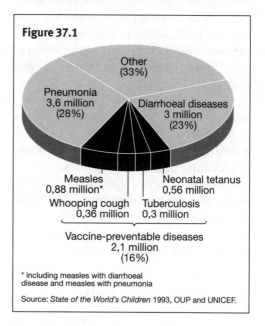

**Figure 37.1**

Other (33%)

Pneumonia 3,6 million (28%)

Diarrhoeal diseases 3 million (23%)

Measles 0,88 million*

Neonatal tetanus 0,56 million

Whooping cough 0,36 million

Tuberculosis 0,3 million

Vaccine-preventable diseases 2,1 million (16%)

\* including measles with diarrhoeal disease and measles with pneumonia

Source: *State of the World's Children* 1993, OUP and UNICEF.

Most deaths from ARI are due to pneumonia. Lung puncture studies in developing countries indicate that severe pneumonia is mostly bacterial, usually *Streptococcus pneumoniae* or *Haemophilus influenzae*. This contrasts with the situation in developed countries, where the great majority are due to viruses. Many of these deaths are therefore potentially preventable by the appropriate administration of antibiotics. This forms the basis for the World Health Organization's initiatives to lower the number of deaths from ARI. These initiatives will be briefly described here (WHO/ ARI/90.5). Acute respiratory infections – classified as cough or cold, or pneumonias of graded severity – are a major component of the UNICEF IMCI strategy.

ARI is also a major contributor to the burden of disability through the chronic sequelae of pneumonia (suppurative lung disease and bronchiectasis), otitis media (hearing loss), and rheumatic fever.

The term ARI embraces a number of conditions affecting the respiratory tract from the nasal cavity to the lungs. The common mode of infection is by droplet spread, hence their greater frequency in overcrowded environs and cold conditions. Viruses causing the common cold (rhinoviruses and coronaviruses) are spread by hand-to-face contact as well as by exhaled droplets.

However, ARI has other important modes of transmission. For example, young infants may be infected via the birth canal by Group B beta haemolytic streptococci, *Chlamydia trachomatis, Ureaplasma urealyticum,* and *Mycoplasma hominis,* resulting in pneumonia; staphylococcal pneumonia is commonly acquired from skin or nasal carriage; cytomegalovirus infection in young infants may be transmitted by blood transfusions.

# Clinical profile of ARI

ARIs are traditionally divided into upper and lower respiratory tract infections. Moffet (1981) introduces a third category, classifying ARI as upper, middle, and lower respiratory syndromes based on the clinical problems produced (*upper:* nose, sinuses, ears, throat;

*middle:* larynx to the terminal bronchi; *lower:* alveoli and lung substance), and the recognition of a 'middle respiratory' category is useful to embrace the common conditions of croup, bronchitis, and bronchiolitis. However, the aetiological agents, of which there are over 300 known antigenic types of virus and other micro-organisms, show little correlation with this classification.

## UPPER RESPIRATORY SYNDROMES

The term 'upper respiratory tract infection' may include any of the conditions listed here:

*The common cold.* This is characterized by sneezing, watery nasal discharge, and nasal obstruction in the absence of significant fever. The most common causative organisms are coronaviruses and rhinoviruses. In older children and adults simple colds are also caused by a range of other viruses.

*Purulent nasal discharge.* Thick yellow or green discharge, often with excoriation around the nose, is particularly common in poor environments; an indication of the greater prevalence of pathogenic bacterial colonization of the upper respiratory tract in these communities. Beta-haemolytic streptococci, *Streptococcus pneumoniae* or S*taphylococcus aureus* are most commonly responsible.

*Pharyngitis* and/or *tonsillitis.* This is indicated by a sore throat with clear evidence of inflammation of the pharynx such as erythema, exudate, follicles or ulceration, and cervical adenitis. Viruses are mainly responsible but bacterial throat infections may be clinically indistinguishable, and the most important of these is Group A streptococcus. Possible complications of streptococcal pharyngotonsillitis are rheumatic fever and acute glomerulonephritis. Suspect streptococcal pharyngitis if (a) the throat is very inflamed with white pharyngeal exudate, (b) there are no 'cold' symptoms, and (c) tonsillar lymph glands are enlarged and tender. Viruses that cause pharyngitis include adenoviruses, measles, herpes simplex, Coxsackie, ECHO, para-influenza, influenza, and Epstein-Barr virus. Other agents causing pharyngitis are *Neisseria gonorrhoeae* (but rarely in children) and *Corynebacterium diphtheria*. Suspect diphtheria if a grey, adherent pharyngeal membrane is seen.

## Suppurative complications of pharyngitis include:

- cervical abscess – a greatly enlarged tender lymph node that can attach to skin and suppurate;
- quinsy (peritonsillar abscess) – a very enlarged inflamed tonsil, pushing the uvula to one side; and
- retropharyngeal abscess – a large abscess in the back of the throat. It may cause stridor and a hyperextended neck.

*Stomatitis*. Here there is reddening of the buccal mucosa with ulceration or exudate and often with inflammation of the gums or tongue. Herpes simplex is the usual cause while, less commonly, Coxsackie A or B virus are causative agents.

*Influenza-like syndromes*. This is characterized by fever, cough, headache, sore throat, fatigue, and muscle pains. While influenza is the usual cause of these symptoms, adenoviruses, para-influenza, and Coxsackie viruses, *Mycoplasma pneumoniae* and Group A streptococci may also be responsible.

*'Fever without localizing signs'*. High fever with constitutional symptoms such as headache and abdominal pain is often referred to as upper respiratory infection (URI). A variety of agents may cause this picture.

*Acute otitis media*. This is an infection of the middle ear. The common pathogens are

*Streptococcus pneumoniae* and *Haemophilus influenzae*, which are also the main causes of bacterial pneumonia. It is characterized by persistent ear pain, and by an ear drum that is red and shows lessened mobility. The ear drum readily ruptures in young children causing a perforation and ear discharge.

*Chronic otitis media*. In developing countries, children who present with a long history of discharge from one or both ears are a major problem, leading to long-term morbidity and hearing loss. Such cases result from neglect or inadequate care of the initial attack of otitis media. When the ear drum has been ruptured for more than two weeks, secondary infection with fungi, yeasts, *Pseudomonas, Proteus*, or other enteric organisms usually occurs. This makes antibiotic therapy less effective. Complications of chronic otitis media may be mastoiditis, meningitis, or brain abscess.

*Sinusitis*. Infection of the nasal sinuses may follow ARI. Symptoms may include any or all of the following: persistant purulent nasal discharge, facial pain, fatigue, or fetid breath.

## MIDDLE RESPIRATORY SYNDROMES

*Cough only*. This applies when a cough is present without fever, stridor, wheeze or any other objective signs. Cough of short duration is generally due to viral infection around the larynx and/or postnasal discharge. When of longer duration a variety of other possible causes must always be considered – in particular, tuberculosis, pertussis, asthma or an inhaled foreign body.

*Pertussis*. The classic case has a protracted paroxysmal cough followed by an inspiratory whoop. Complications are frequent and include pneumonia, atelectasis, encephalopathy, and fatal apnoea in young infants (see Chapter 24: Vaccine-preventable infectious diseases).

*Croup.* Stridor is a harsh inspiratory noise caused by inflammation of the larynx, trachea, or epiglottis. Croup is the clinical syndrome characterized by the acute onset of stridor, harsh, barking cough, and a hoarse voice. Croup is most commonly caused by viruses, para-influenza, influenza, respiratory syncytial virus, or measles. Croup may also be caused by diphtheria or other bacteria. Bacterial croup can involve the epiglottis (acute epiglottis usually due to *Haemophilus influenzae*) or the trachea (bacterial tracheitis), where *Staphylococcus aureus* is the usual cause.

Viral croup is an extremely common and important paediatric emergency. It may be categorized as 'mild croup' if there is a hoarse voice and barking cough, but no stridor when calm. In 'severe croup' there is stridor in a calm child, indrawing of the chest, and hoarseness. When croup complicates measles, superinfection with herpes simplex results in a particularly severe and lethal form of the condition. Intubation or tracheostomy are often required, and months of treatment may be needed, placing a great burden on hospital services.

Persistent stridor may also be caused by congenital malformation, foreign body, and pressure on the trachea from tuberculous glands.

*Acute bronchitis.* Here there is coughing with wheezes or coarse crackles that clear with coughing. Bronchitis is common in children, especially in those living in smoky environments, and it is usually associated with an upper respiratory infection. Some children have recurrent attacks of bronchitis whenever they get a cold. Many of these later develop asthma, but this is by no means inevitable, and the tendency to wheeze is often outgrown.

*Asthma.* It is worth emphasizing the part played by ARI in the induction of lower airway obstruction in asthma-prone children. Episodes of bronchitis or bronchiolitis often precede the recognition of true asthma, and a viral infection is the most frequent precipitating factor in asthma in the early years of life. The prevalence of asthma is rising, now affecting 10 to 15 per cent of children in urban areas. Overcrowding, indoor air pollution, rapid climatic changes, and high pollen counts are all aggravating factors (see Chapter 45: Childhood asthma).

*Acute bronchiolitis.* Acute bronchiolitis is a common cause of wheezing and cough in the first two years of life. It is distinguished by an inflammatory reaction in the walls of the tiny bronchioles and surrounding tissues with sparing of the alveoli. Plugging of the bronchioles gives rise to lower airway obstruction. Winter epidemics of bronchiolitis are generally caused by *respiratory syncytial virus* with the following characteristics:

- occurrence under the age of two years;
- usually the first such episode;
- acute general peripheral airway obstruction – tachypnoea, chest wall recession, decreased breath sounds; and
- typical air trapping on X-ray.

However, many other respiratory viruses may cause a similar picture.

## LOWER RESPIRATORY INFECTIONS

Infections of the lung parenchyma fall, in practice, into three broad groupings.

- *Acute lobar or segmental pneumonia.* Fever above 39 °C is usually present together with tachypnoea, flaring of the nostrils, chest wall indrawing, and often grunting. Pleuritic pain may be noted. The most common cause is *Streptococcus pneumoniae*, while *Haemophilus influenzae* is also a frequent pathogen. However, viruses account for many cases in this category.

- *Bronchopneumonia.* The terms 'bronchopneumonia' and 'interstitial pneumonia' are often used where there are bilateral or ill-defined radiological signs. The illness may be acute or sub-acute; viruses, *mycoplasma pneumoniae*, chlamydia, and a variety of other organisms may be responsible. Bronchopneumonia may also result from secondary infection in bronchiolitis, pertussis, measles or tuberculosis, and is a particular hazard in malnourished and immune-comprised infants.
- *Progressive or fulminating pneumonias.* These become clinically or radiologically worse despite normally effective anti-biotic therapy. *Staphylococcus aureus* and *Klebsiella pneumoniae* are particularly frequent and dangerous causes, as is *Pneumocystis carinii* in HIV-infected individuals. Mycobacterium tuberculosis always requires exclusion. Adenovirus and Legionella are two of the many other possibilities.

Pleurisy, effusion, or empyema may complicate any form of pneumonia.

Recurrent chest symptoms or chronic suppurative lung disease can follow acute middle and lower respiratory tract infections, when there has been lung collapse from bronchial obstruction or unresolved pneumonia. Measles virus, *B. pertussis*, respiratory syncytial virus, adenovirus, and *M. tuberculosis* are the infectious agents most often responsible (Wesley, 1991).

## Indirect results of ARI

Finally, there are the conditions that may result from an idiosyncratic response to a respiratory infection, such as rheumatic fever, acute glomerulonephritis, and the Guillain-Barré syndrome. The most important of these

in terms of its long-term costs to families and communities is rheumatic fever, which is still common in southern Africa. Guillain-Barré syndrome, a cause of acute flaccid paralysis in children, more commonly follows a bowel infection due to *Campylobacter jejuni*.

## Programmes for controlling ARI

An outline of management of some of the above problems is discussed in Chapters 46: Medications for common ailments; and 48: Common paediatric emergencies. For detailed clinical management, the reader is referred to standard paediatric texts. The principles of management of ARI as a community problem have already been outlined in Chapter 36: Integrated management of childhood illness. It has been estimated that up to 98 per cent of infant and childhood deaths due to ARI might be prevented if case fatality ratios could be reduced to those observed in the industrialized world (Stansfield, 1987). However, the heterogeneity of clinical presentations and the variety of organisms has hampered efforts to address this leading cause of death among children.

Much can be done to lessen the number of unnecessary attendances at health centres, while at the same time ensuring that really sick children are seen timeously. Following research in various countries, the World Health Organization initiated policies for a concerted attack to lower mortality and morbidity from ARI in the developing countries (WHO, 1985). The most immediate practical aspect is a case management system that relates the severity of disease to a particular management regime. This is based on the premise that the majority of life-threatening (mainly lower respiratory) illnesses in developing countries are due to bacterial infections and are therefore amenable to chemotherapy.

Shann et al (1984) studied the criteria for selection of patients for antibiotic therapy and hospital admission. They concluded that, while crepitations on auscultation and infiltrates on chest X-ray suggest the need for antibiotics, tachypnoea is the best available indicator of need for antibiotic therapy in a primary care situation. Rapid breathing reported by the mother correlated relatively well to the objective observation of tachypnoea.

The management scheme is based on flow charts using easily recognizable symptoms and signs. For example, mild ARI (cough, but no tachypnoea or recession) would be treated with simple supportive measures at home. Moderate ARI would be diagnosed by tachypnoea but no recession or chest indrawing, and requires oral antibiotics and supportive home treatment; while severe disease would be treated with parenteral antibiotics and oxygen in a hospital. Pharyngitis associated with enlarged lymph glands and earache or acute otorrhoea should also be treated with antibiotics.

Supportive home measures should include continuing breast-feeding, ensuring adequate hydration but not excessive feeding of the child with pneumonia, neutral temperature (using antipyretics if temperature is greater than 38,5 °C), clearing of air passages, clearing away ear discharge, using steam to soothe and clear air passages, and postural drainage.

An important aspect of the control programme is the health education of both parents/caregivers and health care workers. The prime messages are as follows:

- If a child with a cough is breathing much more rapidly than normal, then the child is at risk. It is essential to get the child to a clinic quickly. Rapid breathing is age dependent. A rate above 60 per minute in infants under 2 months, above 50 from 2 to 12 months, and above 40 per minute over 12 months should be regarded as rapid.

- Families can prevent pneumonia by making sure that babies are breast-fed for at least six months of life and that all children are well nourished and fully immunized. They should minimize the child's exposure to cigarette and other smoke.

- A child with a cough or a cold should be helped to eat and to drink plenty of liquids.

- A child with a cough or a cold should be kept warm but not hot, and should breathe clean, non-smoky air.

Tables 37.1 and 37.2 describe the recommended management of the infant and young child in a small hospital.

# Broader preventive strategies

Deaths from five vaccine-preventable diseases – measles, pertussis, diphtheria, tuberculosis, influenza – account for 25 per cent of total mortality from ARI. Immunization is thus the most important of the related child survival activities that could lessen mortality. In addition, infections due to the encapsulated Group B strain of *Haemophilus influenzae* (but not non-encapsulated strains) can be prevented by immunization with HiB vaccine. Undernourished children are more prone to ARI and such infections are more often fatal. The promotion of breast-feeding and better nutrition in young children is clearly also a key issue. A beneficial role for vitamin A in lowering mortality from infection in developing countries has also been shown (Sommer & West, 1987; Hussey & Klein, 1990). Smoke reduction, both from cigarettes and cooking stoves, should also be the focus for prevention. However, relatively little is known about the cost effectiveness of such interventions (Stansfield, 1987).

**Table 37.1** Management of the young infant with cough or difficult breathing at the small hospital (based on WHO, 1994)

For the young infant aged less than 2 months

| Clinical signs | Classify as | Summary of treatment instructions |
|---|---|---|
| • Stopped feeding well<br>• Convulsions<br>• Abnormally sleepy or difficult to wake<br>• Stridor in calm child<br>• Wheezing<br>• Fever (38 °C or more) or low body temperature (below 35,5 °C)<br>• Fast breathing[a]<br>• Severe chest indrawing<br>• Central cyanosis<br>• Grunting<br>• Apnoeic episodes<br>or<br>• Distended and tense abdomen | *Severe pneumonia or very severe disease* | • Admit<br>**Give oxygen[b] if:**<br>• Central cyanosis<br>• Not able to drink<br><br>**Give antibiotics:**<br>• Ampicillin plus gentamicin<br><br>Careful fluid management<br><br>Maintain a good thermal environment<br><br>Specific management of wheezing or stridor |
| • No fast breathing<br>• No signs of pneumonia or very severe disease | No pneumonia:<br>Cough or cold | *Advise mother to give the following home care:*<br>• keep young infant warm;<br>• breast-feed frequently; and<br>• clear nose if it interferes with feeding.<br>Return quickly if:<br>• breathing becomes difficult;<br>• breathing becomes fast;<br>• feeding becomes a problem; and<br>• the young infant becomes sicker. |

[a]Fast breathing is 60 breaths per minute or more in the young infant (age less than 2 months) – repeat the count.
[b]Oxygen should be given to a young infant with:
• restlessness (if oxygen improves the condition);
• severe chest indrawing; and
• grunting.

**Table 37.2** Pneumonia management at the small hospital

For the child age 2 months up to 5 years with cough or difficult breathing (who does not have stridor, severe undernutrition, or signs suggesting meningitis)[a]

| Clinical signs | Classify as[b] | Summary of treatment instructions |
|---|---|---|
| • Central cyanosis<br>or<br>• Not able to drink | *Very severe pneumonia* | *Admit*<br>• Give oxygen[c]<br>• *Give an antibiotic:* (see EDL*)<br>• Treat fever, if present<br>• Treat wheezing, if present<br>• Give supportive care<br>• Reassess twice daily |
| • Lower chest indrawing and<br>• No central cyanosis and<br>• Able to drink | *Severe pneumonia*<br>If child is wheezing, assess further before classifying. | *Admit*<br>• *Give an antibiotic:* (see EDL*)<br>• Treat fever, if present<br>• Treat wheezing, if present<br>• Give supportive care<br>• Reassess daily |
| • No lower chest indrawing and<br>• Fast breathing[d] | *Pneumonia* | *Advise mother to give home care*<br>• *Give an antibiotic* (at home): cotrimoxazole or amoxycillin<br>• Treat fever if present<br>• Treat wheezing, if present<br>• Advise mother to return in two days for reassessment, or earlier if the child is getting worse |
| • No lower chest indrawing and<br>• No fast breathing. | *No pneumonia:*<br>*Cough or cold* | • If coughing more than 30 days, assess for causes of chronic cough<br>• Assess and treat ear problem or sore throat, if present<br>• Assess and treat other problems<br>*Advise mother to give home care*<br>• Treat fever, if present<br>• Treat wheezing, if present |

[a]If the child has stridor, follow the treatment guidelines in Chapters 46 and 48

If the child has severe undernutrition, admit for nutritional rehabilitation and medical therapy. Treat pneumonia with appropriate antibiotic.

If the child has signs suggesting meningitis, admit and treat with antibiotic.

[b]These classifications include some children with bronchiolitis and asthma.

[c]Oxygen should be given to a child with:
• restlessness (if oxygen improves the condition);
• severe chest indrawing; or
• breathing rate of 70 breaths per minute or more.

[d]Fast breathing is:
• 50 breaths per minute or more in a child age 2 months up to 12 months; and
• 40 breaths per minute or more in a child age 12 months up to 5 years.

* Essential Drugs List and Treatment guidelines, 1998

# References and further reading

DIXON RA. 1985. Acute respiratory infections in the under fives. *Lancet.* 952.

HUSSEY GD & KLEIN M. 1990. A randomised, controlled trial of vitamin A in children with severe measles. *New England Journal of Medicine.* 323:160–4.

MOFFET HL. 1981. *Pediatric infectious diseases,* 2nd ed. Philadelphia, Toronto: JB Lippincott Company.

NATIONAL DEPARTMENT OF HEALTH, RSA. 1998. *Standard Treatment Guidelines and Essential Drug List.*

SHANN F, HART K, and THOMAS D. 1984. Acute lower respiratory tract infections in children: Possible criteria for selection of patients for antibiotic therapy and hospital admission. *Bulletin of the WHO.* 62(5):749–53.

SOMMER A & WEST KP JNR. 1987. Impact of vitamin A on childhood mortality. *Indian Journal of Pediatrics.* 54:461–3.

STANSFIELD SK. 1987. Acute respiratory infection in the developing world: Strategies for prevention, treatment and control. *Pediatric Infectious Diseases Journal.* 6:622–9.

WESLEY AG. 1991. Prolonged after effects of pneumonia in children. *South African Medical Journal.* 79(2):73–6.

WORLD HEALTH ORGANIZATION. 1985. *Basic principles for control of ARI in children in developing countries: A Joint UNICEF/WHO Statement.* New York: WHO.

WORLD HEALTH ORGANIZATION. 1994. ARI – Programme for controlling acute respiratory infections. 6th program report 1992–1993.

WORLD HEALTH ORGANIZATION. *Acute respiratory infections in children: Case management in small hospitals in developing countries.* WHO/ARI/90.5

# 38 Diarrhoeal disease

## H SALOOJEE

Childhood gastroenteritis remains one of the greatest killers of children in developing countries (between 2,4 and 3,3 million deaths in under-fives annually) despite the discovery and use of what the *Lancet* in 1978 hailed as 'potentially the most important medical advance this century'– oral rehydration therapy (ORT).

Some successes of ORT and the global Diarrhoeal Disease Control programme have been spectacular. ORT is said to save one million lives annually. By 1998, 69 per cent of the world's population were using ORT. During the International Drinking Water Supply and Sanitation Decade (1981–1990), some 1 600 million people were served with safe water and about 750 million with adequate excreta disposal facilities. However, more than one billion people around the world still lack safe water and some 2,9 billion (over half the world's population) do not have adequate excreta disposal facilities. Rapid population growth and lagging rates of coverage expansion have left more people without access to basic sanitation today than in 1990.

## Definitions

Diarrhoea is one of the commonest symptoms in childhood and infectious causes are very common in young children. Despite this there remain disagreements about definitions. Currently accepted definitions are summarized opposite.

## Epidemiology

Diarrhoeal disease remains a major cause of morbidity and mortality in children in South Africa, accounting for 28 per cent of deaths in children under five years of age (Yach et al., 1989). In a Northern Province district, communicable disease and malnutrition (diarrhoea and kwashiorkor predominantly) were responsible for over half of the deaths in under-fives (Kahn et al., 1999).

The group at highest risk of diarrhoea are children under the age of one year living in poor socio-economic conditions. In these conditions, a marked seasonal cycle is evident in diarrhoeal disease mortality rates with peaks occurring from December to March. No seasonal effect on mortality is evident in more

## Definitions of different types of diarrhoea

*Acute diarrhoea* means the passage of abnormally loose or fluid stools more frequently than normal (this depends on perception by parents about what is 'normal'). The passage of three or more loose stools daily after infancy is generally considered abnormal.

*Persistent diarrhoea* means that the diarrhoea started acutely but the stools have been abnormally loose for 14 days or more irrespective of the nature of the stools, i.e., watery, mucoid, bloody, or pasty, and requiring hydration support.

*Chronic diarrhoea* is defined as diarrhoea continuing for longer than 14 days, but not requiring additional fluids to maintain hydration. It is usually due to non-infectious causes, such as sensitivity to gluten or inherited metabolic disorders.

*Dysentery* refers to diarrhoea with visible blood in the faeces. The term 'bloody diarrhoea' is preferred.

affluent communities. In a rural South African community, 16 per cent of 4- to 24-month-old children (under-twos) experienced an episode of diarrhoea during a two-week period (Faber & Benade, 1999). World-wide, children under five experience an average of 3,3 episodes each year, but in some areas, the average exceeds nine episodes per year. Rates among children in child care centres are three times higher. Most episodes of acute gastro-enteritis resolve within three to seven days.

Individual risk factors for diarrhoea in young children living in urban and peri-urban areas of South Africa include not having an inside tap or a flush toilet in the homes, not owning a refuse receptacle, not being connected to an electricity supply, low household income, crowding (more than two people per room), and maternal education less than Standard five (von Schirnding et al., 1991).

# Aetiology

Despite improved microbiologic methods and the recognition of 'newer' aetiologic agents, causative agents are identified at best in about 70 per cent of episodes of infectious diarrhoea. Unfortunately, most reported studies concentrate on one possible infectious agent or group of such agents, e.g., rotavirus or E.coli, rather than providing a comprehensive assessment of possible causes. Figure 38.1 presents a composite picture combining results of multiple studies from different regions and different settings.

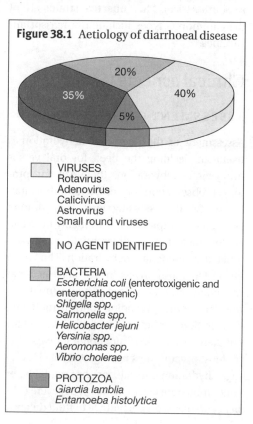

**Figure 38.1** Aetiology of diarrhoeal disease

VIRUSES
Rotavirus
Adenovirus
Calicivirus
Astrovirus
Small round viruses

NO AGENT IDENTIFIED

BACTERIA
*Escherichia coli* (enterotoxigenic and enteropathogenic)
*Shigella spp.*
*Salmonella spp.*
*Helicobacter jejuni*
*Yersinia spp.*
*Aeromonas spp.*
*Vibrio cholerae*

PROTOZOA
*Giardia lamblia*
*Entamoeba histolytica*

The pathogens most strongly associated with disease in developing countries are rotavirus (16 per cent of cases), *Shigella spp.* (11 per cent), and enterotoxigenic and enteropathogenic *Escherichia coli* (16 per cent). *Campylobacter jejuni* and Salmonella are also of importance in South Africa. World-wide, *Vibrio cholerae* 01 and *Shigella dysenteriae* type 1 cause major epidemics in which morbidity and mortality in all age groups may be high.

A recent review has confirmed the importance of rotavirus in Africa. It was detected in a quarter of children who were hospitalized for diarrhoea and in the same percentage of outpatients. This makes it the single most important cause of diarrhoeal disease in African children. Infants account for 81 per cent of cases. Rotavirus is detected year round in Africa with distinct peaks in the dry months (April to June in South Africa). Most infective strains are of the common G types included in reassortant vaccines.

## Clinical aspects

### ASSESSMENT OF DEHYDRATION

Assessment of the degree of dehydration is useful in deciding the need for oral versus intravenous rehydration, the need for prolonged observation, or occasionally, hospitalization. Because assessing signs of dehydration is inherently imprecise it is probably unrealistic to expect precise differentiation between 'mild' and 'moderate' dehydration. The World Health Organization has, in fact, suggested that hydration status be judged as 'none' (no dehydration), 'some' (including mild to moderate dehydration), or 'severe' (properly reserved for children with shock or impending shock).

Most practitioners use a system of classifying dehydration into categories of mild (<5 per cent), moderate (5 to 9 per cent) or severe (≥10 per cent) based on percentage of fluid deficits,

using subjective and objective clinical parameters. Studies have proven this schemata to correlate poorly with actual weight loss. Table 38.1 presents the diagnostic performance of 10 individual clinical findings (Liebelt, 1998).

**Table 38.1** Predictive value of 10 clinical signs of dehydration

| Clinical finding | Sensitivity | Specificity |
|---|---|---|
| Decreased skin elasticity | 0,35 | 0,97 |
| Capillary refill >2 sec | 0,48 | 0,96 |
| General appearance (ill-appearing, irritable, apathetic) | 0,59 | 0,91 |
| Absent tears | 0,67 | 0,89 |
| Abnormal respiration | 0,43 | 0,86 |
| Dry mucous membranes | 0,80 | 0,78 |
| Sunken eyes | 0,60 | 0,84 |
| Abnormal radial pulse | 0,43 | 0,86 |
| Tachycardia (heart rate > 150) | 0,46 | 0,79 |
| Decreased urine output | 0,85 | 0,53 |

- Of the 10 findings, no single finding is sufficiently accurate to be used alone.
- The presence of fewer than 3 signs corresponds with a fluid deficit of less than 5 per cent.
- Children with a fluid deficit of 5 to 9 per cent generally have 3 or more clinical findings.
- At least 6 to 7 findings should be present to diagnose a deficit of 10 per cent or more.

### RISK FACTORS

The risk of dehydration is highest in infants (<12 months of age). Other risk factors in children include frequent vomiting (> twice/day) and passage of stools (>8/day), watery diarrhoea, failure to use ORT, breast-feeding being stopped during the illness, and severe undernutrition.

### DIFFERENTIAL DIAGNOSIS

Before the diagnosis of acute gastroenteritis is made, other disease states that present with symptoms that resemble acute gastroenteritis should be carefully excluded. The list of possible conditions is long and includes infections (e.g., septicaemia, pneumonia, urinary tract infection, acute otitis media), surgical disorders (e.g., intussusception, necrotising enterocolitis, acute appendicitis), acute food intolerance (cow milk protein) and others (e.g., coeliac disease, ulcerative colitis, inborn errors of metabolism, etc.). In southern Africa, the possibility of the use of traditional therapies should also be considered.

## LABORATORY EVALUATION

Children who present with mild or moderate dehydration do not need laboratory studies and can be managed using a combination of clinical parameters. Electrolytes, urea, creatinine, and glucose should only be checked in a child with severe dehydration and in moderately dehydrated children whose histories and physical examination are inconsistent with each other or with a straightforward gastroenteritis illness. Stool examination is usually only required for bloody or persistent diarrhoea.

Stool microscopy is helpful to distinguish infectious (presence of pus cells, blood or mucus) from non-infectious causes. Routine culturing of the stool is of little value because many invasive bacteria require special culture media, unusual growth conditions, or diagnostic antisera that are often unavailable.

## MANAGEMENT

The World Health Organization (WHO, 1993) case management strategy for children with diarrhoea, subsequently incorporated in IMCI, consists of the following elements:

- prevention of dehydration through early administration of appropriate fluids available in the home;
- treatment of dehydration with oral rehydration solution (ORS);

- treatment of severe dehydration with an intravenous electrolyte solution;
- continued feeding during, and increased feeding after, the diarrhoeal episode; and
- selective use of antibiotics and non-use of anti-diarrhoeal drugs.

# Fluid management

## ORAL REHYDRATION THERAPY

### Composition of ORS

While the success of ORT is unquestioned, controversy continues as to the ideal composition of ORS and whether the formulation should be standardized for universal use or allow for local modifications. The composition of WHO-ORS and some other common fluids used for rehydration in acute diarrhoea are shown in Table 38.2. Because fluids with high concentrations of simple carbohydrates such as sweetened fruit drinks and soft drinks have a high osmolarity (more than 300 mOsm/L) they can worsen gastrointestinal fluid losses and are not recommended for fluid therapy in acute diarrhoea. Other fluids, such as soup, may have inappropriate amounts of sodium. Home-prepared sugar and salt solution should contain eight teaspoons of sugar and half a teaspoon of salt added to one litre of boiled water.

### SODIUM

The sodium content of ORS recommended by WHO (90 mmol/l) was set to approximate the sodium losses in stools in children with cholera. The common pathogens causing diarrhoea in developed countries and in South Africa, however, cause much lower stool sodium losses (e.g., 40 mmol/l in rotavirus diarrhoea and 50 to 60 mmol/l for *Shigella* and *Escherichia coli*). This fact, together with a few reported cases of hyper-natraemia following the use of WHO-ORS, has led to the recommendation that a solution containing 60 mmol/l or less of sodium be used to manage diarrhoea in Europe and in South Africa. Clinical trials have shown this solution to be safe and effective in acute non-cholera diarrhoea.

## POTASSIUM

WHO-ORS and most other solutions contain at least 20 mmol/l of potassium. This is adequate for well-nourished children but may be problematic for dehydrated, malnourished children. One study, for example, showed that a third of the children treated with ORS containing 20 mmol/l of potassium developed hypokalaemia compared with none in the group receiving ORS with 35 mmol/l of potassium.

## BASE

Bicarbonate or base precursors (e.g., citrate) have been included in ORS with the rationale that they help correct any metabolic acidosis and enhance sodium and water reabsorption. There is little clinical evidence to support their routine inclusion in ORS. In all but the most severe cases, correction of the acidosis with base-free ORS is slower but as effective as with bicarbonate-containing solutions. Citrate, when added to ORS, increases its shelf life, but gives similar results to bicarbonate-containing ORS with respect to correction of acidosis and dehydration.

## CARBOHYDRATE SOURCE

Glucose was the first substrate shown to be effective for ORT and is still the most widely used world-wide. The process of coupled glu-

**Table 38.2** Composition of ORS and other fluids used for acute diarrhoea

| Solution | Sodium (mmol/l) | Chloride (mmol/l) | Potassium (mmol/l) | Base (mmol/l) | Glucose (mmol/l) | Osmolality (mosmol/kg) |
|---|---|---|---|---|---|---|
| WHO-ORS | 90 | 80 | 20 | 30 (B) | 111 | 331 |
| WHO-citrate | 90 | 80 | 20 | 10 (C) | 111 | 311 |
| Sorol | 64 | 54 | 20 | 10 | 110 | 278 |
| Rehidrat | 50 | 50 | 20 | 20 (B) | 90 ^ | 336 |
| ReSoMal# | 45 | 70 | 40 | 7 (C) | 125 | 300 |
| Rice-based ORS | 50 | 45 | 25 | 10 | 0 * | 200 |
| Maize-based ORS | 81 | 81 | 4 | 0 | 194 | 360 |
| Hypotonic ORS | 60 | 50 | 20 | 10 (C) | 84 | 224 |
| **Clear liquids (not recommended)** | | | | | | |
| Cola | 2 | 2 | 0,1 | 13 (B) | 730 | 750 |
| Apple juice | 3 | 30 | 28 | 0 | 690 | 730 |
| Chicken broth | 250 | 250 | 8 | 0 | 0 | 450 |
| Tea | 0 | 0 | 0 | 0 | 0 | 5 |

WHO= World Health Organization, B=bicarbonate, C=citrate
* Rice-syrup solids 30 g/l
^ also contains sucrose 94 mmol/l and fructose 2 mmol/l
# ReSoMal = Rehydration Solution for Malnourished children. Also contains magnesium, zinc, and copper.

cose/sodium absorption remains intact in diarrhoeal states resulting in increased water absorption when ORT is given. Current evidence suggests that the optimal glucose concentration is between 70 and 100 mmol/l, which is lower than that present in WHO-ORS (111 mmol/l). While this lower concentration does not reduce sodium absorption, it significantly increases water absorption, which is related in part to the lower osmolality of these solutions.

WHO has recommended sucrose (sugar) for home-based rehydration therapy ('sugar and salt solution') when glucose-ORS or formulated brands are unavailable. Trials show that, in equivalent concentrations, sucrose can be at least as effective as glucose.

## OSMOLALITY

The osmolality of ORS is an important factor influencing water absorption. Optimal water absorption can be obtained by using a hypotonic solution with a sodium concentration of 50 to 60 mmol/l and a glucose concentration of 50 to 100 mmol/l. Low-osmolality ORS (osmolality 224 mosmol/kg) has been shown to reduce the stool output and the mean duration of illness as compared to standard WHO solution (osmolality 311 mosmol/kg). WHO is reconsidering its recommendations for the formulation of ORS in the light of these results.

## CEREAL-BASED ORS

Cereal-based ORS (containing rice, wheat, maize, lentils, etc.) has been used successfully in many developing countries. The advantage of cereal-based ORS (ORS-CB) lies in the availability of the ingredients in almost every home, cultural acceptance, and higher nutritional value. Anxious parents demand that the diarrhoea be stopped rather than the imaginary threat of dehydration prevented.

Cereal-based ORS has the advantage of reducing stool output and the duration of diarrhoea when compared to standard ORS. Its main benefits, however, appear to be in patients with cholera.

On the negative side, preparation of ORS-CB at home requires cooking, which means time and fuel. Commercial packets of pre-cooked cereal powder have been developed and are available in developed countries. They can be mixed with cold water to give an instant ORS-CB. However, it is feared that packaging will medicalize ORS-CB and the cost of packets (thrice that of standard ORS) can be prohibitive.

In South Africa, as in most of southern Africa, maize (mielie meal) rather than rice is the common staple. Maize gruel may be recommended as an appropriate home-available fluid for the management of acute diarrhoea at the community level. (Recipe: boil 50 g of maize flour in 1 litre of water while stirring for 5 to 8 minutes and add 5 g [1 teaspoon] of common salt to the gruel on cooling.)

## ORAL REHYDRATION SOLUTION FOR SEVERELY MALNOURISHED CHILDREN (ReSoMal)

WHO has proposed that a special ORS be provided to severely malnourished children. This solution has a higher concentration of potassium and less sodium compared to standard WHO-ORS. It also contains magnesium, zinc, and copper to correct deficiencies of all these minerals in these children. ReSoMal is available commercially. ReSoMal can also be made by diluting one packet of standard WHO-ORS in two litres of water, instead of one litre, and adding 50 g of sucrose (25 g/l) and 40 ml (20 ml/l) of mineral mix solution (a WHO-recommended preparation).

# Rehydration

## PREVENTION OF DEHYDRATION

A child who has diarrhoea, but is not dehydrated, may be given ORS in addition to his or her regular diet, to replace stool losses. Special solutions are, however, not necessary as long as the well-hydrated child can consume an age-appropriate diet and is encouraged to drink more than the usual amounts of the usual fluids in his or her diet.

## MILD TO MODERATE DEHYDRATION

In all but the most seriously ill patients, rehydration is possible using ORT. Mildly or moderately dehydrated children should receive ORT at 15 ml/kg/hour, offered in frequent small quantities and increased to 25 ml/kg/hour, if the child wants more, until hydration has improved (usually four to six hours). This should ideally be done under medical supervision. At this stage the child should immediately re-commence her/his normal diet. Depending on the child's thirst, 5 to 15 ml/kg of ORS may be offered after feeds. Replacement of stool losses (at 10 ml/kg for each stool) and of vomitus (estimated volume) will require adding appropriate amounts of solution to the total. Breast-feeding should not stop during rehydration. Use of cola, undiluted fruit juice, and sports beverage is discouraged.

## SEVERE DEHYDRATION

Severely dehydrated children who are in a state of shock must receive immediate and aggressive intravenous (IV) therapy. It should begin with an isotonic solution (e.g., normal saline, Ringer's lactate, or Plasmalyte B, 20 ml/kg over 20 to 30 min). Thereafter, the child should receive half-strength Darrow's solution with 5 per cent dextrose at a rate of 10 ml/kg/hour until oral fluids can be re-introduced. The rate may be increased to 15 ml/kg/hour for 4 to 6 hours if there are large ongoing losses (e.g., in stool). The goal of IV rehydration is not necessarily to completely rehydrate the child but rather to rehydrate the child to the point where oral rehydration is feasible. As soon as the child can tolerate an ORS, it should be used to complete rehydration.

## MANAGING THE VOMITING CHILD

Both parents and health professionals view the child with protracted vomiting as the most challenging clinical situation. Indeed, truly intractable vomiting (along with ileus and altered consciousness) is one of the few contra-indications to oral rehydration therapy. Nevertheless, experience in a variety of settings has shown that slow, steady administration of oral fluids (i.e., as little as a teaspoonful of solution every two to five minutes) is often the key to success in children with vomiting. Giving ORS at low rates reduces the chances of vomiting by both preventing over-distention of the stomach and helping to correct acidosis. Administering ORS by nasogastric tube is cheaper and associated with shorter hospital stays than management with IV therapy.

## NUTRITIONAL MANAGEMENT

Until recently, the major emphasis of diarrhoeal disease control programmes was the appropriate management of dehydrated children, primarily through the use of ORT. Little attention was directed to the proper dietary management of children with diarrhoea. This may not have severe consequences in well-nourished children but a delay in reintroducing feeds may have devastating effects in undernourished children. Many studies have found significant relationships between poor growth in children and the prevalence and duration of diarrhoea. Diarrhoea and malnutrition combine to form a vicious cycle, which, if not broken, can eventually result in death. The final event may be a particularly severe or prolonged episode of diarrhoea or another serious infection such as pneumonia. Deaths from diarrhoea are, in fact, usually associated with malnutrition. In hospitals where good management of dehydration is practised, virtually all mortality from diarrhoea is in malnourished children.

## TIMING OF REINTRODUCTION OF FEEDS

Traditionally, children with diarrhoea were routinely starved for 24 hours or longer in the belief that this would decrease the duration and severity of the illness. Present evidence favours the early reintroduction of feeds as soon as the child is rehydrated, ie., within four to six hours. Early feeding enhances enterocyte regeneration, reduces intestinal permeability and promotes recovery of brush border disaccharidase production. Complete resumption of the child's normal feeding, including lactose-containing formula, does not result in worsening or increased duration of diarrhoea, increased vomiting, or lactose intolerance. Indeed, earlier feeding results in decreased stool output with improved nutritional results. Children are more comfortable and their caregivers are more likely to comply with therapy when feeding is continued.

## MILK-CONTAINING AND MIXED DIETS

Transient lactase deficiency secondary to brush border injury is common, particularly after rotavirus gastroenteritis. Unabsorbed lactose could conceivably worsen the diarrhoea by an osmotic effect. However, the majority of children with acute diarrhoea can safely continue receiving undiluted, lactose-containing, non-human milks. Only in the presence of severe diarrhoea and dehydration, or persistent diarrhoea, should evidence for lactose intolerance be sought. A lactose-free formula may then be considered if the stool pH is less than 5 and it contains more than 0,5 per cent reducing substances.

Continuation of breast-feeding during diarrhoeal illness is unanimously accepted, although breast milk contains more lactose than cow milk. Available evidence shows that continued breast-feeding results in reduced severity of purging and a decrease in the duration of illness. There is no role for the dilution of milk feeds. Even in high-risk malnourished infants less than six months of age, the rapid reintroduction of full-strength milk formula during gastroenteritis results in no more treatment failures than in those in whom feeds are regraded over 48 hours. In general, the foods that should be given during diarrhoea are the same as those the child should receive when he or she is well. Energy-dense, locally available staple foods (e.g., maize, rice, millet, wheat, sorghum, or potato) have consistently reduced the duration of diarrhoea in studies. This may be related to the fibre contained in these diets. Other appropriate foods include fresh fruits, vegetables, yoghurt, and lean meats. Mothers need to be specifically encouraged to resume feeding with these foods and to provide an extra meal per day for the two weeks following the onset of diarrhoea.

## NUTRITIONAL ADVICE

The mother may better understand and accept dietary advice if she is given a dietary prescription. This can be prepared as a printed pamphlet that shows pictures of various foods along with their names and the amounts of each usually given at different ages. If specific staple foods, vegetables, fruit, meats, and oils are circled and the amount of each to be given is indicated, the mother has a handy reminder of how her child should be fed. When dietary advice is provided in this form it is also more likely to be taken seriously by the mother.

## DRUG THERAPY

In 1990, WHO published a seminal report on the use of drugs in the management of acute diarrhoea in children. The book emphasized the primacy of ORT and concluded that there was no role for commonly used drugs (WHO,1990). At least 13 developing countries banned, deregistered, or restricted the use of products containing loperamide, kaolin, pectin, or diphenoxylate because of the WHO report.

*Adsorbent agents* such as kaolin, pectin, and charcoal act by binding to unbound bacterial toxins and adsorbing water. Clinical trials show that their effect is purely cosmetic and they cause no change in stool weight and water. More disturbingly, they interfere with the absorption of concurrently administered medication such as antibiotics.

*Antimotility drugs* such as loperamide and diphenoxylate slow transit time, shorten the duration of diarrhoea, and reduce stool output. However, they can have important side effects in children including nausea, vomiting, drowsiness, respiratory depression, and ileus. Loperamide was reported to be the cause of 18 cases of severe abdominal distention and at least six deaths in children. Diphenoxylate can prolong diarrhoea and toxicity associated with infections like shigellosis.

*Antisecretory drugs* attempt to decrease intestinal secretion, which is the major cause of a watery stool. Some promote sodium absorption while others act by inhibiting chloride secretion. Agents studied in this class of drugs include prostaglandin synthetase inhibitors such as bismuth subsalicylate.

Bismuth has been proven to be beneficial in reducing the duration and severity of diarrhoea. However, difficulties with its administration and costs are limiting factors to its widespread use.

## ANTIMICROBIALS

Most diarrhoeal episodes are self-limited and do not require or benefit from antimicrobial therapy. Antibiotics may be indicated in the neonate, in immunocompromised patients (particularly those with severe malnutrition), and in those who are systemically ill. Both gram positive and negative cover should be provided (Ampicillin and Gentamicin) for five to seven days. There is good evidence to treat *Shigella* dysentery – it shortens the duration of diarrhoea and the duration of pathogen excretion. WHO also recommends that suspected cholera, amoebiasis, and giardiasis be treated with antimicrobials (WHO,1990).

## Other therapies

- Zinc supplementation results in a reduction in the number of watery stools in children with diarrhoea.
- Folic acid has no value in treating acute diarrhoea.
- Regular vitamin A supplementation has been shown to reduce the severity of diarrhoea. Its effects on the prevalence or duration of diarrhoea have been variable.
- Lactobacillus GG, a probiotic, given daily over 15 months , prevents diarrhoea in undernourished non-breast-fed infants, but is of little value in breast-fed infants.
- Homeopathic medication may have a role in managing gastroenteritis, but there is little convincing evidence of its benefits in scientific literature.

# Prevention

Various interventions have been proposed for preventing diarrhoea in young children, most of which involve measures related to provision of safe water, safe disposal of faeces, fly control, infant feeding practices, personal hygiene, and immunization. Effective implementation of these preventive strategies requires involvement of a range of sectors (e.g., agriculture, public works, and environmental health).

## WATER AND SANITATION

Most infectious agents that cause diarrhoea are transmitted by the faecal–oral route. This includes transmission by contaminated drinking water or contaminated food, and person-to-person spread. A plentiful supply of clean water helps to encourage hygienic practices, such as hand washing, cleaning of eating utensils, and cleaning of latrines. These practices can interrupt the spread of infectious agents that cause diarrhoea.

To facilitate good hygiene, it is more important that the water supply be abundant than clean, although both qualities are desirable. Clean water is essential, however, for drinking and for preparing food. Improvements in sanitation reduce the risk of diarrhoea to the same, or greater, extent than improved water supplies. The greatest benefit occurs when improvements in sanitation and water supply are combined and education is given on hygienic practices.

Water supply and sanitation (WSS) interventions are highly cost effective for the control of diarrhoea among under-five-year olds, on a par with oral rehydration therapy.

WHO estimates that it costs an average of US$ 105 per person to provide water supplies in urban areas and US$ 50 in rural areas, while sanitation costs an average of US$ 145 in urban areas and US$ 30 in rural areas.

WSS infrastructure is generally built and operated by public works agencies and financed by construction grants, user fees, and property taxes. Health sector agencies can assist in project design, hygiene education, social marketing of good hygiene practices, and water quality regulation. Sustainability of WSS projects has been of some concern in South Africa and internationally, i.e., there is concern about the ability of communities to maintain and repair the WSS facilities that have been constructed.

## FLY CONTROL AND WASTE DISPOSAL

Studies done in the Gambia and Pakistan have confirmed that fly control can have an impact on diarrhoea incidence similar to, or greater than, that of the interventions currently recommended by WHO for inclusion in diarrhoeal disease control programmes. There was virtual elimination of flies and 22 to 26 per cent less childhood diarrhoea in villages where insecticides, such as deltamethrin, were used, compared with controls. Technologies and practices that interrupt disease transmission by flies need to be developed and promoted.

## HYGIENE

Behavioural practices associated with occurrence of diarrhoea include disposal of faeces around the house, careless handling of cleaning material, use of feeding bottles, purchase of cooked food from food vendors, and the presence of domestic animals in food preparation places. A consistent relationship between almost all non-hygienic practices and diarrhoea has been detected.

Washing of hands, domestic cleanliness (kitchen, living room, yard) and the use of a napkins or underclothing by the child have the strongest protective effect. Hand washing is particularly effective for preventing the spread of *Shigella*, which is the most important cause of dysentery. More schooling (more than three years of primary school) and a better economic position (e.g., possession of a radio) have a positive influence on general hygiene behaviour. Individual hygiene behaviour appears to be highly variable in contrast with the consistent behaviour of communities as a whole. Hygiene promotion campaigns are most likely to be successful if they target a single activity, e.g., handwashing, rather than marketing multiple messages.

## HEALTH EDUCATION

The available evidence suggests that health education programmes may be a cost-effective intervention on diarrhoeal morbidity, with a median reduction of 33 per cent. Information on the prevention of diarrhoea can be provided in a variety of ways, e.g., at community meetings, through schools, during home visits, and during visits to a health centre. Improved health education should focus on the benefits of exclusive breast-feeding, early signs of dehydration, the quantity of ORT needed and address mothers who have no prior knowledge of ORT. Management of diarrhoea may also be improved by a more liberal distribution of ORS sachets, as it has been shown that the availability of ORS sachets at home at the onset of diarrhoea is the strongest predictor of their use.

## BREAST-FEEDING

Studies have consistently shown the beneficial effects of breast-feeding in preventing morbidity and mortality from diarrhoea in infants. Breast-fed babies have fewer episodes of diarrhoea, less severe episodes, and have a lower risk of dying from diarrhoea than babies who are not breast-fed. For example, during the first six months of life, the risk of having severe diarrhoea that requires hospitalization can be 30 times greater for non-breast-fed infants and the risk of dying is 25 times greater than for those who are exclusively breast-fed. The protective effects of breast-feeding do not appear to continue after the cessation of breast-feeding.

## WEANING EDUCATION

It is possible, even in poor communities, to improve substantially the nutritional status of infants and young children by weaning education. It is estimated that, through its effects on nutritional status, weaning education may reduce the diarrhoea mortality rate, among children under 5 years of age, by 2 to 12 per cent. Mothers should be taught ways of preparing, giving, and storing weaning foods that minimize the risk of bacterial contamination. They also need to be taught about the importance of breast-feeding, the nutritional value of common foods, and the importance of regular feeding in childhood. Face-to-face communication by locally recruited workers, reinforced by radio and other mass media, may be the most effective channels for weaning education.

## IMMUNIZATION

While the list of pathogens causing diarrhoea is large, just a few bacteria and viruses combine to cause a substantial proportion of diarrhoeal illness. Because of the strong relationship between measles and serious diarrhoea, measles immunization is a very cost-effective measure for reducing diarrhoea morbidity and deaths. Measles vaccine given at nine months of age can prevent up to 25 per cent of diarrhoea-associated deaths in children under 5 years of age. A tetravalent rotavirus vaccine was licensed in the USA in 1998 and in the European Union in 1999, but routine use has been suspended because it appears to cause intussusception. The vaccine is most effective

(67 to 100 per cent) in preventing severe diarrhoea. There are good prospects of developing practical and effective vaccines within the next few years against cholera, *Shigella* and enterotoxigenic *E. coli*. Two Salmonella typhi vaccines have been licensed for high-risk groups in high-income countries.

## MICRONUTRIENT SUPPLEMENTS

This has become the new frontier in the battle against childhood gastroenteritis and many trials are being or have recently been completed in this area. . How these different micronutrients should best be integrated into a uniform strategy to combat childhood diarrhoea has yet to be established.

Zinc supplementation in children in developing countries is associated with substantial reductions in the rates of diarrhoea and pneumonia, the two leading causes of death in these settings. Vitamin A supplementation in young children results in average reductions in all-cause mortality of 23 per cent and 30 per cent with a reduction of deaths from diarrhoeal disease by 39 per cent.

# Persistent gastroenteritis

With improved management of acute episodes of infectious diarrhoea, increased attention is now being given to persistent diarrhoea and its nutritional consequences and associated mortality. A total of 3 to 23 per cent of cases of acute diarrhoea in developing regions progress to persistent diarrhoea (diarrhoea for more than 14 days). Yet, in some areas, it causes 30 to 50 per cent of all diarrhoea-associated deaths, and as many as 15 per cent of episodes of persistent diarrhoea result in death.

There is no single microbial cause, although enteroadherent *E. coli* may play a greater role than other agents. *Cryptosporidium* may also be important in severely undernourished or immunodeficient persons. A number of other pathogenic bacteria and protozoa are found with nearly equal frequency in cases of acute and persistent diarrhoea, but their role in causing this problem is unclear. Irrespective of its cause, persistent diarrhoea is associated with extensive changes in the bowel mucosa, especially flattening of the villi and reduced production of disaccharidase enzymes. These cause reduced absorption of nutrients and may perpetuate the illness after the original infectious cause has been eliminated.

Risk factors for the development of persistent diarrhoea include young age, malnutrition, impaired immune function, recent introduction of milk feedings, prior antimicrobial therapy, and infection with pathogenic strains of *E. coli* or *Cryptosporidium*. Late consultation (after 48 hours) has been associated with persistent diarrhoea, reflecting that these episodes were initially less acute. The use of ORS does not appear to impact on the development of persistent diarrhoea, whereas home medication tends to increase the risk of persistent diarrhoea.

Persistent diarrhoea is largely a nutritional disease. It occurs more frequently in children who are already undernourished and is itself an important cause of malnutrition. A single episode of persistent diarrhoea can last three to four weeks or longer and cause dramatic weight loss, sometimes rapidly leading to severe malnutrition. Proper feeding is the most important aspect of treatment for most children with persistent diarrhoea. The aims of nutritional therapy are to:

- Temporarily reduce the amount of animal milk (or lactose) in the diet. The use of milks in which the lactose content has been lowered, e.g., by hydrolysis, can reduce diarrhoea and improve retention of dietary carbohydrate, protein, and energy.

Lactose and sucrose-free formulas are commercially available;

- Provide yoghurt (or a similar fermented milk product), which reduces by half the amount of lactose in the child's diet. It is a useful carbohydrate source that is better tolerated in children with chronic diarrhoea. In many cases, this step will cause the diarrhoea to subside rapidly;
- Ensure a full energy intake for the child (i.e., about 110 kcal/kg/day) to facilitate the repair process in the damaged gut mucosa and improve nutritional status. Offer a cereal with added vegetable oil; mix this with other foods, such as well-cooked and mashed pulses, vegetables, and, if possible, meat or fish. Avoid low-energy foods that are dilute or bulky. At least half of the child's energy intake should come from foods other than milk or milk products. A traditional diet and yoghurt combination can be used satisfactorily for nutritional rehabilitation in over 80 per cent of children;
- Give food in frequent small meals, at least six times a day; and
- Provide supplementary vitamins and minerals, in particular zinc, vitamin A, folate, vitamin B12, and iron, if possible. Zinc supplementation (20 mg/day) in persistent diarrhoea has been proven to significantly reduce the length of the recovery period in malnourished children.

In some centres antibiotics (gentamicin) and cholestyramine (the 'bowel cocktail') have long been used. It may have particular advantage in patients with bacterial overgrowth. There is no role for 'antidiarrhoeal' drugs (including antimotility and antisecretory drugs and adsorbents).

Patients with bloody stool or a stool culture positive for *Shigella* should receive an antibiotic for shigellosis. If stool culture yields another bacterial pathogen, e.g., enteropathogenic *E.*

*coli*, an oral antibiotic to which that agent is sensitive must be given. If *giardia* cysts, or trophozoites of either *giardia* or *E. histolytica* are seen in the faeces, a course of appropriate antiprotozoal therapy should be prescribed.

## BLOODY DIARRHOEA (DYSENTERY)

About 15 per cent of all diarrhoeal episodes in children under five years are dysenteric, but these cause up to 25 per cent of all diarrhoeal deaths. The clinical diagnosis of dysentery is based solely on the presence of visible blood in the diarrhoeal stool. Patients with bloody diarrhoea frequently have fever, but sometimes the temperature is abnormally low, especially in the most serious cases. Cramping, abdominal pain, and rectal pain during defecation, or attempted defecation (tenesmus), and mucoid stools are common. However, young children are unable to describe these complaints.

Children with bloody diarrhoea should be presumed to have shigellosis and treated accordingly. This is because *Shigella* cause about 60 per cent of dysentery cases seen at health facilities and nearly all cases of severe, life-threatening disease. Resistance of *Shigella* to cotrimoxazole is increasing world-wide. There is widespread resistance of *Shigella* to ampicillin and cotrimoxazole in South Africa too, and nalidixic acid is presently recommended for outpatients. If the child is hospitalized, IM ceftriaxone (100 mg/kg) once daily for five days is recommended.

Although treatment is recommended for five days, there should be a substantial improvement after two days, i.e., less fever, pain, faecal blood, and loose stools. If this does not occur, the prescribed antibiotic should be stopped and a different one used (e.g., ciprofloxacin). Children who are improving should continue the treatment for five days. If microscopic examination of the stool is performed and trophozoites of *E. histolytica* containing erythrocytes are seen, metronidazole should also be given.

## CHOLERA

Cholera should be suspected when a child older than five years develops severe dehydration from acute profuse, painless, watery diarrhoea (usually with vomiting), or when a child above the age of two years has acute watery diarrhoea in an area where there is an outbreak of cholera. Symptoms appear within six hours to five days (usually two to three days) following exposure. Death is usually the result of hypovolaemic shock. Asymptomatic carriers of the disease are common and may be infectious for months. Diagnosis is made by isolation of the bacteria in a stool culture.

Rehydration and maintaining adequate hydration (as described earlier) is the mainstay of effective management. An effective antibiotic can reduce the volume of diarrhoea in children with severe cholera. Unfortunately, recent strains of *Vibrio cholerae 01* in South Africa have been resistant to all conventional antibiotics, for example, tetracycline, doxycycline, cotrimoxazole, etc. The organism remains sensitive to nalidixic acid and ciprofloxacin. Use of these antibiotics should be reserved for children who are severely dehydrated and older than two years (see also Chapter 25: Immunization).

## HIV and diarrhoea

Gastrointestinal disease is a major problem for patients with HIV and AIDS, and diarrhoea is reported in up to 60 per cent of patients with AIDS. Diarrhoea may wax and wane over time, and in at least 30 per cent of patients, an aetiology cannot be determined. In such cases, the diarrhoea is often attributed to HIV enteropathy.

A study done in Soweto comparing diarrhoeal disease in HIV-infected and uninfected children found that HIV-infected children were more likely to be malnourished, to have prolonged diarrhoea, to have an associated pneumonia, and require a longer hospital stay. There was no significant difference in stool pathogens and the degree of dehydration on admission between the HIV-infected and uninfected children (Johnson et al.). The management of diarrhoea in HIV-infected children does not differ from that of uninfected children. Vitamin A has been shown to be effective in reducing mortality in HIV-positive children with diarrhoea and pneumonia.

## Conclusion

There have been important developments in the prevention and management of gastroenteritis over the past decade. The primacy of ORT over all other interventions still stands. However, changes in the formulation of ORS can be expected.

The dietary management of diarrhoeal episodes has assumed increasing prominence in the last decade. Re-establishing usual feeding habits is vital, particularly in developing countries. Foods readily available in the home, such as rice and maize, have an important role to play in both preventing and correcting dehydration and ensuring that the child's caloric needs are satisfied in the recovery period. The role of micronutrient supplementation (e.g., zinc, vitamin A) in national diarrhoeal disease control programmes has yet to be clearly defined. Some newer drugs show promise in reducing the severity of diarrhoea, but the use of drugs in general must continue to be strongly discouraged.

The high mortality and morbidity from childhood gastroenteritis can only be reduced if more efforts are made to prevent it. Improvements in the provision of water and sanitation, better breast-feeding practices, improved fly control, more effective health education, and the promise of new vaccines against gastrointestinal pathogens hold the key to conquering this scourge.

## References and further reading

FABER M & BENADE AJ. 1999. Nutritional status and dietary practices of 4–24-month-old children from a rural South African community. *Public Health Nutrition.* 2:179–85.

JOHNSON S, HENDSON W, CREWE-BROWN H, et al. 2000. The effect of HIV infection on episodes of diarrhoea among children in Soweto, South Africa. *Pediatric Infectious Disease Journal.* 19(10):972–9.

KAHN K, TOLLMAN SM, GARENNE M, and GEAR JS. 1999. Who dies from what? Determining cause of death in South Africa's rural north-east. *Tropical Medicine and International Health.* 4:433–41.

LIEBELT EL. 1998. Clinical and laboratory evaluation and management of children with vomiting, diarrhea, and dehydration. *Current Opinions on Pediatrics.* 10:461–9.

VON SCHIRNDING YE, YACH D, BLIGNAULT R, and MATHEWS C. 1991. Environmental determinants of acute respiratory symptoms and diarrhoea in young coloured children living in urban and peri-urban areas of South Africa. *South African Medical Journal.* 79:457–61.

WHO. 1990. The rational use of drugs in the management of acute diarrhoea in children. Geneva:WHO.

WHO. 1993. The management and prevention of diarrhoea: practical guidelines. Geneva: WHO.

YACH D, STREBEL PM, and JOUBERT G. 1989. The impact of diarrhoeal disease on childhood deaths in the RSA, 1968–1985. *South African Medical Journal.* 76:472–5.

# 39

# HIV infection

## GD HUSSEY

Human immunodeficiency virus (HIV) infection, and its full clinical presentation, the acquired immunodeficiency syndrome (AIDS), are now major public health problems in most countries world-wide. Developing countries, particularly in Africa, have borne the brunt of the HIV pandemic. In 1999, WHO estimated that 67 per cent of approximately 34 million persons living with HIV and 85 per cent of the 2,6 million deaths were from sub-Saharan Africa (UNAIDS, 1999). The HIV epidemic has also had a significant impact on child health, reversing the gains achieved through child survival strategies over the last two decades. During 1999, it was estimated that approximately 500 000 new paediatric infections and almost 400 000 AIDS-related child deaths occurred in Africa. At least 95 per cent of the world's AIDS orphans are African.

South Africa is experiencing one of the fastest-growing HIV epidemics in the world. In 1999, over 50 per cent of all new infections in southern Africa occurred in this country. Currently, in South Africa, it was estimated that three to four million persons were infected with HIV and that approximately 75 000 infants would be born with HIV infection during the year 2000. These data are based on the routine anonymous unlinked screening of pregnant women attending antenatal clinics in South Africa, of whom 23 per cent were estimated to be infected in 1999 (Department of Health, 1999). HIV is also having a major impact on health service utilization in that 20 to 35 per cent of paediatric hospital beds are occupied by HIV-infected children (Zwi et al., 1999).

## Transmission of HIV

HIV transmission may occur during the intra-uterine, intrapartum, or postpartum period. In the absence of breast-feeding approximately 30 per cent of infant infections occur *in utero* and 70 per cent during the intra-partum period (Newell, 1998). In breast-feeding populations, these proportions are reduced to approximately 20 and 60 per cent respectively, while breast-feeding itself is responsible for 15 to 25 per cent of infant HIV infections. Some researchers have suggested that one-third to one-half of all perinatal HIV infections in sub-Saharan Africa may be a consequence of breast-feeding.

Transmission of the virus from an infected mother to the fetus or infant is not invariable.

In the absence of interventions, rates vary from 15 to 25 per cent in Europe and the USA, and 25 to 45 per cent in Africa. Risk factors for transmission have been well defined (Gibb & Tess, 1999). Women who have clinical, virological (high viral load), or immunological (low CD4 count) markers of severe HIV disease have a greater chance of transmission of the virus to their infants. Prolonged labour, vaginal delivery, and prematurity are also significant risk factors. Invasive obstetrical procedures and emergency caesarian section deliveries, which increase the risk of maternal–fetal blood contact, may also be important. Vitamin A deficiency in the mother and clinical or histological evidence of chorioamnionitis have also been associated with increased perinatal transmssion. Transmission rates in Africa tend to be higher than in developed countries, which may be a reflection of more severe disease in mothers.

Parenteral (horizontal) transmission via blood and blood-products is no longer a problem in countries where systematic screening of blood donors has been implemented. Blood transfusions do, however, continue to be an important mode of transmission in poorer countries with no screening facilities. Transmission following sexual abuse has been reported. HIV transmission has also been reported among family members in a household setting, but this is extremely rare and is of no practical importance.

# Natural history of HIV infection in children

HIV has a bimodal presentation in children. One group, the rapid progressors, presents early with severe disease, usually within the first year of life. These children have a poor prognosis and most die within the first three years of life. The other group, the slow progressors, remain relatively healthy, present with minor signs and symptoms by eight to ten years of age, and the disease runs a slower and more benign course. The intermediate group tends to develop signs and symptoms of severe disease by five to eight years of age (Nielsen, 1999).

AIDS mortality rates in the first year of life vary from 5 per cent in Europe and the USA to between 10 and 40 per cent in Africa. The latter may be the result of higher viral load, increased risk of other infections, nutritional factors, lack of medical care, and unavailability of specific anti-retroviral therapy. Studies from Europe and the USA indicate a median survival time of between 8 and 12 years. Data from developing countries suggest a much shorter median survival time of between 3 and 5 years (Hussey et al., 1998).

# Clinical features of AIDS in children

Many of the signs and symptoms are non-specific and are seen in other common childhood diseases such as tuberculosis, malnutrition, and malaria. The important characteristics of these signs and symptoms are that they are frequently recurrent, persistent, and may respond poorly to therapy.

Common presenting syndromes are as follows:

*Wasting syndrome:* Failure to thrive is a prominent feature of childhood AIDS and is usually associated with chronic or recurrent diarrhoeal disease and oropharyngeal or gastrointestinal candidiasis. Diarrhoea may be the result of the direct effect of HIV infection on the gastrointestinal tract or follow opportunistic infections such as cryptosporidium, cytomegalovirus, other viruses, and bacteria.

*Recurrent bacterial infections:* A wide variety of infections of varying severity are seen, including pneumonia, septicaemia, meningitis, osteomyelitis, otitis media, tonsillitis, cellulitis, and urinary tract infections. The organisms causing disease are those that commonly cause infections in normal children such as *S. pneumoniae, H. influenzae, S. aureas,* and Salmonella.

*Pulmonary syndromes:* Two common specific syndromes are *Pneumocystis carinii* pneumonia (PCP) and lymphoid interstitial pneumonitis (LIP). PCP is characterized by a sudden onset with fever, tachypnoea, hypoxaemia, and a diffuse interstitial infiltrate on X-ray. It is associated with a very poor prognosis. LIP is a slowly progressive interstitial lung disease of unknown aetiology, characterized by bilateral reticulonodular infiltrates on the chest X-ray and a prolonged and more benign course. Other common problems are tuberculosis and bacterial pneumonia.

*Persistent generalized lymphadenopathy:* This is often associated with hepatosplenomegaly and parotid gland enlargement.

*Neurological syndromes:* Encephalopathy is probably the result of HIV infection itself and manifests as developmental delay, loss of developmental milestones, convulsions, and behavioural abnormalities.

*Dermatitis:* Severe scabies, seborrhoeic, and other skin rashes are common especially in infants.

*Haematological manifestations:* These include anaemia, thrombocytopaenia, and neutropaenia.

*Opportunistic infections: Pneumocystis carinii, Candida albicans,* cytomegalovirus, *Cryptosporidium, Mycobacterium tuberculosis* and other mycobacteria, and herpes simplex.

Rarer manifestations sometimes seen are hepatitis, cardiomyopathy, renal disease, toxoplasmosis, cryptococcal meningitis, and malignancies (lymphoma and Kaposi sarcoma).

The clinical features of AIDS in children are different from those found in adults. LIP, severe recurrent infections, and encephalopathy are common manifestations in children, while Kaposi sarcoma, lymphoma, and central nervous system opportunistic infections, common in adults, occur rarely in children.

In children hypergammaglobulinaemia, together with the presence of generalized lymphoid hyperplasia, serve to differentiate AIDS from primary immune deficiencies that also present with recurrent and unusual infections in children.

# Diagnostic tests for AIDS in children

Because congenitally infected newborns will have passively acquired anti-HIV antibodies from their mothers, the standard anti-HIV IgG antibody tests cannot be used as diagnostic tests in children under 18 months of age. In these children, tests such as virus culture, detection of HIV, DNA by PCR, or p24 antigen assays are highly specific and virtually 100 per cent accurate by 3 months in the absence of breast-feeding. However, these tests are expensive and not freely available. In the absence of such specific tests, the diagnosis is usually suspected if the child has a positive antibody test and clinical signs compatible with HIV infection. Other laboratory evidence of immune deficiency such as a low total lymphocyte or CD4 count or hypergammaglobulinaemia will provide supportive evidence for the diagnosis. Children over 18 months of age can be diagnosed by the usual serological methods.

Many clinicians in Africa will be forced to suspect or diagnose AIDS in children on clinical criteria alone. Consequently WHO has proposed a clinical case definition for paediatric AIDS for use where diagnostic resources are limited.

# Management

## HIV-EXPOSED INFANTS

Infants born to women who are HIV positive, i.e., HIV exposed, require follow-up to con-

## WHO case definition

Paediatric AIDS is suspected in an infant or child presenting with at least two of the following major and at least two of the following minor signs in the absence of known causes of immunosuppression, such as cancer, severe malnutrition, or other recognized aetiologies.

**Major signs**

- Weight loss or abnormally slow growth.
- Chronic diarrhoea lasting for more than one month.
- Fever lasting for more than one month.

**Minor signs**

- Generalized lymphadenopathy.
- Oropharyngeal candidiasis.
- Repeated common infections (otitis, pharyngitis, etc.).
- Persistent cough.
- Generalized dermatitis.
- Confirmed maternal HIV infection.

These criteria lack sensitivity and specificity and the inclusion of other criteria such as encephalopathy or pulmonary disease should be evaluated to increase the validity of the definition.

firm whether infection has occurred or not. Ideally a PCR test should be done at about four months of age to confirm or refute HIV infection. However, as stated above, these tests are not always available. Conventional ELISA tests will only reliably exclude infection at 18 months of age. HIV-infected mothers must be provided with the information to make informed decisions about breast-feeding. Infants who develop signs of AIDS need close surveillance. The mainstay of therapy is general medical and psychological supportive care with treatment of opportunistic infections.

## NUTRITIONAL SUPPORT

Ensure adequate nutrient intake. Treat dental caries and opportunistic infections, particularly gastrointestinal disorders and oropharyngeal problems, which may impact on nutritional status. In areas of high worm prevalence give albendazole or mebendazole prophylaxis every six months to prevent helminthic infestations. Vitamin A supplementation in HIV-infected children has been associated with reduced morbidity, particularly in relation to diarrhoeal disease, as well as reduced mortality. Use either daily multivitamin supplements or high dose vitamin A supplements every four to six months (Eley & Hussey, 1999).

## PCP PROPHYLAXIS

Trimethoprim-sulphamethoxazole prophylaxis prevents PCP as well as other bacterial infections (WHO, 2000). It is recommended that all HIV-exposed infants be given prophylaxis from six weeks to four months of age. If at this stage the infant is HIV negative then prophylaxis is stopped. If the infant is truly infected then prophylaxis is continued until one year. Older children should be given prophylaxis only if their CD4 count falls below 15 per cent or after an episode of PCP. If CD4 counts are not available, then all symptomatic children should be given prophylaxis. Give the medication as a daily dose three times a week on consecutive days as follows: less than 5 kg – 5 ml; 5 to 9,9 kg – 7,5 ml; 10 to 4,9 kg – 10 ml; 15 to 19,9 kg – 15 ml; greater than 20 kg – 20 ml.

## PCP TREATMENT

Signs and symptoms of PCP may be indistinguishable from other causes of severe pneumonia. Suspect PCP in HIV-infected children under a year of age with severe pneumonia.

- Treat with cotrimoxazole intravenously 10 mg per kilogram of trimethoprim

(TMP) as a loading dose, followed by 20 mg per kilogram per day of TMP given in four divided doses for two to three weeks. Change to oral therapy once there is clinical improvement.

- Prednisone (1 mg per kilogram p.o. in two divided doses for five days, then 0,5 mg per kilogram p.o. in two divided doses for five days, then 0,5 mg per kilogram daily for seven days or until no longer hypoxaemic).

## TUBERCULOSIS PROPHYLAXIS

HIV-infected children who have had household contact with sputum-positive patients or who are positive tuberculin reactors (tuberculin reactions of 4 mm or greater) should be given supervised prophylaxis (Bucher et al., 1999). The South African Tuberculosis Advisory Committee suggests INH for six months or INH, RIF, and PZA for three months.

## MANAGEMENT OF BACTERIAL INFECTIONS

Children with AIDS who present with fever or signs suggestive of a bacterial infection should be investigated appropriately and antibiotic therapy prescribed accordingly. In children with recurrent or persistent infections who are neutropaenic or who do not respond to conventional therapy, consider a resistant organism and give appropriate antimicrobial therapy. High-dose intravenous immunoglobulin (400 mg per kilogram monthly) reduces episodes of infection and improves quality of life and should be used in children who have recurrent bacterial infections if resources permit (National Institute of Child Health, 1991).

## ANTIRETROVIRAL THERAPY (ARV)

This is a complex and evolving field (Nielsen, 1999). ARV therapy has been shown to improve the quality and duration of life of children. Currently, where resources permit, treatment with highly active antiretroviral drugs is recommended for all HIV-positive infants, but only for children over the age of 12 months who are symptomatic or have evidence of immunosuppression. The current preferred regimen is two nucleoside reverse transcriptase inhibitors with a protease inhibitor. Monotherapy is no longer recommended except as prophylaxis to prevent mother-to-child transmission or after exposure following needle-stick injuries.

# Prevention of vertical transmission

## ANTIRETROVIRAL THERAPY

In 1994 the first placebo-controlled efficacy trial of zidovudine (AZT) treatment of pregnant HIV-positive women was completed in the USA and France. In this study, AZT administered to the mother during pregnancy and during labour and given to the newborns for six weeks post-delivery reduced the risk of transmission by 67,5 per cent. Following this trial, AZT has become part of the standard level of care provided to HIV-positive women in developed countries and has resulted in dramatic decline in perinatal transmission (de Kock et al., 2000).

The AZT regimen described above is costly and impractical for developing countries. Subsequent shorter-course regimens in Thailand and Africa have shown efficacy rates of between 38 and 50 per cent. Lower rates were found in breast-feeding populations. A recent study from Malawi reported that a single 200 mg dose of nevirapine given to the mother at the onset of labour combined with a single 2 mg per kilogram dose given to the infant within two to three days of birth was successful in reducing mother-to-child HIV transmission. This is an attractive, cost-effective option for developing countries.

Even though these regimens may be cost effective, many developing countries lack the infrastructure or the resources for implementation of ARV interventions. Critical to any intervention is a system for HIV counselling and testing for women and their partners and a mechanism for following-up mothers and infants who are HIV positive.

## BREAST-FEEDING

Since HIV is transmitted via breast milk WHO has recommended that where resources permit, HIV-infected mothers should not breast-feed. However, in resource poor settings, where infectious diseases and malnutrition are the primary causes of infant mortality and where the risks of artificial feeding may be high, breast-feeding should be recommended (WHO, 1992). These recommendations have been endorsed in a recent randomized clinical trial comparing HIV transmission rates in breast-fed versus formula fed infants in Kenya (Nduati et al., 2000). In this study the HIV transmission rate in exclusively formula-fed infants at three months of age was 13 per cent compared to 25 per cent in those breast-fed. At 24 months of age the rates were 21 per cent and 37 per cent respectively.

In contrast, a recent observational study from Durban indicated that HIV transmission rates in exclusively breast-fed infants at three months of age (15 per cent) was similar to that in artifically fed infants (19 per cent) but significantly lower than in infants who received mixed feeding (24 per cent) (Coutsoudis et al., 1999). These findings have important implications for the prevention of HIV and for infant-feeding policies in sub-Saharan Africa. However, additional research is needed before current policies are changed.

## OTHER INTERVENTIONS TO REDUCE MOTHER TO CHILD TRANSMISSION

*Vitamin* A: Even though vitamin A deficiency has been associated with an increased risk of mother-to-child transmission of HIV (Semba et al., 1994), supplementation with vitamin A in South Africa and Tanzania have shown no impact at all, except possibly in premature infants in the South African trial.

*Obstetric interventions*: Obstetric interventions that prevent infant exposure to infectious material may reduce vertical transmission (VT) rates. Such interventions include vaginal virucidal cleaning and elective cesarean section (CS). In Malawi a trial of chlorhexidine use as a vaginal virucidal agent had no effect on the transmission rate but did have some effect in a subset of women with prolonged rupture of membranes (Rouse et al., 1997). A recent meta-analysis of 15 cohort studies in Europe and the USA reported a 50 per cent reduction of vertical transmission following CS (International Perinatal HIV Group, 1999). These findings have been confirmed in a randomized clinical trial of mode of delivery. CS was associated with a VT rate of 1,7 per cent compared with 10,7 per cent among those randomized to vaginal delivery (European Mode of Delivery Collaboration, 1999). This intervention is clearly not feasible in developing countries.

# Universal blood precautions

The routinely recommended precautions for handling blood and body fluids in all infectious disease patients, as laid down by the hospital authorities, should be followed for HIV-infected children. Children should be cared for in paediatric wards and strict isolation is not required unless they have no control of body secretions, and do not have uncoverable oozing skin lesions, dysentery, or uncontrollable aggressive behaviour. Good handwashing is essential and gloves should be worn during procedures. The doctor in charge of the patient should regularly appraise the risk imposed by such a child to other children and the staff.

The same precautions that apply in hospital apply in the community and children who do not pose a risk of infection to others can be admitted to pre-school facilities and to school. If affected families are assured of support and understanding, they are more likely to have a responsible attitude towards community contacts, and to accept the necessity of confidentially informing those in charge about the child's infection.

# Immunization of HIV-infected children

HIV-infected children, whether clinically normal or symptomatic, should receive all the routine childhood vaccines with due consideration being given to the benefits and potential risks of the use of live vaccines. BCG should be given at birth or soon after but should not be given to the older symptomatic child. Measles and polio live vaccines pose a potential risk for symptomatic children who are immunodeficient. However, in a retrospective survey of HIV-infected children who had received live polio, measles, mumps, and rubella vaccine, there were no reports of serious adverse events following vaccination (McLaughlin et al., 1988). In contrast, severe and fatal cases of natural measles have been reported in children who are HIV infected, and measles vaccination is recommended for all children in developing countries (Epidemiological Notes and Reports, 1988). Inactivated polio virus vaccine is preferable but where it is not available the oral polio vaccine should be used in high-risk communities. Since

infection with encapsulated bacteria is common, immunization with S. pneumoniae and H. influenzae vaccines are recommended, if available. Measles or zoster immune globulin should be given to children following exposure to measles or chicken pox respectively.

# Counselling and support

The diagnosis of HIV infection in a child is a devastating life event for the family unit, since it implies that the mother is infected and in all probability the father as well. It is essential therefore that health and social services provide the necessary support for affected families. Where possible, they should be referred to community-based structures for ongoing support. Care should be taken not to abuse the trust of patients and disclosure of their HIV status to a third party should not be made without their permission.

Women should be advised about the possible risk of HIV infection in their newborn infants. They should be counselled about the potential risk of transmission of the virus via breast milk and be allowed to make an informed choice, considering individual socioeconomic circumstances, on infant feeding practices. Where the child is infected, ensure that the mother's health is considered as well. The stress of looking after a sick child may have adverse consequences to her own health.

# Education in schools about AIDS

Properly conducted programmes for the education of school-age children about health, sex, and AIDS is essential. Young people need to understand the AIDS epidemic and the specific actions they can take to prevent HIV infection, especially during adolescence. Because AIDS is a fatal disease, and educating children about becoming infected during sexual contact is controversial, both local and national guidelines are needed to formulate policies in this regard.

## References and further reading

BUCHER HC, GRIFFITH LE, GUYATT GH, et al. 1999. Isoniazid prophylaxis for tuberculosis in HIV infection: A meta-analysis of randomised controlled trials. *AIDS*. 13:507–510.

COUTSOUDIS A, PILLAY K, SPOONER E, et al. 1999. Influence of infant-feeding patterns on early mother-to-child transmission of HIV-1 in Durban, South Africa: A prospective cohort study. *Lancet*. 354:471–6.

DE COCK KM, FOWLER MG, MERCIER E, et al. 2000. Prevention of mother-to-child HIV transmission in resource-poor countries. Translating research into policy and practice. *JAMA*. 283:1175–82.

ELEY B & HUSSEY G. 1999. Nutrition and human immunodeficiency virus infection in children. *South African Medical Journal*. 89:190–5.

EUROPEAN MODE OF DELIVERY COLLABORATION. 1999. Elective cesarean-section versus vaginal delivery in prevention of vertical HIV-1 transmission: A randomized clinical trial. *Lancet*. 353:1035–39.

GIBB DM & TESS BH. 1999. Interventions to reduce mother-to-child transmission of HIV infection: New developments and current controversies. *AIDS*. 13 (suppl A): S93–S102.

GUAY LA, MUSOKE P, FLEMING T, et al. 1999. Intrapartum and neonatal single-dose nevirapine compared with zidovudine for prevention of mother-to-child transmission of HIV-1 in Kampala, Uganda: HIVNET 021 randomised trial. *Lancet*. 354:795–802.

HUSSEY GD, REIJNHART RM, SEBENS AM, BURGESS J, SCHAAF S, and POTGIETER S. 1998. Survival of children known to be perinatally infected with HIV. *South African Medical Journal*. 88:554–7.

INTERNATIONAL PERINATAL HIV GROUP. 1999. The mode of delivery and the risk of vertical transmission of human immunodeficiency virus type 1: A meta-analysis of 15 prospective cohort studies. *New England Journal of Medicine*. 340:977–87.

NEWELL ML. 1998. Mechanisms and timing of mother-to-child transmission of HIV-1. *AIDS*. 12:831–7.

NDUATI R, JOHN G, MBORI-NGACHA D, et al. 2000. Effect of breastfeeding and formula feeding on transmission of HIV-1. A randomized clinical trial. *JAMA*. 283:1167–74.

NIELSEN K. 1999. Pediatric HIV infection. In HIV Clinical Management – Medscape, Web site. Available at: http://www.medscape.com/medscape/HIV/Clinical Mgmt/CM.v12/public/index-CM.v12.html

ROUSE DJ, HAUTH JC, ANDREWS WW, MILLS BB, and MAHER JE. 1997. Chlorhexidine vaginal irrigation for the prevention of peripartal infection: a placebo-controlled randomized clinical trial. *American Journal of Obstetrics and Gynecology* 176:617–22.

SEMBA RD, MIOTTI PG, CHIPHANGWI JD, SAAH AJ, CANNER JK, DALLABETTA GA, and HOOVER DR. 1994. Maternal vitamin A deficiency and mother-to-child transmission of HIV-1. *Lancet*. 342:1593–7.

SHAFFER N, CHUACHOOWONG R, MOCK PA, et al. 1999. Short-course zidovudine for perinatal HIV-1 transmission in Bangkok, Thailand: A randomised controlled trial. *Lancet*. 353:773–780.

UNAIDS. 1999. *Report on the global HIV/AIDS epidemic*. UNAIDS Web site. Available at: *http://www.unaids.org/publications/index. html*.

WORLD HEALTH ORGANIZATION. Global
  programme on AIDS. 1992. Consensus
  statement from the WHO/UNICEF
  consultation on HIV transmission and
  breast-feeding. *Weekly Epidemiological
  Record.* 67:177–9.

WORLD HEALTH ORGANIZATION. Global
  programme on AIDS. APRIL 2000. Use of
  cotrimoxazole in adults and children
  living with HIV/AIDS in Africa:
  Recommendations and operational
  issues. Available at: *http://www.unaids.org/
  whatsnew/press/eng/geneva050400.html.*

ZWI KJ, PETTIFOR JM, and SODERLUND N.
  1999. Paediatric hospital admissions at a
  South African urban regional hospital:
  The impact of HIV, 1992–1997. *Annual of
  Tropical Pediatrics.* 19:135–42.

# 40 Childhood injuries

## SM KIBEL & N DU TOIT

Injuries to children may be accidental or wilful. Injuries are seldom true accidents: they are not random isolated events but rather the inevitable consequence of a vulnerable child in a hazardous environment. Injuries can be regarded as symptoms, indicators that all is not well either with the child, or with the child's environment.

Poisoning is also a carelessly used term. The transitive verb implies wilful injury to the child. In situations of child abuse this may occasionally be the case, but generally it refers to the unintentional ingestion or administration of a toxic substance.

The impact of childhood injury is increasing world-wide. In part, this is a relative increase as infections and malnutrition become controlled. Children are also increasingly exposed to hazards. Because of urbanization and industrialization, without adequate safety awareness, the motor car is the most notable hazard. In some developing countries, increases in mortality from injuries have been dramatic. For example, deaths from road traffic accidents in Mexico in the 15- to 24-year age group increased by over 600 per cent between the late 1950s and early 1970s (Mauciaux & Romer, 1986).

In the industrialized world, injuries are the greatest cause of death of children over the age of one year. In developing countries where infectious diseases and malnutrition are rife, the impact of injury is felt more by older children and young adults. In South Africa, injuries are the leading cause of death between the ages of 5 and 34 years.

Figure 40.1 shows the complex and interacting causes of injury. The agent is the object that inflicts the injury directly. Some agents, like motor cars with smooth tyres or flammable liquids, are inherently dangerous. Others, like buckets of water, become dangers only in specific situations, e.g., in the presence of small children who are left unsupervised.

Children become vulnerable to particular types of injury at various stages of their development. For example, inquisitive, active toddlers with their lack of co-ordination and inability to perceive danger are particularly vulnerable to poisoning, drowning, and burns. Infants are vulnerable to choking as they have a need to feel objects with their mouths. Children under nine years of age lack the physical and cognitive maturity to assess traffic, and, as a result, those between five and nine years of age have the highest rates of pedestrian injury. Emotional and social stress

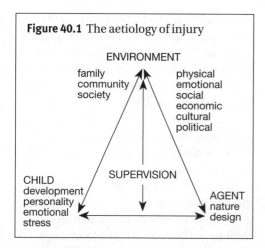

**Figure 40.1** The aetiology of injury

ENVIRONMENT

family
community
society

physical
emotional
social
economic
cultural
political

SUPERVISION

CHILD
development
personality
emotional
stress

AGENT
nature
design

streets. Pedestrian injuries can potentially be prevented through a range of techniques, including traffic calming measures, change in land use, transporting policies, provision of school crossing patrols, speed restrictions and also through educational programmes directed at the child and car driver. Although children in low socio-economic groups are generally more vulnerable to injury, toddlers from privileged homes have the highest drowning rates because of their exposure to domestic swimming pools. Children from lower income groups drown in dams, rivers, or buckets far more frequently than in swimming pools.

within the child or family puts some children at greater risk, while others are considered to have accident-prone personalities, but this concept is controversial. Throughout the world, boys have higher injury rates than girls because of the inherent and sociological differences in behaviour.

Both the child and the agent of injury are influenced by the environment that provides the setting or backdrop to injury patterns. A knowledge of the physical, social, and emotional environment is essential for an understanding of how and why injuries occur. Socio-economic factors are crucial because they determine the type and quality of hazards, the space available for safe play, the quality of adult supervision, and the access to health care. In this way they determine not only the occurrence and type of injury, but also the severity and ultimate outcome. A few examples serve to illustrate this. The incidence of burns is highest in overcrowded areas and the most serious burns (due to fire) are found amongst squatters housed in makeshift shacks. Burn injuries in the informal settlements are commonly caused by paraffin lamps and stoves as well as candles falling over. Pedestrian injuries are most common where children lack the playground and domestic space necessary for safe play, and are forced to play in the

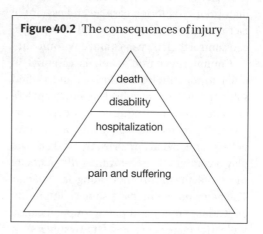

**Figure 40.2** The consequences of injury

death

disability

hospitalization

pain and suffering

Emotional stress makes the child more vulnerable and also distracts the caregiver from providing adequate supervision. Alcohol abuse plays an important role in this regard. As a result of social and cultural factors, many people have a fatalistic attitude to life and believe that injuries are beyond their control. The quality of life, hazards, and health facilities are ultimately all determined by the environment. All aspects of the environment therefore influence the patterns of childhood injury.

This chapter deals only with non-intentional injuries as child abuse/assault is covered in Chapter 61: Child abuse. However, the distinction between intentional and unintentional injuries is blurred, as all injuries occur against the backdrop of a compromised environment.

## Prevention

Although the aetiology is complex, injuries are preventable. Effective control involves changing both the environment and people's behaviour. It is the concern of society as a whole and requires a multifaceted approach will involve the community, professionals of many disciplines (health workers, engineers, teachers, lawyers, etc.), and government. A high priority is to increase awareness of the fact that there is a problem and that people can control their own lives and environment.

Community participation is essential in order to identify local priorities and to find solutions that are most likely to be acceptable and effective. A pre-requisite is in-depth local research that includes the study of customs, beliefs, and behaviour. Health workers can play a central role in informing the public of the problem and in motivating for change. Teachers and the media also have important educational roles, and peer-group education is ideal for increasing the safety awareness.

Safety legislation coupled with adequate enforcement are also essential. Legislation of this sort is intended to either make it compulsory for people to use devices designed for their own protection (motorcycle helmets, seat belts or pool fences) or to stop the production of hazardous items, (cots with bars spaced widely enough to trap a child's head).

Organizations such as the SABS are responsible for establishing and maintaining safety standards. In many cases safety legislation has proved to be effective, but only when it has been appropriate to the needs of the communities at risk and when it could be adequately enforced. Examples of effective safety legislation include child-resistant packaging

of medicines (notably Aspirin) in the United States and the use of motorcycle helmets. There is, however, a limit to the political acceptability of such legislation. In South Africa, legislation governing the safe packaging and sale of paraffin as well as other hazardous products is urgently needed to control poisoning. Child-resistant closures are available to assist paraffin users with safe storage of this product

There are a number of general measures that are likely to prevent many types of injury and minimize their consequences. These include supervision of children, improved socio-economic conditions, control of alcohol abuse, and improved emergency services.

No safety measure can replace *active* supervision. A person who is able to understand danger should watch and be involved in the activities of the child. In many developing countries, parents are forced to leave their children in the care of older siblings while other children may be left unattended to play in the streets. Play groups, crèches, or after-school groups and activities could alleviate this problem.

It is hoped that improved socio-economic conditions will lead to better supervision, improved housing, and less overcrowding, all of which play a role in the prevention of injuries. Another important factor is alcohol abuse, which is a direct cause of traffic accidents and assault, and also plays a part in other injuries.

Improved emergency services, inpatient facilities, rehabilitation services, and well-trained health workers are essential if lives are to be saved and the severity of injuries minimized once they have occurred. Table 40.1 shows some specific interventions for the main types of childhood injury. This list is by no means comprehensive and the interventions mentioned can serve only as examples and must be adapted to the needs of specific communities. Children have a need to

**Table 40.1** Prevention of childhood injury and poisoning

| TYPE OF INJURY | AGE GROUP MOST AT RISK | SAFETY INTERVENTIONS | |
|---|---|---|---|
| | | PREVENT OCCURRENCE | MINIMIZE DAMAGE |
| **High mortality** | | | |
| *Road traffic accidents* | | Control drunken and reckless driving. Speed restrictions & enforcement. Improve road design & street lighting. | Speed restrictions |
| – pedestrian | 5–9 years | Provide enclosed playgrounds. Accompany children under 9 years in traffic. Teach safe road behaviour. Wear reflective clothing. | Improve car designs. |
| – passenger | All ages (under one year most at risk of serious head injury) | Ensure vehicles are roadworthy. Don't overload vehicles. Never hold a young child on an adult's lap – especially in the front seat. | Install and use seat belts and child restraints. Make infant seats available for hire at low cost. |
| *Burns* | Under 5 years | Reduce overcrowding. Provide electricity. | Put burn in cold water immediately (preferably running). Don't use grease or butter on burns. |
| – fluid | | Keep hot substances and objects out of reach of young children. Keep paraffin stove up on table. Turn pot handles in over stove. Keep kettle flex short and out of reach. | |
| – fire (most serious) | | Provide adequate housing (shack dwellers at greatest risk). Keep children away from open fires. Keep matches and flammable liquids away from children. Extinguish candles at bedtime. | If clothing catches alight, roll on ground or smother flames with blanket. In smoke-filled room crawl on ground. |
| *Drowning* – dams – rivers – pools – buckets – sea – any water | 1 to 4 years and older children who cannot swim | Never leave young children near water unsupervised. Provide piped water in houses. Cover buckets. Don't swim in swift rivers. Fence swimming pools. Cover swimming pools with safety nets. Teach children to swim. Never swim alone. Avoid boisterous play near water. Buoyancy aids. | Teach CPR to adults and older children. Reverse hypoxia as soon as possible. |

A young child can die silently within 30 seconds in 4 cm of water.

| TYPE OF INJURY | AGE GROUP MOST AT RISK | PREVENT OCCURRENCE | MINIMIZE DAMAGE |
|---|---|---|---|
| *Poisoning* – pills and medicines – household & garden chemicals (notably paraffin) | 1 to 4 years | Keep all poisons on high shelf or locked in cupboard. Child-resistant containers. Danger labels on containers (e.g., skull & crossbones). Avoid storing poisons in food containers (e.g., soft drink bottles). Use child resistant caps/closures on paraffin containers. | Pills and medicines – induce emesis. Household chemicals – drink milk or water: NO emesis. Get medical advice from 24-hour poison advice centres. |

| TYPE OF INJURY | AGE GROUP MOST AT RISK | SAFETY INTERVENTIONS | |
|---|---|---|---|
| | | PREVENT OCCURRENCE | MINIMIZE DAMAGE |
| *Choking and suffocation* | | | |
| – inhalation | Under one year | Keep small objects, e.g., coins, beans, buttons away from small children. Mash baby food well. Never leave a baby to feed alone. Don't walk or run while eating. | Teach CPR, blow to back or Heimlich manoeuvre. |
| – strangulatory suffocation | | Keep plastic bags, strings, and cords away from young children. Don't put dummies on long strings. | |
| **High morbidity** | | | |
| Falls | | | |
| – on level | All ages Under-one years | Never leave a baby under three months alone on bed or high surface. Put hand rails and gates | Replace tar and cement in playground with grass, sand, |
| – from height | most at risk of serious head injury | on stairs. Put bars on windows. Avoid slippery floors and loose carpets. Put safety rails on double bunks. Don't let children under five years sleep on top bunk. | shells, or rubber. |
| Cuts | All ages | Pick up all broken glass. Recycle glass containers. Keep glass, knives, and scissors away from toddlers. Don't walk or run with sharp objects, e.g., pencil, in mouth. Point knives and scissors down when carrying them. | Clean wound thoroughly with soap and water (purified or boiled and cooled). Stop bleeding with pressure and elevation. |

explore the world in as free a way as possible and it is the responsibility of adults to create a safer environment without hindering the natural curiosity of childhood.

It is important that there be an awareness of the problem of childhood injuries in developing countries. In South Africa, urbanization is progressing very rapidly, and this may well be associated with a growing injury epidemic unless it is accompanied by improved safety awareness and adequate hazard control.

More detailed information can be obtained from The Child Accident Prevention Foundation of South Africa (CAPFSA):

(Cape) P O Box 791, Rondebosch, 7701
Tel. 021-685 5208.
(Gauteng) P O Box 1001, Bromhof, 2154
Tel. 011-792 4332.

## References and further reading

BRADSHAW D, BOTHA H, JOUBERT G, PRETORIUS JPG, VAN WYK R, and YACH D. 1987. *Review of South African mortality, 1984* (Medical Research Council Technical Report No 1).

JARVIS S & TOWNER EML. 1998. Introduction. *Injury Prevention.* 4 (suppl):s7–s9.

KIBEL SM, JOUBERT G, and BRADSHAW D. 1990. Injury related mortality in South African children, 1981–1985. *South African Medical Journal.* 78(7):398–403

MAUCIAUX M & ROMER CJ. 1986. Accidents in young children, adolescents and young adults: A major public health problem. *World Health Quarterly.* 39:227–31.

# 41 Tuberculosis

## P R DONALD

Tuberculosis is responsible for 83 per cent of notifications of infectious disease in South Africa and is thus a major health problem. In childhood, while not an important cause of infant mortality, tuberculosis does give rise to considerable morbidity and may play a complicating role in any situation where immunity is compromised. HIV infection is the most important current example of the interaction of immunosuppression and predisposition to tuberculosis infection and disease.

## The organism

*Mycobacterium tuberculosis* is a rod-shaped acid fast micro-organism with a high lipid cell wall content, which makes it resistant to physical agents and many antibacterial drugs. It is a strict aerobe which divides at a considerably slower rate than other bacteria – approximately once every 10 to 20 hours – and the clinical events following infection stretch over a commensurately longer period than those that follow other bacterial infections. Of great importance to the pathogenicity of *M. tuberculosis* is its ability to survive and multiply within the mononuclear phagocytic

cells. Finally, the antigenic constituents of the organism are powerful inducers of granuloma formation.

The concept of the 'timetable' of tuberculosis is essential to an understanding of the disease processes resulting from tuberculous infections (see Table 41.1).

Infection results from the inhalation of tiny droplets less than 10 μm in diameter containing *M. tuberculosis* and derived in most instances from close contact with an adult who has active, often cavitating, disease. More than 90 per cent of primary infections will be localized in the lungs.

From the primary focus of infection, the Ghon focus, the organism spreads via lymphatics and/or the bloodstream throughout the body and is most likely to be seeded at sites of high oxygen tension, such as the apices of the lungs, the meninges, the bone ends, and kidneys. Approximately two months after infection a cell-mediated immune response and hypersensitivity to tuberculoprotein develop. Spread of *M. tuberculosis* from the primary focus is stopped but caseation (necrosis) may still develop, often with subsequent cavity formation. If cavitation occurs in the lungs, the ideal conditions for the rapid multiplication of

363

**Table 41.1** The timetable of tuberculosis

| Infection | | Period following infection |
|---|---|---|
| Transient fever of initiation | | |
| Ghon focus/complex | | |
| Cellular immunity develops | | |
| Hypersensitivity to tuberculoprotein | | One to two months |
| Tuberculin test positive | | |
| Phlyctenular conjunctivitis | | |
| Erythema nodosum | | |
| **In majority** | **In minority** | |
| Infection is controlled but there is a lifelong possibility of endogenous reactivation | Pleural effusion | |
| | Progressive primary; hilar/paratracheal adenopathy and segmental lesions | Two to twelve months |
| | Miliary tuberculosis | |
| | Tuberculous meningitis | |
| | Bone involvement | One to two years |
| | Renal tuberculosis | Five to ten years |

*M. tuberculosis* are created and with coughing the organism can be spread to uninfected individuals, completing the cycle of infection.

In the majority of cases the events of primary infection pass unnoticed and only the development of a positive tuberculin test will indicate that infection has in fact taken place. Careful observation may detect the occurrence of a transient fever, the so-called fever of initiation, while a minority of individuals may develop allergic phenomena such as erythema nodosum or phlyctenular conjunctivitis.

In most infected individuals, the infection is now controlled by cell-mediated immunity. Viable organisms may, however, remain present within an infected individual's macrophages with a lifelong potential for endogenous reactivation should the immune system be depressed for any reason.

While the infection is controlled and contained in most instances, the first six to twelve months following infection is a period of great danger. It is during this period that disease processes such as pleural effusion, progression of the primary focus to cavitation, and the development of disseminated forms of tuberculosis, such as miliary tuberculosis and tuberculous meningitis are particularly likely to develop. Furthermore, it is important to note from a paediatric viewpoint that the younger the infected individual the greater is this danger. A number of studies indicate that five per cent of children infected before two years of age will develop miliary tuberculosis or tuberculous meningitis. Hence the concern of the paediatrician for the young child with a strongly positive tuberculin test. Other pulmonary complications that are particularly likely to develop during this post-infection danger period are closely related to the enlargement of the regional, hilar, and paratracheal lymph nodes. Not only is the lymphoid tissue more prominent in the young child, but the airways are narrower than in the adult and more likely to be obstructed.

Enlargement and ulceration of hilar nodes may lead to obstruction of an adjacent airway with varying degrees of hyperinflation or collapse with or without consolidation. The histological nature of the resulting segmental lesion seen on chest radiograph may vary from that of a 'tuberculin response' with few mycobacteria present, and little sign of tubercle formation to that of a caseating tuberculous bronchopneumonia.

Age is once again an important determinant in the above course of events and up to 25 per cent of children infected at less than one year of age may develop a segmental lesion.

At a later point in time (one or two years after infection), tuberculosis of the bones may develop while renal tuberculosis is unusual until five to ten years after infection and is consequently not often seen in childhood.

# HIV infection, AIDS, and tuberculosis in children

It is now well established that HIV infection and AIDS in adults predisposes them to the development of active tuberculosis. This, in turn, hastens the progression of HIV infection to AIDS. This unfortunate interaction of two formidable diseases has led to a rising incidence of tuberculosis throughout the world. This interaction is also now being described in childhood, and will considerably complicate the diagnosis and management of childhood tuberculosis as the manifestations of AIDS, uncomplicated by tuberculosis, are clinically, and in many instances radiologically, indistinguishable from those of tuberculosis. Without better diagnostic tests it seems inevitable that many children with HIV infection and AIDS who do not have tuberculosis will receive antituberculosis treatment.

As with adults, extrapulmonary tuberculosis appears to be more common in children with HIV/AIDS. Chronic tuberculous otorrhoea is a striking feature in many young children. Although a tuberculin test may more frequently be negative, it remains a worthwhile investigation. In our experience approximately 60 per cent of children with HIV/AIDS complicated by culture proven tuberculosis will have a Mantoux test with ≥ 15 mm induration.

The treatment of tuberculosis follows the same principles as for immunologically competent individuals. In certain instances it may be necessary to individualize treatment and to extend the continuation phase to six months.

This interaction is also likely to have an as yet unexplored effect on the 'timetable' of tuberculosis, altering many of our longstanding concepts of the pathogenesis of tuberculosis in childhood.

# The tuberculin test

Induration of the skin developing on tuberculin testing arises as the result of hypersensitivity to tuberculoprotein and indicates prior contact with *M. tuberculosis*, *M. bovis*, other atypical mycobacteria such as the *M. avium* complex or BCG immunization.

## MANTOUX TEST

The most accurate manner of tuberculin testing is the Mantoux test during which 0,1 ml of stabilized solution of purified protein derivative (PPD) is injected intradermally. A strength of 5 international units (IU) per dose is most generally used. If PPD RT23 (Statens Serum Institut Copenhagen) is used 2 TU will give a result equivalent to 5IU of other PPD preparations. The test is read after 48 to 72 hours. A transverse induration of 15 mm or more indicates infection with *M. tuberculosis* even if BCG has been given. An induration of 10 mm or more indicates infection with *M. tuberculosis* if BCG has not been given. Induration of from 5 to 10 mm may indicate infection with *M. tuberculosis* but may also result from BCG immunization or contact with atypical mycobateria.

The importance of the tuberculin test in paediatrics will be appreciated when it is recalled that the young child under five years of age who is infected with *M. tuberculosis* is in grave danger of developing disseminated tuberculosis and more complicated forms of pulmonary tuberculosis. For this reason, they should be given prophylactic therapy with INH for six months or, if supervised therapy is possible, isoniazid, rifampicin, and pyrazinamide for three months. Prophylactic treatment is particularly important in children below two years.

## THE TINE AND THE HEAF TEST

PPD is injected into the skin by multiple puncture devices. These tests are ideal for screening of large numbers of children in an outpatient or consulting room situation and a doubtful test can be followed up by the more accurate Mantoux test. As a generalization, a confluence of the papules or ulceration or vesiculation in a multiple puncture test can be regarded as equivalent to a 15 mm Mantoux test results.

The tuberculin test may be used in epidemiological work to determine the annual risk of infection in an area. The number of children of a particular age group who are infected is determined and compared to the proportion infected in other age groups and at other points in time, thus giving an accurate indication of tuberculosis trends.

## NEGATIVE TUBERCULIN TESTS

A negative tuberculin test does not necessarily mean that the individual is not infected, and the possible reasons for negative tests are summarized in Table 41.2. Tuberculin tests

are contraindicated in phlyctenular conjunctivitis, a condition associated with extreme hypersensitivity to tuberculin.

**Table 41.2** Causes of a false negative tuberculin test

- Overwhelming advanced forms of tuberculous disease
- Severe protein-energy malnutrition
- Measles, rubella, and varicella
- Measles, rubella, mumps, and yellow fever live attenuated vaccines
- Steroid therapy
- Malignancies and immunosuppressants used in the treatment of malignancy
- Exposure to high doses of radiation
- Sarcoidosis
- Hyperthyroidism
- HIV infection
- Technical faults in performing the test

# Diagnosis

The diagnosis of tuberculosis in childhood rests firstly upon suspicion on the part of the clinician. Malnutrition or failure to thrive, the finding of lymphadenopathy or hepatosplenomegaly, or a history of contact with an adult with pulmonary tuberculosis should lead to a careful evaluation of the child for possible tuberculosis. Particular care is required in the case of tuberculous meningitis when early diagnosis is essential to a satisfactory outcome. Subtle changes in behaviour, lethargy, and complaints of headache should lead to a lumber puncture and the institution of antituberculous therapy in cases where the possibility of tuberculous meningitis exists.

## CULTURE OF *M. TUBERCULOSIS*

Although culture of *M. tuberculosis* is often unsuccessful in childhood, because of the infrequency of cavitating disease, it should nonetheless always be attempted when facilities are available. Early morning gastric aspirate is cultured in the young child because of the child's inability to produce sputum. Other body fluids – cerebrospinal fluid, pleural aspirate, and ascitic fluid – and biopsy material from lymph nodes, synovium, or bone marrow aspirate should be cultured as the opportunity arises. Nasopharyngeal aspiration has been suggested as an alternative means of obtaining material for culture. This has the advantage that it could be done at any time of day and that hospitalization is not necessary.

## CHEST RADIOGRAPHY

This is the means by which tuberculosis in childhood will most often be diagnosed. The interpretation of a chest radiograph in a young child is, however, fraught with difficulty due to poor inspiratory films, rotation, or underpenetration. In the presence of undoubted lymphadenopathy, tuberculosis may be considered with more confidence. Lymphadenopathy is often more clearly evident on the lateral than the PA film. A lateral should always be taken when tuberculosis is suspected. In cases of doubt, where facilities are available, high kilovoltage films may delineate adenopathy and narrowed airways more clearly. A non-resolving pneumonia should always lead to consideration of possible tuberculosis.

## THE TUBERCULIN TEST

The importance of the tuberculin test in detecting tuberculous infection in the young child has already been discussed. It must however be reiterated that a negative tuberculin test does not mean that a child does not have tuberculosis.

## CONTACT WITH AN ADULT CASE OF PULMONARY TUBERCULOSIS

A diligent persistent search must be undertaken for an adult contact. The grandparents and the extended family with whom many children live must not be forgotten in this search. Resort to chest radiography of those in closest contact with the child may be rewarding in selected cases.

## FAILURE TO THRIVE

Failure to gain weight adequately or, more important, loss of weight (as demonstrated on a Road to Health Chart) will often result from a multiplicity of socio-economic factors but may also result from tuberculosis. Children failing to thrive should be tuberculin tested and enquiries made as to contact with an adult case of tuberculosis. A chest radiograph should be taken if facilities are available. Conversely, it must be realized that many children requiring treatment for tuberculosis actually may be gaining adequately in weight.

# Tuberculous meningitis

Tuberculous meningitis is the most serious complication of tuberculosis and is the commonest cause of death in childhood as a result of tuberculosis. A considerable proportion of the survivors suffer permanent brain damage. Tuberculous meningitis must be suspected in any case of meningitis where another causative organism has not been clearly identified. This suspicion should lead to enquiry as to a household contact suffering from tuberculosis, a chest radiograph, and tuberculin testing. Many children with tuberculous meningitis will have experienced recent failure to thrive or loss of weight.

Typically the cerebrospinal fluid (CSF) will be clear with a relatively low cell count (less than 300 per mm$^3$) and a lymphocyte predominance, raised protein, and reduced glucose concentration. Pandy's Test for excess globulin is easy to carry out and requires only a small amount of CSF. The finding of a + or more of turbidity in a clear fluid should lead to consideration of the possibility of tuberculous meningitis. In a minority of cases a CSF pleocytosis of more than 500 per mm$^3$ may be encountered with a polymorphonuclear leukocyte predominance while CSF protein and glucose concentrations within the range expected for a viral meningitis are not unusual.

A number of other investigations have been proposed for the diagnosis of tuberculous meningitis such as the determination of CSF adenosine deaminase activity, CSF lactate and lactate dehydrogenase concentrations, and the bromide partition test. None of these investigations can be relied on with certainty and new immunologic tests await a thorough evaluation. When in any doubt as to the diagnosis it is better to treat for tuberculous meningitis and then to reconsider the diagnostic evidence when the patient has fully recovered.

## Treatment

All populations of M. tuberculosis in tuberculous lesions will contain a small number of organisms that are resistant to each of the commonly used antituberculous drugs. Treatment, other than chemoprophylaxis, where isoniazid alone may be used, must therefore always be with multiple drugs. Three main populations of M. tuberculosis exist in tuberculous lesions. These are:

- a large metabolically active, rapidly dividing population that lines the walls of cavities. Isoniazid, and rifampicin are active against this population;
- a relatively small intermittently active population found in caseous tissue and within macrophages against which rifampicin has a specific action. Pyrazinamide is also active against these organisms and is helped by the low pH in these lesions; and

- a small number of dormant organisms contained within macrophages. It is doubtful if these organisms are killed by any of our existing antituberculosis agents.

Rifampicin and pyrazinamide have the ability to sterilize caseous tissue and to kill the intermittently active organisms lying within macrophages, and the success of modern short-term chemotherapy rests upon this fact.

The therapy of virtually all forms of tuberculosis can today be undertaken with a six-month supervised regimen of isoniazid, rifampicin, and pyrazinamide. This is given in an intensive initial bactericidal phase whose purpose is to eliminate the majority of actively multiplying organisms and a continuation or sterilizing phase aimed at eliminating all of the less active, persisting organisms remaining in macrophages and caseous tissue.

The initial bactericidal phase consists of isoniazid, rifampicin, and pyrazinamide given for two months and the continuation phase of isoniazid and rifampicin. Should problems be experienced in giving daily supervised therapy (or five days a week), intermittent therapy two or three times weekly may be undertaken during the continuation phase or from the start of treatment. When cavitation is present, it is advisable to follow the recommendations for adult tuberculosis and to add a fourth drug to the regimen. This could be ethambutol, streptomycin, or ethionamide if this can be tolerated. The fourth drug is intended to help prevent the development of rifampicin resistance.

Used in daily therapy the dosages are isoniazid 10 mg/kg body mass daily; rifampicin 12 mg/kg body mass daily; and pyrazinamide 30 mg/kg body mass daily. Used in twice-weekly intermittent therapy during the continuation phase, isoniazid may be given in a dosage of 15 mg/kg mass to a maximum of 900 mg daily and rifampicin in a dose of 15 mg body mass to a maximum of 600 mg daily.

All drugs should as a general rule be given in a single daily dose before breakfast, except streptomycin, which is administered intramuscularly.

Toxicity or allergy is relatively rare in children but can occur. Liver enzymes frequently rise on starting treatment, but, in the absence of jaundice and if less than five times the normal value, therapy may be continued. The development of liver enlargement, tenderness, or jaundice should be a reason for referral for specialist advice.

In *tuberculous meningitis,* the dosages are often increased to ensure entry into the cerebrospinal fluid. Isoniazid 20 mg/kg/day to a maximum of 600 mg; rifampicin 20 mg/kg/day to a maximum of 600 mg; and pyrazinamide 40 mg/kg/day to a maximum of 2 g.

Ethionamide can be added (20 mg/kg/day) but this drug is now difficult to obtain and ethambutol (15–20 mg/kg/day) is an alternative. Treatment is continued for six months (though some still use longer regimens). The inflammatory response that contributes to the basal exudate and associated vasculitis often complicates this disease, and it has been shown that cortico-steroids improve the outcome of *tuberculous meningitis.* Prednisone in a higher dose than normal (3–4 mg/kg/day for one month) may be used. The higher dose is necessitated because of the induction of increased steroid metabolism by rifampicin.

*Chemoprophylaxis.* Children under five years of age in close household contact with a smear-positive case of pulmonary TB, and breast-feeding infants of affected mothers, should be treated with isoniazid once daily for five days a week for three months. Supervised therapy with rifampicin and isoniazid, with or without pyrazinamide, are again considered preferable (see page 366). Combination tablets are available. (For dosages, see Standard Treatment Guidelines and Essential Drug List, 1998.)

# Tuberculosis control and childhood tuberculosis

There can be little doubt that the first priority of tuberculosis control measures must be to treat and cure those tuberculosis sufferers who have smear-positive sputum. Even in this context the detection of young children with tuberculous infection and disease is still important as this should lead to an intensive search for the source of the child's infection, which will often be a smear-positive family member.

Conversely, the diagnosis of tuberculosis in an adult, particularly if smear positive, should lead to an immediate evaluation of all close childhood contacts for signs of tuberculous infection (a positive tuberculin test) or tuberculous disease. The supervised treatment of such children will contribute significantly to a reduction in the number of cases of tuberculous meningitis (which is responsible for the major part of childhood morbidity and mortality resulting from tuberculosis).

The success of tuberculosis control measures may also be gauged by a surveillance of the level of tuberculin sensitivity in children and by determining the incidence of tuberculous meningitis that affects children. A falling level of tuberculin sensitivity reflected as the annual risk of infection and a falling incidence of tuberculous meningitis would indicate that tuberculosis control measures are successful.

# Classification of childhood tuberculosis

Given the difficulties inherent in diagnosis of tuberculosis in childhood, the World Health Organization and workers in Kenya have suggested a graduated approach to better reflect the certainty with which the diagnosis of childhood tuberculosis is made, and to aid epidemiological comparisons between different areas. Cases are designated as suspected, probable, or confirmed tuberculosis.

*Suspected tuberculosis:* The chest radiograph is compatible with a diagnosis of tuberculosis but there is little other evidence to support the diagnosis.

*Probable tuberculosis:* The chest radiograph suggests a diagnosis of tuberculosis, or else a suspicious chest radiograph is accompanied by a strongly positive tuberculin test, a history of contact with an adult case of tuberculosis, or recent loss of weight or failure to gain in weight.

*Confirmed tuberculosis:* The diagnosis is confirmed by culture of *M. tuberculosis* from gastric aspirate, other body fluids or tissues, or acid fast bacilli are identified on histological examination of biopsy material.

In addition to the above-defined groups the clinician may at times feel compelled to institute antituberculous therapy in a malnourished child or a child recovering from another infectious disease, who has no other evidence of tuberculosis.

## References and further reading

BEYERS JA. 1979. The radiological features of primary pulmonary tuberculosis. *South African Medical Journal.* 55:994–7.

CUNDALL DB. 1986. The diagnosis of pulmonary tuberculosis in malnourished Kenyan children. *Annals of Tropical Paediatrics.* 6:249–55.

DONALD PR, FOURIE PB, and GRANGE JM. 1999. *Tuberculosis in childhood.* Pretoria: JL van Schaik.

FOURIE PB. 1983. Patterns of tuberculin hypersensitivity in South Africa. *Tubercle.* 64:167–79.

MILLER FJW. 1982. *Tuberculosis in children.* Edinburgh: Churchill Livingstone.

MITCHISON DA. 1985. The action of anti-tuberculosis drugs in short-course chemotherapy. *Tubercle.* 66:219–25.

ROUILLON A, PERDRIZET S, and PARROT R. 1976. Transmission of tubercle bacilli: The effects of chemotherapy. *Tubercle.* 57:275–99.

SCHAAF HS, BEYERS N, GIE RP, et al. 1995. Respiratory tuberculosis in childhood: The diagnostic value of clinical features and special investigations. *Pediatric Infectious Diseases Journal.* 14:189–94.

STANDARD TREATMENT GUIDELINES AND ESSENTIAL DRUGS LIST, PAEDIATRICS. NATIONAL DEPARTMENT OF HEALTH. 1998.

STARKE JR. 1988. Modern approach to the diagnosis and treatment of tuberculosis in children. *Pediatric Clinics of North America.* 35(3):441–64.

VAN RIE A, BEYERS N, GIE RP, et al. 1999. Childhood tuberculosis in an urban population in South Africa: Burden and risk factor. *Archives of Disease in Childhood.* 80:433–7.

WALLGREN A. 1948. The 'time-table' of tuberculosis. *Tubercle.* 29:245–51.

# 42

# Malaria

M ISAÄCSON &
LH BLUMBERG

## Types of malaria in southern Africa

The malignant tertian form is by far the most prevalent type of malaria. It is caused by *Plasmodium falciparum* and it accounts for approximately 95 per cent of all cases. In South Africa, the most common species among those responsible for the remaining five per cent of cases is *P. ovale*. Quartan malaria, caused by *P. malariae*, is occasionally seen, often having been acquired in Mozambique. Vivax malaria is rare and virtually absent in the black population because of the genetic absence of the *P. vivax* red cell receptor, known as the Duffy factor (see below). Of some clinical importance is the occurrence of mixed infections with *P. falciparum* and one of the other three species. Falciparum malaria is not only the most common, but also the most serious clinical form, frequently associated with severe and often fatal complications in the non-immune population. From a prophylactic point of view, it is also the most troublesome one because of escalating drug resistance. Most of the following discussions will therefore deal with falciparum malaria unless otherwise specified.

## Geographic distribution

The southernmost part of southern Africa is free of malaria, while the southern limits of the malaria affected zone is subject to a seasonally fluctuating prevalence with 'unstable' transmission occurring chiefly during the warm and rainy season. In the latter areas, malaria therefore tends to present in epidemic form. This zone merges to the north with the vast belt of 'stable' malaria transmission which extends across the bulk of tropical Africa until it meets with the arid regions of the Sahel and the Sahara. Transmission of malaria in this holoendemic belt is mostly intense and subject to little or no seasonal fluctuation, resulting in an endemic rather than an epidemic prevalence. These epidemiological factors have a very important clinical bearing because they determine the presence or absence of immunity to malaria in local communities. Therefore, the clinical severity of malaria as well as its mortality are affected. Also affected by the presence or absence of immunity are policies regarding drug treatment and, particularly, drug pro-

**Figure 42.1** KwaZulu-Natal malaria risk

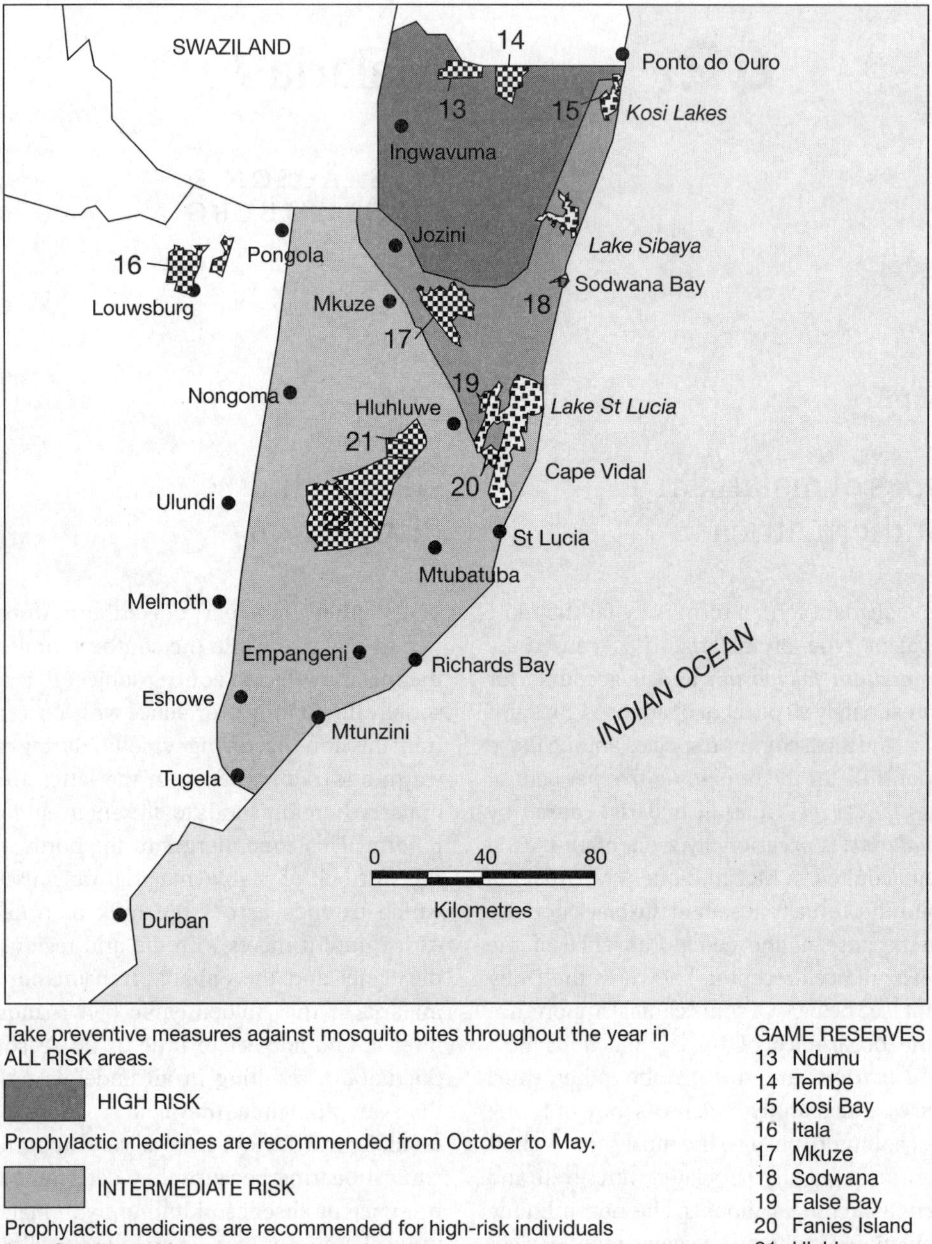

Take preventive measures against mosquito bites throughout the year in ALL RISK areas.

HIGH RISK

Prophylactic medicines are recommended from October to May.

INTERMEDIATE RISK

Prophylactic medicines are recommended for high-risk individuals from October to May.

LOW RISK

No prophylactic medicines are recommended.

GAME RESERVES
13 Ndumu
14 Tembe
15 Kosi Bay
16 Itala
17 Mkuze
18 Sodwana
19 False Bay
20 Fanies Island
21 Hluhluwe
22 Umfolozi

phylaxis. Recommendations for KwaZulu-Natal are shown in Figure 42.1.

# Immunity to malaria

Immunity to malaria is a relative concept, which, because it is not absolute, is usually referred to as 'semi-immunity' or 'premunition'. Such resistance to malaria, which is species specific, is acquired as the result of (and its maintenance is dependent on) frequent reinfections throughout the year. Therefore, while being a prominent characteristic in most of Africa, it does not develop to any significant extent in foci such as Mpumalanga and the Northern Province lowveld where unstable malaria transmission is the rule. In northern KwaZulu-Natal, on the other hand, an element of stable transmission has been noted.

## CONSEQUENCES OF IMMUNITY TO MALARIA

Congenitally acquired clinical malaria (due to transplacental transfer of infected maternal red cells) is extremely rare in infants of semi-immune mothers, although parasites have been found in up to 22 per cent of newborn infants.

Congenital malaria occurs more frequently in infants born to non-immune mothers, but its incidence is still relatively low. The reasons for this are unclear – it is obviously not the result of protection by maternal antibody.

Other factors must therefore play a role in the protection of the newborn against malaria. The inhibitory effect of fetal haemoglobin (HbF) on the parasite is one such factor and this inhibition is further promoted by ageing of the red cells. In infants living in endemic areas, protection lasts for several months, after which parasitaemic attacks start developing with increasing clinical severity. From about three years of age, the clinical severity of malaria attacks declines and children above

the age of four or five years show a marked decrease in malaria mortality. Low-grade asexual parasitaemia without any symptoms then becomes common, and may affect as much as 25 per cent of a given community.

Acute attacks of malaria always cause splenic enlargement, and since such attacks in endemic areas tend to become less frequent in children as they develop immunity, the prevalence rates of splenomegaly, particularly in two- to nine-year-olds, have been used as a measure of malaria endemicity. The following terms are used to indicate the level of endemicity in malaria areas.

**Table 42.1** Splenomegaly rates in children 2–9 years

Hypoendemic: 0–10 per cent
Mesoendemic: 11–50 per cent
Hyperendemic: 51–75 per cent
Holoendemic: more than 75 per cent

Complications, such as cerebral malaria, are rare in semi-immunes, unless their specific immune status has been interrupted by one or other factor (see below).

Immunity to malaria therefore protects against *disease* rather than against *infection*. Benefit to the human host arising from the development of immunity is further reinforced by the fact that mosquitoes feeding in the presence of minimal parasitaemias tend to have lower parasite burdens and so inoculate lower doses into the next human victim. *Severity of illness has been directly equated to the number of sporozoites inoculated.*

The production of gametocytes, the sexual stage necessary for infection of the mosquito and therefore for completion of the parasitic life-cycle, is not directly affected by the immune process. Epidemiologically, this benefits the parasite in that many healthy, ambulant, mildly parasitaemic hosts are con-

## Factors inhibiting or abolishing immunity to malaria

- *Antimalarial chemoprophylaxis.* Unless absolute compliance can be ensured, which is rarely the case, mass chemoprophylaxis may be harmful rather than beneficial. Partly for this reason, and also because of the problems associated with drug resistance, mass chemoprophylaxis is no longer administered to populations in holoendemic areas. However, in the case of smaller communities or individuals, when compliance can be more easily ensured, inclusion of drug prophylaxis in control programmes may still be reasonably successful.
- *Absence from a holoendemic area* for a lengthy period with cessation of the reinfection necessary for the maintenance of immunity.
- *Pregnancy,* especially first pregnancies.
- *Intercurrent disease.*

stantly available to the mosquito for optimal reservoir maintenance.

The absence of immunity in non-malarious areas or in areas with unstable malaria transmission means that individuals of all ages are susceptible to severe clinical malaria, which, unless promptly treated, is frequently associated with a host of serious and potentially fatal complications.

# Some genetic and other factors governing malaria susceptibility

## DUFFY FACTORS

Persons homozygous for FyFy, i.e., whose red cells lack the determinants that act as recep-

tor sites for *P. vivax* attachment and invasion, are resistant to vivax malaria. This is the case with most blacks, especially in West Africa, whereas whites and more than 50 per cent of San people ('bushmen') are Duffy positive. This accounts for the rarity of vivax malaria in sub-Saharan Africa.

## SICKLE CELL TRAIT

Malaria is only slightly less prevalent in children with the sickle cell trait (HbS/HbA), but their parasitaemias are much lower and death due to malaria is rare. The mechanism, formerly thought to be due directly to lowered oxygen tension in HbS/HbA erythrocytes, is known now to be an indirect effect resulting from the loss of intracellular potassium (essential for plasmodial growth) under low oxygen tension.

## GLUCOSE-6-PHOSPHATE DEHYDROGENASE (G6PD) DEFICIENCY

G6PD deficiency is known to protect heterozygous females against the effects of falciparum malaria but the exact mechanism has not yet been elucidated.

# Nutritional factors and malaria

## IRON

Several reports document that administration of iron to iron-deficient patients may result in latent malaria infections becoming clinically overt. It has also been shown that the administration of prophylactic iron to infants in an iron-deficient population has resulted in much higher parasitaemias in these infants than in iron deficient ones (see Chapter 16: Malnutrition).

## PROTEIN-ENERGY MALNUTRITION (PEM)

In general, PEM causes impairment of the immune processes and renders individuals more susceptible to a variety of infections. Numerous observations that severe malaria is most unusual in badly malnourished children, that parasitaemias tend to be lower in the malnourished than in the well nourished, and that children dying of cerebral malaria are usually well nourished, are therefore of great interest. The reasons for this paradoxical protection are uncertain. During the Bengal famine of 1943, there were few deaths due to malaria, but a sharp rise in malaria mortality followed the establishment of feeding centres.

## EFFECTS OF MALARIA ON THE UNBORN CHILD

*Plasmodium falciparum* preferentially parasitizes the maternal blood spaces of the placenta, and, through interference with blood supply to the foetus, may have various results including death *in utero* and low birthweight. The latter is the most common effect in infants of semi-immune mothers, while stillbirths occur much more commonly in the absence of immunity. Low birthweight may also be caused by premature labour induced by malaria.

It has been shown that malaria control programmes have been followed by a substantial increase in mean birthweights (up to 250 g), and an overall reduction in low birthweight prevalence of eight per cent, with as much as a 20 per cent reduction in low birthweights among firstborns.

# Clinical features of malaria

The presenting signs and symptoms of malaria are non-specific and a great awareness of the occurrence of the disease in children returning from known malaria areas and in those living in malaria areas is imperative.

Fever is the most consistent, common, and often first symptom of malaria. Fever may, however, be present intermittently or even absent on presentation to the health care centre. Other important symptoms in children include lethargy, poor feeding, vomiting, and sleepiness. Chills, body pains, sweats, and diarrhoea occur less frequently.

Clinical signs may include fever, anaemia, jaundice, respiratory distress due to fever and/or acidosis, splenomegaly, and varying degrees of impairment of the central nervous system ranging from sleepiness and agitation to convulsions and coma.

Three clinical syndromes account for the majority of deaths in children: severe anaemia (Hb < 6 g /d$\ell$), malaria with impaired consciousness, and malaria with respiratory distress due to metabolic (mainly lactic) acidosis, with the first being the most common syndrome in malaria endemic areas. The poorest outcome is often associated with overlapping of these syndromes.

Important signs of cerebral malaria include agitation, confusion, depressed level of consciousness, and coma. Abnormalities of muscle tone and posture are frequently seen, such as muscular hypotonia or more commonly decerebrate posturing, including opisthotonus. Coma may reflect not only specific cerebral pathology but may result from multiple causes, including severe systemic disease with lactic acidosis. In patients with acute malaria, severe anaemia may contribute to cerebral signs of confusion and restlessness and cardiopulmonary signs.

Hypoglycaemia is an important complication of malaria in children, but renal failure and acute respiratory distress syndrome are rare. Secondary bacterial infection with non-typhi Salmonellae, *Staphylococcus aureus* and *Streptococcus pneumoniae* has been reported.

The differential diagnosis of malaria includes meningitis, encephalitis, tetanus, septicaemia, pneumonia, hepatitis, and typhoid fever.

There is limited information on the impact of HIV co-infection on the occurrence and severity of malaria disease in children. In early studies, malaria was not found to be more frequent or more severe in children with progressive HIV-1 infection and malaria did not appear to accelerate the rate of progression of the HIV disease.

## Diagnosis

The diagnosis and treatment of malaria is an emergency, as death may occur within 48 hours of the first symptom appearing in non-immune children. In many endemic areas, treatment is based on a clinical diagnosis, but, where possible, laboratory confirmation should be sought by microscopic examination of a Giemsa-stained blood smear, or by using a rapid malarial antigen detection method. A single negative smear does not exclude a diagnosis of malaria, and the smears should be repeated until the diagnosis of malaria is either confirmed, the patient has recovered, or another cause is identified. The rapid tests should be used for diagnostic purposes only (mainly *P. falciparum*) and not for monitoring response to treatment, as they can remain positive several weeks after successful treatment. Most patients with uncomplicated malaria will demonstrate thrombocytopaenia of varying degrees.

## Treatment

High-grade chloroquine resistance is widespread in Africa and its continued use has been associated with a significant increase in malaria-related mortality and morbidity. Many countries are now recommending sulpha-doxine plus pyrimethamine as first-line treatment for uncomplicated falciparum malaria in adults and children. A convenient dosing schedule and a favourable safety profile are advantageous, but the drug is slow acting and the emergence of resistance is of concern.

Quinine is at present the mainstay of treatment for malaria in children in Africa. Severe or complicated falciparum malaria and severe vomiting are indications for the use of parenteral quinine, which must be given by slow intravenous infusion. The dose must be calculated by body weight. If the necessary facilities for this are not available, quinine may be given by deep intramuscular injection. Although there has been much concern about the safety of intramuscular preparations in children, the lack of appropriately trained personnel in many rural African clinics precludes the use of safer, slow, intravenous infusion in severely ill young children. In all cases, however, parenteral treatment should ideally be stopped and replaced by oral treatment as soon as this becomes practical. Some oral antimalarials are very bitter, so tablets should be crushed and mixed with syrup or sweetened condensed milk.

Quinine resistance is at present not a significant problem in Africa, but has emerged in South East Asia. Halofantrine and mefloquine are alternative agents, but only for uncomplicated disease.

The artemisinin derivatives – artemether and artesunate – have proved successful and safe in treating both complicated and uncomplicated malaria, particularly in areas where quinine resistance has emerged. They are, however, not registered for widespread use in Africa. Current usage is restricted to cases of quinine resistant malaria, or when quinine toxicity is a problem. Combination therapy using an artemisinin derivative with sulphadoxine-pyrimethamine or mefloquine is being studied for future use. Drug regimes are frequently updated because of changing circumstances.

Revised guidelines are provided by the Department of Health.

Malaria is a progressive disease and complications may develop despite appropriate chemotherapy. The patient should be carefully monitored, and those with any of the following should be referred to a higher level of care:

- any change in the level of consciousness, or convulsions and agitation;
- vomiting or refusal of fluids;
- hypoglycaemia;
- poor urinary output;
- hyperpyrexia > 41,0 °C;
- respiratory rate above 30/minute;
- jaundice;
- severe anaemia; and
- all children less than one year of age.

Supportive treatment includes antipyretics, adequate but not excessive hydration, and blood transfusion if the Hb is less than 5 g/dℓ (if virus-free blood is available). The use of prophylactic anti-convulsants and exchange transfusion is controversial.

## Hyper-reactive malarial splenomegaly

This occurs in children living in malaria endemic areas and presents with massive splenomegaly as a result of an immune response to repeated malaria infections. Raised levels of non-specific IgM antibody, and specific malaria antibody are found but peripheral parasitaemia is rare. The condition is managed by administering long-term malarial chemoprophylaxis.

## Malaria control in childhood

Prophylactic measures include chemoprophylaxis, which prevents diseases but not infection, and measures aimed at avoiding exposure (i.e., preventing infection). The latter have assumed much greater importance in recent years in the light of increasing drug resistance problems, and may be practised alone or combined with chemoprophylaxis.

### CHEMOPROPHYLAXIS

A clear distinction must be made between children in hyperendemic areas and those living in non-malaria areas. The latter group has no specific antimalarial immunity at any age and must, on visiting a malaria area, take prophylactic drugs. This applies to all age groups, including neonates.

However, the prophylactic policy with regard to children born and living in hyperendemic areas is quite different. Education on individual malaria prevention in such areas should be integrated into antenatal care programmes. Since pregnancy, and especially a first pregnancy, can often result in diminished immunity and severe malaria, often with serious complications, a pregnant woman must take antimalarials until about six weeks after parturition. She is thus taught the benefits and the practicalities of her own protection against malaria and will more easily learn to apply malaria prophylaxis to her child.

The newborn child has maternal antibody and is therefore protected until about four months of age. However, the child should receive chemoprophylaxis from four months until at least one year of age. Thereafter, in areas where medical facilities are not readily available, therapeutic drugs may be kept by the mother for treatment of clinical malaria in the child, instead of chemoprophylaxis being continued on a potentially harmful long-term basis.

Schoolchildren are sometimes given regular antimalarials in school, but this protection tends to be interrupted during school holidays when the child may suffer more serious malaria than would have been the case if natural immunity had been allowed to develop. Unless compliance can be ensured during holidays, the benefits of such programmes may be very limited.

Malaria eradication is an unattainable goal within the foreseeable future. Malaria control and individual protection, on the other hand, are practical propositions and should be an integral part of the primary health care system.

## CHOICE OF PROPHYLACTIC ANTI-MALARIALS

Chloroquine resistance has increased during recent years. Current opinion recommends the use of weekly chloroquine combined with daily proguanil. Both drugs and their combined use are considered safe in childhood and in pregnancy. Experience elsewhere has shown that resistance to the combination readily emerges and its usefulness may be expected to decline in due course.

Diarrhoea has been shown to interfere with the intestinal absorption of proguanil, but not chloroquine. The antimalarial protection of children suffering from gastroenteritis while taking proguanil may thus be compromised.

Mefloquine is licensed in South Africa for prophylactic use, but not in children below 5 kg body mass, nor in pregnancy. The malaria chemoprophylaxis situation remains fluid and readers are therefore urged to monitor the literature in this regard.

## OTHER MEASURES FOR INDIVIDUAL MALARIA PREVENTION

These include the use of mosquito repellants, bed nets (which may effectively be impregnated with residual insecticides), door and window screening and protective clothing. Nets for infants' cots are especially important. Currently there is no effective malaria vaccine and trials to date using the Spf66 vaccine have not shown significant benefit.

## References and further reading

ANON. 1984. Prevention of malaria in pregnancy and early childhood. *British Medical Journal.* 289:1296–97.

ANON. 1996. *Guidelines for Treatment of Malaria.* Pretoria: South African Department of Health.

BOETE VAN HENSBROEK M, ONYIORAH E, JAFFER E, et al. 1996. A trial of artemether or quinine in children with cerebral malaria. *New England Journal of Medicine.* 335:69–75.

ENGLISH M & MARSCH K. 1997. Childhood malaria – pathogenesis and treatment. *Current Opinion in Infectious Diseases.* 10:221–5.

GREENBERG AE, NSA W, RYDER RW, MEDI M, et al. 1991. *Plasmodium falciparum* malaria and perinatally acquired human immunodeficiency virus type 1 infection in Kinshasa, Zaire. *New England Journal of Medicine.* 325(2):105–9.

ISAACSON M. 1989. Malaria and its management in pregnancy and childhood. *South African Journal of Continuing Medical Education.* 7:132–7.

TRIGG PI, WERNSDORFER WH, SHETH UK, and ONORI E. 1984. Intramuscular chloroquine in children. *Lancet.* 2 (8397):ii, 288.

WERNSDORFER WH & MCGREGOR I (eds.). 1988. *Principles and practice of malariology.* Edinburgh: Churchill Livingstone.

WHITE NJ. 1996. The treatment of malaria. *New England Journal of Medicine.* 335: 11.

WHITE NJ. 1996. Malaria. In: Cook GC (ed.). *Manson's tropical diseases,* 20th ed. Philadelphia, London, Toronto: WB Saunders Company.

WHITE NJ, MARSCH K, MILLER KD, WILLIAMSON DH, TURNER RC, and BERRY CD. 1987. Hypoglycaemia in African children with severe malaria. *Lancet.* 1 (8535): i, 708–11.

WORLD HEALTH ORGANIZATION MALARIA ACTION PROGRAMME. 1990. Severe and complicated malaria, 2nd ed. *Transactions of the Royal Society of Tropical Medicine and Hygiene.* 84 (supp 2):1–65.

# 43

# Parasitic infestations of the gut

## MD BOWIE & MA KIBEL

Protozoa (single-celled organisms) and helminths (worms) may parasitize the gut and are related to poverty and undernutrition. They are found primarily in populations living in poor sanitary conditions and lacking a basic understanding of hygiene. Most of these infestations are transmitted via soil contaminated with human faeces, but some are transmitted by ingestion of polluted water. Some are associated with diarrhoea (e.g., giardiasis), but it is not a feature of the symptomatology of others (e.g., ascariasis).

Two kinds of nutritional interaction may be seen in parasitic infestations. Firstly, they may impair nutritional status in a variety of ways. Parasites can cause functional or structural changes of the intestinal mucosa, including inflammation and ulceration with an increased loss of nutrients from the gut. They may stimulate hypermotility, obstruct the pancreatic or bile ducts, or compete directly with their host for certain nutrients. Anorexia induced by infestation is probably also a significant factor. Secondly, malnutrition per se may alter the severity of the infestation. Reduced resistance leads to larger parasite loads, increased severity of disease, and further deterioration in nutritional status.

The control of parasitic infestations in a community will only be successful when there is a holistic approach and the simultaneous employment of a number of different interventions. Gastrointestinal parasitic disease prevention requires the provision of effective waste disposal, safe and sufficient water supplies, and health education in the use of these facilities.

Only the most common protozoal and helminthic infestations of the gastrointestinal tract will be considered.

## Amoebiasis

This infection occurs throughout the world but is most common in tropical regions. In Africa, invasive disease is reported particularly from KwaZulu-Natal and the West African coast (Coulter, 1998). Transmission of the parasite occurs by means of relatively non-resistant, but abundant, cysts in contaminated food and water. Following the ingestion of cysts, the trophozoites excyst in the small intestine. *Entamoeba histolytica* (the pathogen) tends to inhabit the colon. The trophozoites may be excreted in diarrhoeic stools, but in formed stools they are excreted as cysts, which are better able to survive in the external environment.

*Entamoeba histolytica* is often found in symptomless carriers. There are probably many factors that induce pathogenicity, but amoebic colitis appears to start with the adhesion of the trophozoites to the epithelial cells of the colon. Necrosis of the cells follows, but initially there is little evidence of tissue inflammation; subsequent infiltration of inflammatory cells may be a response to secondary bacterial infection. Tissue invasion by amoebae induces specific antibody formation and later cell-mediated immune reactions but, despite this, the observation of frequent reinfections suggests that little or no protective immunity develops.

Symptomatic intestinal amoebiasis varies in severity from mild intermittent diarrhoea lasting for weeks to a severe fulminant dysentery. The onset is usually gradual in adults but may be abrupt in children. Constitutional symptoms (fever, toxicity) are usually absent or slight. Abdominal discomfort and tenderness over the colon and liver may be found, even in the absence of hepatitis. Sigmoidoscopy commonly reveals discrete ulcers with a yellow exudate, while the intervening bowel appears normal.

Complications may be local and the most common are perforation and peritonitis. Strictures, amoeboma, severe haemorrhage, and post-dysenteric colitis also occur. Systemic spread may complicate the infection, and, of these, amoebic liver abscess is the most common. Fever, toxicity, and leucocytosis with pain and tenderness in the right upper quadrant suggest this diagnosis. In childhood, amoebic liver abscess tends to occur in the first three years of life and multiple abscesses are common. Jaundice is rare. Extension of the abscess and rupture may occur into the peritoneum, the pleura, or pericardium. Rare extra-intestinal complica-

tions are perianal cutaneous amoebiasis or amoebic abscess of the brain or lungs.

Diagnosis is by identifying the haematophagous *E. histolytica* in stool or by aspiration of a liver abscess. Ultrasonography and radioactive scintigraphy are useful when identifying liver abscess. Serological tests (gel diffusion) provide supportive evidence for systemic complications as they are more commonly positive in young children with hepatic amoebiasis than in those with dysentery. In the older child the presence of antibodies does not distinguish present from past amoebiasis.

*Treatment:* metronidazole 50 mg/kg/day in three divided doses for seven days is effective in the majority of cases.

## Giardiasis

Giardiasis is found in both temperate and tropical regions and is common in South Africa. Humans are the major reservoir of infection and *Giardia lamblia* is transmitted in cyst form by direct personal contact and contaminated water supplies. Children in crèches are frequently infected.

Giardia trophozoites live mainly in the upper small bowel and a variety of mechanisms have been postulated as the means by which these parasites impair the host's absorption of nutrients. Histologically a variable degree of partial villous atrophy is seen. Giardia trophozoites induce an immune reaction which results in both secretory IgA and cell-mediated responses. The response produces a protective immunity and this is underlined by the frequent association of giardiasis with common variable immunodeficiency and isolated IgA deficiency. The immune response may be responsible for the pathological changes in the small intestinal mucosa and clinical disease.

Giardiasis presents a broad clinical spectrum. Many individuals are asymptomatic carriers. In children exposed to the organism for the first time, it frequently presents as a sudden explosive watery diarrhoea with abdominal discomfort and distension, nausea, and anorexia. It may resolve spontaneously or subside into a low-grade chronic or recurrent diarrhoea with weight loss and debility. The stools may become pale, bulky, and offensive, with a picture typical of a malabsorption syndrome.

The diagnosis is made by finding the trophozoites or cysts in the stool, or trophozoites in the duodenal content. The appearance of trophozoites or cysts in the stools may be intermittent and diagnosis difficult. A therapeutic trial with an antiparasitic drug may support the diagnosis.

*Treatment:* metronidazole, 25–50 mg/kg/ day in three divided doses, for five days.

# Cryptosporidiosis

Cryptosporidiosis is found in a variety of animals, including mammals, birds, and reptiles. Person-to-person transmission occurs and can cause outbreaks in day care centres. Water-borne outbreaks have been recorded. This parasite occurs in South Africa and appears to be fairly common.

Common clinical manifestations are frequent watery diarrhoea, but abdominal pain, anorexia, and weight loss have also been recorded. Immunocompetent individuals have a self-limited diarrhoeal illness but the immunocompromised can develop chronic or protracted diarrhoea with malnutrition. It is thus a particular problem in HIV-infected children and adults.

Diagnosis is made by identifying the oocysts in the stool with an acid-fast stain.

*Treatment:* no specific treatment is available.

# Ascariasis

Ascariasis is widespread throughout both temperate and tropical regions. It is prevalent in areas where sanitation is poor and particularly where human faeces (humus) is used as fertilizer. *Ascaris lumbricoides* is acquired by ingestion of soil or food contaminated with embryonated eggs. The larvae hatch in the small intestine, penetrate the mucosa, and pass to the lungs via the bloodstream. They enter the alveolar spaces and migrate up the airways to be swallowed again, after which they mature into adults in the bowel.

The clinical manifestations of *Ascaris lumbricoides* infestation can be related to the life-cycle. The migration of the larvae through the lungs may be associated with pulmonary infiltration (flitting pneumonitis) and eosinophilia. Episodes of wheezing can occur, particularly when transmission of infestation is episodic or seasonal. Most older individuals with adult worms in the bowel are asymptomatic or have ill-defined abdominal discomfort. In young children with heavy infestation a bolus of worms may cause intestinal colic or even intestinal obstruction. Such a bolus may rarely form the lead point for intussusception or the fulcrum for an intestinal volvulus. Adult worms may migrate up the common bile duct, causing an obstructive jaundice and biliary colic. More rarely they may obstruct the pancreatic duct with all the signs of an acute pancreatitis. Ascaris have been found in a variety of aberrant sites (including the liver parenchyma, and pulmonary artery) but such events are extremely rare.

The effects of ascariasis on nutritional status is controversial but heavy infestations probably have a deleterious effect.

The diagnosis is made by finding eggs in the faeces or by noting the passage of adult worms.

*Treatment:* piperazine citrate, 120 mg/kg (max. 4 g) as a single dose, or mebendazole

100 mg twice daily for three days, or albenda-zole as a single dose (200 mg under two years, 400 mg over two years).

## Trichuriasis (whipworm)

Trichuriasis is found in warm, moist regions and is widespread in South Africa. It is acquired by the ingestion of eggs from soil contaminated by human faeces. The egg develops directly into an adult worm that attaches to the mucosa of the large bowel.

The majority of infected persons are asymptomatic. Diarrhoea, rectal blood loss and prolapse may occur in heavy infestations. Some may present with a gross iron deficiency anaemia, distended abdomen, failure to thrive and clubbing of the fingers. With the advent of more effective treatment this mode of presentation has become very uncommon.

The diagnosis is made by finding typical eggs in the faeces, or by seeing the worms on sigmoidoscopy.

Treatment: mebendazole, 100 mg twice daily, for three days, or albendazole as a single dose (200 mg under two years, 400 mg over two years).

## Enterobius vermicularis (threadworm)

Enterobius is widespread throughout the world. The adult worm inhabits the lower small bowel and colon and the female migrates out of the anus to lay her eggs in the perianal folds. Infection is acquired either by scratching the perianal region, or by ingestion of the eggs that have been dislodged and found in house dust.

There are usually no gastrointestinal symptoms and the main clinical presentation is pruritis ani. This may be further complicated by secondary infection and the development of perianal impetigo. In girls, vulvovaginitis and urethritis may result from egg deposition in the lower genito-urinary tract.

Diagnosis is made by picking the eggs off the perianal folds with transparent adhesive tape. They are rarely found in the stool.

*Treatment:* should be of the whole family with mebendazole 100 mg twice daily for three days, or albendazole as a single dose (200 mg under two years, 400 mg over two years).

## Taeniasis (tapeworms)

Both *Taenia saginatum* and *T. solium* are widespread throughout the world, humans being the definitive host and cattle and pigs the respective intermediate hosts. The infection is acquired when meat containing cysts with viable scolices is ingested. The head attaches to the small intestinal mucosa and develops into an adult worm which may be several metres long with many proglottids (segments). Proglottids containing the eggs break off and are passed in the faeces. When ingested by cattle or pigs, the larvae hatch, penetrate the mucosa and spread throughout the tissues to develop into cysts. In the case of *T. solium*, eggs ingested by humans behave like those in the gut of pigs and cysts develop in the human. The human then becomes the intermediate host (see Figure 43.1).

Most patients are asymptomatic and the most obvious sign is the spontaneous passage of the white, stamp-like, motile proglottids. They may cause intestinal colic and some patients have constitutional symptoms such as fever, sweating, and loose stools. When the human becomes the intermediate host of *T. solium* (cysticercosis) the cysts lodge in various tissues (skin, muscle, liver, lungs, eyes, brain, or meninges).

Central nervous system involvement – neurocysticercosis – is an important community health problem in South Africa. It appears

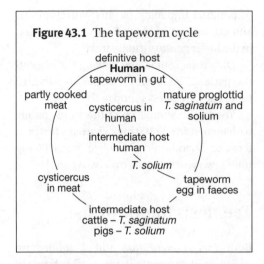

**Figure 43.1** The tapeworm cycle

definitive host
**Human**
tapeworm in gut

partly cooked meat

cysticercus in human

mature proglottid
*T. saginatum* and solium

intermediate host human

*T. solium*

cysticercus in meat

tapeworm egg in faeces

intermediate host
cattle – *T. saginatum*
pigs – *T. solium*

to be most common among the Xhosa people in the Eastern Cape, because of their free-ranging pigs. The most common clinical manifestation is recurrent convulsions. It is estimated that 30 per cent succumb as a result of the 'malignant' form of the condition (Thomson, 1990). Active cerebral cysticercosis can be successfully treated with praziquantel by mouth (50 mg/kg/day as a single dose or in divided doses for 15 days) or albendazole (15 mg/kg/day in three divided doses for at least eight days). Dexamethasone is added in order to control cerebral oedema.

Diagnosis of taeniasis is made when proglottids or eggs are seen in the stool. The diagnosis of neurocysticercosis has been greatly simplified by CT scanning.

*Treatment of intestinal taeniasis:* niclosamide 2 g by mouth on an empty stomach, or mebendazole 100 mg twice daily for five days.

# Hookworm

Hookworm infestation is widespread in warm, moist regions and is particularly common in northern parts of KwaZulu-Natal. In such areas, it is an important cause of anaemia. Infection is prevalent where sanitation is poor and people walk barefoot. Infective larvae penetrate the intact skin and pass via the bloodstream to the lungs, from where they migrate up the airways to be swallowed. They mature in the small intestine and attach themselves to the mucosa, causing loss of blood. Eggs are produced and excreted in the faeces. Humans are the reservoir of the common parasites *Ancylostoma duodenale* and *Necator americanus.*

Most infestations are asymptomatic. Skin penetration by the larvae may cause an irritating papulovesicular dermatitis, commonly on the feet. Larval migration through the lungs is usually asymptomatic, but occasionally pulmonary infiltrates, wheezing, and eosinophilia occur. Patients with heavy infestations may have abdominal pain and diarrhoea with blood and mucus in the stools. Symptoms and signs of iron deficiency, anaemia, and hypoproteinaemia may be the presenting features.

Diagnosis is made when eggs are found in the faeces.

*Treatment:* Mebendazole 100 mg twice daily for three days or albendazole as a single dose (200 mg under two years, 400 mg over two years). The iron deficiency anaemia must be treated.

The dog hookworm, *A. braziliense*, is one cause of the intensely itchy 'sandworm' (cutaneous larva migrans). This responds well to thiabendazole cream or to a cream made up with crushed mebendazole tablets.

# Strongyloides

*Strongyloides stercoralis* is widespread in tropical areas but also occurs in some temperate areas. The life-cycle is similar to that of the hookworms. Unlike the hookworm, auto-infection can occur with the infective larvae developing in the gut of the human host and penetrating the intestinal mucosa to reinvade the circulation. This explains the persistence of the parasite for long periods in the human.

Many patients are asymptomatic. A creeping eruption, red and irritating, is often found in the perianal region or buttock. Urticarial eruptions and oedema may occur elsewhere and the skin lesions tend to recur for many years. Intermittent attacks of diarrhoea, weight loss, and abdominal distension may be present. Shock, Gram-negative septicaemia, pneumonia, and meningitis may supervene.

The diagnosis is made by finding larvae in faeces or duodenal fluid.

*Treatment:* thiabendazole 50 mg/kg/day in two divided doses orally for three days. Albendazole is reported to be effective in a dose of 400 mg on three consecutive days.

For both hookworm and strongyloides infestations, the wearing of shoes and improved sanitation may help to reduce the incidence in highly endemic areas.

# Mass deworming

The long-term solution of intestinal helminthiasis as a community problem lies in improved sanitation and living conditions, but there is evidence to show that the mass delivery of helminthic treatment to children is an important public health option. The *World Development Report* of the World Bank includes mass deworming in its 'essential package of health interventions' (1993), and school-based mass delivery is singled out as one of the most cost-effective measures. At the present time albendazole is probably the drug of choice but may not be readily available in all areas. While results can be achieved quickly with chemotherapy, they are only temporary, and in the absence of other control measures, prevalence rates and worm loads can only be kept low by repeated doses, usually three or four times during a year. In this regard, see also the role of chemotherapy in Chapter 44: Schistosomiasis. As with any control programme, efforts to impose a helminth control programme on a population that is unaware of the reasons for it, or unwilling to accept it, is doomed to fail (Vince, 1991).

## References and further reading

COULTER JBS. 1998. Amebiasis. In: AGM Campbell & N McIntosh (eds.). *Forfar and Arneil's textbook of paediatrics*, 5th ed. Edinburgh: Churchill Livingstone.

THOMSON AJG. 1990. Neurocysticercosis. *South African Medical Journal.* 77:119–20.

WORLD BANK. 1993. *World Development Report: Investing in health.* Oxford: Oxford University Press.

VINCE J. 1991. In: P Stanfield, M Brueton, M Chan, M Parkin, and T Waterston (eds.). *Diseases of children in the tropics and subtropics*, 4th ed. London: Edward Arnold.

# 44

# Schistosomiasis

## M ISAÄCSON & J FREAN

## Occurrence

The main species of Schistosoma responsible for human pathology are *S. haematobium* and *S. mansoni,* and their principal target organs are the genito-urinary and gastrointestinal tracts respectively. The prevalence of schistosomiasis (bilharzia) in schoolchildren is as high as 95 per cent in some areas, but its geographical distribution in southern Africa is largely confined to the north-eastern regions, tailing off in a south-easterly direction. In South Africa, *S. haematobium* is much more widespread than *S. mansoni,* which is mainly found in low-lying areas. *Schistosoma mattheei,* a bovine schistosome that may also be found in humans has a distribution similar to that of *S. haematobium,* but its role in human pathology has not been completely elucidated. Some doubt exists as to whether it is capable of causing human disease on its own; a hybrid form between it and *S. haematobium* may be a pre-requisite.

## Epidemiology

Ova excreted in urine or faeces must gain access, directly or indirectly, to surface water.

The larval form, a ciliated miracidium, hatches from the ovum in water and enters an aquatic snail where it undergoes further development. In due course, numerous cercariae emerge, which swim around until a human host is encountered. Entrance is gained through the skin. This needs to be accomplished within a matter of hours, before cercarial infectivity is lost. In the human host, the worms mature and can remain alive and sexually productive for many years.

Environmental temperature is crucial to the development and shedding of the cercariae by the snail. The viability of cercariae and snail hosts is affected by water temperature and velocity.

The time of day when cercariae are shed by the snails varies according to the species of schistosomes involved and has an important bearing on the epidemiology of schistosomiasis. Cercariae of *S. haematobium* are predominantly shed around midday, those of *S. mansoni* somewhat earlier, while *S. mattheei* cercariae are shed in the early morning and early evening, coinciding with the usual drinking time of cattle and wild animals. The midday peak of *S. haematobium* cercarial shedding favours the infection of persons who habitually cool off by swimming during the heat of the day. These are usually children, which is at least partly the reason why S. haematobium is so highly prevalent in the young. The optimal time for S. haematobium egg deposition in the vascular bed of the bladder is also during the hours around noon. Since these eggs dry out and die if shed on soil, the swimming habits of rural children affect not only their own infection by cercariae but also the infection of snails by hatched miracidia. The incidence of S. haematobium egg deposition as well as the number of eggs passed decreases as children mature to adulthood.

The epidemiology of S. mansoni differs significantly. Of prime importance is the fact that ova are excreted in human faeces, which, unlike urine, are almost exclusively deposited on land. Mansoni eggs survive longer than haematobium eggs (up to a week), being protected by moist faeces. They are dependent on rain for their ultimate survival and further development in an aquatic environment. S. mansoni infection is therefore likely to be more prevalent in communities situated close to a body of water. This is frequently the case with, for example, irrigation projects. The prevalence of intestinal schistosomiasis, unlike that of the urinary form, is thus related to faecal pollution of water.

# Immunity and morbidity

There is a gradual build-up of infection during childhood and adolescence, which, from the age of about 25 years, is often followed by a steady decrease in the number of eggs passed. Immune processes play a major role in this. It has been postulated that antigens released from the ova form the main immunogenic stimulus in young children. These antigens, however, elicit blocking antibodies, while the predominantly protective immune responses develop much later. This hypothesis may explain why heavily exposed children are often very slow in developing immunity.

There is evidence that IgE is the important effector antibody isotype in protective immunity. The cellular regulation of the protective IgE response is not completely defined, but it is at least partly related to the cytokines associated with the CD4+T helper 2 (TH2) subset of lymphocytes. In experimental mouse schistosomiasis there is a switch from a predominantly TH1 cytokine response (IFN-gamma, IL-2) to a TH2 response (IL-4, IL-5, IL-10) at the onset of egg production, and there is evidence that infections in humans also follow this pattern.

Changes in cytokine balance can be linked to inflammatory events as well as to the pattern of antibody isotype production. It is not known whether these immune responses are modulated by schistosomes to prolong their survival or restrict acquisition of new schistosome infections by the host (the latter is well recognized and is called 'concomitant immunity'). One strategy that adult schistosomes are known to use to evade the immune system is to acquire host antigens on the tegument. These include histocompatibility antigens, immunoglobulins, intercellular substance antigens, and blood group glycolipid antigens.

Immunity is, however, not the only factor in the declining intensity of infection with age. As shown above, a reduction in water contact during adolescence may result in a greatly reduced exposure to infection. Such a change in lifestyle must be an important contributing factor to the declining worm load noted in the majority of affected adults in some areas, especially those people with S. haematobium infections. However, age-related decreasing worm loads do not always occur. For example, studies in KwaZulu-Natal, where there was little reduction in water-related activities during adolescence, showed no significant changes in prevalence.

While it is generally agreed that the worm burden as seen by the number of eggs passed is an important determinant of the degree of morbidity likely to be experienced, geographical differences have been noted in respect of the severity of schistosomiasis and its effect on physical and intellectual performance. It has been suggested that such differences may reflect variations in the virulence of different geographic strains within a schistosomal species. On the other hand, it has been shown in Brazil that host factors such as blood groups or race may also be important in this context. In Egypt, some haplotypes of the HL-A system have been correlated with severity of *S. mansoni* pathology. In southern Africa, marked regional differences have also been noted and a study of Eastern Caprivi schoolchildren showed a remarkably high prevalence of hepatosplenomegaly due to *S. mansoni* infection. This is unlike the findings in other endemic areas of southern Africa. Again, there was a positive correlation in this study between parasite load as determined by egg counts, and severity of infection.

# Effects of schistosomiasis on physiological performance

Numerous studies have been done to assess the effect of schistosomiasis on physiological performance levels in both adults and children. These studies have yielded contradictory findings. A recent, carefully controlled and standardized investigation involving 153 Zimbabwean schoolchildren was designed to evaluate the effect of heavy schistosome burdens on physical performance. The results showed a statistically significant difference between infected children and non-infected controls and, in the former, a significant improvement in performance following successful treatment of schistosomiasis.

# Factors relevant to the control of schistosomiasis

From the foregoing it is clear that schistosomiasis is an important problem in childhood. Especially in the case of *S. haematobium*, childhood activities are the very factors that promote reservoir maintenance and parasite transmission. It is therefore at this level that the appropriate control measures must be directed. In any given schistosomiasis focus, the design of a control programme must be based on locally obtained surveillance data.

## A schistosomiasis control programme

The following principles govern a total schistosomiasis control programme:

*Snail control*
- molluscicides, e.g., niclosamide;
- biological methods, e.g., fish;
- habit eradication, including eradication of the vegetation to which snails attach themselves and measures to prevent its regrowth; and
- exclusion of features that promote snail breeding in new irrigation schemes.

*Prevention of exposure to infected snails*
- access to bilharzia-affected surface water should be hindered by fencing – by canals being constructed with steeply sloping concreted banks, by dense reed banks being planted, etc.;
- snails should be prevented from becoming infected;
- faecal contamination of soil near surface waters should be prevented; and
- urinary contamination of surface waters should be prevented.

# Enviromental aspects of control

Implementation of the first principle (snail control) can be very expensive and may carry the potentially serious risk of harmful ecological imbalances being created, particularly with regard to natural food chains. This line of attack has therefore become less popular, especially since the advent of safer, single-dose chemotherapeutic agents. Snail control should not be dismissed, however. Well-planned, focal snail control schemes have been successful.

Prevention of access to bilharzia-infested water is part and parcel of the protection of snails against infection. The provision, therefore, of human waste disposal facilities and of safe domestic and recreational water supplies is crucial for the protection of both snails and humans. This requires the installation of latrines, laundry facilities, and swimming and paddling pools. Health education programmes must include advice on the dangers of exposure to natural surface waters and on the benefits and conveniences of using sanitary facilities. Self-help schemes are very important in the establishment of some of these facilities, especially the construction of economical latrines. As far as the provision of clean water supplies is concerned, the role of government agencies in providing both expertise and funds is indispensable.

# The role of chemotherapy

Effective and safe agents are now available (praziquantel for all forms, metrifonate for *S. haematobium*, oxamniquine for *S. mansoni*). Ideally, chemotherapy should be just one of the tools in a multi-targeted control programme. In reality, the latter often fails to be implemented, mainly for lack of the necessary funds and other resources. A lower level of priority than, for example, malaria control, is another common constraint. Various schemes based mainly on some form of mass chemotherapy have therefore been applied. A great deal has been published on the limitations of mass chemotherapy, but if the principal objective of schistosomiasis control is the reduction of morbidity rather than of prevalence per se, chemotherapy assumes a key function.

With respect to the selection of candidates for chemotherapy, at least five possible regimens have been described:

- *Mass population chemotherapy.* Treatment of the entire population without diagnostic procedures;
- *Selective population chemotherapy.* Treatment of all persons with positive stool/urine microscopy;
- *Selected mass chemotherapy.* Treatment of all individuals in a selected young age group;
- *Selected selective chemotherapy.* Treatment of all infected individuals in a selected age group; and
- *Targeted chemotherapy.* Treatment limited to persons with a defined high egg output.

The relative cost-effectiveness can be calculated, but it will vary regionally according to several factors such as the cost of diagnostic tests and drugs, compliance, etc.

Macroscopic and reagent-strip-defined haematuria were used as criteria for a selective population chemotherapy approach in Tanzanian schools. This approach was dictated by the lack of trained staff and funds at the primary health care level. It was found that the reagent strip method had a sensitivity of 90 per cent which increased to 98 per cent among those with heavy worm burdens, and for whom chemotherapy was especially important. After only one year, gross haematuria was reduced by 94,5 per cent and micro-haematuria by 69 per cent. Both teachers and pupils were motivated and, with a staff of only five rural health assistants, it was possible to screen and treat 26 000 children in less than a month.

Treatment regimens need to be repeated at intervals of six months to a year to be of lasting benefit.

## Vaccination

In the long term, vaccination against schistosomiasis may be a realistic control measure if and when drug resistance becomes a major problem. However, an emerging view is that even an effective vaccine would probably have to be used in conjunction with chemotherapy and other control methods. A great deal of work is currently in progress and vaccination against this infection is considered to be an achievable goal. Examples of schistosomal molecules under investigation as candidate vaccines include enzymes (glutathione S-transferase, triose-phosphate isomerase), muscle proteins (paramyosin), and membrane antigens.

## References and further reading

BUTTERWORTH AE & HAGAN P. 1987. Immunity in human schistosomiasis. *Parasitology Today*. 3:11–15.

GEAR JHS & PITCHFORD RJ. 1988. *Bilharzia in South Africa*. Pretoria: Government Printer.

LIESE B. 1986. The organization of schistosomiasis control programmes. *Parasitology Today*. 2:339–45.

NDAMBA J. 1986. Schistosomiasis: Its effects on the physical performance of school children in Zimbabwe. *Central African Journal of Medicine*. 32:289–93.

PRESCOTT NM. 1987. The economics of schistosomiasis chemotherapy. *Parasitology Today*. 3:21–4.

SAVIOLI L & MOTT KE. 1989. Urinary schistosomiasis on Pemba Island: Low-cost diagnosis for control in a primary health care setting. *Parasitology Today*. 5:333–7.

WALKER ARP. 1977. The health handicap of schistosomiasis to children in southern Africa. *South African Medical Journal*. 51:541–4.

WARREN KS & MAHMOUD AAF (eds.). 1990. *Tropical and geographical medicine*. New York: McGraw-Hill.

# 45

# Childhood asthma

## EG WEINBERG

In any industrialized country 5 to 15 per cent of the childhood population is affected by asthma. Boys are more often affected than girls (by a ratio of 2:1), but in adolescence the sex incidence becomes equal. The prevalence of childhood asthma is increasing very rapidly. As there is considerable misunderstanding about the principles of its management, the clinical aspects will be dealt with in some detail.

Although it is generally agreed that asthma is a condition in which there is reversible airways obstruction, it remains impossible to reach agreement on a precise definition which can be applied to all. This is particularly so in children, as many have recurrent wheezing and coughing attacks in the first year of life but do not respond to bronchodilators.

The narrowing of the airways may be mild or severe and may improve spontaneously or require intensive therapy to reverse. A very important component of the problem is the 'twitchiness' or hyper-reactivity of the airways, which occurs in response to a variety of irritants. This is thought to be due to the presence of inflammation.

Clinically, asthma is characterized by wheezing, a high-pitched expiratory sound

## A definition of asthma

A definition that would be acceptable to many experts in the field of childhood asthma is as follows:

'Asthma is a condition characterized by recurrent episodes of breathlessness, coughing or wheezing caused by variable or intermittent narrowing of the intra-pulmonary airways.'

generated from partially obstructed airways, and by coughing. Asthma may also occur without obvious wheezing and the diagnosis may be missed, especially in children. Many young children with wheezing are labelled as having wheezy bronchitis or bronchiolitis. Follow-up studies have shown that these children are indistinguishable from other asthmatic children. It is not surprising that, with all the difficulties of definition and the often confusing clinical presentation, asthma is underdiagnosed and undertreated in most countries.

# Pathology and pathophysiology

Asthma is a disease in which large and small airways are intermittently narrowed in varying degrees, but in the majority of cases the disease process is confined to the bronchial wall. The only conditions commonly associated with asthma are allergic and inflammatory conditions of the upper respiratory tract and atopic eczema.

Our understanding of the pathophysiological abnormalities is still rather poor but some aspects are well known. The tracheobronchial tree may either change its calibre or alter the amount of glandular secretion produced. Bronchial narrowing is accompanied by an increase in secretions, coughing, and breathlessness and may be due to three separate processes:
- bronchial smooth muscle contraction;
- inflammation and swelling of the bronchial mucous membrane; and
- accumulation of bronchial secretions within the lumen.

These three processes cause obstruction to different degrees in each individual. Many factors are known to be capable of causing contraction of the bronchial muscle in asthmatics, who differ from non-asthmatics in that they are highly sensitive to a wide variety of bronchoconstricting stimuli. This tendency is referred to as 'bronchial hyper-reactivity'.

## BRONCHIAL HYPER-REACTIVITY

Bronchial hyper-reactivity (BHR) is an exaggerated sensitivity of the airways to physical, chemical, and pharmacological stimuli. A history of chest symptoms related to non-specific stimuli such as viral respiratory tract infections, exercise, and emotional stress are all suggestive of increased BHR, as are nocturnal symptoms of coughing and wheezing and a typical diurnal variation in the peak expiratory flow rate (PEFR). The PEFR can be easily measured on a simple and cheap Mini-Wright Peak Flow Meter. The diurnal changes will be clearly seen if the patient records morning and evening PEFR readings on a diary card.

If there is any doubt about the diagnosis, a standard exercise challenge test will settle the issue in most cases. Here, a baseline PEFR reading is taken and the child told to run as fast as possible on level ground for six minutes. The exercise should be of sufficient intensity to raise the heart rate to about 160 beats per minute. After the six-minute run the child rests for five minutes. Following this, another PEFR reading is taken. In asthmatics the post-exercise value will typically have fallen 15 per cent or more from the pre-exercise reading. The bronchospasm produced by this test can easily be reversed by using any of the common beta-agonist metered dose inhalers (MDI).

Where the exercise challenge test has been negative, but asthma is still suspected, more sophisticated inhalation challenges using histamine or metacholine may be used to confirm the diagnosis. This should only be performed in centres where they are done regularly.

Non-specific bronchial hyper-responsiveness is virtually universal in asthma and is of profound importance in the pathophysiology of the condition. The underlying cause of bronchial hyper-reactivity is uncertain. Viral infections increase this response but the effect disappears after six weeks. The sustained reactivity of asthmatics has been attributed to an imbalance of autonomic control, increased permeability of the airway epithelium, and intrinsic differences in the action of smooth muscle.

## PRECIPITATING FACTORS AND RELATED MANAGEMENT

### Exercise

Vigorous exercise produces narrowing of the airway in most asthmatic subjects and, as noted above, may be used as a diagnostic test. Asthma occurring during or after exercise is most likely to be a clinical problem for children whose games at school may be affected. The type of exercise influences the response and most asthmatics find that swimming is the activity least likely to induce asthma. Exercise-induced asthma can usually be prevented by prior inhalation of a beta-agonist bronchodilator, sodium cromoglycate, or recently the use of leukotriene antagonists taken orally. Such treatment will normally allow a child to take part in games at school. General fitness and activity should be encouraged, and many asthmatics do, in fact, excel at sport.

### Housedust mites

The housemite, *Dermatophagoides pteronyssinus*, is thought to be the most common allergen responsible for asthma attacks in susceptible individuals. This applies especially to the coastal regions of southern Africa, but mites may be found in many inland areas where there is a temperate climate and relatively high humidity. Mites feed on human skin scales and are widely distributed in bedding, carpets, furniture, and on soft toys. Only very rigorous avoidance measures, such as the use of special mattress and pillow covers, washing bedding in warm water, removal of carpets from bedrooms and regular vacuum cleaning of rooms, are effective; unfortunately these may be unaffordable for many parents in Southern Africa. In poorer homes exposure of mattresses and bedding to sunlight is an alternative option.

### Pollens and spores

Seasonal asthma is very rare in southern Africa. Most cases are perennial in nature, but possibly with some seasonal flare-ups. Grass pollen is by far the most common sensitizing pollen, and the long grass seasons account for the perennial nature of symptoms. On the Highveld and in the natural grasslands of the country, very high grass pollen counts are found throughout the year with a tapering only in May, June, and July each year. Tree and weed pollens seldom affect young children. Fungal spores are a common cause of sensitization in all parts of the country – even in relatively dry areas. The common allergenic spores occur throughout the year with a slight increase in the autumn and winter months.

### Pets

Parents of asthmatic children often worry about household pets. Cats cause the greatest problem but most domestic animals can on occasion trigger asthma. Patients with severe asthma should be advised not to acquire any new pets. Pets already in the house should be kept out of bedrooms; and certainly never allowed to sleep on the children's beds.

### Food allergy

Food allergies usually affect young children, especially those under two years of age, and cause eczema and gastrointestinal symptoms rather than asthma. Intolerance to foods may be related to naturally occurring pharmacological agents, such as histamine or tyramine, or be provoked by food additives such as tartrazine. Where there are definite allergies to foodstuffs, milk, egg white, wheat, soya, and peanuts are most commonly implicated.

A common precipitator of acute asthma attacks of short duration is sulphur dioxide used as a preservative in cold drinks. A total of 20 per cent or more of childhood asthmatics react adversely to this additive.

## Emotional factors

Psychological factors on their own do not produce asthma. They may, however, aggravate established asthma, especially where there is poor control. Asthma associated with laughing or crying may be related to breathing in cold or dry air, rather than the emotion itself.

## DIAGNOSIS OF CHILDHOOD ASTHMA

This is perhaps the most important step in good management. Recent studies have shown that asthma is grossly underdiagnosed even in highly developed countries. Underdiagnosis is a particular problem for children who subsequently miss significant amounts of schooling because of recurrent wheezing episodes. Many are erroneously diagnosed and treated for recurrent respiratory infections.

Most asthmatic children present with recurrent episodes of wheezing and cough, although some may complain of cough alone. The majority of children who are going to develop asthma do so before they are five years of age. A careful history, especially when accompanied by a positive family history, is helpful in the diagnosis. As asthma is very often an intermittent disease, the child may be quite well when presenting to the doctor. Only in the more severe cases will there be features such as very marked hyperinflation of the chest with a pigeon chest deformity, bowing of the sternum, and Harrison's sulcus formation. These children will usually also suffer from stunted growth and delayed puberty. Wheezing that is mainly expiratory is heard in the milder cases only when there is exacerbation of their asthma, but it is commonly present in the more severe cases.

The diagnosis is strengthened by showing that the child has an allergic or atopic background, and by the presence of bronchial hyper-reactivity (BHR).

### PRESENCE OF ATOPY

Atopy may be defined as the predisposition to develop Immunoglobulin E (IgE) antibodies to common environmental allergens, and the presence of the combination of diseases asthma, allergic rhinitis, and atopic eczema.

About 95 per cent of children with asthma are atopic. In an individual child, evidence of an atopic background is supported by a positive family history of allergic disorders and a personal history of illnesses such as eczema or rhinitis.

Clinical examination may show the typical 'allergic' facies, which is pale with mild periorbital swelling. The so-called 'allergic shiners' refer to blue discoloration of the lower eyelids. The conjunctivae are often congested and the nasal mucous membrane is pale and swollen, with an associated clear watery mucous discharge. A transverse nasal crease is often seen where the bridge of the nose and the cartilaginous portion meet. These features are usually due to the presence of allergic rhinitis.

Further confirmation of atopy can be obtained by demonstrating positive reactions to one or more common allergens on skin-prick testing. Only three allergens need to be used: housedust mite, grass pollen, and cats with positive and negative controls. The measurement of total IgE levels is probably not useful in the southern African environment, because of the common presence of parasitic infestation. The Phadiotop screening test may be of greater value as a pointer to atopy in this region.

### DIFFERENTIAL DIAGNOSIS

Not all children wheeze because of asthma, and sometimes other causes of wheezing need to be considered and a chest X-ray taken. The more important possibilities are listed in Table 45.1. Remember the old maxim 'not all that wheezes is asthma'.

**Table 45.1**  Some other causes of wheezing and coughing

| | |
|---|---|
| • Mechanical obstruction | Foreign body |
| | Enlarged lymph nodes |
| | Cysts |
| | Pneumothorax |
| • Familial diseases | Cystic fibrosis |
| | Immunodeficiency diseases |
| | Alpha1-antitrypsin deficiency |
| | Immotile cilia syndrome |
| • Developmental causes | Anomalies of the upper airway, trachea, great vessels, and bronchi |
| • Secondary to other disease | Tuberculosis |
| | Pulmonary oedema |
| | Oesophageal reflux |
| • Parasites | Ascaris infestation |

# Management of childhood asthma

In every case it is important to tailor treatment to the individual, but some measures do apply in all cases.

It is important to allay anxiety about the disease. This is best done by thoroughly explaining about asthma, what to do if an attack occurs, why medicines are used and how they work, and especially by emphasizing the importance of their regular use. Time spent on this initial explanation and advice is well rewarded by the future well-being and correct use of medicines. Regular follow-up of patients, preferably by the same doctor, is very important.

## AVOIDANCE OF TRIGGER FACTORS

Some of these have been discussed. Allergen avoidance is a valuable way of helping to decrease the severity of a child's asthma but it may be more difficult than is often appreciated. Airborne allergens such as pollens and fungal spores may be impossible to avoid.

Housedust mites are by far the most common allergen to which most asthmatic children react and simple control measures will help a lot.

If patients move to environments free of housedust mites (such as the Karoo), their symptoms may improve considerably. This can also be achieved in hospitals. Relocating a family is a major upheaval and should not be undertaken without careful assessment of the associated consequences. Where possible, there should be a trial period to establish benefits. Regular cleaning of bedrooms and attention to dust control help to reduce mite counts. Expensive methods to reduce mite infestation are usually not justified.

Removal of pets such as cats from the child's home is also not as simple as may be thought. Many families are very reluctant to get rid of the favourite pet. Even where cats are removed from the home, the remaining cat allergen may take many months to clear and symptoms may continue to occur. Unjustified removal of favourite pets without good reason may often provoke more problems because of the emotional aspects.

Avoidance of non-specific triggers such as cigarette smoke is very important. Care should also be taken when children go from warm rooms into the cold outside air. Cooking in bedrooms and the use of paraffin stoves should be discouraged. Parents must not smoke in the child's presence, especially in bedrooms. It is usually futile to try to prevent the child from being exposed to viral infections but sometimes removal from a crèche may be advisable if infections are frequent and troublesome. As far as possible the child should be encouraged to live a normal life and to participate fully in all activities.

## DRUG TREATMENT

Effective use of the correct drugs forms the mainstay of modern asthma management. These drugs can be divided broadly into those which relieve symptoms at once (bronchodilators) and those which prevent symptoms (prophylactic drugs). Some preparations may fall into both of these categories.

## Bronchodilators

The beta-agonists such as salbutamol (Ventolin) and fenoterol (Berotec) are very valuable bronchodilator drugs. They are effective in children over 18 months of age and offer immediate relief of symptoms. Side effects include a fine tremor of the hands and slight increase in heart rate. These preparations are available in oral, inhaled, and injectable forms, and can be used according to the age of the child and the situation being dealt with. Inhaled forms are preferable.

The anticholinergic drug ipratropium bromide (Atrovent) is also an effective bronchodilator, especially when combined with a beta-agonist. It is available for inhalation as an aerosol or as a nebulizer solution. It is especially recommended for infants under 18 months of age, or where coughing does not respond to other forms of bronchodilator.

## Theophyllines

The theophylline preparations have been used for the treatment of asthma for many years. It is possible to determine the therapeutic level of theophylline required to promote and maintain adequate bronchodilation in the majority of patients. This, together with the production of slow-release long-acting theophylline preparations, has given a new lease of life to these drugs. Another factor of importance is that theophyllines are relatively cheap and only need to be administered twice a day in most cases. This helps to achieve adequate patient compliance.

The therapeutic response to theophyllines and the emergence of side effects are very closely related. Best control is achieved at serum concentrations of between 5 and 20 mg/$\ell$ and side effects usually begin to emerge from 20 mg/$\ell$ upwards.

The main side effects of theophylline are caused by its effects on the cardiovascular, central nervous (CNS), and gastrointestinal systems. CNS toxicity may present with fits, although irritability, insomnia, and headache are more common.

Certain factors may interfere with the normally very effective clearance of theophylline from the child's system. Fever and the use of macrolide antibiotics, such as erythromycin, are the most important of these.

The most successful application of the slow-release theophylline preparations has been in the management of night asthma and of those children affected by early morning symptoms (the so-called 'morning dippers').

Intravenous aminophyllines (theophylline plus ethylene diamine) are useful for patients admitted to hospital for acute severe asthma. Great caution must be exercised when treating children who have recently taken oral theophylline. Serum levels should be determined and it is always best to administer the drug only when the child is in a high care unit where the staff are capable of managing the possible severe side effects, such as cardiac arrest, gastric haemorrhage, and convulsions.

Rectal theophylline preparations should not be used in children because of their unpredictable absorption.

## Prophylactic drugs

Sodium cromoglycate (Lomudal) is an extremely safe so-called mast-cell stabilizing drug for the prevention of asthma attacks. Its mode of action is poorly understood but its discovery was the catalyst for a tremendous upsurge in research into the mechanisms of asthma, with special emphasis on what is now regarded as mucosal inflammation. Sodium cromoglycate is poorly absorbed when taken orally, and is only effective by inhalation. It is highly effective in the management of childhood asthma, but apparently less so in adults. It is best employed in mild persistent asthma, especially where allergic and exercise triggers play an important role. This preparation is available as a nebulizer solution for use in very young children, as a powder administered via a spinhaler for the majority of children and in aerosol form for older children and teenagers. Ketotifen, an orally administered mast-cell stabilizing drug, appears to be most effective in mild to moderate young asthmatics.

## Corticosteroids

Corticosteroid drugs have been used in the treatment of asthma for many years. These are very potent drugs which can control virtually all severe cases of asthma, but, as is well known, these drugs may cause many unwanted side effects when taken orally for prolonged periods.

The introduction of inhaled steroid preparations using an extremely small dose has revolutionized the treatment of many childhood asthmatics. The best known of these preparations are beclomethasone dipropionate (BDP) (Becotide) and budesonide (Pulmocort, Inflammide). Side effects are extremely rare unless an excessive dosage is employed and the most common complication is that of oropharyngeal candida infection, which is easily treated. In children, the growth retardation caused by systemic steroids does not occur with standard doses of BDP therapy (below 400 ug daily). As asthma may in itself cause growth retardation, some children actually improve their

growth on inhaled steroids, especially when their asthma is brought under control.

Several forms of BDP are now available for inhalation. These range from dry inhalers such as Accuhalers to the well-known MDI. In spite of their apparent lack of side effects, inhaled steroids are powerful drugs which should be restricted to children with symptoms inadequately controlled by other means. The lowest effective dose should always be used.

In recent times, groups of experts on the treatment of childhood asthma have met in several countries in efforts to formulate an approach to the treatment of asthma that could be applied in most countries, irrespective of the standard of their health services.

## PROTOCOL FOR ASTHMA TREATMENT

There have been considerable changes in the prevailing attitudes to asthma prevention and therapy over the past decade. The South African treatment scheme is outlined in Figure 45.1. Treatment depends on the severity of symptoms and on the age of the child.

## Severity of symptoms

Mild occasional symptoms may be treated with intermittent bronchodilators. In this situation, continuous use of bronchodilators is not only expensive and wasteful but has no advantage over intermittent use. The decision as to when such treatment is inadequate varies with the individual but in general terms regular preventive treatment should be introduced if a bronchodilator is needed more than twice a week or if the child has a regular or frequent night symptom or exercise-induced wheezing. In those children who have only occasional symptoms, prophylaxis can be given during the bad season and stopped during the good ones.

Regular inhaled sodium cromoglycate, which may have a dramatic effect, is a sec-

**Figure 45.1** Stepwise approach to management of chronic asthma in children

| CLASSIFY SEVERITY AT PRESENTATION | | | | |
|---|---|---|---|---|
| | Intermittent | Persistent | | |
| | | Mild | Moderate | Severe |
| Category | 1 | 2 | 3 | 4 |
| Daytime symptoms<br>Night-time symptoms<br>PEFR (predicted) | ≤ 2 / week<br>≤ 1 / month<br>≥ 80 % | 2 – 4 / week<br>2 – 4 / month<br>≥ 80 % | > 4 / week<br>> 4 / month<br>60 – 80 % | continuous<br>frequent<br>< 60 % |

**Start treatment at any step depending on the level of severity.**

**ALL CATEGORIES**
→ Short-acting ß₂ agonist as needed (reliever)
→ Environmental control
→ Education / Self management

**STEP 1 : *Intermittent***
→ No daily preventer or controller medication needed

**STEP 2 : *Mild persistent***
*Daily medication:*
→ Low dose* inhaled corticosteroid
→ Secondary options:
  • cromoglycate/nedocromill
  • sustained release theophyline
  • leukotriene receptor antagonist

**STEP 3 : *Moderate persistent***
*Daily medication:*
→ Medium dose* inhaled corticosteroid
→ And if needed
  • long-acting inhaled ß₂ agonist or sustained release theophylline
  • consider adding leukotriene receptor antagonist

**STEP 4 : *Severe persistent***
*Daily medication:*
→ High dose* inhaled corticosteroid
→ And if needed
  • long-acting inhaled ß₂ agonist or sustained release theophylline
  • consider adding leukotriene receptor antagonist
*If still not controlled*
→ Add
  • prednisone long-term (preferably alternate days) – reduce to lowest dose that controls symptoms

**Increase treatment**

→ If control is not achieved, consider step up. First review medication technique, adherence, environmental control.
→ A short course of oral steroids may be required to achieve control. (Prednisone 1–2mg/kg/day for 7–14 days)

**Reduce treatment**

→ Review treatment every 3–6 months. If control is sustained, reduce treatment.
→ Reduce or stop controllers before reducing dosage of inhaled steroids

**Choice of spacer devices**

< 3 yrs MDI + spacer with mask
> 3 yrs MDI + spacer with mouthpiece or DPI/breath actuated MDI

**\* Recommended daily dosages of inhaled corticosteroids**

| STEROID | LOW DOSE | MEDIUM DOSE | HIGH DOSE |
|---|---|---|---|
| Beclomethasone | 100 – 200 µg | 200 – 400 µg | > 400 µg |
| Budesonide | 100 – 200 µg | 200 – 400 µg | > 400 µg |
| Fluticasone | 50 – 100 µg | 100 – 200 µg | > 200 µg |
| Triamcinolone | 100 – 200 µg | 200 – 400 µg | > 400 µg |

**Figure 45.2** An asthma diary

## ASTHMA DIARY

Name .................................................................................  Age ......................................  Height ...........................cm

**MONTH**..................................................................... Day

**WHAT SORT OF NIGHT DID YOU HAVE?**    Write down the appropriate number for each night

Good night. No coughing or wheezing ................................. 0
Slept well but coughed or wheezed once or twice................... 1
Woke up two or three times due to cough or wheeze.............. 2
Awake most of the time due to cough or wheeze .................... 3

**ACTIVITY DURING THE DAY**    Write down the appropriate number for each day

Quite normal ........................................................... 0
Only able to run short distances ............................................. 1
Limited to walking.................................................................. 2
Too breathless to walk .......................................................... 3

**PEAK FLOW METER READING (best of three readings)**    Record the reading for each category

(Normal range for size ......................... to ........................... )
On waking, before medicine ........................................................
Midday, before lunch or sport ....................................................
Before evening medicine ...........................................................

**MEDICATION**    Record the number of doses used in the last 24 hours

Name of medicine          Dose

**COMMENTS**    Write down your comments on anything that may be related to the asthma
ie., to what do you attribute the attack?
What causes the wheeze (weather? diet? cold? dog? exercise? etc)
Lots of phlegm? Is phlegm coloured?
Nebulization? Hospital admission?

Use this diary to keep a record during the month.    Try and be as regular as you can in recording the score,
You can photocopy this page and show it to your doctor at your next    but don't worry if you cannot complete all the information.
appointment.    The diary will help your doctor to see how you are
Write the score in the box provided.    progressing.

ondary option in mild persistent asthma. Regular inhaled steroids in graded dosage are used in these cases and in those with moderate persistent and severe persistent childhood asthma.

Where night or early morning asthma is a great problem, or when the child cannot manage inhaled preparations, use may be made of slow-release theophyllines. The long-acting beta-agonist salmeterol is another possible choice. Inhaled beta-agonist bronchodilators are added during exacerbations of asthma. If control of symptoms is still inadequate, then inhaler technique, compliance, theophylline dose, and blood levels must all be reviewed.

Regular oral steroids may be needed in a very few cases with uncontrollable symptoms. These children are best managed by an experienced paediatrician. Oral steroids are always reduced to the lowest effective daily dose which produces asthma control. The drug is then given on alternate mornings to minimize side effects. These children need very careful monitoring and should be provided with a diary card to record symptoms and drug use. In addition, regular PEFR measurements at home with a mini-Wright Peak Flow Meter are strongly advised. An example of a simple diary card is given in Figure 45.2.

## Age of child

Under 18 months of age, symptoms usually arise in association with viral respiratory infections. The children are not usually very distressed but may wheeze quite loudly. Symptoms usually disappear within three to five days, but coughing, particularly at night, may be a persistent symptom. Antibiotics do not influence the illness nor do these children obtain much benefit from using beta-agonists. The effects of theophylline, sodium cromoglycate, and inhaled steroids are also limited at this age. Ketotifen may occasionally be of use, especially in those children with associated allergic rhinitis and/or atopic eczema. Children who are very distressed may require hospital admission where oxygen therapy, fluid management, and oxygen blood gas monitoring are required. Ipratropium bromide may transiently relieve wheezing in many of these children, and when all else fails intravenous steroids may be required. However, children over the age of 18 months begin to respond to drugs in a far more satisfactory manner. The age of the child then begins to influence the manner in which the various drugs should be administered.

## Route of administration

Inhalation is the preferred route for the administration of drugs for asthma. Obvious advantages include the fact that much lower doses are used than if the drug were to be given orally and the fact that the drugs are delivered directly to the lungs. Side effects are also considerably less likely to occur with inhaled drugs. Even children under four years can now use simple inhalers. Children under eight to ten years of age may have trouble using MDIs and simple spacer devices can improve the effectiveness of inhaled beta-agonist bronchodilators and require no inhalation skills. These spacer devices are usually plastic commercial pear-shaped devices. Almost as effective and far cheaper is the use of an empty plastic soft drink bottle with a hole in the end of it to incorporate the opening of the MDI. Although this device does not have the one-way valve of the commercial devices, it is quite adequate. With all types of inhalers and spacers, it is essential to educate the child and the parents in their correct use. Regular review of the technique is essential and careful attention to compliance and use should be maintained. Oral drugs are usually limited to night symptoms and are suitable when the child cannot use an inhaler device of any kind.

Leukotriene antagonist drugs such as montelukast and zafirlukast have recently become available. They are the first new class medicines to be introduced for persistent asthma treatment in 25 years. Their main role is likely to be for mild to moderate asthma and for exercise-induced bronchospasm. Their role as steroid-sparing agents for moderate to severe asthma is not established.

# Emergency therapy

## ACUTE SEVERE ASTHMA

Prompt treatment of acute severe asthma is very important. Parents and children must have a clear idea of what to do when an acute asthma attack occurs and must know when to seek medical help. This is especially important if the child is using a home nebulizer, as many parents are inclined to continue administering dose after dose of bronchodilator mediation and fail to realize that their child's asthma attack is very severe.

In all children old enough to use a peak flow meter, the response to treatment should be measured. Initially the child is given a nebulized beta-agonist bronchodilator. Failure to improve after an adequate dose of bronchodilator or a peak flow that is less than 25 per cent of the expected level are indications for admission to hospital. Steroids should not be withheld. Hydrocortisone (4 mg/kg) should immediately be administered intravenously. Nebulized salbutamol, fenoterol, or ipratropium bromide should be continued every two or three hours. Oxygen is very important and should be given via intra-nasal prongs.

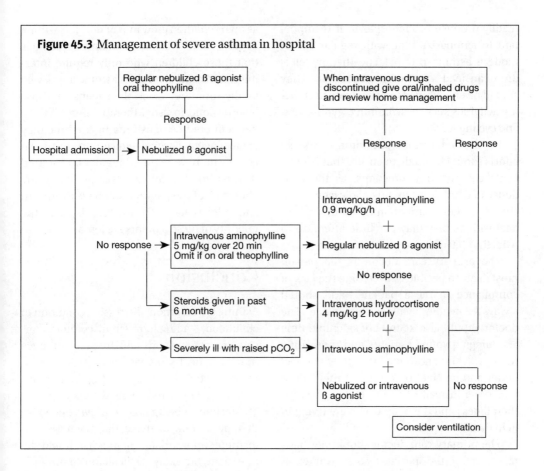

**Figure 45.3** Management of severe asthma in hospital

Dehydration may occur because of poor fluid intake, sweating, and hyperventilation, and must be corrected, but there is always the risk of overhydrating children. The wisest course is to administer only normal fluid requirements, usually in the form of five per cent dextrose water.

A management algorithm is shown in Figure 45.3. This can be applied in most centres. If there are any difficulties then the child should be referred to a specialist centre for further treatment.

*The warnings given previously about the use of intravenous aminophylline should be noted.*

No child should be discharged from hospital until recovery is adequate and the peak flow meter rate is at least above 80 per cent of the predicted value.

# Education of patients

With any chronic disease, patient education is extremely important, and this applies equally to the parents, who cannot be expected to follow a restrictive routine that involves much effort, administration of drugs, and expense unless they understand what they are to do and why they are doing it. Even the problem of environmental control requires a great deal of work in many cases and unless those involved understand the need for it, they are most unlikely to comply with directions.

The fact that asthma is a disease characterized by irritable airways must be explained to patients and parents. They must be made aware that people with asthma are different from others in that a great many factors may readily produce bronchospasm. It is important to emphasize that, with regular use of modern asthma prophylactic therapy, children can lead a virtually normal life. They should be encouraged to participate in sporting activities such as swimming, gymnastics, and cycling.

In the education programme special efforts should be made to ensure that adolescents comply with directions, as the incidence of death in asthmatic adolescents is of concern. These patients may be difficult to deal with as they may pay little attention to what they have been told over the years.

The primary care doctor is the person most likely to be able to overcome the lack of compliance in these patients, and should always be readily available for advice. The doctor should also spend considerable time encouraging young patients and motivating them with the knowledge that they will feel better and be able to do more if they follow directions instead of trying to fight against their illness and the people who are trying to help them.

The primary care doctor should not hesitate to call in the specialist, social worker, or psychologist to help in the more difficult cases.

## Asthma prognosis

There is a great deal of controversy as to whether asthmatic children 'outgrow' their asthma or not. Conflicting conclusions have been drawn from studies that have examined this question. Some authorities maintain that

as many children grow into or develop asthma as grow out of it. What is certainly apparent is that those children who only require intermittent treatment for their asthma are all well by the time they reach their teens. Of those who respond to usual therapy more than 50 per cent are free of asthma by the time they are teenagers. The worrying group consists of those who have required regular oral steroid therapy to control the symptoms. Here, almost all of the patients still have asthma in late adolescence. Of interest is that the majority of these patients are female.

## Conclusion

Asthma is a common, distressing condition in childhood, leading to much discomfort, concern, hospitalization, and frequent absence from school. Its management is simple in most affected children, allowing them to live normal, full lives and giving the doctor much satisfaction in being able to provide effective therapy. Failure to make the diagnosis and institute appropriate treatment should be rare today, but sadly is still all too common in many parts of southern Africa.

## References and further reading

THE BRITISH THORACIC SOCIETY, THE NATIONAL ASTHMA CAMPAIGN. 1997. The British guidelines on asthma management: 1995 review and position statement. *Thorax.* 52(1):s1–s2.

# 46

# Medications for common ailments

## GH SWINGLER

The following list covers some medications used in the *ambulatory* management of common paediatric ailments. It is consistent with the Standard Treatment Guidelines and Essential Drugs List for Primary Health Care (1998). This chapter should be read in conjunction with other texts, as it does not offer guidance on diagnosis, assessment of severity, or referrral criteria.

## ANAEMIA, IRON DEFICIENCY

- *Elemental iron* 3–4 mg/kg/day, i.e., Ferrous sulphate: 15 mg/kg/day, in 2–3 doses *or* Ferrous gluconate: 25 mg/kg/day, in 2–3 doses.
- Consider treatment for whipworm or hookworm.

## ASTHMA

### Acute severe

(See also Chapter 45: Childhood asthma; and Chapter 48: Common paediatric emergencies.)
- *Oxygen* via nasal cannula (4 L per min).
- *Salbutamol*: 0,5% solution by nebulization, 0,03 ml/kg, in 2–3 ml saline.

Repeat every 20 minutes for the first hour, if no relief. Thereafter 4 hourly.
- *Ipratropium bromide (Atrovent)*: 0,025% solution by nebulization, 0,5–1 ml mixed with salbutamol solution. Repeat 4 hourly.
- *Prednisone*: 1–2 mg/kg orally daily.

Bacterial infections are uncommon in acute severe asthma. Antibiotics are not indicated unless bacterial superinfection is strongly suspected.

### Chronic

See Chapter 45: Childhood asthma, p. 398, Figure 45.1.

## COMMON COLD

This can be managed at home. Advise the mother to give home care. This includes:
- feeding the child through the illness;
- Increasing fluids;
- clearing the nose with saline drops if it interferes with feeding; saline nosedrops (1/2 teaspoonful of salt, 1 teaspoonful of bicarbonate, in 300 ml of water);
- watching for signs indicating pneumonia;

and

- giving paracetamol for high fever or pain (Paracetamol*: 4–6 hourly, maximum of 4 doses per 24 hours).

Decongestants are of questionable effectiveness in children, especially if repeated doses are given. The side effects of symptomatic medications will usually outweigh any relief they might bring.

## *Paracetamol dosage:

3 mths–1 yr: 2,5–5 ml (60–120 mg)
1 yr–5 yrs: 5–10 ml (120–240 mg)
5 yrs–12 yrs: ½–1 tab (250–500 mg)
Over 12 yrs: 1–2 tab (500–1 000 mg)

## COUGH

- Cough mixtures are ineffective in children, and can be harmful. Soothe the throat with a safe remedy (tea with sugar or home-made cough syrup: hot water (1 cup) with honey (one teaspoonful) and lemon juice (1–2 squeezes).
- An exception is cough due to asthma, where bronchodilators help.
- Avoid in particular all remedies that contain atropine, alcohol, promethazine, or high doses of antihistamines generally.
- Cough and/or wheezing lasting for more than 2 weeks must be investigated for the cause.

## CROUP

### Mild

- Treat at home.
- Antibiotic therapy should not be given.
- Advise the mother to give home care.

- Paracetamol*: 4–6 hourly, maximum of 4 doses per 24 hours.

### Severe

See Chapter 48: Common paediatric emergencies.

## DIARRHOEA

(See also Chapter 38: Diarrhoeal disease)
- *Oral rehydration*: 1 sachet oral rehydration powder (e.g., Sorol, Gastrolyte) in 1 litre of clean water *or* 8 level teaspoons sugar and 1/2 level teaspoon salt in 1 litre of clean water.
- If there is fever and blood-streaking of the stools: *Nalidixic acid*: 50 mg/kg/day in 4 doses × 5 days (or an antibiotic, as indicated by local sensitivity patterns).
- If ill looking or under 3 mths, *Ceftriaxone* in hospital.

## ECZEMA

- Use aqueous cream for washing or bathing, and apply to dry areas as a moisturiser.
- For severe eczema, 1% hydrocortisone cream twice daily. Apply sparingly to face, and not at all around eyes, and maintain treatment with aqueous cream.
- Chlorpheniramine: twice daily (6 mths–1 yr: 1 mg; 1–5 yrs: 1–2 mg).

## FEVER AND 'FLU-LIKE' SYNDROMES

- Paracetamol*: 4–6 hourly, maximum of 4 doses per 24 hours.

## HIV INFECTION

*Pneumocystis carinii prophylaxis*
*Cotrimoxazole*: 3 doses per week (under 6 mths: 2,5 ml; 6 mths–5 yrs: 5 ml; over 5 yrs: 10 ml).

## IMPETIGO

- It is advisable to give an oral antibiotic (amoxycillin **) even for the mildest cases, but be guided by local antibiotic sensitivity patterns.
- For the lesions: 10% povidone iodine cream, three times a day *or* zinc oxide ointment, three times a day.

### **Amoxycillin dosage:

0–6 mths: 62,5 mg
6 mths–10 yrs: 125 mg
Over 10 yrs : 250 mg

## NAPPY RASH

- Good hygiene and exposure of the nappy area to sunlight are helpful.
- Apply 15% zinc oxide ointment with each nappy change.
- *Vioform* (3%) combined with *hydrocortisone* (1%) cream is very helpful for severe rashes.
- If there is no response or if skin folds are involved, suspect candida, and treat with *nystatin* ointment three times a day for 14 days after healing.
- If nystatin fails, 2% miconazole cream, three times a day for 14 days after healing.

## OTITIS MEDIA

### Acute

- Give an antibiotic for at least 5 days (preferably 10 days): oral cotrimoxazole, or amoxicillin**.
- Give paracetamol* for pain or high fever.
- Dry the child's ear by wicking if discharging.
- Antihistamines and decongestants are ineffective.

### Chronic

- If an antibiotic has not been given recently, start with a 10-day course.
- Wash out ear and keep dry.
- Demonstrate to the mother how to dry the child's ear by wicking at home.
- Reassess weekly and check for the development of complications. These require specialist treatment.
- Amoxicillin**
- Paracetamol*: 4–6 hourly, maximum of 4 doses per 24 hours.

## PAIN

- *Mild to moderate*: Paracetamol*: 4–6 hourly, maximum of 4 doses per 24 hours.
- *Severe*: Morphine: 6 mths–12 mths: 0,02 mg/kg; 1 yr–5 yrs: 2,5–5 mg; 6–12 yrs: 5–10 mg.

## PAPULAR URTICARIA

- Calamine lotion.
- Chlorpheniramine: twice daily (6 mths–1 yr: 1 mg; 1–5 yrs: 1–2 mg).
- Try to get rid of fleas and bed-bugs!

## PERTUSSIS

- Erythromycin: 25–50 mg/kg per day 6 hourly for 5 days.
- Salbutamol: 0,15 mg/kg as necessary 4 times a day for cough.

## PNEUMONIA

- Amoxycillin**: 3 times daily.
- Paracetamol*: 4–6 hourly, maximum of 4 doses per 24 hours.

## PURULENT NASAL DISCHARGE

Purulent nasal discharge alone or with cough is not an indication for antibiotic therapy.

Cotrimoxazole, ampicillin, or amoxycillin** should be considered only if the child has definite signs of bacterial sinusitis – persistent fever, sinus tenderness, swelling of the face or around an eye.

## RINGWORM

- For scalp and nail infections, use griseofulvin orally: 10 mg/kg (125 mg tabs) for 4–6 weeks.
- For ringworm of body, use Whitfield's ointment, 6% benzoic acid and 3% salicylic acid, 2–3 times daily. Do not use in sensitive areas.
- On face, in groin, or other sensitive areas, or if above treatment is unsuccessful, 2% miconazole cream.

## SCABIES

- After hot bath and scrubbing, apply 12,5% benzyl benzoate. Reapply to any areas that must be washed. Wash off after 24 hours.
- In infants under 6 mths: sulphur ointment 2,5%.
- 5% monosulfiram soap may be used.
- If benzyl benzoate unsuccessful, use 5% permethrin cream.

## SEIZURES

(See also Chapter 38.)

- *To stop a seizure*: Diazepam: rectal (under 10 kg: 5 mg [1 ml]; over 10 kg: 10 mg [2 ml]) *or* IV: 0,2–0,3 mg/kg (max 10 mg) over 3 minutes (NOT IMI).
- *If no response*: Phenytoin 10–20 mg/kg at 1–3 mg/kg/minute (NOT IMI) *or* Phenobarbitone: 10–20 mg/kg IVI.

## Epilepsy

- Generalized tonic clonic. and complex partial (focal, with loss of consciousness):

Phenobarbitone: orally 3–5 mg/kg at night.
- Review behaviour and academic performance.
- If deterioration on treatment, change to carbamazepine. Carbamazepine: orally, 2–3 times daily (first 2 weeks: 8 mg/kg/day; then 10–15 mg/kg/day; max dose: 20 mg/kg/day).

## STOMATITIS

This is most commonly due to herpes virus, which causes painful mouth ulcers and swollen gums.
- Ensure good fluid intake (cold fluids are best).
- Mouthwashes or paints are ineffective.
- Give sips of water to keep mouth clean.
- Give paracetamol* for the discomfort: 4–6 hourly, maximum of 4 doses per 24 hours.
- Give an extra feed a day for a week after recovery.

## TONSILLITIS AND PHARYNGITIS

Most sore throats should not be treated with antibiotics as they are of viral origin. If streptococcal pharyngitis is suspected, give penicillin V or amoxycillin (125–250 mg three times daily) by mouth, only if compliance can be assured as it must be administered for 10 days. Otherwise give benzathine penicillin as a single injection (0,6–1,2 million units). Cotrimoxazole is not effective.
- Penicillin V: 6 hourly for 10 days (5–10 kg: 62,5 mg; 10–30 kg: 125 mg; over 30 kg: 250 mg).
- Benzathine penicillin: under 30 kg: 600 000 IU; over 30 kg: 1 200 000 IU.

## Suppurative complications

Several weeks' treatment with antibiotics that are effective against *S. aureus* may be required. Drainage of an abscess may be necessary.

## URINARY TRACT INFECTION

Antibiotics should be used according to local bacterial sensitivities. In some areas of South Africa, common pathogens are almost all resistant to cotrimoxazole and amoxicillin.
*For children over 3 months*:

- Amoxycillin: orally
  - under 20 kg: 20–40mg/kg/day in 3 divided doses for 7–14 days.
  - over 20 kg: 250–500 mg 8 hourly for 7–14 days.
  *or*
- Cotrimoxazole: orally
  - 6 wks–5 mths: 2,5 ml, twice daily for 7–14 days.
  - 6 mths–5 yrs: 5 ml twice daily for 7–14 days.
  - 6 yrs –12 yrs: 10 ml or 1 tab (80/400 mg) twice daily for 7–14 days.
  *or*
- Cefadroxil: orally, 25 mg/kg/day in two divided doses for 7–14 days.
  *or*
- Nalidixic acid: orally, 50 mg/kg/day in 4 doses for 5–14 days.
- Paracetamol*: 4–6 hourly, maximum of 4 doses per 24 hours.

## URTICARIA

- Chlorpheniramine: twice daily (6 mths–1 yr: 1 mg;1–5 yrs: 1–2 mg).

## WHEEZING

- Administer a rapid-acting bronchodilator, such as nebulized salbutamol, and assess response after 15 minutes.
- If central cyanosis or child not able to drink: admit, give oxygen, give antibiotic, treat fever, supportive care.
- If respiratory distress persists, but none of the above: admit, continue bronchodilator, give antibiotic, treat fever, supportive care.

- If no respiratory distress, no central cyanosis, child is able to drink, but breathing fast: treat as pneumonia (see above).
- If no respiratory distress, no central cyanosis, child is able to drink, and no fast breathing: Give oral salbutamol at home.
- *Cough and/or wheezing lasting for more than 2 weeks must be investigated for the cause.*

## WORMS

- Mebendazole: orally, twice daily for 3 days (1–2 yrs: 100 mg; over 2 yrs: 100 mg) *or* 500 mg as a single dose.
  *or*
- Albendazole: as a single dose (1–2 yrs: 200 mg; over 2 yrs: 400 mg).

## References and further reading

ESSENTIAL DRUGS PROGRAMME. 1998. *Standard treatment guidelines and essential drugs list for South Africa. Primary health care.* Pretoria: Department of Health.

DEL MAR CB & GLASSZIOU PR. 2000. Antibiotics for the symptoms and complications of sore throat. (Cochrane Review). *The Cochrane Library.* Issue 1. Oxford: Update Software. Updated quarterly.

TAVERNER D, BICKFORD L, and DRAPER M. 2000. Nasal decongestants for the common cold. (Cochrane Review). *The Cochrane Library.* Issue 1. Oxford: Update Software. Updated quarterly.

# 47

# Childhood Poisoning

IT HAY & MA KIBEL

Poisoning is fully preventable, and it is the caretaker's responsibility to ensure a safe environment. The medicines and chemicals in the child's environment will determine the different poisoning profiles that occur in traditional, transitional, and modern communities. Paraffin, plants, rodent poisons, agricultural remedies, and household substances are important causes of unintentional poisonings in rural communities, whereas medicinal drugs and household substances are the most common offenders in urban environments. As soon as the child becomes ambulant he or she is 'at risk', and accidental poisoning is particularly a problem for the under-five-year old.

Knowledge of the local poisoning profile is essential to the health professional practising in any area. Accidental ingestion of paraffin, for example, is primarily a summertime problem caused by thirsty children mistaking paraffin for water. Insecticides are used during specific agricultural seasons, and berries and seeds are also seasonal poisonings.

Traditional healers utilize herbs, roots, bark, and seeds in the preparation of their medicines. Whilst many of these are harmless, or indeed useful, some are very toxic.

Not much is known about the medicinal and toxic properties of these preparations and an attempt should be made to contact the traditional healers to identify and analyse the active substances in their medicines, so that the clinical effects can be described and the body of knowledge extended. Until this is available, symptomatic management will remain the mainstay of treatment.

Deaths involving poisoning, including paraffin and herbal, are not natural and the death certificate should not be completed. In these cases the reverse side of the death certificate should be completed for legal and forensic review. Keep detailed clinical notes on all poisoning cases (as is good clinical practice) as they have a tendency to reappear in court!

Health care workers sometimes overlook underlying disease when making the diagnosis of 'traditional medicine intoxication', and so miss the opportunity to treat curable disease.

## Specific prevention

Labelling information on medicines must include the name, concentration, and amount dispensed.

## Health promotion

The following points should be emphasized in poison prevention programmes aimed at parents, children, the public and manufacturers of potentially toxic substances:

- keep cleaning supplies, medicines, garage products, and insecticides out of reach of children;
- store food away from these products. Do not store dangerous solutions in food or beverage containers;
- insist on safety closures and know how to use them;
- always call medicine by its proper name; do not take it in your child's presence as children love to imitate;
- heed cautions and instructions on labels. First aid and treatment of poisoning should be included on the label;
- if you are interrupted while using a hazardous product, store it safely and out of reach of children. Safely discard and dispose of unnecessary toxic substances after use;
- know what your child can do. Store substances securely out of reach;
- don't eat seeds and berries from unknown plants;
- know the phone number of your clinic, doctor, and poison information centre.

Blister packaging and child-resistant containers have been effective in reducing the incidence of accidental medicine poisonings, but one must remember that they are not 'child-proof'! Lock-up medicine cupboards are ideal but expensive, and children are expert climbers and key-finders. Children must be taught about the hazards of playing with, and ingesting, unknown substances.

# Early diagnosis and management

(For a full description the reader is referred to a recognised reference on poisoning).

### FIRST AID

## Ingested poison

- The range of toxic substances and medications is today so huge, and the management of poisoning so complex that the best first aid measure is to telephone the nearest poisons centre for advice.
- Activated charcoal (to diminish poison absorption) can be given before transfer to a medical facility (1g/kg in 50–100 ml water). It is favoured over induction of vomiting and gastric lavage.
- Syrup of Ipecacuanha to induce vomiting is no longer in favour, and should be abandoned (Terebein, 1999). At best, its action is unpredictable, and an overdose can have toxic effects.
- Never use salt solutions or cathartics.
- Lay persons should not attempt treatment if the patient is convulsing or unconscious.
- Transport the child to a medical facility where gastric lavage can be performed under controlled conditions
  - if a life-threatening dose has been taken
  - if within 60 minutes of ingestion.
- Multi-dose activated charcoal (to absorb residual poison) is of proven benefit if the child has ingested life-threatening amounts of certain drugs (e.g., carbamazepine, phenobarbitone, quinine, theophylline).

## Inhaled poison

- Carry the victim to fresh air immediately.
- Give artificial respiration if breathing is depressed.

409

## Skin contamination

- Apply a stream of water to the skin while removing clothing.
- Cleanse skin thoroughly with soap and water.
- Do not attempt to use chemical antidotes.

## Eye contamination

Holding the eyelids apart, wash the eye for five minutes with running water.

## Snake bite

Immobilize the patient and transport to a treatment facility as soon as possible. Try to remember the snake's colouring, appearance, and behaviour for later identification – amateur snake collectors are generally more useful to consult than doctors!

Do not apply a tourniquet but apply a firm crepe bandage to the whole limb, regardless of the site of the bite, in order to delay lymphatic absorption of the venom and to diminish pain and swelling.

Observe the patient's breathing very carefully; this should be done for at least 24 hours in a health care facility. Give artificial respiration if the patient's breathing is depressed.

Use antivenom immediately if one is certain that the bite was due to a mamba or cobra. The dose is four 10 ml ampoules of polyvalent antivenom given intravenously. Give chlortrimetron (antihistamine) concurrently to prevent mild horse serum reactions. Adrenaline must be available to administer in cases of severe hypersensitive reactions. Corticosteroids have no place in the emergency treatment of snakebite.

Large amounts of intravenous fluids, carefully monitored, are mandatory in the case of puff adder bites.

## Paraffin

Accidental ingestion of paraffin is the most common form of childhood poisoning in South Africa. This problem will escalate with increased paraffin usage and will only diminish when affordable electricity becomes widely available.

Paraffin is mistaken for water by thirsty toddlers and is accidentally ingested from carelessly stored household containers. It is predominantly a summertime problem. Paraffin is easily volatized during swallowing or vomiting and the risk of aspiration and chemical pneumonitis is very high, even with small amounts. Hypoxia makes oxygen therapy the most important therapeutic modality. Emetics are absolutely contra-indicated. Limit intravenous fluids to twice the insensible fluid loss (i.e., $2 \times 25$ ml/kg/day) as overhydration may aggravate pulmonary oedema. Antibiotic usage is controversial but may be indicated. Pyrexia for one or two days is a normal feature in the acutely poisoned child. Morbidity is high and case fatality rates for hospitalized children are around 2 per cent.

Prevention of the problem is clearly where attention is needed. Child-resistant containers are effective. Safe storage of household paraffin must be included in health education messages to both adults and children. As paraffin is also used for various domestic cleaning purposes, this not infrequently results in the use of intermediate containers, which constitute a further hazard for children.

# Substance identification

Remind the enquirer to bring the poison to the health care facility for identification, or send someone to fetch it.

## General measures

There are six important principles to remember:
- give first aid advice, instruct the caretaker to bring the poison for identification, and arrange for the safe transport of the patient to a medical facility while monitoring the respiratory depression;
- maintain respiration and control shock;
- identify poison if possible but do not delay life-supporting treatment in this process;
- remove poison to minimize further absorption;
- give the specific antidote if available. (Remember that *very few* poisons have specific antidotes.) Toxic antidotes should not be used unless poison identification is certain;
- give specific treatment. The important principle here is to *consult*. Telephonic contact with poison information centres is generally available; these are listed in Table 47.1.

These centres will provide detailed information on the symptoms and signs of the poisoning, as well as details on toxic doses, general and specific treatments, and access to the manufacturers for very specific information. If one is uncertain about the poison identification, the centre will be able to assist with probable identification based on symptoms and signs. A good handbook (such as Dreisbach's *Handbook of Poisoning*) should always be available.

**Table 47.1** Poison information centres in South Africa

**BELLVILLE**
Pharmacology & Toxicology Consultation Centre
Tygerberg Hospital
Tel: (021) 931-6129 (all hours)
*SPECIAL INTEREST IN BITES & STINGS*

**BLOEMFONTEIN**
Department of Pharmacology
Poisons Control & Medicines Information
Tel: 082 491 0160 (all hours)

**CAPE TOWN**
Poisons Reference Service
Red Cross War Memorial Children's Hospital
Tel: (021) 689-5227 (all hours)

**DURBAN**
St Augustine's Trauma & Poison Unit
St Augustine's Hospital
Tel: (0800) 333-444 (all hours)

**JOHANNESBURG**
Garden City Clinic
Tel: (011) 495-5112

MRI (Medical Rescue International)
Tel: (011) 403-7080 (all hours)
Toll free: 0800 111 997

## Notification

Notification enables local authorities to investigate the circumstances surrounding accidental poisonings so as to prevent recurrences. It also enables passive surveillance by the health authority.

The following poisonings are notifiable:
- lead (ICD Code E866);
- agricultural and stock remedies registered in terms of the Fertilizers, Farm Feeds, Agricultural Remedies and Stock Remedies Act (No 38 of 1947) (ICD Code E863);

- food poisoning, where four or more cases occur (ICD Codes 003, 005, E865).

# Limitation of disability

Utilize available information as provided by the information centre. Supportive management requires that attention be given to pain treatment, fluid and electrolyte imbalance, acidosis, body temperature regulation, and nutrition.

The impact of the poisoning on specific organ systems must be carefully evaluated.

*Respiratory tract:* Examine for an adequate airway, hypoxaemia, and respiratory depression.

*Central nervous system:* Examine for coma, convulsions, delirium, hyperactivity, and hypoglycaemia.

*Cardiovascular system:* Examine for signs of circulatory failure.

*Genito-urinary tract:* Examine for signs of renal failure. Remember that the onset of renal failure may be very insidious.

*Gastrointestinal tract:* Vomiting and diarrhoea generally aid in the removal of the poison but, if prolonged, may lead to fluid imbalance.

Hepatic cell damage and cholestasis may result from poisoning and expert help must be utilized.

*Haematopoietic system* involvement may result in methaemoglobinaemia, haemolysis, or agranulocytosis.

Regional hospitals and academic hospitals will be able to provide specific therapies such as heavy metal chelation, forced osmotic diuresis, haemoperfusion, and dialysis, should these be required according to management guidelines provided by the poison information centre. These hospitals also have access to pharmacokinetic study laboratories if needed.

# Rehabilitation

Medical rehabilitation will occasionally be required. Parents frequently need to be counselled as the poisoning episodes generally cause a great deal of anxiety. Specific advice, as outlined in the sections on health promotion and specific prevention, needs to be emphasized.

Children who ingest poisons on a number of occasions are called 'poison repeaters'. Special attention must be given to these children. They may live in disorganized homes or be particularly adventurous. On the other hand this may be purposeful behaviour suggesting that careful attention be given to emotional problems.

## References and further reading

DREISBACH RH & ROBERTSON WO. 1987. *Handbook of Poisoning,* 12th ed. Lange Medical Publications.

HARRISON VC (ed.). 1999. *Paediatric handbook,* 5th ed. Cape Town: Oxford University Press.

KEMPE H et al. 1987. 9th ed. *Current paediatric diagnosis and treatment,* 9th ed. Lange Medical Publications.

POLNAY L & HULL D. 1993. *Manual of community paediatrics,* 2nd ed. Edinburgh: Churchill Livingstone.

TEREBEIN M. 1999. Consensus statement; Recent advances in Pediatric Toxicology. *Paediatric Clinics of North America.* 46(6):1179–88.

# 48

# Common paediatric emergencies

## GH SWINGLER & JD DAUBENTON

This chapter provides an overview of common paediatric emergencies and their management. It highlights important general principles and specific aspects of management, but does not offer detailed 'recipes' for managing specific conditions. The reader is referred to standard texts for further details. Practical training in paediatric emergencies is available from the Resuscitation Council of South Africa, PO Box 1555, Northcliff, 2155, Tel (011) 4781874; or PO Box 15652, Panorama 7506, Tel (021) 928390.

## General principles

### RECOGNIZE SERIOUSLY ILL CHILDREN EARLY

Early recognition of seriously ill children is of utmost importance. It enables earlier treatment, which is much simpler and more effective than heroic efforts on a pre-terminal child. To achieve this, all children should be triaged on arrival at a health facility, and monitored while waiting to be seen. All staff in a health facility (including clerical and cleaning staff) should have basic training in the identification of children who are seriously ill.

### Serious illness

Apart from cyanosis, unconsciousness and convulsions, other signs which suggest a very ill child who needs immediate attention include:
- failure to make eye contact with the mother;
- lethargy;
- floppiness;
- severe lower chest wall indrawing;
- stridor in a calm child;
- dehydration; and
- purpura or petechiae.

### GET THE BASICS RIGHT

It is of utmost importance to get the basics right. Most of the benefits of paediatric emergency management come from ensuring an adequate airway, appropriate oxygen administration, intravascular volume replacement, correction of hypoglycaemia, and early antibiotic administration (if an underlying infection is present). Even if more advanced techniques are necessary, they will not be effective if this basic management is not attended to.

## Priority attention

Children who are less ill but who neverthe-less need priority attention (i.e., should jump the queue) include those who have none of the above signs but who are:
• not feeding;
• vomiting everything;
• have fast breathing;
• have a history of toxin ingestion; and
• infants under seven days of age.

Even if they look well, children with diarrhoea need to be observed and given oral rehydration solution while they are waiting to be seen.

### COMMUNICATION

If a child needs transfer to another facility, communication with the receiving facility is very important. Initial on-site treatment can be optimized, management during transfer planned, and arrangements made at the receiving hospital for the child's arrival.

### FLUID THERAPY IN SHOCK

This includes severe dehydration due to gas-troenteritis.

Hypovolaemia is by far the commonest cause of shock in children.

Early recognition of shock is very impor-tant. The first sign is tachycardia. This is fol-lowed by cold hands and feet with a pro-longed capillary filling time, and peripheral pulses that are weaker than central pulses (e.g., brachials). *A fall in blood pressure is a late and pre-terminal sign.*

### Management

• Oxygen by face mask or nasal prongs.
• Intravenous plasma volume replacement

(Ringers lactate, Plasmalyte B): 15–20 ml/kg as fast as the drip will run.
• Then re-assess the circulation.
• If signs of shock persist, give another 10 ml/kg.
• Identify the cause of the shock. In southern Africa diarrhoeal disease is the commonest cause. Other important causes that may not be obvious include septicaemia and internal haemorrhage.

### IF AN IVI LINE CANNOT BE PUT UP

When a drip cannot be set up, an intra-osseous infusion is easier to set up than an IVI line. It is a suitable alternative in an emergency in a *child under five years* (see VC Harrison, 1999, chapter 37, for details of the technique).

### REHYDRATION IN GASTROENTERITIS

Use half-strength Darrow's solution in five per cent dextrose, and give 10 ml/kg for each one per cent of clinical dehydration (i.e., if a child is 10 per cent dehydrated, the rehydra-tion fluid required = 100 ml/kg). The total rehydration volume is calculated to run in over 6 to 12 hours. In patients who are mal-nourished, who are hypernatraemic, or who have significant respiratory disease, it may be safer to give the rehydration slowly over 24 hours. Whichever method is used, frequent re-evaluation of the hydration status (every three to four hours) and adjustment of the fluid rate is essential. In the absence of shock or persistent vomiting, rehydration may be given orally or by infusion via a nasogastric tube.

The WHO recommendations for the more rapid correction of severe dehydration – 70 ml/kg in 2,5 hours (age 12 months to 5 years) or five hours (age under 12 months) – can also be used but may be hazardous in patients

414

who are malnourished, hypernatraemic, or have significant respiratory disease. With rapid rehydration the patient's state of hydration must be checked every one to two hours.

## MAINTENANCE FLUIDS

Maintenance fluid in diarrhoeal disease should be given in the form of the child's usual milk feed. With severe or persistent vomiting the volumes for rehydration and maintenance may need to be given intravenously until the vomiting has settled.

*Requirements:*
- Under one year: 120 ml/kg/24 hours.
- Older than one year: 80–100 ml/kg/24 hours.

An additional amount of fluid may be necessary if ongoing losses are large.

## SEIZURES

The three aspects of management are life support, stopping the seizure, and finding the cause of the seizure:

## Life support

- *Airway:* lie the child on her side, extend the neck, and hold the jaw forward. Do not try to force anything into the mouth.
- *Breathing:* give oxygen.
- *Circulation:* check for shock or hypertension, and correct when necessary.

## Stopping the seizure

- Diazepam (Valium): rectally (under 10 kg: 5 mg (1 ml); over 10 kg: 10 mg (2 ml). Use a 1-ml syringe (keep a supply with the diazepam ampules).
  *or*
- IVI 0,3 mg/kg (max 10 mg) IVI over 10 minutes.

- If response is unsatisfactory, repeat once after 15 minutes.
- Diazepam given intramuscularly is *not* effective.
- Diazepam is very short acting – following multiple or prolonged (more than 30 minutes) seizures, give phenobarbitone 20 mg/kg IMI or IV over 5 minutes, to a maximum of 200 mg.
- *If the seizure continues:* Phenobarbitone as above (if not already given).
- *If no response after a further 15 minutes:* Phenobarbitone: 10 mg/kg IVI slowly.
- *If no response after a further 15 minutes:* Phenytoin (Epanutin): 15–20 mg/kg in normal saline IVI over 15 minutes (with ECG monitoring, if available). *Never give phenytoin IMI.*

These drugs (particularly given intravenously) may depress respiration, and therefore the means to resuscitate/ventilate must be available.

## Finding the cause

The likely causes of seizures depend on age (see Table 48.1). It is particularly important to exclude hypoglycaemia, meningitis, and hypertension. The younger the child the more important it is to look for a treatable cause for a seizure.

## DECREASED LEVEL OF CONSCIOUSNESS/COMA

- *Airway:* ensure that airway is patent. This is usually achieved by turning the child on his/her side (but not if trauma suspected).
- *Breathing:* ensure and maintain adequate ventilation.
- *Circulation:* correct shock or hypertension.
- *Then evaluate for:*
  - raised intracranial pressure;
  - focal neurological deficit;

415

**Table 48.1** Likely causes of seizures

| Neonate | One month–five years | Over five years |
|---|---|---|
| Hypoglycaemia | Febrile (over 6 months) | Epilepsy |
| Electrolyte disturbances | Meningitis/ encephalitis | Meningitis/encephalitis |
| Birth injury | Encephalopathy, e.g., shigella | Tuberculoma/abscess |
| Birth asphyxia | Hypoglycaemia | Brain damage/defects |
| CNS infections | Electrolyte disturbances | Toxins/metabolic |
| Cerebral malformations | Brain defects/ damage | Tumour |
| Drugs | Toxins | Vascular |
| Inborn metabolic errors | Epilepsy | |

  - meningism;
  - signs of trauma; and
  - hypoglycaemia.
- *If raised intracranial pressure:*
  - elevate the head;
  - treat shock, if present;
  - treat convulsions, if present; and
  - treat the cause.
- *Consider:*
  - mannitol 0,5–1 gm/kg IV;
  - hyperventilation; and
  - dexamethazone 0,2-0,4 mg/kg IV
    (doubtful value).

Common causes of coma in children include a post-ictal state, shock, drugs and toxins, meningitis, hypoglycaemia, and head injury. The differential diagnosis depends on the presence or absence of focal signs and the intracranial pressure (ICP).

## Decreased level of consciousness: no focal signs

| Normal ICP | Raised ICP |
|---|---|
| CNS infection | CNS infection |
| Concussion (trauma) | Trauma |
| Post-ictal state | Hydrocephalus |
| Drug intoxication | Tumour |
| Most metabolic | Some metabolic |
| encephalopathies | encephalopathies |

## Decreased level of consciousness: focal signs

| Normal ICP | Raised ICP |
|---|---|
| Post-ictal with | |
| Todd's paralysis | CNS infection |
| CNS infection | Trauma (subdural, etc.) |
| Vascular disease | Tumour |
| Cerebral contusion | Vascular malformation |

### MENINGITIS

The diagnosis of meningitis is very difficult in infants and young children. *Suspicion* is the key to the diagnosis. The early presenting complaints are vague. The younger the child, the more non-specific the signs and symptoms. Newborns may present with poor feeding, lethargy, apnoea, a full fontanelle, and fever or hypothermia. *Neck stiffness is usually absent.* In older infants symptoms are irritability, drowsiness, poor feeding, high-pitched cry, high fever, and a full fontanelle. *Vomiting* is an important clue, especially if it is severe or lasting longer than a day or two, or getting worse. Toddlers and older children have a similar presentation to adults with fever, headache, vomiting, photophobia, and neck stiffness. Seizures may be a presenting feature at any age.

Lumbar puncture is the only way to make a diagnosis of meningitis and should be done on *suspicion* of meningitis, unless there is a contra-indication (depressed level of consciousness, petechiae or 'focal' neurologic signs). If there will be a delay before a lumbar puncture can be done, or if it is contra-indicated, do a blood culture and start antibiotic treatment immediately.

- Ceftriaxone 100 mg/kg/dose IMI daily. In children under three months add ampicillin 200 mg/kg/day IVI in four divided doses.
- Dexamethasone 0,15 mg/kg IVI, preferably before the first dose of antibiotic, and then six hourly for four days.

Remember that meningococcal infections are notifiable, and close contacts require prophylaxis with rifampicin:

- adults: 600 mg 12 hourly for two days;
- children over one year: 10 mg/kg, 12 hourly, for two days;
- children under one year: 5 mg/kg, 12 hourly, for two days.

## ACUTE SEVERE ASTHMA

Peak expiratory flow rate is the most important measure of the severity of the attack (and the response to treatment) in children over five years. Every clinic and GP should have a peak flow meter and a chart or tables for predicted values for height. A peak flow rate of 70 to 90 per cent represents a mild attack, 50 to 70 per cent a severe attack, and less than 50 per cent a very severe attack. In children under five years, the respiratory rate is the most helpful single measurement. A rate of more than 40/min is cause for concern. A silent chest or unexplained restlessness at any age are very serious signs.

- *Oxygen:* hypoxia is the mode of death in acute severe asthma. Oxygen is the priority. Give 100 per cent oxygen by face mask (4 ℓ/min) or nasal catheter (2 ℓ/min).
- *Bronchodilators:* a metred dose inhaler

with a spacer is at least as effective as a nebulizer, and is probably safer.

- – *Salbutamol* (Ventolin) by metered dose inhaler. In children of five years and under, use a spacer with a mask. In older children, use a spacer without a mask. Give four to five puffs (one puff at a time) into the spacer, allowing the child to breathe normally for 20 seconds after each puff.

    *and*

- – *Ipratropium* (Atrovent). Administer as for salbutamol, but with the first dose only.

  Measure the peak flow rate before and after bronchodilator use.

  If no response, repeat salbutamol after 20 minutes, but do *not* repeat ipratropium.

- *Steroids:* Prednisone 2 mg/kg orally stat (max dose 40 mg). If vomiting, use dexamethasone 0,3 mg/kg IM instead.

*Patients in extremis* with a very severe attack should be given adrenalin 0,3 ml subcutaneously immediately, and salbutamol (4 ug/kg IV) if they are unable to use a nebulizer. Intravenous theophylline should not be used in children outside an intensive care unit. Rectal theophylline should never be used in children.

## SEVERE LOWER RESPIRATORY INFECTION

Signs of severe lower respiratory infections include not feeding, grunting, lethargy, severe lower chest wall indrawing, and cyanosis.

- Give 100 per cent oxygen by face mask (4 ℓ/min), nasal prongs, or nasal catheter (2 ℓ/min).
- Start ampicillin (100 mg/kg/day in four doses) IVI. If under three months of age, severely malnourished, or if very severe or extensive pneumonia, consider adding gentamicin (3–6 mg/kg/day) IV daily.

417

- Treat wheeze, if present. The place of bronchodilators is uncertain in bronchiolitis and bronchopneumonia. If used, use a beta-2 agonist (e.g., salbutamol) rather than theophylline. If there is no response, do not continue. If the bronchodilator does work, consider asthma.

## STRIDOR

*Viral croup* is by far the commonest cause of stridor. Features that suggest another cause are:
- the dramatic onset of severe obstruction (foreign body);
- drooling, or the patient prefers a sitting position (epiglottitis, retropharyngeal abscess);
- systemic 'toxicity' (bacterial infection, including epiglottitis);
- following measles (herpes); and
- ulcers in the mouth (herpes).

Assessment of severity *of viral croup*:
- Grade I: Inspiratory stridor only.
- Grade II: Inspiratory and expiratory stridor and/or prolonged expiration
- Grade III: Active expiration (i.e., visible or palpable contraction of abdominal muscles) or palpable pulsus paradoxus.
- Grade IV: Marked retractions, apathy, cyanosis.

*Remember: Stridor becomes softer as the obstruction becomes worse.*

## Management of viral croup

### Grade I obstruction
Observe at home, provided that the condition is not getting worse and home circumstances are favourable.

### Grade II obstruction
- Hospitalize.

- Keep the child comfortable (crying makes the obstruction worse).
  - support the mother;
  - continue oral feeding;
  - avoid painful procedures; and
  - give paracetamol if the child is febrile.
- Nebulized adrenalin:
  Mix 1 ml of 1:1000 adrenalin with 1 ml saline and nebulize (with oxygen, if possible). Repeat every 15 minutes until the expiratory obstruction is relieved.
- Steroids:
  Prednisone 2 mg/kg orally or dexamethasone 0,5 mg/kg IMI or IVI as a single dose. Repeat after 12 to 24 hours if no improvement. Give steroids to all patients except those with recent measles or oral Herpes.
- Antibiotic:
  Use amoxycillin (Amoxil) if bacterial croup is suspected, i.e., if there is 'toxicity' or fever > 38 °C or purulent sputum or pneumonia.

### Grade III obstruction
- As for grade II.
- If no improvement within one hour, intubate or perform tracheostomy under general anaesthesia.

## POISONING
See Chapter 47: Childhood poisoning.

## ANAPHYLAXIS
This is commonly due to drugs (i.e., penicillin), vaccines, sera, and insect bites and stings.

## Management

- Adrenaline (1:1000): 0,3–0,5 ml IMI;
- Promethazine (phenergan): 0,25–0,5 mg/kg IMI;
- IV fluids if shocked;

- Oxygen; and
- Hydrocortisone: 5–10 mg/kg, IVI 4–6 hourly, for 24 hours.

## ACUTE HYPERTENSION

It is important to measure blood pressure in any child routinely, but this is essential in children with coma or convulsions.

If symptomatic/severe acute hypertension:
Nifedipine (Adalat): 0,3–0,5 mg/kg/dose sublingual.
Puncture the capsule and squeeze out under the tongue. Use only if fluid overload, e.g., in acute glomerulonephritis.
   *or*
Hydralazine (Nepresol): 0,1–0,3 mg/kg/dose IM or slow IV, max 20 mg/dose.
With severe fluid overload, such as occurs in acute glomerulonephritis, furosemide (Lasix): 2 mg/kg should be given orally or IV in severe cases.

## CARDIAC FAILURE

- Digoxin (Lanoxin): initial dose: 0,005 mg/kg/dose eight hourly for three doses only. Maintenance dose: 0,005mg/kg/dose 12 hourly orally.
- Furosemide (Lasix): 1–2 mg/kg/day IV or oral.
- Potassium supplements: 50 mg/kg/day.
- Restricted fluid: 70–80 ml/kg/day.
- Oxygen if patient is in significant respiratory distress.
- Salt restriction/low-salt infant formula.

## References and further reading

HARRISON VC (ed.). 1999. *Handbook of paediatrics*, 5th ed. Cape Town: Oxford University Press.

# 49 Sudden Infant Death Syndrome

## MA KIBEL

The Sudden Infant Death Syndrome (SIDS), commonly referred to as 'cot death' was first defined by Beckwith in 1969 as 'the death of an infant or young child, which is unexpected by history and in whom a thorough necroscopy examination fails to reveal an adequate cause of death'. Unexpected infant deaths have occurred since biblical times and have gone under several different names. The classical belief was that these deaths were due to overlaying or suffocation. In fact, the official title for the condition in the USA until the early 1950s was 'accidental mechanical suffocation'. In the developed world, SIDS is the commonest cause of death between one week and one year of age. It occurs in all countries and socio-economic groups, but rates vary widely, from well below one to over six per thousand live births.

A careful autopsy will fail to demonstrate an adequate cause of death in the majority of infants. Many, however, show changes indicative of a mild, 'non-lethal' respiratory or bowel infection. In a minority, frank pathology will be found, such as pneumonia or meningitis, intracranial trauma, or significant cardiac anomaly. In these cases, death may indeed have been totally sudden and unexpected; more often there have been prior symptoms that have been unrecognized by the mother or caregiver.

## Epidemiology

Regional comparisons of SIDS incidence rates have limitations, as there is still considerable controversy over the definition of SIDS and little consensus between forensic and paediatric pathologists about what constitutes 'an adequate cause of death' (Rambaud et al., 1994). Some insist that a death-scene examination or review must be included to exclude accidents, infant neglect, or abuse. There is little consistency also as to whether sudden deaths under one month are included, or whether infants who die suddenly and unexpectedly with underlying disorders such as bronchopulmonary dysplasia should be regarded as SIDS. The method of classification suggested by Arneil et al. (1982) is still useful to facilitate meaningful regional comparisons:

- group 1: cause of death definitely established;
- group 2: minor findings which may be related to death or a contributing factor;

- group 3: no abnormal findings which would account for death; and
- group 4: autopsy not performed, and no explanation forthcoming.

It is not surprising then that in southern Africa, and in developing countries generally, the incidence of SIDS is difficult to establish. This is because:

- detailed autopsies by paediatric pathologists are only available at larger centres;
- the majority of infants who are reported as dying suddenly show advanced disease at autopsy, such as gastroenteritis or meningitis, which was inadequately treated; or no medical treatment had been sought or was available; and
- doctors and pathologists often prefer to ascribe causes such as bronchopneumonia or gastroenteritis rather than the more honest 'cause unknown' or SIDS.

Accurate estimates of incidence are thus impossible to obtain unless special population studies are carried out. In a Cape Town study of deaths below the age of four years in 1983, cot death was listed as the diagnosis in 29 infants in a total of 19 463 births (an incidence per 1 000 live births of 1,06 for whites and 1,57 for coloured infants). However, when circumstances surrounding death and post-mortem data were analysed, it was considered that 58 infants could be so classified, the respective incidences remaining the same for whites, but rising to 3,41 for coloured infants (Sinclair-Smith & Kibel, 1986). A recent prospective study from Zimbabwe reported an incidence of only 0,2 per thousand in a black township community (Wolf & Ikeogou 1996), and South African data show a relative risk for black infants, which is one-third that of whites (Davies & Kibel, 2000).

# Risk factors

SIDS is commonest in infants between the ages of two and four months, but may occur in younger and much older infants, and even in childhood. It is commoner in the winter months, in lower socio-economic strata, and in crowded environments. Boys are more often affected. Infants of low birthweight, whether because of prematurity or intra-uterine growth failure, are at greater risk, as are multiple births. There are reports of twins dying simultaneously of SIDS. A total of 20 per cent of deaths are below 2 500 g at birth. The 'typical' mother is young (below 25 years) and already has other young children. Later babies are more at risk than firstborns, risk increasing with birth order. Smoking during pregnancy increases the risk of SIDS by a factor of two or three, and abuse of illegal drugs is associated with even higher rates. Studies of recurrence of SIDS in families in the USA, Norway, and Sweden do not provide evidence that genetic factors play an important role (Smedby et al., 1993).

*Sleeping position.* A role for unintentional suffocation or overlaying by the mother in the causation of SIDS has been repeatedly rejected over the past 20 years. However, there is now clear evidence that the infant's position during sleep is of importance (Beal & Finch, 1991). Studies from New Zealand, Australia, the UK, Holland, and Norway show an increased risk of SIDS in infants who sleep in the face-down (prone) position. Intervention studies in which the supine or lateral sleeping position has been recommended have been followed by significant decreases in incidence (Mitchell et al., 1994; Smedby et al., 1993).

*Clothing and bedding.* Studies by Nelson in New Zealand have provided evidence that overheating may be a factor in some cases. When thick clothing and bedding are used, the infant's head becomes the main route for heat loss. This could be compromised in the face-down position (Nelson, 1996).

*Bed-sharing.* In many African and Asian cultures, it is normal practice for the infant to sleep close to the mother (co-sleeping) (Potgieter & Kibel, 1992). Whether this is a risk factor for SIDS or actually protective remains an important but as yet unanswered question. Certainly, unintentional suffocation or overlaying of the infant by the mother does occasionally occur, generally in an unsuitable sleeping environment such as a sofa. Yet SIDS rates are lowest in Asian communities where co-sleeping is the norm. Parental sleep contact provides constant stimulation to the infant through vocalizations, body movements, radiant heat, and respiratory sounds. In fact, infants who share the parents' bed exhibit synchronous arousal and co-ordination of sleep stages with the parent (McKenna & Mosko, 1994). These authors therefore consider that parent–infant contact throughout the night may help some vulnerable infants to override the deficits that result in SIDS.

## Pathogenesis

Although the risk factors just discussed have been clearly identified, much remains to be learned about why these infants die. The most popular hypothesis is that they succumb during a period of extreme vulnerability when breathing control is in transition between the fetal and the 'adult'. Studies on infants who have been resuscitated from 'near-miss' episodes suggest that many such infants have poorly developed control of respiration similar to that seen in premature infants. Breathing during sleep is shallow and instead of regular breathing a periodic pattern is seen with a tendency to prolonged apnoeic pauses. Southall (1988) believes that the commonest mechanism of death in the SIDS victim is prolonged expiratory apnoea, the infant developing bradycardia, progres-

sive anoxia, hypotension, and sinking irreversibly without a struggle.

In those with lesser degrees of impairment, an added noxious stimulus may be required to precipitate lethal apnoea. This could be a 'mild' viral infection, especially one causing upper or middle airway obstruction. It should be emphasized, however, that the great majority of babies dying of 'cot death' do so without any previously recognized apnoeic episodes, or abnormal breathing patterns.

Most controversial is the hypothesis that gases emitted by plastics could accumulate and rise to levels toxic to the infant. Richardson (1994) published experimental evidence that fungi present in or on old mattresses could generate the poisonous gases stibine, arsine, or phosphine, from the elements antimony, arsenic, and phosphate, often present in plastic materials. Sprott (1996) pointed out that many of the risk factors associated with SIDS could be explained on this environmental basis. He mounted a campaign in New Zealand to promote the use of impermeable polythene mattress covers to prevent egress of toxic cases, and claimed that no infant sleeping on such a mattress had died of SIDS. The experimental evidence on which this hypothesis is based has been disputed (Limerick Final Report 1998).

There is, nevertheless, good evidence that a small minority of SIDS cases are due to a mixed bag of rare disorders, for example infantile botulism, inborn errors of metabolism, cardiac conduction disorders (prolonged QT interval), certain disorders of respiratory control, and filicide (non-accidental injury). These together do not constitute more than 0,5 cases per thousand live births (Nelson, 1996).

*Filicide.* Before recognition of sudden infant death as an entity, many parents were accused of killing their infants either deliberately or accidentally. Recently the role of willful suffocation has again come to the fore as a factor in some cases. It must be realized that it is difficult to distinguish post-mortem between sudden death and smothering by a soft pillow and undoubtedly instances of infanticide do occur in this fashion. *Nevertheless, awareness of this possibility must not be allowed to interfere with the sympathetic approach to the shocked and grief-stricken parents, the vast majority of whom are totally innocent.*

While the pathogenesis of SIDS remains a fascinating enigma, three aspects of the condition are of immediate practical importance to health professionals. Firstly, there are preventive measures that may lessen the risk of SIDS, particularly in households that have already sustained such a loss. Secondly, there is the efficient handling of the event that will respect the feelings of the bereaved parents and family and provide maximum support to them. Thirdly, there is the management of real or alleged near-miss events, which, with greater public awareness, have become a common community concern.

# What to do in the event of a sudden infant death

The Foundation for the Study of Infant Deaths in Great Britain has provided a series of helpful guidelines to be adopted by various personnel who may have first contact with the dead or moribund infant and his/her parents.

In the usual course of events, the infant is rushed by car or ambulance to the casualty department of a hospital. Ambulance and casualty staff need to be well informed as to the nature and special problems of cot death. Every effort should be made to ensure privacy for the parents. A brief perinatal history and details of events leading up to the death should be taken before the news of the infant's death is broken. Unless there has been a prior history of illness, obvious signs of injury, or suspicious behaviour on the parents' part,

## Preventive measures

The evidence on which preventive advice is based has been thoroughly reviewed by Henderson-Smart et al. (1998).

- *Put your baby on the back to sleep.* The prone sleeping position of infants should be avoided; from birth, infants should be put to sleep on their sides or back, unless there are specific indications against this. The supine sleeping appears to be preferable to side sleeping, because of the greater likelihood of the infant rolling face down when on the side.
- *Make sure your baby's head remains uncovered during sleep and avoid overheating and tight wrapping.*
- *Cover the mattress with polythene sheeting.* Many new mattresses are fitted with such covering; used mattresses should be wrapped in a sheet of thick polythene (125 microns) which is folded and taped underneath. The evidence for toxic gases is still incomplete, but the practice has been shown to be safe, and is recommended in the UK and New Zealand. The best underblanket to use on a wrapped mattress is fleecy cotton.
- *Keep your baby smoke free – before birth and after.* Mothers should be warned of the dangers of smoking and drug taking.
- *Is immunization linked with SIDS?* A number of studies have shown that immunization does *not* increase the risk of SIDS, and in fact may be protective.
- *Breast-feeding.* The commonly held belief that breast-feeding is protective against SIDS has been negated in several studies, but the many advantages of breast-feeding need no emphasis. It is the mothers who are socially at risk of SIDS who would be least likely to breast-feed in developed settings.

they should be informed that the cause of death is probably SIDS. A minister of religion should be called if baptism is requested; they rank high as sources of comfort and support at this time and later. The parents should be informed of the great desirability of a post-mortem examination in all circumstances, and of its legal necessity if prior circumstances or lack of a regular medical attendant merit this. Parents should be offered the opportunity to see and hold the baby before its removal to the mortuary.

The family doctor, if there is one, should be informed immediately, as he or she can be a key figure in the support of the family. A subsequent meeting should be arranged with the parents to discuss the results of the post-mortem examination and to allay the many feelings of guilt and self-blame that they will experience. A drug to induce sleep may be prescribed, but anti-depressants should be avoided. Suppression of lactation must also be considered. An interview with a paediatrician with a good understanding of the problem may be desirable.

There is a special poignancy in the tragedy of a cot death. The parents are generally young and may have had no prior contact with death. The mother is in a particularly vulnerable period emotionally, following pregnancy and puerperium. Great happiness and elation over the normally healthy baby is transmuted overnight into shock, bewilderment, and guilt. Often lack of understanding of the nature of cot deaths and confusion with child abuse lead to stigmatization of the parents. Death-shy society tends to shun them just when the greatest support is needed. Mothers vary in the extent of their reaction to such a tragedy. Some seem to be well adjusted initially and may suffer much longer with the internal suppression of their grief. There may be psychosomatic symptoms such as aching in the arms or hallucinations of hearing the baby crying. Such manifestations often

## 'Near-miss' episodes

Brief apnoeic spells or a few seconds of ineffectual breathing due to airway closure are commonly seen in normal infants during sleep. More prolonged attacks, and especially those associated with pallor, cyanosis, or a long recovery period, are more important. With increased public awareness, such 'acute life-threatening events' – ALTEs – have become a major problem for paediatricians, but the great majority of such reported episodes are benign and simply represent normal sleep pauses or brief choking spells. It should be stressed that in the majority of cot deaths there is no antecedent history of such events.

There are, nevertheless, a few infants who will go on to suffer recurrent apnoeic episodes leading to death or neurological damage. It is very important that an accurate and detailed description of the episode be obtained. An attack that occurs when the infant is awake is less likely to be serious than one that occurs during sleep. Extreme pallor or definite cyanosis is obviously significant, whereas mere flushing is less likely to be important. The resumption of normal, quiet breathing during sleep after stimulation would be reassuring, while delayed onset of crying after resuscitation or gasping respiration would cause concern. In such cases, admission to hospital and further evaluation are mandatory. There is a place in some cases for pharmacological stimulation of breathing with theophylline or caffeine citrate, and the use of apnoea monitors (see Southall, 1988).

decrease with time, but there may be occurrences of feelings of isolation and remorse for months and years afterwards, engendered by anniversaries or recollections of the dead child, often long after sympathetic support has been withdrawn by those about her.

Psychological reactions are not confined to the mother. The father may also suffer severe disturbance and be badly affected by the loss. There have been many instances of serious family disruption and divorce as a result of cot deaths. Siblings may also show behavioural expressions of loss and insecurity, such as reversion to infantile behaviour, bedwetting at night, and nightmares.

It has been found that an unhurried visit by a doctor or health visitor a week or so after the infant's death will allow parents to unburden themselves. They need to ventilate all their imagined errors of omission or commission which they feel may have contributed to the child's death, and thus mitigate feelings of guilt.

Contact with those who have suffered similar tragedies can be a major source of support. Parents should be put in touch with a Cot Death Society, if available, or other appropriate resources. A pamphlet titled *Information for the parents of a child who has died unexpectedly* has proved helpful. Copies may be obtained from the above (see Chapter 30: Community support groups).

## References and further reading

ARNEIL GC, BROOKE E, GIBSON AAM, HARVIE A, MACKINTOSH H, and PATRICK WJA. 1982. Post-perinatal infant mortality in Glasgow, 1979–1981. *Lancet.* 18(2):649–51.

BEALE SM & FINCH CE. 1991. An overview of retrospective case-control studies investigating the relationship between prone sleeping position and SIDS. *Journal of Paediatric Child Health.* 27:334–339.

DAVIES M & KIBEL MA. 2000. *Should the baby sleep with mother?* Proceedings of the Sixth SIDS International Conference, Auckland, New Zealand.

GILBERT R. 1994. The changing epidemiology of SIDS. *Archives of the Diseases of Children.* 70:445–9.

GOLDING J, LIMERICK S, and MACFARLANE A, 1985. *Sudden Infant Death.* Berkeley, California: Open Books.

MCKENNA J & MOSKO S 1994. Sleep and arousal, synchrony and independence, among mothers and infants sleeping apart and together (same bed): An experiment in evolutionary medicine. *Acta Paediatric.* (397):94–102.

HENDERSON-SMART DJ, PONSONBY AL, and MURPHY E. 1998. Reducing the risk of sudden infant death syndrome. *Journal of Paediatric Child Health.* 34:213–19.

LIMERICK FINAL REPORT MAY 1998. Expert group to investigate cot death theories. British Department of Health.

MITCHELL EA, BRUNT JM, and EVERARD C. 1994. Reduction in mortality from sudden infant death syndrome in New Zealand 1986–1992. *Archives of the Diseases of Children.* 70:291–4.

NELSON EAS. 1996. *Sudden Infant Death Syndrome and Child Care Practices.* ISBN 962-85089-1-1. 151–68.

POTGIETER ST & KIBEL MA. 1992. Sleeping positions of infants in the Cape Peninsula. *South African Medical Journal.* 81:355–7.

RAMBAUD C, GUILLEMINAULT C, and CAMBELL P. 1994. Definition of the sudden infant death syndrome. *British Medical Journal.* 308:1439.

RAMOS V, HERNANDEZ AF, and VILLANUEVA E. 1997. Simultaneous death of twins. *American Journal of Forensic Medicine and Pathology.* 18(1):75–8.

RISK FACTORS OF SUDDEN INFANT DEATH IN CHINESE BABIES. 1997. *American Journal of Epidemiology.* 144:1070–3.

SINCLAIR-SMITH CC & KIBEL MA. 1986. Sudden infant death. *South African Journal of Continuing Medical Education.* 4:13–17.

SMEDBY B, IRGENS L, and NORVENIUS G. 1993
Consensus statement on epidemiology.
*Acta Paediatric Supplement.* 389:42–3.

SOUTHALL DP. 1988. Role of apnoea in the
sudden infant death syndrome. *Pediatrics.*
81:73–84.

SPROTT TJ. 1996. *The cot death cover-up?*
Auckland, London: Penguin Books.

WOLF BHM & IKEOGU MO. 1996. Is sudden
infant death syndrome a problem in
Zimbabwe? *Journal of Tropical
Paediatrics.* 1996:150–3.

# PART THIRTEEN

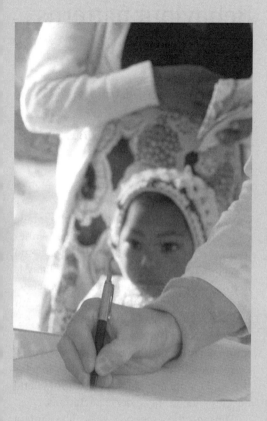

# Child mental health

'Difficult' behaviour in childhood is often simply difficult in the eye of the beholder. Such problems extend through the entire spectrum from behaviour appropriate to the phase of development to serious psychiatric disorders. Parental understanding of what is normal, and appropriate guidance, can do much to prevent small problems becoming large ones.

# 50

# Behaviour patterns in pre-school children

**PM LEARY & MA KIBEL**

Someone once said that there are no problem children, only problem parents! This joke contains more than a grain of truth. It is the parent and not the child who sees behaviour as abnormal, and therefore problematic. Most parents have had little adult exposure to young children before they have their own first offspring, and so they are largely ignorant of the stages of a child's normal social, emotional, and intellectual development. This lack of understanding leads to unrealistic expectations, failed recognition of predictable behaviour patterns, anxiety, and, frequently, consultations with doctors and psychologists. Much of this can be avoided if parents are better informed. Doctors who wish to help those troubled in this way will find that a genuine liking for small children is their greatest asset. They must also be familiar with all the phases of normal childhood development, and must appreciate that parental concepts of acceptable behaviour vary widely.

## Normal social and emotional development

The principles have been outlined in Chapter 6: Emotional and cognitive development.

During the first year of life, the infant is totally dependent on the mother or caregiver. A one-to-one relationship exists, which makes no demands on his or her person. The baby is free to sleep, cry for food, posset, eructate, urinate, or defecate at whim. All his or her needs are met without question and no reasonable mother will expect adherence to a time schedule or observance of any social convention. She is quite satisfied as long as the child appears healthy and grows and develops according to her expectations.

During the second year, the infant becomes a toddler. The first inklings of personal identity and personal volition are felt. Increased mobility brings a measure of vulnerability and the first demands for conformity. The first prohibitions are encountered in the form of exclusions from hazardous areas – the kitchen, the workshop, and the fire – and summary confiscation of intriguing objects encountered during household explorations. Former total acceptance is replaced by the need to comply with maternal requests to at least a certain extent. The sense of security that is engendered by familiar domestic surroundings is tested as environmental exposure extends to include the street, the park, the shops, and the beach. New and unfamiliar faces are encountered and, as the second birthday approaches, the potty appears on the scene. At this stage the child's view of the world is egocentric and immediate personal gratification is the only motivating force. Thus, the stage is set for confrontations. Clashes of will produce temper tantrums and maternal disapproval engenders anxiety, for the toddler still depends on a one-to-one relationship for peace of mind. In moments of conflict, maternal appeals to reason are ineffective, for there is as yet no sense of reason.

Jealousy and competitiveness are added to the emotional profile in the third and subsequent years. These are fired by growing possessiveness. The combination produces illogical acquisitiveness, a disinclination to share, fierce competition for individual attention, and aggressive acts in defence of perceived territorial rights. The sense of personal identity is now well developed but self-gratification remains the overriding motivational force. Only as he or she learns to postpone immediate wish fulfilment is the toddler able to wait for a turn, to allow others to be the centre of attention and to share toys and consumables with his or her peers. Two-year-olds in a playground do not play together. They play in parallel, all doing their own things. All is well as long they keep to their own activities. A simultaneous desire for the same diversion will immediately produce conflict with potential for violence. Only in the fourth year does emotional development reach the stage at which co-operative play can take place – turn and turn about at pushing and riding in the kiddie cart or on the swing. In the third year, there is the first realization that human beings come in two patterns. Genital differences become a source of considerable attention and future attitudes are strongly influenced by the manner in which parents handle this normal and healthy interest. During this period and subsequently, there is also an increasing appreciation of the differences between socially acceptable and unacceptable actions and between 'mine' and 'thine'. The child's conscience stems from this awareness and in time it becomes a potent source of anxiety. During pre-school years any surfeit of anxiety is likely to produce behaviour regression, sometimes to infantile forms long since discarded.

# Normal cognitive development

In the first six months of life, healthy infants are little cocoons of personal sensations. They are unable to distinguish their own inner world of 'self' from the outer world round about. One kindly disposed person is not distinguishable from another and the baby will smile in toothless fashion at all comers. All this changes at about six months. Mother is recognized as someone very special, and separation from her is traumatic. This in turn may produce anxiety in the mother who believes that she has 'spoilt' the child through too much attention. Separation anxiety is a normal phenomenon and parents must be reassured about its cause. Attention from strangers is not well received and they must work hard for their smiles. This stranger response persists throughout much of the toddler period and should not be construed as unnatural shyness or a sign of insecurity.

In pre-school years the child's thinking is directed by four strong psychological influences: egocentricity, animism, logic, and morality.

*Egocentricity* remains a powerful factor, and activity that does not manifestly serve self-interest is likely to have little appeal.

Approach to life is *animistic*. Trees, plants, furniture, vehicles, the sun and moon, and all animals are invested with human faculties, virtues, and vices. There is easy acceptance of stories about animated cars, trains, and animals. The household object on which the child is hurt is vindictive. Fairies may live at the bottom of the garden and witches and dragons may menace at bedtime and intrude into dreams.

Thought processes are not influenced by considerations of *logic*. A plausible explanation is accepted without question even though it may be frankly unscientific and false. Thus, the Father Christmas myth does not evoke questions about the logistics of Christmas Eve activities, nor indeed does the multiplicity of Father Christmases found in shopping centres during the month of December!

*Morality* is authoritarian and defined by mother. Transgressions that are discovered carry penalties, and all disagreeable, unpleasant, and painful experiences are construed as punishment for wrongful acts, whether or not they are consciously perceived by the child as such.

## ENVIRONMENTAL FACTORS

Professionals working with children soon recognize the environmental circumstances that attend complaints about behaviour.

## IGNORANCE OF NORMAL DEVELOPMENT

Reference has already been made to parental ignorance of normal social, emotional, and intellectual development.

## DOMESTIC INSECURITY AND DISHARMONY

Abnormal behaviour patterns frequently occur in children who are exposed to *domestic insecurity* and *disharmony*. Frequent exposure to parental arguments and violence may lead to sleep disorders, bedwetting, and a range of socially unacceptable attention-seeking activities. Such aberrations are common when there is parental alcohol abuse. The presence in the home of a critical, interfering, and perhaps infirm grandparent may severely disrupt healthy family dynamics and be the root cause of disordered behaviour in the child. A whole range of abnormal behaviour patterns may be found in the siblings of a physically or mentally disabled child who makes heavy demands on maternal time and emotional resources.

## SINGLE PARENTS

Complaints are often registered about children who live in a single-parent situation. The parent, almost always the mother, is usually obliged by her circumstances to work full-time outside her home. In consequence, she is likely to be tired and not able to give of her best during evening and weekend hours spent with the child, who in turn misses her after spending long days with a hired caregiver or in a crèche. In consequence, sustained maximal attention is demanded during the hours spent in mother's company, and the pejorative 'hyperactive' label is readily but incorrectly applied. Social contacts by the single parent with members of the opposite sex may be a catalyst for unacceptable behaviour. The child perceives the parent's friend as an interloper who attracts attention and affection which is the child's by right. This leads to exacerbation of attention-seeking behaviour and even to aggressive acts directed at the visitor.

A variant of the single-parent situation occurs when the father's work keeps him from his family for weeks and months at a stretch. His absence generates a degree of insecurity in the whole family and the mother may have difficulty in consistently maintaining a home atmosphere that is conducive to acceptable behaviour.

## PERSONALITY AND TEMPERAMENT

A further important dimension that determines children's behaviour is their individuality and personality. This affects the manner in which they will pass through the developmental stages, settle into a routine, and deal with sleeping, feeding, and frustration.

# Troublesome behaviour in young children

Whether or not 'normal behaviour' becomes 'problem behaviour' will thus depend on the interaction between the child's personality, parents' knowledge and acceptance, and the extent of the environmental stresses present. *Infantile colic, waking at night, separation anxiety, normal exploratory behaviour, negativism, poor appetite,* and *resistance to toilet training* are the seven most important potential problem areas. For the child living in a high-risk family, these innocent behaviours can cause severe tensions and even trigger physical abuse. Schmitt (1987) has suggested simple ways in which these problems can be pre-empted or dealt with and these ideas are incorporated in the following sections.

## INFANTILE COLIC

In Western countries, the term 'infantile colic' has come to be associated with the regular occurrence of paroxysmal bouts of vigorous loud crying in infants aged between two weeks and three months. Attacks are most common in the late afternoon or early evening. During the spells, the infant cries persistently, cannot be placated, thrashes about, and draws up the legs or arches backwards as though in pain. In all other respects, the infant is healthy and thriving. The spells diminish after the age of three months and the infant shows no after effects.

Studies by Brazelton (1962) provide information on the duration and regularity of crying during early infancy. Even when all needs in terms of food, physical comfort, and close human contact have been met, many otherwise normal infants spend a considerable portion of the waking hours fretting and crying. As with infantile colic, such crying is most frequent between 18h00 and 22h00, at a time when the infant has accumulated a surfeit of stimuli from the environment – perhaps this accounts for the irritability.

It seems likely that the so-called 'colicky' infant simply represents the extremity of a continuum of what is really normal behaviour. These infants have a low threshold for frustration and discomfort. They gulp air during feeds and cry when wind or a normal stool is passed. Painful spasm of the bowel may occur. The behaviour is as common in breast-fed as in bottle-fed infants. Allergy does not appear to play a role in the great majority, atopic symptoms being neither more frequent in family members, nor more common subsequently in these babies than in the 'non-colicky'. An improvement in colic by eliminating cow milk from the diet of breast-feeding mothers has been claimed, but disputed by others.

Prolonged crying can be unnerving and exhausting for parents, whose inability to console their baby leads to frustration, anxiety, and loss of self-esteem. Sometimes the difficulties in the mother–infant relationship may be primarily maternal. The infant is keenly sensitive to the mother's reaction, and lack of confidence and tension on her part may lead to excessive irritability in the infant. Less commonly, there may be more serious causes such as postpartum depression or difficulties with bonding.

This pattern of behaviour in infancy is universal, being just as common in unsophisticated as in sophisticated communities.

However, it appears to be perceived as a problem far more often among more educated parents. On questioning mothers and experienced health visitors in Cape Town child health clinics, it is evident that this pattern of early evening crying is just as common in black infants as in white or coloured ones. But these mothers seldom seek advice for this behaviour, regarding it as perfectly normal and accepting it with a relaxed attitude. They do not seem to associate it with the concept of pain or colic. It is of interest that the Xhosa word for such screaming in the evenings, *uyazilinda*, means 'the child is guarding himself'. Infants are not offered the breast during attacks, but are either nursed against the mother's chest in the prone position or carried around on her back. On the other hand, studies by Richter (1994) in Soweto show that black mothers often make the assumption that their milk is not enough, or is bad for the baby and they offer solids or the bottle.

*Rule out organic causes!* The diagnosis of infantile colic cannot be considered if there is any deviation from normal physical or developmental progress. Underfeeding is another common reason for excessive crying.

Parental anxiety and anger, though clearly not causes of colic, do seem to aggravate the condition, as does rough handling. In the majority of cases there seems to be no family tension or disharmony.

## Management

Once the normality of the infant has been established, full explanation of the behavioural and benign nature of the crying, coupled with simple advice on handling, will generally go a long way towards allaying fears, improving parents' confidence, and easing the situation.

- Attention to feeding techniques and the mother's method of bringing up wind may be fruitful.
- Overfeeding should be eliminated. Some parents get into a pattern of feeding the child every time it cries.
- Parents often need to be reassured that sucking a dummy or, better still, fingers or thumb, is a harmless and useful pacifying measure as long as hygiene is adhered to.
- A harness or sling to carry the infant on the mother's back or in front of her is a further very helpful measure.

Parents need to be advised that, if these recommendations are unsuccessful, they should leave the baby's room and walk away. Medications containing dill and bicarbonate of soda – gripe water – and the surface-tension-lowering agent polysiloxane are of value only for their placebo effects. *The prescribing of atropine-containing medication is to be vigorously discouraged because of potentially harmful side effects.* Many turn readily to soya formulae or other formula changes in such infants. This is, however, seldom justified – unless there is a strong history of food allergy in the family or if symptoms persist past the age of four months.

The mother needs the opportunity to catch up on her own sleep. A friend or relative may be needed to help her mind the family during these periods.

Colic can cause a serious crisis in the family and doctors should be on the lookout for vulnerable families. They should then keep in regular contact until the troublesome behaviour improves.

## SLEEP DISORDERS

A healthy baby will wake every three to four hours and lustily demand a feed. Most infants do, however, sleep for one uninterrupted period of six to eight hours, and happy the mother whose child chooses for this period the conventional sleeping hours of 22h00 to 06h00! She will be much less likely to complain to her family doctor than the mother whose infant is restless and disturbs the peace through the night hours and then sleeps soundly from 07h00 to 14h00. Alleged sleep disorders at this age may thus be no more than an inconvenient time choice. There are, however, other possible causes – underfeeding, wet nappy irritating a sore bottom, a blocked nose, teething and, of course, any painful infection. These causes of sleeplessness must be sought and eliminated. Sometimes an infant who is sleeping poorly requires nothing more than increased cuddling. Black mothers who look after their babies in the traditional fashion seldom, if ever, complain of sleep disorders.

Suitable advice to parents of young infants who cry regularly at night is listed below:
- eliminate long daytime naps;
- if the cot is in the parents' bedroom, move it;
- put the child to bed awake;
- if the child wakes, wait five minutes before going in;
- if crying continues, go in for one minute or less – don't remove the child from the cot; and
- if crying continues, stay away, but recheck every 20 minutes for one minute or less.

Sleeping problems in healthy toddlers and older pre-school children may take one of two forms. The child may go to sleep as required and then wake at an abnormal time, or refuse to go to sleep until a very late hour. Either pattern may arise if the child is allowed to sleep excessively during the day. A daytime nap after the second birthday should never exceed one hour and for many children is not necessary at all. Sleep refusal in children who are at crèche all day is the result of a combination of enforced daytime resting and a desire to extend contact time with the mother to the maximum. Rough-and-tumble with the father and other high jinks just before bedtime may cause excitement that precludes sleep for several hours. Violent and frightening television and video films viewed before bedtime may also prevent sleep or induce nightmares that wake the child. Anxiety induced by bedroom isolation, darkness, and strange window shadows may all keep the young child from sleep, as may a noisy environment, loud music, and barking dogs.

In most instances the cause of the sleep disorder can be identified by careful history-taking. Elimination is achieved by simple adjustments in routine and there is no call for hypnotic drugs. When a sleep disorder is prominent in a brain-damaged or intellectually disabled child, however, there should be little hesitation in resorting to chloral hydrate or trimeprazine in appropriate doses. An unbroken succession of disturbed nights has a profoundly demoralizing effect on the parents of such a child, and timely introduction of a bedtime hypnotic encourages the child to develop reasonable sleep habits.

## SEPARATION ANXIETY

Fear or anxiety about the absence of the mother begins to show itself at about six months of age. Infants becomes alarmed when their mothers leave their field of vision and go into another room of the home. This aspect usually resolves by 18 months or so, but in certain children it may persist longer, especially if there have been periods of enforced separation such as hospitalization. During this period the child's sense of security is closely linked to the presence of the mother. Parents who do not understand the reason for the fear and clinginess that are part of this phase may consider that the child is spoiled and punish inappropriately.

## NORMAL EXPLORATORY BEHAVIOUR

Children around a year of age become extremely interested in their environment.

Having just learned to walk, they are able to explore and to discover the contents of drawers, cupboards, and table tops. This healthy curiosity can get them into considerable trouble, both from dangerous objects and from irate adults. Exploration of their surroundings should be encouraged, but priority must be given to rendering them safe (see Chapter 40: Childhood injuries).

## Advice for normal exploratory behaviour

The following advice should be given to parents in order to encourage normal behaviour in a safe environment:
- safety-proof the home;
- keep valuables out of reach;
- distract with toys, old newspapers, etc.;
- be firm on safety issues; and
- permit as much exploration as possible.

## Advice for separation anxiety

The following advice is appropriate for parents whose children suffer from separation anxiety:
- clarify the cause;
- offer reassurance, not punishment;
- rehearse separations before leaving;
- don't leave the room quickly;
- don't leave the child with unfamiliar people; and
- don't leave the child alone for punishment.

## NORMAL NEGATIVISM, TEMPER TANTRUMS, AND AGGRESSION

An outline has been given of the emotional and psychological forces that influence toddler behaviour. Normal negativism, temper tantrums, and aggressive acts must be seen against this background. Negativism is a normal healthy phase seen in most children between 18 months and three years. They delight in refusing suggestions such as to take a bath or go to bed.

This is an important phase in the child's progress towards self-determination, but is misunderstood by some adults who may then punish inappropriately. Temper tantrums must be recognized and managed in a consistent fashion. It is incorrect to make any attempt to comfort or commiserate with a child who is having a temper tantrum. The parent should immediately distance him- or herself physically from the child, who should be completely ignored, if at all possible. This will soon end the behaviour, as tantrums do not occur in the absence of an audience. Consistently applied, this action will signal to the child that such behaviour has no positive yield and temper tantrums will cease. Commiseration and capitulation on the other hand serve to reinforce and perpetuate the behaviour.

The child should not be punished for saying 'no'. The parents should avoid unnecessary demands and instead give extra choices and alternatives to increase the child's sense of control. However, he or she should not be given a choice when no choice exists – taking a bath and going to bed are non-negotiable. Diversion is useful as a means of obtaining compliance in negative situations.

Aggressive acts are often eliminated or much reduced in two- and three-year-olds by the simple provision, if this is feasible, of greater living space so that the offender no longer feels threatened by siblings or peers. Ideas of sharing and toleration will take root if supported by incentives and positive reinforcement.

*Aggressive acts should never be managed by physical punishment.* This only reinforces the concept that 'might is right'.

## Advice for normal negativism

The phase is important for normal development and can be managed with the following tactics:
- don't punish for saying 'no';
- reduce rules;
- give the child extra choices. 'Let's do this or that' not 'do this or else';
- don't give non-choices, however;
- state requests positively; and
- give transition time.

*The breath-holding attack* is a common and harmless spell, which has its highest frequency in the age range of one to three years. A tendency to breath-holding, however, may be evinced at a much earlier age, even from the early days of life. In the classical attack, children take in breath to cry, let out a single cry and then hold the breath in expiration. They are then unable to breathe in again because of glottic spasm, and no sound emerges. Children become progressively more suffused, the eyes turn up, and neck and back extend with pronation of the upper limbs. The heart slows markedly as cyanosis develops and it is this slowing that results in a loss of consciousness. This lasts only a few seconds, after which the child relaxes and begins to breathe normally. Very occasionally, a proper clonic seizure will follow. Crying is induced by frustration in a determined child. However, the episode is *not* induced voluntarily, and it is a widely held misconception that the breath is held purposefully in inspiration. Unlike true seizures, attacks are always precipitated by physical hurt or frustration.

An association with anaemia – particularly due to iron deficiency – is sometimes found, and there is improvement when this is corrected. However, drug treatment is seldom necessary. A full explanation emphasizing the good prognosis is all that is required.

'*Reflex anoxic spells*' are less common and invariably induced by sudden pain as when the toddler bangs his or her head against the edge of a table. The child gives a cry and then abruptly loses consciousness. The face becomes ashen. Colour improves after 10 to 15 seconds and consciousness returns. These spells are due to a pain-induced surge of vagal tone. They seldom recur after the age of four and may be controlled in severe cases with small oral doses of atropine.

## POOR APPETITE

The appetite of many children falls off between 18 months and 3 years and, in the perception of many anxious parents, they eat almost nothing. A power struggle develops at mealtimes, and the forcing of food may further diminish appetite. Parents need reassurance that their toddler is eating less than he or she used to because growth is occurring at a slower rate. The child should be encouraged to feed him- or herself.

The oft-given advice to 'leave him; he'll eat when he's hungry' is misleading as many toddlers do not feel hungry as they drink too much milk, tea, or juice. Because toddlers are often in conflict as a result of negativism and frustration, they are likely to resort to comfort habits like frequent demands for the breast or

## Advice for 'normal' poor appetite

The child is usually healthy, but the problem can be managed with the following tactics:
- keep milk below 500 ml per day;
- limit fruit juices and snacks;
- let the child feed him- or herself; and
- make mealtimes pleasant.

435

they walk around all day sucking tea, fruit juice, or milk from a bottle. This serves to diminish the appetite for solids. The lack of suitable solids is also likely to result in iron deficiency anaemia with all its effects. Iron deficiency must be corrected, any parasitic infestation treated and the right kinds of foods introduced (see Chapter 15: Infant and child nutrition).

## RESISTANCE TO TOILET TRAINING

This is discussed in Chapter 51: Common functional problems.

## ATTENTION SEEKING

The young child realizes that he or she is small, totally dependent, and insecure away from mother. Increasing ego development moves the child at the same time to seek recognition as an individual. Attention-seeking behaviour or acting out is the predictable outcome of this emotional conflict. It is likely to be exhibited whenever the child feels he or she is not the centre of attention, as when the mother is talking to a friend, guests visit the home, or a sibling is receiving notice. Attention-seeking behaviour takes many forms. The toddler may climb up onto mother's lap or tug at her dress. Objects may be deliberately broken or knocked over. Shelves in shops may be disarranged. Some young children run away at crucial moments in the sure knowledge that mother will drop everything and join frantic pursuit.

The successful management of attention-seeking behaviour calls for insight and an understanding of the child's needs. Scolding, chiding, and physical punishment will serve to perpetuate undesirable behaviour. The child's need for attention must be recognized and parents should be advised to acknowledge their child's need and incorporate him or her into whatever they are doing. The child

should be encouraged to 'help' mother in simple domestic tasks and his or her advice should be given due consideration. 'Help' cleaning the car and in the garden should be acknowledged with gratitude, and praise expressed in front of the whole family. This policy should be followed for all good and desirable actions.

## SIBLING RIVALRY

Though essentially an expression of normal emotional development, sibling rivalry may cause considerable distress within a family. An only child who has never had to compete for attention feels displaced when a new baby arrives on the scene and apparently becomes the centre of parental interest. This new situation is interpreted as rejection and, at the stage of authoritarian morality, is attributed to wrongdoing. Resentment is displayed towards the newcomer and unacceptable actions instigated in attempts to regain parental attention. The middle child in a family may encounter especially difficult circumstances. He or she is constantly made to feel inferior by older siblings who by virtue of size and developmental status can excel over him or her at every turn. The middle child is also constantly put out by the greater maternal attention enjoyed by younger and less independent siblings. Hence misery and acting-out are common in the pre-school middle child. Mature parents see each one of their children as an infinitely precious individual, but children often cannot comprehend this emotion, and see family life as a competition for attention and acknowledgement. Thus, praise and reward accorded to one child may be construed by the others as implied criticism and rejection. Animosity towards the favoured sibling is the outcome.

Parental insight is all-important in the successful management of sibling rivalry. Careful explanation should enable parents to handle the situation with understanding and to make adjustments in domestic routine so that each child receives an adequate quota of parental time, preferably on a one-to-one basis. The talents of each sibling should be recognized and acknowledged by all members of the family. A useful ploy is to assign one or two special responsibilities within the home to each child. Each then becomes the family expert in the area designated and derives satisfaction and self-esteem from this status. Suitable duties include caring for domestic animals, watering pot plants and fetching in the post.

## LYING

Reference has been made to the animism and absence of logical reasoning which characterize the thinking of pre-school children. This leads to blurring in the child's mind of the boundaries between fact and fantasy. Coupled with a vivid imagination, this situation predisposes to statements and claims that adult ears immediately recognize as transparently false. Pre-school children who generate tall stories in this way should not be berated as liars. The child's motive is usually to draw attention rather than to deceive, and the mature adult to whom the tale is told should express surprise, wonder, astonishment, and gentle disbelief, rather than snub the child.

Older children tell lies for a variety of reasons. An obvious one is to achieve a desired but otherwise unattainable goal. Another incentive is the avoidance of punishment. When these motives are evident and lying is uncovered the child should be left in no doubt that such behaviour is not acceptable.

## STEALING

Young toddlers who have no appreciation of property rights will take any object that they encounter. This cannot be labelled as theft. In impoverished communities, theft is often a means of survival and pre-school children from underprivileged backgrounds may follow the example of their elders and lift food and property that they would otherwise have to go without. It is well recognized that some parents encourage shoplifting by young children in the knowledge that discovery will not be followed by prosecution.

When thefts are perpetrated by children from better-off homes, two altogether different reasons must be suspected. When the first pertains, thefts are usually confined to the child's own home and involve the property or money of one person, usually the mother. There may be little attempt to conceal the theft, though commission is strongly denied. The child's parents are often busy, successful people who provide their offspring with every material need, but have little time or inclination for prolonged personal contact or leisurely family diversions. The child steals to draw attention to him- or herself and thefts usually cease if parents can be persuaded to make adjustments to their lifestyle which will meet the child's emotional need for attention.

The second reason for thefts is a burning desire for peer approval. The child, often the smallest in his or her peer group, buys popularity by distributing sweets, ice creams, cakes, and other attractive consumables among friends. This lifestyle is financed by stealing money or the items themselves. Splurgestealing, as it has been called by American authors, is less common in the pre-school group than it is among school children.

# Conclusion

Complaints about the behaviour of pre-school children stem from a failure to appreciate the child's perception of his or her environment and the need for recognition in addition to love and security. The parents of problem children may be poor at recognizing when and how to act. Response to attention-seeking behaviour may be excessive, and erratic and inconsistent to bad behaviour. Insufficient praise and encouragement may be offered and communication between spouses may be poor. Successful intervention demands, above all else, the attainment of parental insight and the achievement of appropriate modifications to the child's domestic routine. These should be our primary goals. There is little place for the summary prescription of medications.

Self-discipline has been described by Penelope Leach as 'a slow growing plant that roots in children's identification with parents or parent substitutes'. Children need to be shown what they should do and prevented from doing what they should not, and they need honest explanations for each piece of everyday advice and instruction, praise, and reproof, so that clusters of behaviour are gradually incorporated into a vast jigsaw puzzle of values that is building up inside them (Leach, 1994). Physical punishment and other methods of summary humiliation are poor and potentially damaging substitutes for these positive methods, but are deeply ingrained in our child-rearing heritage. This is discussed further in Chapter 61: Child abuse.

## References and further reading

BRAZELTON TB. 1962. Crying in infancy. *Pediatrics*. 24:579–85.

GABEL S (ed.). 1981. *Behavioral problems in childhood: A primary care approach*. New York: Grune & Stratton Inc.

ILLINGWORTH RS. 1987. *The normal child: Some problems of the early years and their treatment*, 9th ed. Edinburgh, London: Churchill Livingstone.

LEACH P. 1994. C*hildren first – what our society must do – and is not doing – for our children today*. London: Michael Joseph.

RICHTER L. 1994. *The early introduction of solids: An analysis of beliefs and practices among African women in Soweto*. Proceedings of the Congress of the South African Paediatric Association.

SCHMITT B. 1987. The seven deadly sins of childhood. *Child Abuse and Neglect*. 11:421–32.

WOLFF S. 1973. *Children under stress*. Harmondsworth: Penguin Books Limited.

# 51

# Common functional problems

MA KIBEL, PM LEARY &
CJ SCHOEMAN

## Problems in bladder and bowel control

### BLADDER CONTROL

Most children achieve day and night continence by the age of three to five years. Generally they are dry by day earlier than by night. At the age of five years, 10 to 15 per cent of children still wet their beds at least once a week, the majority never having been dry at night. Boys outnumber girls.

Bedwetting or nocturnal enuresis is the most common developmental disorder. Daytime wetting or diurnal enuresis is less common, but may accompany bedwetting. Bedwetting is rarely more than a nuisance, but daytime wetting may be indicative of potentially serious disease.

Several factors have been suggested as being causative in nocturnal enuresis:
- Physical causes are rare and most children with enuresis have no demonstrable physical abnormality except for small bladder capacity.
- Genetic factors seem to play a part in at least some cases. It is common to obtain a history of bedwetting in childhood in one or other parent or older sibling.
- Deep sleep has been said to contribute to the condition but satisfactory evidence is lacking.
- A widely held view is that delayed maturation of nervous control is an important factor.
- Environmental causes may play a part and there is an association between enuresis and emotional disorders, especially in secondary enuresis.

The term 'secondary nocturnal enuresis' is applied if there has been a period of more than six months of dryness. The condition is often precipitated by psychosocial stress. Urinary tract infection or other pathology should, however, be carefully excluded in such cases.

## Clinical assessment

An accurate history is important. Clinical examination should be thorough, with particular attention being paid to the abdomen, external genitalia, perineum, and lower spine to exclude possible organic causes. The urine should be tested for protein, sugar, blood, nitrite, and leucocyte esterase. If abnormalities are found, a specimen should be sent for microscopy, culture, and sensitivity. Radiological investigation of the urinary tract is unnecessary in the child who only wets the bed and has no urinary abnormalities.

## Management

Treatment should only be considered after the age of five years and is worthwhile if bedwetting occurs more than twice a week. Commonsense advice and reassurance of the parents and child are the mainstays of treatment. Bedwetting should not be seen as a permanent disorder as it resolves before puberty in almost all children. Commonly, the problem is aggravated by parental lack of understanding and undue coercion to use the potty or punishment.

Interest and encouragement by a sympathetic health worker and a supportive family are most important. Dry nights should be praised and rewarded while wet nights should be ignored, and punishment avoided. Fluid restriction after supper and emptying the bladder before going to bed are commonsense measures. 'Bladder exercises' are considered by some to be effective, if only as a psychological boost to confidence. The child is encouraged to increase fluids during the day and to hold the urine in for progressively longer periods. During micturition, the stream should be interrupted for half a minute before resuming. Responsibility for the child's own well-being is reinforced by getting him or her to keep a 'star chart' of dry nights, which serves both as encouragement and as a progress record.

In the older child alarm-conditioning therapy has the highest success rate, provided the child is able and willing to participate and the family is well motivated. The bedwetting alarm should be sufficiently loud to wake the child, but not the whole family! If not available, a simple expedient is a straightforward alarm clock, which the child uses to wake him- or herself to pass urine.

Drug therapy generally should be avoided. Anticholinergic drugs such as oxybutynin and tricyclic antidepressants like imipramine are often prescribed and have a reasonable success rate, but side effects are common and relapses frequent when treatment is discontinued. The danger of accidental poisoning is a major drawback. In very resistant cases, intranasal desmopressin (DDAVP) can be used to restrict urine output, but this form of therapy is expensive.

## CONSTIPATION

Constipation may become a problem during the period of toilet training. It is often initiated by a small anal tear (fissure) caused by a hard stool, resulting in painful defecation and faecal retension. Treating the fissure with an anaesthetic ointment and faecal softeners usually results in rapid improvement. In more protracted cases of constipation, the principles of treatment include education of the parents to increase the fibre content of the child's (and family's) diet and encouragement of the child to evacuate at regular intervals with positive reinforcement if necessary. Short-term use of laxatives may prove helpful.

## BOWEL CONTROL: SOILING AND ENCOPRESIS

A child is normally continent of faeces by the age of three. Some normal children do not achieve continence until a little later, but incontinence after the age of four years should be regarded as abnormal. Some authors differentiate between soiling and encopresis. 'Soiling' means the involuntary leakage of stool secondary to faecal loading. The apparently purposeful passage of stool of normal consistency into underclothes or in abnormal places is termed 'encopresis'. As with enuresis, these conditions may occur in primary or secondary forms.

Soiling is more commonly encountered, occurring in about 1,5 per cent of kindergarten children. It is approximately six times more common in boys than in girls. These children intermittently retain stools and are constipated. The physical and rectal examination may be normal or accumulated stool may be palpable. A plain abdominal radiograph will reveal considerable faecal retention. Some children defecate every day, but produce bowel movements that are incomplete. Simple constipation is more usual in the under-five-year old group whilst soiling tends to present in children older than five years. Abdominal pain or discomfort can occur in both groups.

As stool retention increases, sensory feedback from the bowel becomes impaired. The rectal wall is stretched and unable to contract forcefully enough. There is increased water absorption from the faecal material and painful defecation may follow. The result is further avoidance or economy of toilet use, thereby making the constipation worse. Soon the anal canal becomes stretched and shortened and the function of the sphincter is compromised, allowing the passage of soft faeces and mucus around the impaction.

There is no doubt that such problems in bowel control have a serious negative impact on the lives of affected children. They feel humiliated, self-esteem declines, and they become anxious and socially withdrawn.

## Management

Explanation of the problem to the parents and children is of the utmost importance. The child will often have stigmatized and blamed for his 'dirty habits' and these attitudes must be corrected. Initial complete clearance of the bowel can be achieved by the use of enemas. An effective method for severe cases is a balanced polyethylene glycol electrolyte solution such as Golytely, generally given orally or by stomach tube. Once the bowel has been fully cleared, a less invasive but persistent training routine can be established as far as dietary and bowel habits are concerned. There must be emphasis on regular and unhurried use of the toilet at a fixed time each day. Additional dietary fibre is recommended in the form of wholewheat bread, fruit, and vegetables. Stool softeners are indicated (Milk of Magnesia, sorbital, lactulose) and, if needed, a vegetable laxative (Senokot). This should be given daily for two weeks or longer. Ongoing family involvement is necessary and medical support with long-term follow-up is mandatory.

Encopresis is far less common. It generally signifies cognitive impairment or serious psychological disturbance. Children with encopresis usually need to be referred to a clinical psychologist or psychiatrist. It is important to bear in mind that children who have been sexually abused may present with disturbances of bowel control.

# Recurrent pains

Recurrent abdominal pains, headaches, and limb pains without 'organic' causes are common complaints in childhood. They are seen in all communities, but obviously receive more attention in the industrialized world, where visits to health professionals are more regular, and where there is less serious illness. These pains tend to be found in families who react 'somatically' to stress. In some children, they may well be the result of modelling behaviour. In others, the problem is perpetuated by hidden anxieties about serious pathology, either in the child or in family members; someone in the family may have died of an illness with similar symptoms. In others again, the symptoms may be a sign of significant stress at school, within the peer group, or in the home; and in a minority, they are an indication of serious depression or other mental disturbance.

The unravelling of such problems can be one of the most fascinating and rewarding aspects of primary care, but the practitioner must be prepared to take a comprehensive history and devote time and patience to the problem. If not, he or she will simply feel let down by not being able to find an organic cause for the complaint. The reader is referred to the classic publications of the late John Apley for a full discussion.

## RECURRENT ABDOMINAL PAIN

About 10 to 15 per cent of schoolchildren experience recurrent abdominal pain at some point. It is rarely seen before five years of age and has its peak incidence between ten and 12 years. Discomfort occurs over a period of months or even years, frequently interfering with daily routine, but usually resolving completely between episodes. The nature of the pain varies but is generally vague and peri-umbilical. Most children have difficulty in describing the pain. It follows no consistent pattern of time, duration, intensity, location, or associated symptomatology and may be described as dull, crampy, or sharp. Functional pain rarely disturbs a child from sleep. If this should occur, an organic cause can be strongly suspected. Organic illness is also more likely if the pain is not central, and the further from the umbilicus, the more likely this is to be the case.

Complaints of abdominal pain are significantly more common in the families of affected children and occur more frequently in highly strung, anxious children. Traditionally, recurrent abdominal pain in children has been classified as either organic or psychogenic in origin. An organic cause is found in less than seven per cent of the cases. A more recent and useful model divides children with recurrent abdominal pain into three groups: organic, psychogenic, and dysfunctional. 'Dysfunctional' refers to normal or slightly aberrant physiological phenomena in the child, which are not in themselves pathologic, but which are are largely responsible for the problem. Examples are lactase deficiency, intestinal gas syndromes, spastic colon, and chronic stool retention. The part played by these 'dysfunctional' mechanisms remains controversial.

## 'THE PERIODIC SYNDROME'

Some young children (one to five years) experience clearcut paroxysmal attacks of ill-defined abdominal pain, with or without vomiting, at intervals of weeks or months. With advancing age, the classic symptoms of migraine appear. In these children a history of migraine in other family members is often obtained (see below). Paroxysmal attacks of profuse and repeated vomiting in an otherwise healthy child also fall into this category (cyclical vomiting). For some reason this diagnosis seems to be made less often today than in former years.

## Clinical assessment

When the child is first seen, a careful history and thorough physical (including rectal) examination are essential. Laboratory tests should be ordered judiciously: a full blood count, sedimentation rate, urinalysis, and abdominal X-ray film are justifiable as the initial and only baseline tests. If, at this stage, it is possible to distinguish between organic and psychogenic causes, these avenues must be pursued. The occurrence of vomiting, pain at night, or relief of pain on eating would justify further investigation for gastritis or peptic ulceration, in both of which Helicobacter pylori infection is known to play a causative role (Gormally et al., 1995). For the majority of cases, however, there will be no such explanation, and a provisional diagnosis of dysfunctional pain must be made.

## Management

Discuss the problem with the parents and child, mentioning that this phenomenon is common and not serious. The physician should emphasize that the pain is real and not 'in the child's head'. It should be unequivocally stated that the negative physical and laboratory findings make serious illness extremely unlikely. This reassurance usually goes a long way to relieving often unexpressed anxieties. It is most important to uncover any possible stresses involving the home, school, or peer group. Follow-up visits are important to demonstrate the physician's continued interest in the child's problem. It is useful to have the parents and child keep a diary of pain episodes, diet, bowel habits, and stressful events to be reviewed during return visits. Most of these symptoms decrease in frequency and eventually remit in time. The use of medications should be strongly discouraged, but, in certain circumstances, a placebo can be helpful (e.g., a multivitamin mixture).

### LIMB PAIN (GROWING PAINS)

Limb pain is a common occurrence in normal children during mid-childhood. An organic aetiology is present in less than four per cent of these children. There are clues in the history and initial observations that can suggest an organic rather than a non-organic aetiology for the pain. Children with organic pathology generally localize their pain to a joint or to a well-defined area between two joints. Discomfort will usually be severe enough to interfere with play and other normal activities. It will occur during the day and night and is often unilateral. Constitutional signs and symptoms may be evident, especially limping. When the pain is non-organic, the patient's description of the pain may not fit any logical anatomic or physiological process. The pain will occur especially on school days or during unpleasant situations. Weekends are generally pain-free and there is very little interruption of normal activities. No suggestion of constitutional signs or symptoms should be evident and the physical examination will either be normal or abnormal in a fashion inconsistent with organic dysfunction.

A specific type of 'growing pain' consists of deep-felt pain, usually in the lower limbs, that is severe enough to awaken the child from sleep. The pain occurs intermittently, is mostly bilateral, and resolves by the morning. The pains are exacerbated by excessive exercise during the day and improved by heat, massage, and aspirin.

The pathophysiology of growing pains is unknown. It is now accepted that they do exist, do not progress to serious organic disease, and always resolve with time. It is essential to exclude organic causes such as low-grade rheumatism and leukaemia before diagnosing functional limb pain. A normal full blood count and sedimentation rate would be reassuring in this regard.

## Other functional body pains

Recurrent chest and back pains without organic basis are also encountered, particularly in older children. They appear, however, to be far less common complaints in southern African children than in their North American counterparts.

### HEADACHE

Headache – pain in the cranial vault – is, along with fatigue, anxiety, hunger, and thirst, a discomfort experienced from time to time

443

by every individual. The symptom is common in childhood but should never be lightly dismissed as it may be the only indication of serious disease.

History is all-important in elucidating the cause of headache. Pain that is of recent onset and that wakes the patient from sleep is likely to reflect serious pathology. On the other hand, an organic lesion is unlikely when the symptom has been present on a daily basis over months and years with no change in the child's physical condition.

## Pathophysiology

Head pain arises in areas and structures that are sensitive to mechanical distortion – parts of the dura at the base of the brain and arteries within the dura mater and pia arachnoid, intracranial venous sinuses, their tributaries and the delicate structures of the eye, ear, and nasal sinuses. The periosteum of the skull and superficial tissues of the scalp are clearly also pain-sensitive. The parenchyma of the brain, much of the pia mater, dura mater, and the bony skull itself are without specific pain sensitivity. Posterior fossa lesions may cause pain in the occipito-nuchal region.

Supratentorial lesions cause fronto-temporal pain which may be confined to the side of a unilateral lesion. Pain that originates in paranasal sinuses, teeth, an eye or upper cervical vertebrae is not usually sharply localized, but is felt characteristically in a regional distribution.

The pain of migraine has been attributed to intense cerebral vasodilatation following a period of vasospasm that coincides with prodromal symptoms such as visual disturbances and paraesthesiae. Isotope studies during the prodromal phase have shown that cerebral blood flow is reduced by as much as 50 per cent in corresponding brain areas. Other studies have demonstrated cerebral oligaemia that begins posteriorly and spreads

## The types of headache

The headaches of childhood fall naturally into four categories:
- *Acute headache* is a symptom of current viral or bacterial infection. Onset is fairly rapid and pain may be intense. The child is usually feverish. There may be signs of upper respiratory tract infection, otitis media, or meningitis. The symptom subsides as the acute phase of the infection is overcome;
- *Paroxysmal headache* is the characteristic feature of classic migraine, common migraine and cluster attacks;
- *Chronic non-progressive headache* occurs in children subject to tension, depression, chronic eye strain, and nasal sinusitis; and
- *Chronic progressive headache* reflects increasing intracranial pressure. Initially pain may be present for only a few minutes at a time. Over days and weeks there is an increase both in duration and intensity. Vomiting without nausea is often an associated feature, and the child may be awakened from sleep by the pain. Physical examination reveals signs such as papilloedema, cranial nerve palsies, and evidence of sutural separation. Headaches of this nature occur in children with intracranial tumour, abscess, or increasing hydrocephalus. Springing (opening) of sutures may result in the temporary relief of symptoms, followed by recurrence.

anteriorly at a rate of 2 mm/minute. This is independent of vascular patterns and appears to relate to neuronal cyto-architecture. It is recognized that migraine attacks may be precipitated in sensitive subjects by strong emotion and hypoglycaemia. Attacks may also

444

follow the ingestion of foods containing tyramine, phenylethylamine, nitrites, or mono-sodium-glutamate. These substances cause the release of vaso-active amines, which, in turn, trigger the headache.

Infants and young children are unable to identify or localize the area of their discomfort; headache is evidenced simply by irritability, disinclination to feed and play, or vomiting.

## Special features

'Classic migraine' occurs at intervals of weeks or months. Onset occurs during the day and may be preceded by an aura of tingling, flashing lights, and other phenomena that the individual comes to recognize. Pain is usually throbbing in nature and may be bilateral in children. Peak intensity is reached over 30 minutes and may be accompanied by nausea and vomiting. Symptoms persist for hours to several days and are relieved by sleep. A strong family history of migraine is usual. A variety of syndromes, such as hemiplegic migraine and basilar artery migraine, are described. In these, transitory dysfunction is induced by ischaemia resulting from vasospasm.

'Common migraine' is of more gradual onset than classic migraine. There is daytime onset of throbbing bilateral pain, which may persist for several days. Aura is characteristically absent and family history less prominent than in classic migraine. Sleep does not always bring relief.

'Cluster headaches' are very uncommon in childhood. An affected individual wakes for one or two hours after going to sleep with unilateral non-throbbing pain in the orbital and peri-orbital region. There is associated nasal congestion and lacrimation on the affected side. The headaches tend to occur nightly for days or several weeks on end, and then remit completely for several months or more.

'Tension headaches' may be present on waking, but they more commonly build up during the course of the day. This headache characteristically persists for days and weeks despite manifest good health and does not prevent the victim from sleeping normally. Questioning will reveal domestic or school circumstances that generate tension in the life of the child. When these circumstances are confined to the school situation, there may be freedom from headache at weekends and during school holidays.

'Nasal sinusitis' causes dull pain in the frontal and facial bones. This pain is present on first waking and is intensified if the individual bends over so that the head is lower than the trunk. Drainage proceeds when the upright position is maintained and there is gradual diminution in pain. Pain of a sharper nature may return in the later morning. This is induced by pressure changes and a suction effect on the walls of the sinuses. Sinus X-rays reveal fluid levels and thickening of mucosa.

'Eye strain' induces headache in children with hypermetropia and astigmatism. Such children make good the refractive error by sustained strong action of intra- and extra-ocular muscles and are not aware of the disability. The effort involved induces headache, which builds up during the day. Eye strain headache is seldom found in myopic children.

The headache of depression closely resembles that caused by tension. It is found in children of limited ability on whom excessive scholastic or physical demands are made. It is also found in children who fail to measure up to parental expectations. Domestic disharmony is often an exacerbating factor.

## Management

The management of headache in childhood is the management of the underlying cause. Thus, accurate diagnosis is all important. Acute headache will resolve as the child's infection comes under control. During the acute phase symptomatic treatment with paracetamol or codeine is appropriate. Children with chronic progressive headache need the diagnostic and therapeutic resources of a neurosurgical unit. No time should be lost in arranging referral when headache is of this nature and there are corresponding physical signs.

Migraine is recognized by a classic history and the absence of abnormal physical signs between attacks. Management is multi-faceted. Though not essential, a normal CT scan will provide doctor, parent, and patient with the assurance that there is no tumour or other structural abnormality. When attacks are infrequent, no prophylactic treatment is necessary. During acute episodes the child should be placed at rest in a darkened room and given paracetamol or codeine in appropriate doses. Ergotamine preparations are not recommended for children but may be used in adolescents. When migraines occur at short intervals and impair the child's quality of life, active steps must be taken to decrease their frequency. Missed meals, excessive fatigue, and undue tension should be avoided. Substances known to trigger attacks should be eliminated from the diet. Among these are cheeses, chocolate, nuts, all cola-containing drinks, tea, coffee, oranges, tomatoes, certain spreads (Bovril, Marmite), preserved meats, and Chinese foods. It is advisable at the outset to eliminate all these foodstuffs from the child's diet. If this measure is followed by a period free of migraine, items can be reintroduced one at a time. A return of attacks will serve to identify the offending foodstuff. A number of drugs have been shown to be effective in the prophylaxis of migraine. Most widely used are diazepam administered as a small bedtime dosage and the beta-blocker, propranolol, given two or three times a day. Other drugs include the antihistamine, cyproheptadine, the alpha blocker, clonidine, and the anti-serotonin agents pizotifen and methysergide. Success has been achieved with all of these despite their differing modes of pharmacological action. This is an indication of our, as yet, incomplete understanding of the mechanisms of migraine.

Relief of tension headaches and those that attend depression will follow the recognition of their aetiology, and the introduction of steps to alleviate stress and unhappiness in the child's life.

## References and further reading

APLEY J. 1975. *The child with abdominal pains*, 2nd ed. Oxford: Blackwell.

APLEY J. 1975. *The child and his symptoms*, 3rd ed. Oxford: Blackwell.

BOLLARD J & NETTELBECK T. 1989. *Bedwetting: A treatment manual for professional staff.* London: Chapman & Hall.

GORMALLY SM, PRAKASH N, DURNIN MT, DALY LE, CLYNE M, KIERCE MB, and DRUMM B. 1995. Symptoms in children before and after treatment of Helicobacter pylori infection. *Journal of Pediatrics.* 126:753–6.

LEVIN MD. 1982. Encopresis. *Pediatric Clinics of North America.* 29(2):315–30.

# 52

# Serious psychological disorders

## BA ROBERTSON

## Classification and aetiology

In this section, serious psychiatric disorders in the pre-pubertal child will be described according to their classification in the *Diagnostic and Statistical Manual of Mental Disorders*, 4th edition (*DSM*-IV, 1994). The *DSM*-IV defines a psychiatric disorder as being a clinically significant behavioural or psychological syndrome that is associated with present distress or impairment of functioning. For most psychiatric disorders, there is no unitary aetiological agent, so their classification is made on descriptive grounds.

It is important to know which aetiological factors are likely to have interacted in the causation of a psychiatric disorder, as they will determine its management. Aetiology is always multifactorial and can be divided into biological, psychological, and social components. Examples of some important aetiological factors are given below:

## Biological

- genetic transmission of psychiatric disorder;
- intellectual disability;
- congenital anomalies;
- diseases of the nervous system; and
- male sex.

## Psychological

- low self-esteem;
- poor coping skills;
- lack of schoolreadiness; and
- poor social skills.

## Social

### Family
- young unmarried mother;
- psychiatric disorder in mother;
- death of mother;
- family suicide or homicide;
- family dysfunction;
- marital discord;
- stressful family break-up;
- violence, child abuse and neglect;
- alcohol and drug abuse; and
- poverty.

### Community and environment
- stressful school environment;
- inadequate educational opportunities;
- bad neighbourhood;

447

- urbanization;
- breakdown of traditional way of life; and
- war, migration, and displacement.

# Epidemiology

During any one year 5 to 15 per cent of all children and adolescents will have a psychiatric disorder. The rate of serious disorders is at the lower end of the range. A community study in an informal settlement in South Africa found a prevalence rate of 15,2 per cent for psychiatric disorder with impairment (Robertson et al., 1999).

Many psychiatric disorders of childhood resolve spontaneously, although they may recur. Serious disorders are those that recur and/or persist into adult life causing serious personal, social, and occupational dysfunction. The following factors influence the prognosis:

- the type of disorder, e.g., autistic disorder is always serious;
- the severity of the disorder, e.g., major depression is more serious than dysthymic disorder;
- how long the disorder has been present prior to treatment;
- the presence of significant biopsycho-social stressors; and
- the availability of treatment.

The aim of child and adolescent mental health care services is to prevent the occurrence and/or persistence of psychiatric disorders. Many psychiatric disorders have their origins in early childhood, making early identification possible, ideally before the start of formal schooling.

# Principles of assessment, diagnosis, and management

A disturbance of emotions or behaviour in a child or adolescent significantly affects and is affected by his or her family functioning so that assessment within the context of the family is essential.

The major components of the diagnostic assessment are:

- history – including collateral information;
- examination – physical examination of the child, and mental status of the child and family members;
- special investigations;
- aetiology – the role of biopsychosocial factors; and
- differential diagnosis.

The most important areas of the history are:

- presenting complaints;
- current functioning, including at school;
- developmental history;
- family history, functioning, and relationships; and
- environmental stress.

The following are the main areas to investigate when assessing the mental status of a child or adolescent:

- relationships;
- functioning;
- intelligence;
- mood; and
- behaviour.

The principal special investigations used are:

- class teacher's report – academic ability and behaviour;
- relevant medical investigations;
- psychological testing – IQ, projective tests;
- occupational therapy assessment – perceptual, motor, and neuro-developmental assessment; and
- speech therapy assessment.

The main types of treatment available to health workers who are not mental health specialists are:

- parent counselling;
- marital counselling;
- individual counselling;
- environmental change; and
- medication.

General health workers should be able to manage all mild disorders and emergencies. Only unresolving cases and serious or complex disorders need be referred to mental health specialists. When prescribing psychotropic medication for children, larger doses than expected by body weight are needed because of the higher rate of metabolic breakdown and elimination of these drugs.

# Serious psychiatric disorders in pre-pubertal children

## ATTENTION-DEFICIT/ HYPERACTIVITY DISORDER (ADHD)

### Definition

The essential feature is a persistent pattern of inattention and/or hyperactivity–impulsivity that is more frequent and severe than typically observed in children at a comparable level of development. Some symptoms that cause impairment must have been present before the age of seven, and the impairment must be present in at least two settings, for instance, home and school.

Many of the following behaviours are evident:
- difficulty in remaining seated;
- easily distracted;
- difficulty in awaiting turn;
- difficulty in sustaining attention or finishing tasks or play; and

- shifting from one uncompleted activity to another;
- talking excessively or playing loudly; and
- interrupting or intruding on others.

Prevalence rates vary between one and five per cent. ADHD is more common in boys, but has been reported less frequently in African children. Affected children often also show low self-esteem, mood lability, poor frustration tolerance, soft neurological signs, and perceptuo-motor difficulties. Genetic or antenatal factors are considered to play an important role in the aetiology, with dysfunction of the prefrontal cortex and the noradrenergic and dopaminergic neurotransmitter systems. Chronic stress such as prolonged hospitalization or child abuse may contribute. There is little evidence to support the hypothesis that lead in the environment or additives in the diet cause hyperactivity, except possibly in a minority of cases. The differential diagnosis is from an anxiety, mood, or conduct disorder; or from hyperactivity secondary to intellectual disability, learning disorder, or a stressful environment.

In severe cases, ADHD persists into adolescence and adulthood, where the main features are problems with peer relationships, school failure, conduct disorder, occupational maladjustment, substance abuse, and antisocial personality disorder.

The nature, management, and prognosis of ADHD need to be fully explained and its impact on child, family, and school addressed. Support groups are often helpful. Treatment involves the use of behaviour modification techniques to help the child improve his or her concentration span and control impulsiveness and motor activity.

Medication is also often required in addition. The medication of choice is methylphenidate, which is effective in about 75 per cent of cases. The recommended dose is 5 to 20 mg at breakfast, and a further 10 to 20 mg may be given at noon in older children. In severe cases, methylphenidate may be added in the afternoon or evening, although this increases the risk of insomnia and weight loss. Some suppression of appetite is usual, even in children receiving the medication only at breakfast, with concomitant flattening of the growth curve. Normal growth resumes once the medication is stopped, so that 'drug holidays' are not necessary if continuous medication is indicated. Other side effects include dysphoria, skin reactions, and headaches. The medication may exacerbate pre-existing tics, but this is usually short-lived. Addiction does not occur.

Alternative medications are pemoline and imipramine. Clonidine may be helpful in children who show a rebound phenomenon when methylphenidate is discontinued. Thioridazine may be used in children with severe intellectual disability, who often do not tolerate methylphenidate well. The prescriber should be familiar with the medication used, and its precautions and drug interactions. Medication should be reviewed from year to year.

Identification in the pre-school years may improve the prognosis, as effective treatment will reduce the likelihood of secondary problems developing. Support and guidance of child, family, and school often needs to continue into early adulthood, and special education may be required in some cases.

## CONDUCT DISORDER

This is one of the commoner psychiatric disorders of childhood and adolescence. A significant proportion of the more serious cases are likely to become 'juvenile delinquents' and continue into adult life as antisocial personality disorders.

Several of the following behaviours are usually present:

- stealing on more than one occasion;
- running away from home overnight;
- frequent physical aggression;

### A definition of conduct disorder

The essential feature of the disorder is a repetitive and persistent pattern of behaviour, lasting at least twelve months, in which the basic rights of others and major age-appropriate societal norms or rules are violated.

- truancy;
- destructive to property, firesetting;
- physically cruel to animals or people;
- substance abuse, such as glue sniffing; and
- mugging, housebreaking, and car theft.

The disorder is more common in boys. Conduct-disordered children are usually impulsive, and have poor frustration tolerance and low self-esteem. Coexisting learning disorders and ADHD are common. Those who display less serious antisocial behaviour may have symptoms of anxiety and depression, and show remorse. Those with the most serious antisocial behaviour often show little remorse and are committed eventually to schools of industry and reformatories.

An aetiological association has been demonstrated between conduct disorder and parental rejection, inconsistent management with harsh discipline, and either the absence of a father or the presence of a father with alcohol dependence. In the most severe cases one finds chaotic or disorganized families, family violence and criminality, physical and sexual child abuse, alcohol and drug abuse, and social disadvantage. Street children have usually come from such families.

The nature, management, and prognosis of conduct disorder need to be fully explained and its impact on child, family, school, and community addressed. Support groups such as 'Tough Love' may be helpful in the more severe cases. Concerted efforts often need to be made to engage and retain the child and family in treatment. Parents and teachers will need advice about how to maintain communication and a supportive relationship with the youngster, and about limit-setting and methods of behaviour modification. In the more severe cases, parent-training courses and social skills training for the youth yield the best results. Medication is indicated only when there is a comorbid psychiatric disorder that might respond to pharmacotherapy. The most frequently used medications are methylphenidate, antidepressants, and carbamazepine. The more severe cases should be referred to a mental health professional or a social welfare agency.

Because of the known association between conduct disorder, social disadvantage, and severe family psychopathology, social action and community work aimed at uplifting and improving opportunities for disadvantaged communities are important preventive measures.

## SCHOOL FAILURE

The causes of school failure are complex and often multiple. They include physical factors such as hunger, malnutrition, ill-health, and central nervous system disease, as well as specific psychiatric disorders such as anxiety, depression, conduct disorder, and attention-deficit/hyperactivity disorder. Other important factors are family dysfunction, such as alcoholism and child abuse, and educational factors, such as lack of pre-school stimulation, unsatisfactory conditions for studying at home, overcrowding in the classroom, a variable standard of teaching, and inadequate special educational facilities. The subject is discussed further in Chapter 56: Specific learning problems.

## DISORDERS OF MOOD

The most commonly occurring mood disor-

ders in pre-pubertal children are major depression and dysthymic disorder.

## MAJOR DEPRESSION

The essential features of a *major depressive episode* are the onset of either depressed or irritable mood or loss of interest in former pleasurable activities lasting for a period of at least two weeks, accompanied by several of the following:
- increased or decreased appetite;
- insomnia or hypersomnia;
- increased or decreased motor activity;
- difficulty concentrating with fall-off in school work;
- feelings of worthlessness or guilt;
- fatigue or loss of energy;
- suicidal thoughts; and
- auditory hallucinations.

Depressed mood is not reported spontaneously by children and therefore this disorder is sometimes not detected until suicidal behaviour occurs. Alternatively, depression may be discovered when investigating a coexisting condition such as conduct disorder, substance abuse, or sexual abuse. A depressed mood in older children is usually obvious when looked for and if the child is sensitively questioned. Depressed mood in pre-school children is often expressed non-verbally in angry, aggressive, and destructive behaviour, while in infants it is expressed in severe apathy, irritability, and failure to thrive.

Major depression may be superimposed on a dysthymic disorder. Anxiety disorders are also common in children with major depression, and there is often a family history of anxiety or depression. Genetic factors are important in the aetiology of depression, and the disorder is associated with noradrenergic and serotonergic neurotransmitter dysfunction. Depression can also be associated with hypothyroidism and with viral illnesses such

451

as infectious mononucleosis. Psychosocial factors – lack of parental loving care, loss of a loved parent-figure, loss of health, and chronic stress – play significant roles in the onset and maintenance of depression. Major depression may resolve spontaneously after several months or it may continue in milder form as a dysthymic disorder only to recur again in the future. It predisposes to recurrent major depression and bipolar illness in adult life.

Completed suicide is rare in pre-pubertal children, but suicidal thoughts and wishes are frequently found even in young children and should not be regarded lightly or brushed aside. Children who have attempted suicide should be referred to a mental health professional for assessment of their suicide potential.

The nature, management, and prognosis of depression need to be fully explained, and its impact on child and family addressed. Treatment of major depression is directed primarily at the causative and maintaining factors, and at providing emotional support for the child. Therefore, the family will always need to be involved in the treatment, and the child may also need individual psychotherapy. Social skills training, in groups if available, is effective in older children and adolescents. Medication is usually prescribed in cases of more severe depression, e.g., 25 to 75 mg of a tricylic antidepressant such as imipramine in a single dose at bedtime, and continued for three or four months before being tailed off, to avoid withdrawal effects. Tricyclic antidepressants in doses over 100 mg a day, although sometimes indicated, may be cardiotoxic in children (Gutgesell et al., 1999), and they are potentially lethal in overdose. The newer antidepressants, for instance, the selective serotonin reuptake inhibitors (SSRIs) like fluoxetine, do not appear to have these properties. Children whose major depression is related to severe and longstanding family pathology or stress should be referred to a mental health professional for more comprehensive management.

## Dysthymic disorder

The essential feature of *dysthymic disorder* is a mildly depressed mood for most of the time over the course of at least one year, accompanied by some of the symptoms listed for major depression (with the exception of hallucinations).

Low self-esteem is always present, and these children may initially respond with a negative reaction to kindness and attempts to help them. Dysthymic disorder is sometimes a sequel to chronic physical or psychiatric disorders, and is closely associated with major depression.

Dysthymic disorder usually occurs in the context of chronic stress and/or the emotional unavailability of the parents. Intra-familial stresses include chronic psychiatric or physical disorders in the parents, marital discord, and physical and sexual abuse, and neglect. Extra-familial factors include social disadvantage, prolonged hospitalization and long-standing stress at school. Children may be predisposed to major depression and dysthymic disorder by early experiences of separation and loss, such as significant changes of caregiver, environment, or school.

The management of dysthymic disorder is challenging as the predisposing or maintaining factors may not be easily remedied. Medication is not usually indicated. Making a supportive adult available to the child when there is little support at home is essential, and for this purpose a suitable neighbour, relative, or teacher is best. It is also important to provide emotional support for the parents to ensure some stability in the home life. Vigorous efforts must be made to build up the child's self-esteem, and parents or teachers can be helped to do this. The child can also be helped to develop better ways of coping with stress.

# Anxiety disorders

## SEPARATION ANXIETY DISORDER

The essential feature of this disorder is excessive and persistent anxiety (lasting for at least four weeks) about separation from those to whom the child is attached. The reaction is beyond that expected for the child's developmental level.

It manifests itself by reluctance to sleep alone, unrealistic and persistent worries about harm befalling the parents, or refusal to go to school. Attempts to enforce separation result in stomach aches, vomiting, or temper tantrums. Older children often also have other anxiety disorders or are depressed. The parents themselves frequently suffer from anxiety, depression, or are overprotective. Separation anxiety disorder may be precipitated by a stressful event either at school or at home, for instance, a marital crisis. Besides psychoeducation, management consists mainly of counselling the parents and teacher about how to handle the separation anxiety and of addressing any identified stressors. In general, these children should be helped to cope with increasing degrees of separation according to their capacity.

## SCHOOL REFUSAL

School-refusing children in their first year of primary school should usually be taken to school in a firm but supportive way. More serious cases should be referred to a mental health professional. School refusal in the older child is often indicative of severe psychopathology in both child and family and therefore it is usually not possible to get the child back to school immediately. It is advisable to obtain medical exemption for the child until treatment has been given. These children often have severe anxiety or depressive disorders but occasionally also have a learning disorder or conduct disorder. Even so, it is usually easy to distinguish them from truants who have no difficulty leaving home in the morning but do not attend school. Truants are always conduct disordered, often have a history of learning difficulties and school failure, and often come from homes where there is either lack of supervision or harsh discipline. By contrast, the parents of school-refusing children usually provide a caring home, although there may be severe marital discord (not always acknowledged), parental depressive disorder, or some other family stress. A crisis in the family is the usual precipitator of school refusal in the older child, but there may be stress at school as well.

These children and their families usually require specialist treatment and it may be several weeks before the child is able to return to school. During this time the child should be kept as occupied as possible with constructive tasks. Homework should be obtained from the teacher, ideally by the child after school. As much contact as possible should be kept up with school and peers. When the child is feeling better, he or she may be able to begin attending school for a few hours a day. Parents and school need to understand that school refusal is a problem that requires co-operation from both and is not the responsibility of one or the other. Tricyclic antidepressants may be indicated in severe cases.

## GENERALIZED ANXIETY DISORDER

The essential feature is excessive or unrealistic anxiety or worry for at least six months. The children worry about achieving, and about future events such as wars or world catastrophes. They are often perfectionistic and may have feelings of religious unworthiness. Individual therapy as well as parent counselling are usually required. Medication may be indicated in severe cases.

## PANIC DISORDER

Panic disorder is rare in young children and difficult to diagnose. It is characterized by recurrent panic attacks in which intense fear is accompanied by acute somatic symptoms of anxiety. Antidepressant medication is usually indicated. Besides adult-type panic disorder, panic states occasionally occur in young children accompanied by visual and/or tactile hallucinations. Once a medical cause has been excluded it is important to identify the underlying psychosocial stress that precipitated the attack. The stress, which may not be obvious, is often a real or imagined threat of separation or abandonment. The panic state tends to be self-limiting provided the stress is dealt with. If sedation is needed, oral or intravenous diazepam can be administered: 2 to 10 mg.

## POST-TRAUMATIC STRESS DISORDER (PTSD)

Post-traumatic stress disorder is frequently undetected, or presents late. The likelihood of children who have been exposed to a very traumatizing experience developing the disorder depends on the severity of the trauma, the vulnerability of the child, experience of past trauma, and the availability of support from the environment, particularly the parents. The disorder is diagnosed if acute stress symptoms persist for more than a month, but frequently symptoms present for the first time only months or years after the traumatic experience. The symptoms involve recurrent, distressing, and intrusive images or flashbacks of the traumatic experience; marked avoidance of particular people, places, or other reminders of the experience; and symptoms of anxiety or increased sympathetic arousal as manifest, for example, by difficulty sleeping, poor concentration, exaggerated startle response, and restlessness.

Affected children do not usually report their symptoms spontaneously, and parents are frequently unaware of the full extent of the symptoms or traumatization, or do not connect the symptoms with traumatic experiences. It is advisable to inquire routinely about possible traumatic experiences in any child presenting with unexplained symptoms or a change in behaviour.

Depression, anxiety, and conduct disorder may accompany PTSD, or be an alternative outcome to traumatic experiences. The management of PTSD involves psychoeducation of child and family, individual counselling, and the use of antidepressant medication such as imipramine or fluoxetine. The short-term use of intermediate acting benzodiazepines such as lorazepam or alprazolam may be helpful for acute symptoms. More severe cases should be referred to mental health specialists. Untreated or unresolving severe PTSD can lead to chronic psychological, occupational and social impairment. Early debriefing of children and families involved in disaster situations or any major trauma is advised in order to reduce the likelihood of PTSD.

# Other anxiety disorders

Specific phobias such as excessive fear of animals do not usually present for treatment. Parent counselling and desensitization of the child in a supportive manner is the recommended treatment. Social phobia, or the excessive fear of social or performance situations, presents more commonly in adolescence and adulthood. Individual therapy, desensitization, and the use of antidepressant medication in severe cases are indicated. *Obsessive-compulsive disorder* is marked by the presence of obsessions or compulsions or both, and is relatively rare. Common obsessions centre around fear of contamination by germs or dirt, while common compulsions involve handwashing or checking. Cognitive behaviour therapy is indicated, and in the more severe cases, the SSRIs (like fluoxetine) relieve many of the symptoms.

## Psychosis

The term 'psychosis' has been dropped from the child psychiatry classifications as none of the disorders have the characteristic features of the adult psychoses. Infantile autism has been renamed 'autistic disorder' and falls into the category of pervasive developmental disorders. It is doubtful whether schizophrenia occurs in pre-pubertal children. When a child presents with symptoms resembling schizophrenia, it is more likely to be a pervasive developmental disorder or a mental disorder due to a general medical condition such as cerebral cysticercosis. Occasionally the underlying medical disorder may not be demonstrable until several months after presentation.

## Pervasive developmental disorders (PDD)

The best-documented PDD is autistic disorder, whose essential features are:
- onset before the age of three;
- qualitative impairment in social interaction as manifest, for example, by:
  - lack of awareness of the existence or feelings of others; and
  - impaired comfort-seeking; impaired social play and peer relationships;
- qualitative impairment of verbal and non-verbal communication as manifest, for example, by:
  - delayed or absent verbal communication;
  - lack of spontaneous make-believe play; and
  - speech abnormalities such as echolalia;

- disturbed motor behaviour or activities as manifest, for example, by:
  - stereotyped body movements;
  - preoccupation with parts of objects; and
  - insistence on sameness with marked reaction to change.

Autistic disorder is extremely rare, although many children may have some autistic features. The diagnosis must be confirmed by a hospital team. Intellectual disability and epilepsy are frequently associated with the disorder. Autistic disorder appears to be an organically based heterogeneous neurodevelopmental disorder involving core psychological deficits. Secondary behavioural symptoms commonly occur. The prognosis is poor. Severe cases often need to be institutionalized, otherwise special schooling is beneficial, if available. Parental psychoeducation, support, and counselling is essential, and palliative medication may be necessary for behaviour control. Major tranquillizers such as haloperidol or thioridazine may be used.

## Tourette syndrome

The essential features of this rare disorder are motor tics which progress to multiple complex movements, including vocal and respiratory tics. Coprolalia (the uttering of obscenities) is present in a small number of cases. Attention-deficit hyperactivity disorder and obsessive-compulsive disorder may also be present. It appears to be transmitted in an autosomal dominant pattern, but is more prevalent in males. However, stress and other psychological factors also play an important role in precipitating and exacerbating the symptoms. Physical examination is usually negative and the disorder is easily distinguished from chorea, myoclonic epilepsy, and stereotypies. The condition may be difficult to cure completely. Because of the poor prognosis and the significant role of psychological factors, these children and their families should receive a comprehensive treatment programme. Haloperidol usually relieves many of the symptoms. Pimozide and clonidine are also used. Stimulant medication (such as methylphenidate) may aggravate the condition.

# Somatoform disorders

The essential features of this group of disorders are symptoms suggesting physical disorder for which there are no demonstrable medical findings and for which there is evidence of psychological factors.

*Conversion disorder* is an alteration or loss of physical functioning such as nausea, vomiting, sensations of movement inside the body, watering eyes in the classroom or inability to see the blackboard, aphonia, seizures, or paralysis. For symptoms that are school or examination related, some African countries have coined the term 'school anxiety'. In such cases treatment will involve exploration of the causes of the child's school-related stress or pressure to achieve. More severe symptoms such as aphonia or paralysis of the lower limbs indicate the presence of serious psychological problems in the child and family, and may require the child's admission to hospital for an intensive treatment programme with concomitant treatment of the family. Conversion symptoms represent an unconscious attempt to avoid an intolerable situation. However, concomitant medical pathology is found in a significant percentage of cases so that the possibility of a mixed aetiology must always be borne in mind.

## References and further reading

DIAGNOSTIC AND STATISTICAL MANUAL OF MENTAL DISORDERS OF THE AMERICAN PSYCHIATRIC ASSOCIATION, 4th ed. 1994 (*DSM-IV, 1994*). Washington: American Psychiatric Association.

GRAHAM PJ. 1991. *Child psychiatry: A developmental approach*, 2nd ed. Oxford: Oxford University Press.

GUTGESELL H, ATKINS D, BARST R, BUCK M, FRANKLIN W, HUMES R, RINGEL R, SHADDY R, and TANBERT KA. 1999. AHA scientific statement: Cardiovascular monitoring of children and adolescents receiving psychotropic drugs. *Journal of the American Academy of Child and Adolescent Psychiatry*. 38:1047–50.

ROBERTSON BA. 1996. *Handbook of child psychiatry for primary care*. Cape Town: Oxford University Press.

ROBERTSON BA, ENSINK K, PARRY CDH, and CHARLTON D. 1999. Performance of the diagnostic interview schedule for children version 2.3 (DISC-2.3) in an informal settlement area in South Africa. *Journal of the American Academy of Child and Adolescent Psychiatry*. 38:1156–64.

# 53

# Adolescence and its related psychology and psychiatry

## CW ALLWOOD

## From childhood to adulthood

Adolescence is a complex period encompassing the transition from childhood to adulthood. When problems present in adolescence they may be due to unresolved childhood disorders, problems relating to puberty and adolescence (e.g., eating disorders and suicidal behaviour), adult type psychiatric disorders arising in adolescence, or a combination of these.

Adolescence is a time of rapid physiological and psychological change. It is a time of adjustment to a new body image, a more specific gender role and to different relationships with parents, siblings, and friends.

Adolescents feel very actively the enormous pressure of the *peer group*. Adjustments are required to school, work, and social life as a preparation for adult roles. Specific developmental tasks have already been outlined in Chapter 6: Emotional and cognitive development.

The establishment of *gender identity* and sex role is most important during this period and can be a source of significant emotional upheaval. This is ideally worked through in relationships with both mother and father. Passionate relationships and hero worship contribute to self-discovery. Experimentation

of all kinds and degrees is frequently part of the learning maturing process. Adolescence does not have to involve a crisis or be traumatic to be normal – either for parents or the adolescent. It is a time of renegotiation, a time when any unresolved conflicts may re-emerge and have to be worked through. Such conflicts may include those arising out of death, divorce, adoption, rape, or incest. This is understandable since gender identity, sex role, and ideas about marriage and parenting are still all being formulated.

For both parent and child the resolution of the *dependence–independence–interdependence conflict* can be difficult. A second weaning is taking place. Parents may have great difficulty adjusting to the emotional fluctuations of the adolescent, who at the same time is going through the painful process of challenging all family and societal norms. Any set limits are questioned or stretched as the adolescent strives for autonomy. *Parenting* requires information, self-knowledge, understanding, and patience (just to be able to 'hang in there'). In difficult cases, professional advice should be sought early rather than late. Eventually, after a period of difficulty and some rebellion, adolescents will probably discover themselves to be comfortable with adult norms not very different from those of the parents or community from which they originated.

The adolescent negotiates many developmental hurdles in the move from childhood to adulthood: finding identity, self-knowledge, independence, and autonomy; finding a place in society; relationships with peers and family; a gender role, matching ideology and ideals with reality and behaviour, and taking adult responsibility in matters of planning and future security.

## Factors that may cause diagnostic confusion in adolescents

- Parents or caregivers may not be objective. They may be rejecting, angry, or guilt-ridden and feel helpless.
- The adolescent may have difficulty trusting others when needing to report on facts and feelings.
- Adolescent behaviour may be paradoxical and confusing, an expression of inner turmoil.
- Personality disorder may be wrongly diagnosed on the basis of temporarily exaggerated behaviour. The message of the behaviour must be correctly heard.
- Clinicians may too frequently attribute aberrant behaviour to growing up or adolescent crisis, thus missing a significant and possibly treatable problem, e.g., depression.
- Significant specific learning problems at school, which may not have been previously detected, emerge for the first time in adolescence, coinciding with the change to high school. This can cause great stress, resulting in behavioural changes or drug taking. This scenario is particularly true when the quality of primary schooling has been poor.

# Serious psychiatric disorders

For classification, aetiology, and epidemiology see Chapter 52: Serious psychological disorders. Epidemiological studies reveal an increased prevalence of boys compared to girls, particularly in the 12 to 16 year group.

## UNRESOLVED CHILDHOOD PROBLEMS

Some of these disorders have been dealt with already and, though their presentation may change with adolescence, the approach is essentially the same. Common conditions are:

- Attention-deficit disorder;
- school failure and developmental disorders;
- anxiety disorders;
- mood disorders;
- pervasive developmental disorders; and
- Tourette syndrome.

# Disorders related to adolescence

## ADOLESCENT CONDUCT DISORDER AND DELINQUENCY

Antisocial behaviour in adolescents may have started in this period or it may have continued from childhood. Adolescents commonly manifest transient deviant behaviour and poor impulse control, which must be distinguished from the persistent and pervasive symptoms of antisocial behaviour that constitute conduct disorder (see Chapter 52: Serious psychological disorders). Throughout history the idealist teenager has been easily caught up in a wide range of 'protest movements', which express discontent with the establishment, and whose activities may even constitute antisocial or criminal behaviour. The involvement of the adolescent is a response to a combination of group pressure, internal conflict resolution, and the need for excitement. During the course of 'protest activity', youth are sometimes responsible for horrifying actions but because of the transient nature of their activity and the highly charged emotions most individuals could not be described as having 'antisocial personalities' or 'conduct disorders'. Similar statements may be made even of adult football hooligans or vandals.

By definition, 'delinquency' implies that the person has been in conflict with the law – in other words, he or she has committed a crime and been caught. Therefore, when describing a behaviour syndrome, 'delinquency' is not especially useful.

*DSM*-IV does not apply *antisocial personality disorder* to people below the age of 18 years. Antisocial personality disorder may be strongly suspected where there has been a pervasive pattern of disregard for and violation of the rights of others since the age of 15 years. It is more probable if there has been evidence of conduct disorder before the age of 15.

*Conduct disorder* may be suspected where there has been a history of truancy, running away from home, fighting, using a weapon, forcing sexual activity on someone, cruelty to animals or people, fire-setting, etc. For conduct disorder to be diagnosed, there needs to be a sustained pattern of irresponsible and antisocial behaviour and acts, and a pattern of poor relationships. It is important that conduct disorder in the adolescent be correctly diagnosed. *Affective disorders* are frequently wrongly diagnosed as being personality (antisocial) or conduct disorders. Patients who later present with schizophrenia were often diagnosed as conduct disorder when they were adolescents. Antisocial behaviour and conduct disorder often go together with abuse of drugs beginning in childhood and continuing into adult life (see Drugs of abuse below). Treatment is generally not very satisfactory, but the degree of antisocial behaviour will dic-

tate the level of intervention required. The law, social services, the family and psychological interventions (especially behaviour modification) may all have a place. It appears that those who survive having had antisocial personality disorders may become more functional and less disruptive in middle age.

## DRUG TAKING (SUBSTANCE-RELATED DISORDERS – *DSM*-IV)

'Drug' is a term that refers to a multitude of substances. There is a wide range of psychoactive substances used by people to alter their moods and their perceptions of reality. Psychoactive drugs range from those that are legally and widely available, such as caffeine, alcohol, tobacco (nicotine), to substances such as cocaine, cannabis, barbiturates, amphetamines, LSD, inhalants, and opiates.

The distinction between the use and abuse of drugs may be socially defined in some cases. Factors that affect the use or abuse of a drug include the form of the drug taken, the circumstances and setting in which it is used, the purpose for which it is used, and finally the effects on the person's function in his or her occupation or in social interaction.

The *prevalence* of drug taking in the child and adolescent populations of southern Africa is uncertain. Indications that it constitutes a very large and increasing problem can be gained from the numbers of street children, and the incidence of drug-related criminal offences, sexual offences, school problems, and family problems related to taking drugs. The incidence of drug taking appears to be greatest in the large cities and to be associated with social deprivation, lack of recreational facilities, peer group pressure, and the availability of drugs. Use of drugs by the middle classes may be escaping detection and social sanction.

*Drugs of abuse*: Pre-adolescent children tend to use inhalants, generally the substances most readily available: petrol, benzine, thinners, acetone, and various glues. Adolescents more commonly use alcohol and cannabis. In the more affluent communities, mandrax, cocaine, and the opiates are used by older children.

The use of psychoactive substances goes back to the beginnings of humanity. Predisposing causes to drug abuse include non-conforming ideologies and attitudes, a desire to improve or escape from reality, and freely available psychoactive substances – including prescribed and over-the-counter medication. The fact that the drug abuser is in some way vulnerable to becoming dependent on drugs is also a factor. This vulnerability may be emotional (needing the drug for special effects), biochemical, or a combination of the two. Patients may be psychologically or physically dependent on a drug.

Drug abusers tend to have poor relationships with their parents and to come from broken homes. Examples of drug use by parents or peers appear to have a very strong influence on the young person. A causal relationship between delinquency and drug-taking is not clear, but drug-taking may be implicated in antisocial acts such as sex crimes, homicide, or damage to property. Alternatively, abusers may turn to crime in order to pay for the habit.

When it comes to diagnosing drug abuse, a high index of suspicion is needed, as the condition is so common.
- *History.* There may have been a change in the patient's school performance, behaviour, or personality. The deterioration may have been fairly subtle or slow, and collateral histories from parents, school, and social worker are essential. The patient is often making an effort to conceal the drug abuse, and without collateral history the correct diagnosis may not be made.
- *Physical examination* may have to be repeated. This may reveal the physical effects of the drug or stigmata of use by

injection. Tests of blood and urine may be helpful. As a baseline, the urine can be screened for cannabis and mandrax use.

Ultimately, the diagnosis can only be made if the patient admits to abuse of the drug or if the drug is positively identified in blood or urine.

*Drug dependence* (*DSM*-IV) is indicated when the person cannot control the use of the drug despite adverse consequences, and where there are physiological symptoms of tolerance (increased dosing) and withdrawal.

The following are *indicators of dependence*:
- the person needs to increase the dose to overcome a diminishing effect;
- the person has attempted to cut down or control the use of the drug;
- the use of the drug affects social relationships and/or work; and
- the drug continues to be used despite physical problems or contra-indications.

The *treatment* of drug abuse is generally very difficult and yields poor results. Every effort should be made to prevent drug abuse and to address social, community, family, and personal factors that predispose to drug abuse – a major mental health problem.

The following treatment guidelines are useful:
- the abuser needs to acknowledge that there is a problem and be willing to participate in a treatment programme;
- a problem analysis must include biological, psychological, educational, and social aspects;
- a holistic treatment programme must include the family and, if possible, the community;
- rehabilitation requires major changes in attitudes, interactions, and lifestyle; and
- physical problems connected with drug withdrawal may be life-threatening and need medical intervention.

Finally, drug abuse is a world-wide problem. It is also an increasing mental health and public health hazard in southern Africa. The drug addict can frequently trace a stepped progression that begins with the intermittent and controlled use of relatively innocuous, freely available drugs, progressing through increasingly higher doses and potency until an uncontrolled dependence is reached. Treatment of drug abuse is difficult and energies should be directed towards prevention programmes, public awareness, and the early detection of experimentation with drugs by young people.

Drug abuse is a complex problem best understood in a socio-cultural context and best treated holistically within that context.

## Some drugs of abuse

### Tobacco
Smoked or chewed. Nicotine is powerfully addictive, but widely advertised and readily available to young people.

### Alcohol
Drunk as beer, wine, and distilled spirits. Causes physical and psychological dependence. It is widely abused and introduced to children in families.

### Cannabis products
Includes marijuana, hashish, 'hash oil', 'dope' etc. Smoked in cigarettes, 'joints', and pipes. Intoxicant and euphoric. Causes psychological dependence, is relatively cheap, readily available, and circulates in schools.

### Stimulants
Includes amphetamines, 'speed', methylphenidate. Taken orally or intravenously. Cause feelings of well-being and increases energy. May cause psychoses. Dependence is common, mainly psychological.

### Hallucinogens
Includes LSD (acid), mescaline, phencyclidine (PCP, angel dust). Taken orally. Cause altered consciousness, hallucinations, and unusual subjective states. They often result in psychological dependence.

### Barbiturates
Taken orally or intravenously. They have a sedative effect and may be used to counter effects of stimulants. Can cause serious dependency.

### Tranquillizers
Especially benzodiazepines ('Valium', 'Halcion', 'Librium'). Taken orally, rarely intravenously. Result in lightheadedness and relief of tension. Used for 'coming down' after using cocaine, amphetamines, and other stimulants. Can result in psychological dependence.

### Narcotics
Heroin, morphine, methadone, codeine, and related compounds are taken intravenously and orally. They cause feelings of well-being, pleasant drowsiness, and contentment. Major physical dependence may occur.

### Cocaine
Inhaled as powder, smoked ('freebasing'), or taken intravenously. A stimulant producing great euphoria briefly, and stimulation of heart and other organs. May cause psychotic state and severe psychological dependence.

### Inhalants
Includes solvents in glue etc., petrol. They are inhaled, often from plastic bags. Cause brief euphoria and confusion. Psychological dependence may occur. May also cause brain damage.

## SIGNS AND SYMPTOMS OF ALCOHOL ABUSE

The first warning signs of a *developing alcohol problem* are:
- an increase in the frequency of drinking;
- an increase in tolerance for alcohol, which leads to an increase in the amount of alcohol consumed; and
- a need to get intoxicated or to feel the effect of alcohol on most drinking occasions.

As the condition progresses any number of the following may manifest:
- *Psychological/emotional symptoms*
  - Relief drinking
  - Feelings of anxiety and tension
  - Feelings of remorse
  - Feelings of self-hatred
  - Feelings of guilt
  - Suspiciousness
  - Flattening of emotions
  - Personality changes
  - Illusions
  - Use of defence mechanisms
  - Black-outs and faulty memory recall
  - Irrational jealousy
  - Hallucinations
  - Alcoholic dementia
- *Behavioural symptoms*
  - Secret drinking
  - Inappropriate drinking
  - Gulping
  - Drinking alone
  - The use of 'regmakers'
  - Compulsive drinking
  - Binge drinking
  - Change of drinking companions
  - Attempts at going on the wagon
  - Repeated drunkenness
  - 'Driving while intoxicated' offences
  - Attempts at geographical escape
  - Sexual difficulties
  - Anti-social behaviour
  - Aggression toward self and others
  - Irrational behaviour
  - Child abuse
  - Sleep disturbances
  - Irritability
  - Family arguments
  - Marital disharmony
  - Job absenteeism and tardiness
  - Accidents at work and at home
  - Job changes and loss of jobs
  - Financial problems

(Galanter et al., 1994; Desjarlais et al., 1996)

## SEXUAL PROBLEMS AND TEENAGE PREGNANCY

Changing social patterns and the breakdown of traditional sex education programmes frequently leave teenagers to cope with sexual development in silence and loneliness. Premarital sex and how to obtain contraceptives are not easy to discuss with parents. Sexual experiences, whether heterosexual or homosexual (commonly transient among boys), may arouse profound guilt and anxiety and have an effect on the adolescent's day-to-day functioning. Anxiety disorders, obsessions, depression, and even eating disorders may emerge at this time and may be related to anxieties about sexuality.

*Teenage pregnancy* is a major problem. The causes are many: incest, sexual abuse, rape, early unprotected regular sexual intercourse, teenage parties where cannabis and alcohol encourage sexual activities, and child and teenage prostitution. Family breakdown and the loss of parental control are also often linked to teenage pregnancies. Gang-raping has become a difficult problem resulting in no woman or girl being safe, even in a group. Sexual assault, largely performed by older teenage boys in gangs, is a major cause of family stress and of post-traumatic stress disorder in the victim.

A teenage pregnancy is seldom *not* a catastrophe, and usually has sequelae well into the future for both the mother and the child. Teenage pregnancy may be reduced by:

- active promotion of good *family life* and all that goes with it, socially and economically;
- *education* for parents and children about sex and contraception, encouraging openness. (It is hoped that the fear of AIDS and continuing education about AIDS is having some effect in this area.);
- *post-coitus intervention.* Pregnancy can be prevented in cases of unprotected sexual intercourse by treating within 48 hours with Ovral. The dose is two tablets, to be repeated 12 hours later. This brings on menstruation; and
- *legal abortions.* Under the new South African law, a pregnant girl may quite easily procure an abortion provided the pregnancy is less than 20 weeks. For the adolescent who carries an unwanted pregnancy, the abortion needs to be very sensitively worked through with the girl, the family, and, if possible, the father of the baby. There are many religious and cultural problems connected with the issue. A minor does not need to have the consent of her parents to obtain an abortion (5(3) Act No 92 of 1996).

Should it be decided that the teenager should go ahead with the pregnancy, then adoption is a possibility. The family should be helped with this decision, as the teenager is often rebellious, feels guilty and defiant, while the parents feel angry and rejecting. They frequently need professional help to move beyond these negative emotions in order to be able to make those decisions that will be best for the unborn child, the teenage mother, and the family. In some cultures adoption out of the family is not an acceptable option.

The teenage mother (or new parents) need a great deal of help and support during and after the pregnancy. Every individual will have different personal needs and the dynamics of the wider family may warrant considerable professional input if positive relationships, acceptance, understanding, and support are to be achieved.

All health programmes should seriously address the issues of teenage sexuality and parental responsibility, aiming to help people to develop satisfying stable relationships that counter past disadvantages and break the cycles of destructive maladaption. Sound family structures are fundamental to a healthy society and, in turn, to healthy people.

## EATING DISORDERS

Eating disorders are characterized by gross disturbances in eating behaviour. They range from refusal to maintain minimal normal body weight by rigid self-control (anorexia nervosa) to little self-control, the patient being impulsive and unpredictable (bulimia nervosa).

The essential features of *anorexia nervosa* (*DSM*-IV) are:

- refusal to maintain bodyweight over a minimal normal weight for age and height (bodyweight 15 per cent or more below normal);
- intense fear of gaining weight or becoming fat, even though underweight;
- a distorted body image with declarations by the patients that they feel fat even when emaciated; and
- amenorrhoea in females.

Weight loss is usually accomplished by a reduction in total food intake with extensive exercising. The patient does not truly have a lack of appetite. Frequently there is self-induced vomiting or the use of laxatives or diuretics. Some patients have intermittent loss of control with eating binges followed by vomiting. Other behaviours concerning food are common. Often patients will have a need to prepare elaborate meals for others, but limit themselves to small amounts of low-calorie foods. Most people with this disorder minimize the severity of their illness and are resistant to therapy. Many adolescents have delayed psychosexual development. The differential diagnosis of anorexia nervosa is physical illness, depression, schizophrenia, and bulimia nervosa, where there may be an intense fear of obesity.

Since anorexia nervosa is potentially life threatening, treatment in hospital or by a specialist team may be necessary. The programme should include refeeding with concurrent behavioural controls and rewards, individual psychotherapy and family counselling, medication if indicated, and long-term follow-up.

The essential features of *bulimia nervosa* (*DSM*-IV) are recurrent episodes of large amounts of food being rapidly eaten in a discrete period of time (binge eating), a feeling of lack of control over eating behaviour during binges, self-induced vomiting, the use of laxatives or diuretics, strict dieting or fasting, vigorous exercise in order to prevent weight gain, and persistent over-concern with body shape and weight. To be diagnosed as bulimic, the person must have averaged at least two eating binges a week for more than three months. People with bulimia nervosa are usually within a normal weight range.

Bulimics may have a concurrent depressive disorder and some may abuse drugs such as tranquillizers, amphetamines, alcohol, or cocaine. The age of onset is often in adolescence and the course is chronic and intermittent over a number of years. The differential diagnosis includes other conditions that may give unusual eating patterns: schizophrenia, some neurological conditions (epilepsy, Kluver-Bucy-like syndromes, Kleine-Levin syndrome), and some cases of borderline personality disorder in females.

Treatment is by appropriate combinations of behaviour modification and individual and group psychotherapy. Any medication that may be addictive should be avoided.

Eating disorders are found in all races and cultures.

## SUICIDE BEHAVIOUR IN ADOLESCENTS

Accurate figures for *adolescent suicide behaviour* for all population groups in southern Africa are not available. It seems that suicide attempts by males are more violent than those by females and have a higher potential lethality. Successful suicides are frequently related to school anxiety and poor performance. In all population groups, attempted suicides (parasuicides) are common. Females predominate and most commonly at about 13 years of age. The methods used vary, depending on those commonly available for self-destruction. More affluent adolescents tend to use tablets of various kinds and to slash their wrists. The less affluent adolescents tend to use household cleaners, benzine, thinners, and rat poison. Young children (six to eight years) have been known take rat poison, apparently in serious suicide attempts.

Family and interpersonal stress continue to precipitate a steady stream of parasuicides, potentially perilous cries for help. During the 1985 to 1986 protests in Soweto, there was a great increase in the number of adolescents admitted after making suicide attempts – an indication of a desperate response to environmental stress.

Most adolescents who make suicide attempts do not show signs of depression. It is commonly an unplanned, impulsive act, a desperate attempt to escape from an untenable family situation or a response to stress.

The practitioner needs to maintain a high index of suspicion. A suicide attempt must always be taken seriously. Management must begin with an assessment of suicidal intent: 'Have you ever thought seriously about killing yourself?' Assessment must be made of the further risk of suicide: 'How do you see the future?'; 'Have you ever felt that life is not worth living?'

Underlying psychiatric disorders such as major depression or schizophrenia, with self-destructive command hallucinations must be considered.

Generally, the treatment of adolescent suicide behaviour must address the precipitating as well as the predisposing factors. The patient must be helped towards appropriate problem-solving techniques. All this may necessitate a major investment of time and effort. Suicide behaviour in adolescents with personality disorders may be very difficult to manage (see conduct disorder).

## ADULT-TYPE PSYCHIATRIC DISORDERS ARISING IN ADOLESCENCE

Any of the major psychiatric disorders of adult life may arise during adolescence, but because this may be a time of emotional upheaval and uncertainty both for patients and families, and because the form of the disorder is not fully developed, the diagnosis may not be clear. A strong family history of mental disorder should help with early diagnosis and treatment.

On the other hand, unusual phenomena (e.g., hearing voices) experienced in times of heightened anxiety or stress do not necessarily indicate major disorders and there is some merit in conservative management. The aim is to provide support, understanding, and guidance for a usually very anxious teenager and his or her even more bewildered and worried family. Both affective disorders (depression and bipolar disorders) and schizophrenia become more common as adolescence proceeds.

## Affective disorders

Affective disorders are very common in adolescence, with depression being found most frequently.

*Depression:* Tearfulness and feelings of hopelessness may be part of a reaction (adjustment disorder) to a severe psychosocial stress that occurred not more than three months previously.

Management of a depressed mood is usually conservative support for the patient and family.

*Dysthymic disorder* (*DSM*-IV) 'depressive neurosis': The essential feature is a chronically depressed mood, but in children or adolescents it may be an irritable or explosive mood. This needs to have lasted almost continually for more than a year. There may also be associated increase or decrease in eating or sleeping, low energy level, poor concentration, difficulty in making decisions, and feelings of hopelessness. The presence of hallucinations or delusions would indicate a major depressive disorder or schizophrenia.

Dysthymic disorder may be secondary to a physical illness or disorder such as bulimia nervosa or anorexia nervosa. The onset may be a response to chronic stress factors or unresolved issues. The course of dysthymia is often chronic and may have a superimposed major depression. Treatment must address biological, psychological, and social issues. Medication may be effective, especially if there is a major depression as well.

*Major Depressive Disorder* (*DSM*-IV) (single episode or recurrent): The essential features of major depression have been outlined for pre-pubertal children (Chapter 52: Serious psychological disorders). Adolescents may show irritable mood and explosive behaviour rather than classical depression. Other age-specific features of depression may be negativism or frankly antisocial behaviour with abuse of drugs. Feelings of aggression, being unwanted and unloved are common, with the adolescent withdrawing from family and friends and becoming isolated. School difficulties are likely. The use of alcohol and/or cannabis may compound the problem. The teenager may become more sloppy in dress and be emotionally labile. Delusions and hallucinations may be present.

Treatment must involve the patient and family in psychotherapy. Antidepressants are useful. The risk of suicide can be a hazard.

*Bipolar disorder* (manic episode): The essential features of a manic episode include:
- a distinct period of elevated, expansive, or irritable mood;
- during the mood disturbance several of the following are present: grandiosity, decreased need for sleep, pressured speech, flight of ideas, distractibility, agitation, overspending, or hypersexuality;
- delusions or hallucination with the mood disturbance; and
- impairment of function.

'Hypomania' is an episode of elevated mood without impairment of function. A manic episode in adolescence may be short and pass unrecognized. Treatment is with antipsychotic medication, but repeated episodes may require long-term prophylaxis with lithium.

## Schizophrenia disorders

Most of the features of the schizophrenic illnesses to be found in adults also apply to adolescents.

Whatever the clinical presentation in children or younger adolescents may be, only the passage of time will enable the distinction from affective disorders to be made with certainty. 'Organic' causes (possibly toxic or medical) must always be considered. Thought disorder can occur commonly in the turbulence of ideas and feelings of normal adolescents. A lack of communication skills in some adolescents may suggest schizophrenia wrongly. In this age group, symptoms that strongly suggest the diagnosis of schizophrenia are:
- experiences of passivity, thoughts controlled by or broadcast to others;
- auditory hallucinations; and
- primary delusions (the delusions and hallucinations not being part of a mood disorder).

The diagnostic criteria for schizophrenia are:
- the presence of psychotic symptoms (hallucinations or delusions or both), lasting at least a month;
- the patient's level of function is lowered;
- the signs of mental illness and lowered function have lasted more than six months;
- a mood disorder with psychotic features has been ruled out; and
- organic causes (e.g., drug abuse) have been ruled out.

The course of the illness is usually chronic with remissions and relapses and, although patients may retain a normal measurable IQ, their motivation, interpersonal skills, insight, and judgement have deteriorated enough, apart from any florid symptoms of psychosis, to prevent them returning to their full potential of pre-morbid function.

Long-term antipsychotic medication is the cornerstone of treatment, added to which are therapies that will maximize function and family counselling.

## Stress and psychiatric disorders

It is becoming increasingly clear that stress has an important part to play in the aetiology of psychiatric disorders. Although the exact nature of the pathology caused by the stress has not yet been fully worked out, it is apparent that stress may be implicated in the precipitation of mild and major disorders, which must mean that stress causes changes in brain systems which in turn are the cause of mental disorders. (Similarly, stress may result in changes to the immune system of the body.) It is clear that some people are more vulnerable to the effects of a given stressor than others. Certain people may have a specific vulnerability to stressors, which may be biological, environmental, or psychosocial, or a combination of the three.

As a result of severe, possibly life-threatening, stress, a person may suffer from an acute stress disorder characterized by numbing, withdrawal, and avoidance; or may have a more chronic, slower onset post-traumatic stress disorder where the traumatic event is re-experienced in dreams or when there are events that remind the person of the trauma. The result is intense psychological distress and withdrawal from anything that may act as a trigger.

Apart from the above disorders, stress seems to be at least partly responsible for precipitating disorders such as mood disorders, schizophrenia, anxiety disorders, and substance abuse. Attention needs to be paid to helping adolescents to cope with stress in healthy and constructive ways. Teaching living skills should be part of every educational curriculum. In addition, special attention must be given to people caught up in extraordinary stress. It would appear that if people who have experienced severe trauma have immediate treatment in the form of counselling and possible medical treatment, it may be helpful in preventing the more severe and chronic effects of the trauma.

## References and further reading

DESJARLAIS R, EISENBERG L, GOOD B, and KLEINMAN A. 1996. *World mental health.* Cape Town: Oxford University Press.

DIAGNOSTIC AND STATISTICAL MANUAL OF MENTAL DISORDERS, 4th ed. 1994. (*DSM*-IV). Washington DC: American Psychiatric Association.

GALANTER M & KLEBER HD (eds.). 1994. *The American Psychiatric Press textbook of substance abuse treatment.* Washington DC: American Psychiatric Press.

GREEN WH. 1995. *Child and adolescent clinical psychopharmacology,* 2nd ed. Baltimore: Williams & Wilkins.

RUTTER M, TAYLOR E, and HERSOV L. 1994. *Child and adolescent psychiatry – Modern approaches,* 3rd ed. Oxford: Blackwell Scientific Publications.

SCHATSBERG AF & NEMEROFF CB (eds.). 1998. *The American Psychiatric Press textbook of psychopharmacology.* Washington DC: American Psychiatric Press.

# 54

# Child mental health services

## BA ROBERTSON

## Background

Child mental health services in South Africa were established largely in relation to local clinical and academic needs and resources. The result is a very uneven distribution of services with highly developed hospital-based clinics in some major urban centres and few services in peri-urban and rural areas. National child and adolescent mental health policy guidelines are currently being formulated by the Directorate of Mental Health and Substance Abuse. Some provinces have already drawn up provincial guidelines, and are in the process of setting up child and adolescent mental health programmes.

Children and adolescents with mental health problems may be referred to public sector services provided by a range of departments, including Health, Education, Welfare, Justice, and Correctional Services. Many are treated by medical practitioners, psychologists, and other professionals in the private sector. Historically, child mental health services are among the most underdeveloped, due in large part to the low status afforded to women, children, and mental health issues, and to the late development of the discipline.

## Present and future developments

Existing child mental health services in South Africa are being transformed according to two major principles, namely, the primary health care policy, and the integration of mental health into general health care. The primary health care policy emphasizes the role of promotion and prevention, and divides health care into primary, secondary, and tertiary levels. A third important consideration is inter-sectoral collaboration, in order to maximize limited resources, and reduce fragmentation.

Promotion should focus on promoting mentally healthy families, schools, and communities. Public awareness about the concept of mental health, its importance, and how to achieve it should be increased. Public knowledge about key child mental health problems, and their detection and management, should be promoted. The stigma surrounding mental health and psychiatric problems and their treatment needs to be actively addressed.

Prevention programmes will focus on national, provincial, or local priorities such as

Fetal Alcohol Syndrome, child abuse, and other forms of violence involving children, substance abuse, and HIV/AIDS. Early detection and intervention is important as many relatively common serious psychological problems that are associated with significant long-term impairment of functioning remain undetected and/or untreated for years: examples are depression, anxiety disorders including post-traumatic stress disorder, and conduct disorder. It is essential that emotional and behavioural problems are included in developmental screening programmes. Psychological problems are commonly associated with developmental disorders, physical or intellectual disability, and chronic illness, and need to be addressed as part of the comprehensive package of care.

Primary health care staff need to be adequately trained in detecting and assessing serious psychological and other mental health problems in children and adolescents, including evaluating the impact of the problem on the family. They must be able to provide information about the aetiology, treatment, and prognosis of the problem (psychoeducation), and to provide basic counselling around parenting, communication and behaviour management in the home. They need to liaise with other services in the community such as education and welfare services and NGOs (e.g., Mental Health Society) in order to obtain collateral information and/or assistance with management, and to monitor the course of the problem. Primary health care staff need to know where and how to refer mental health problems which they do not have the competence to treat. In many instances, this will be a psychiatric nurse attached to a PHC clinic who is a member of the regional community mental health team. These teams fall under the directorates of Comprehensive Health Care and ideally include a general psychiatrist and other mental health professionals. They work in the community with patients of all ages, and may also provide some services in district and regional hospitals.

At the time of writing, mental health services have not been established for either children or adults at the secondary level of care, with a few exceptions. Emergency care and limited in- and outpatient services (all ages) are planned for district and regional hospitals as resources become available. Only children and adolescents who require more intensive or specialized psychiatric treatment should be referred to tertiary child and adolescent psychiatric units.

## References and further reading

ROBERTSON B. 1996. Handbook of child psychiatry for primary care. Cape Town: Oxford University Press.

DAWES A, ROBERTSON B, DUNCAN N, ENSINK K, JACKSON A, REYNOLDS P, PILLAY A, and RICHTER L. 1997. Child and adolescent mental health policy. In: D Foster, M Freeman, and Y Pillay (eds.). Mental health policy issues for South Africa. Cape Town: Medical Association of South Africa Multimedia Publications.

# PART FOURTEEN

# Children with special needs

Children with any impairment of function are further disadvantaged if their special needs are not met. This is likely to impact directly on the degree to which a disability becomes a handicap for the individual, the family, and the community. Assessment and management of these issues are discussed in this part.

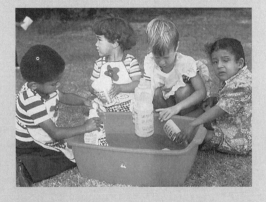

# 55

# Intellectual disability

## CD MOLTENO & J WAGNER

Some form of intellectual disability is found in two to three per cent of the population. More severe forms (IQ <50) are said to occur in at least three or four out of every thousand people in any population. Estimating the population at 40 million, there are thus at least 150 000 severely intellectually disabled people in South Africa, but it is probable that only a small percentage of these have been properly assessed or offered adequate help.

Facilities for people with severe intellectual disability are largely inadequate, though there has been much improvement in the past 20 years.

All health professionals should have some idea of the ways in which these people can be helped, and of the facilities which they need.

Children with intellectual disability are found in every race, religion, and nationality as well as at every level of educational, social, and economic background. They vary considerably in physical characteristics, in degrees of dependency, in levels of intelligence, emotional stability, academic achievement, and social adjustment.

## Terminology

It is widely accepted that terms or labels can have potentially damaging effects on people. Not only do terms cause stigmatization due to the effect of discrediting the person, but labels can also give rise to self-fulfilling prophesies. For example, a child described as 'ineducable' will be denied educational opportunities and then become less competent, thus justifying the original label.

It is hoped that the terms 'idiot' and 'imbecile' have disappeared from use. The term 'mental deficiency' gave way to 'mental retardation' in the USA and 'mental handicap' in the UK. Since 1981, 'disability' and more recently 'learning disability' have come into general use in the UK. Unfortunately, this term causes confusion in many countries as it usually refers to specific learning disabilities, including dyslexia. Criticisms with 'mental handicap' arise because the word 'mental' is considered derogatory to many and 'handicap' implies 'a disadvantage resulting from the effects of a disability which limit the fulfillment of a role'. This signifies a lack of appropriate intervention and is a negation of the 'normalization principle'.

There has recently been considerable support for the term 'intellectual disability' internationally. In a survey conducted by the South African Federation for Mental Health, this was the term that enjoyed most support in South Africa. 'Intellectual disability' should therefore replace the term 'mental handicap'.

# Definition

According to the American Association on Mental Retardation, intellectual disability is characterized by subaverage intellectual functioning, associated with limitations in a number of adaptive skill areas and has an onset before 18 years of age. Subaverage intellectual functioning implies an IQ level greater than two standard deviations below the mean (< 70). Adaptive skill areas include communication, self-care, home living, social skills, community use, self-direction, health and safety, functional academics, and leisure and work.

## Degrees of intellectual disability

Intellectual disability differs in degree and the World Health Organization classifies these degrees as follows:
- *Mild intellectual disability:* Socially competent; may need guidance and assistance during periods of stress.
- *Moderate disability:* Basic self-care skills; need some supervision and guidance.
- *Severe disability:* Some self-care skills; need full supervision.
- *Profound disability:* Minimal self-care skills; need constant nursing care.

# Causation

Intellectual disability may be divided into two groups. The one group represents the lower

**Table 55.1** Degrees of intellectual disability

| Degree | IQ | Prevalence per 1000 |
|---|---|---|
| Mild | 50–75 | 20–30 |
| Moderate | 35–50 | 3 |
| Severe | 20–35 | |
| Profound | 0–20 | 1 |

end of the normal distribution curve of intelligence. Because heredity plays an important role in intellectual ability, this group is often referred to as *familial*. However, the environment, particularly environmental deprivation, also has an inpact in this group. People in the familial/environmental group are usually mildly disabled. The other group is referred to as *organic*, because the causes reflect organic brain damage or dysfunction. Causes in the organic group can be classified according to the timing of the pathology. Prenatal factors arise from the time of conception to the onset of labour. The perinatal group causes are derived from problems occurring during labour, the birth process or in the adaptation to extrauterine life. Postnatal causes originate after this period. There are also cases where, despite a careful history, examination, and relevant investigations, no cause can be found. These fall into the idiopathic group.

# Categories of causes

## PRENATAL

Chromosomal abnormalities account for a significant number of cases and Down syndrome is the commonest identifiable cause of intellectual disability. Trisomy resulting from non-disjunction during meiosis accounts for 95 per cent of cases, while translocations and mosaics make up the rest. Trisomy is associated with increasing maternal age, whereas translocations are not related to maternal age, but may be directly inherited. Because trisomies account for the majority of cases of Down syndrome, even those children born to younger mothers are more likely to have trisomy. The commonest inherited cause of intellectual disability is the fragile X syndrome. This is associated with the presence of a fragile site on the X chromosome resulting from the inheritance of an unstable region of DNA. It occurs in both sexes, although it is more common and more severe in males. Turner syndrome is probably more common than both Down syndrome and the fragile X syndrome, but most cases abort during the first trimester of pregnancy. Those that survive are usually less severely disabled as are the other sex chromosome abnormalities such as Klinefelter syndrome and the triple X syndrome. Autosomal abnormalities include trisomies, translocations, and deletions. Inborn errors of metabolism, resulting from single gene abnormalities give rise to biochemical disorders. For example: organic acidurias (e.g., propionic acidaemia) disorders of amino acid metabolism (e.g., phenylketonuria), disorders of carbohydrate metabolism (e.g., galactosaemia), disorders of lipid metabolism (e.g., Tay-Sachs disease) and disorders of purine metabolism (e.g., Lesch Nyhan syndrome). There are also a number of recognizable syndromes that do not have identifiable chromosomal or gene abnormalities. Congenital abnormalities of the brain give rise to intellectual disability. These include congenital hydrocephalus and absent corpus callosum. Some cases of disability are thought to result from disorders of neuronal migration. Acquired causes arising prenatally are intra-uterine infections of the TORCH group, toxins, especially alcohol, and complications of pregnancy, particularly if they interfere with fetal growth.

## PERINATAL

Most perinatal causes can be related to prematurity and its complications and asphyxia in the full-term infant. The pre-term infant is at risk for perinatal asphyxia, hyaline membrane disease, and septicaemia. The mechanism of brain damage is usually anoxia, haemorrhage, or hypotension. The haemorrhage is classically periventricular, but may be associated with an intraventricular haemorrhage leading to hydrocephalus. The asphyxia in the full-term infant is frequently difficult to predict and presents as fetal distress followed by asphyxia neonatorum leading to the clinical condition of hypoxic-ischaemic encephalopathy. Other mechanisms of brain damage in the neonate are hypoglycaemia, hypocalcaemia, and hyperbilirubinaemia.

## POSTNATAL

Postnatal causes are infections (meningitis and encephalitis) and trauma (both accidental and non-accidental, child abuse). Any severe childhood illness may progress to brain damage. Status epilepticus may preceed a state of chronic disability and some cases of severe disability follow specific types of seizures, for example, infantile spasms.

Attempting to find the cause is important for the following reasons:
- because treatment is occasionally possible;
- for family counselling; and
- for genetic counselling.

**Table 55.2** Causes of intellectual disability in a review of over 1 000 cases in the Western Cape

| Cause | Number (%) |
| --- | --- |
| Prenatal | 406 (40%) |
| Perinatal | 177 (18%) |
| Postnatal | 171 (17%) |
| Idiopathic | 247 (25%) |

# Screening

Because of the importance of early detection of disability, population screening is mandatory. The screening process is outlined in Chapter 21: Health surveillance. Infants detected by the screening process are referred for developmental assessment, which is carried out by a multidisciplinary team.

# Assessment

The results of an assessment will reveal the developmental age in a number of domains – gross motor, fine motor, language and communication, and social. These ages are then compared with the chronological age and if all four levels are low, the child is most likely to be globally retarded. If one level is low and the others normal, an explanation, such as deafness causing a low speech level, or cerebral palsy causing a low motor level, should be considered.

# Multi-disciplinary team

This consists of a paediatrician, speech therapist, physiotherapist, occupational therapist, a social worker, and if available a psychologist. The paediatrician should take an adequate history and examine the child fully, including a nervous system examination, a search for dysmorphic features and abnormal skin markings. He or she should assess the child's mental age and arrange for appropriate investigations. The therapists assess the area of their discipline: gross motor (physiotherapy), fine motor (occupational), and speech. Ideally, a social worker should meet all family members. Referrals to a psychologist, psychiatrist, or other appropriate medical specialist may be indicated. Following the assessments, a team meeting is held to discuss the findings and plan a management programme.

The team method approach has obvious advantages. It is the most accurate method and each therapist will be able to state whether or not therapy is indicated. An important advantage is that those who have worked in a team soon learn what other team members are doing and can then assess more accurately when working on their own. This concept is important in South Africa, which is so short of trained professionals. The obvious drawback is that so few of the intellectually disabled people in South Africa have access to a multi-professional team. Team assessments are available in major teaching hospitals and cerebral palsy schools.

# Treatment of intellectual disability

Treatment of the child and family must follow the assessment and diagnosis of intellectual disability. Whenever possible, he or she should remain in the community with the family or a suitable substitute. Professionals must be able to help the child, the parents and the family, and therefore be familiar with the facilities that are available.

## HELPING THE CHILD

Intellectually disabled children need to be loved and wanted by family and peers, and to be encouraged by praise for their achievements. To be loved, they need to be lovable; and this is one of many reasons why such children should be reasonably disciplined and behaviour made as acceptable as possible. Expectations of the child and the disciplinary measures used must always be appropriate to the mental age rather than to the chronological age.

General health must be promoted and everyday sicknesses treated appropriately.

Problems such as toothache, constipation, and urinary tract infection must not be forgotten. In severely disabled children, presenting symptoms of these conditions may be unrelated to the site of the problem. For example, pain may be expressed by bad behaviour.

The child must be given every chance to reach his or her full potential. Early intervention should be offered from the time of diagnosis in infancy. A suitable day care centre or nursery school should follow from three to four years and special schooling from six to seven. Sadly, such facilities are not available for many disabled children. Adequate assessment and keeping of records will help promote awareness of the need for facilities.

## HELPING THE FAMILY

Helping the parents to cope is of great importance and should start at the time of diagnosis. Telling parents that their child is disabled must be done with great sensitivity, and with as much time as is necessary. Wherever possible, both parents should be present. The diagnosis must be given with gentleness and empathy, but strongly enough for the message to be understood. Two or three meetings may be needed because, in their initial state of emotional shock, parents often take in very little of what is said, and certainly will not be able to discuss any plans for helping the child. Most parents go through the stages of grieving, perhaps for the normal child they have 'lost'. These are the stages of *denial, anger, depression, bargaining,* and finally *acceptance* and *planning*. In counselling, the extended family, especially siblings and grandparents, must always be remembered.

The family of an intellectually disabled child needs ongoing support. Their grieving may recur or be accentuated every time their affected child fails to reach a milestone or achieves less than normal children of similar age.

Counselling can be undertaken by the doctor, social worker, community nurse, therapist or a member of a parent support association such as the Down Syndrome Association. It must include comfort, allowing the parents to understand what is wrong and what the various investigations are likely to involve. The interpretration of the results and the meaning of all medical terms need to be discussed, and plans formulated together.

## GENETIC COUNSELLING

This is a vital part of parent counselling. Services are freely available through university or health departments. However, all doctors should be able to offer an opinion and can obtain help by phone or letter if necessary. Thus, all parents of disabled children should be able to obtain advice on the likelihood of subsequent children having the same problem.

# Facilities

## EARLY INTERVENTION

Disabled pre-school children benefit from stimulation programmes in movement, play, and speech. Parents or caregivers are taught to offer these programmes by attending therapy sessions at a hospital, through the community sister, or through trained home counsellors. Counselling is an important part of early intervention. Parents benefit by the feeling that they are involved, and the children undoubtedly improve in ability and motivation. If available, attendance at a toy library is beneficial.

## EDUCATION

Traditionally in South Africa, a system of segregated education was used with disabled children attending special schools depending on the nature of their disability. In practice, because of the previous racial segregation in education, most special schools were designated for white children only. Black disabled children attended mainstream schools or remained at home. Recently, the trend worldwide has been to move from a segregated system of special education to one of inclusion. The Salamanca Statement, proposing an inclusive education system, was adopted at an international UNESCO conference in Spain in 1994. Inclusion is felt to be important because it breaks down prejudices towards people with disabilities, reinforces the need to value one another, to expose children to a broader experience of life, and to give children the opportunity to help one another. However, to make inclusion work there needs to be a commitment to the philosophy of inclusion, enlightenment of communities, a creative and flexible body of teachers, participation between parents and teachers, and funding to ensure its success. The bill of rights in the South African constitution guarantees an equal right to education for all. The South African Schools Act of 1996 requires public schools to admit all learners and serve their educational requirements without unfairly discriminating in any way. The National Commission on Special Needs in Education and Training and the National Committee on Education Support Services were established in 1997 to investigate and make recommendations on all aspects of special needs and support services. Children with disabilities are now referred to as 'learners with special needs' (LSEN) and special education as 'education for learners with special needs' (ELSEN). It would seem prudent in South Africa, because of financial constraints, to operate a system that retains the ELSEN facilities, but moves progressively towards a fully inclusive system. ELSEN schools should not only continue to educate disabled children, but they should also be seen as resource centres, which extend their expertise into the mainstream schools. Currently, children with an IQ of less than 30 are denied an education. They are placed in special care centres, which fall under the health department. These centres receive some funding but rely largely on parent support. This means that the children in this special care category are not receiving education and are therefore being discriminated against which is in breach of the constitution

## RESIDENTIAL CARE

This can be temporary or permanent.

'Temporary' or 'respite' care is freely available in many overseas countries. It is a facility in a home for intellectually disabled people, or in a hospital, which will provide care in time of crisis, such as mother's illness or confinement, or simply as a means of family relief, once or on a regular basis. If respite care helps the family to cope better, the disabled child can be kept at home for longer periods than might otherwise have been the case.

'Permanent care' was once the usual solution to the presence of an intellectually disabled person in the family, but in the past two decades it has been less and less recommended. If the family is unable to care for the child, if there is no family, or if the harm to the family caused by having a disabled child at home is greater than the benefit to the child, then permanent residential care should be sought. It must be remembered that it is often hard to find places, that waiting lists are long, and sometimes costs are very high.

Alternatives that should be considered are foster care and adoption of disabled children. There are some child-minder schemes for both normal and disabled children, and these should be extended to residential care. Such schemes need careful monitoring by social workers, and the child-minder needs adequate pay for services. The money can be paid by the parents, by some subsidized schemes, and hopefully one day by government grants.

**Table 55.3** Ideal long-term management of children with intellectual disability (J Hollingshead)

MILD DISABILITY

| | |
|---|---|
| 0–3 years | Diagnosis |
| 3–6 years | Diagnosis; nursery school |
| 6–12 years | Normal school; remedial teaching; special class |
| 12–18 years | Normal school; special senior secondary school; technical high school |
| 18 plus years | Post-school education; open labour market |

MODERATE DISABILITY

| | |
|---|---|
| 0–3 years | Diagnosis |
| 3–6 years | Diagnosis; physiotherapy; speech and occupational therapy, nursery school |
| 6–12 years | Mainstream school, or ELSEN school |
| 12–18 years | ELSEN school |
| 18 plus years | Sheltered employment; protective workshop; disability grant from 16 upwards; community-based living |

SEVERE DISABILITY

| | |
|---|---|
| 0–3 years | Diagnosis; physiotherapy; speech and occupational therapy; toy library; parent guidance |
| 3–6 years | Diagnosis; physiotherapy; speech and occupational therapy; play group; parent guidance |
| 6–12 years | ELSEN school |
| 12–18 years | ELSEN school |
| 18 plus years | Protective workshop; disability grant from 16 upwards; community-based living |

PROFOUND DISABILITY

| | |
|---|---|
| 0–3 years | Diagnosis; physiotherapy; speech and occupational therapy; toy library; parent guidance |
| 3–6 years | Diagnosis; physiotherapy; speech and occupational therapy; play group; parent guidance, single care grant |
| 6–12 years | Special care unit – day or residential long-/short-term therapy; care dependency grant |
| 12–18 years | Special care unit – day or residential long-/short-term therapy; care dependency grant (16) |
| 18 plus years | Day or residential care; disability grant from 16 upwards; community-based living |

# Grants and financial aid

Care dependency grants are available for intellectually disabled children. The single care grant is available for 'profoundly disabled' children whose parents have a low enough income.

Disability grants are available for disabled people of 16 or over. Centres can obtain a grant from the Department of Health for 'special care' children. Considerable tax relief for the care of a disabled child can be obtained.

In conclusion, the outlook for children with intellectual disability is changing as the deficit model, which emphasized things that the child was unable to do, is replaced by a developmental model, which recognizes and strives to achieve the full potential of each child. The adoption of the inclusion principle and help and support of professionals should lead to an improved quality of life for all children with intellectual disability and their families.

## References and further reading

GILLHAM B (ed.). 1986. *Handicapping conditions in children.* London: Croom Helm.

ILLINGWORTH RS. 1985. *Development of infant and young child: Normal and abnormal.* Edinburgh: Churchill Livingstone.

LEA S & FOSTER D (eds.). 1990. *Perspectives on mental handicap in South Africa.* Durban: Butterworth.

SUNSHINE CENTRE AND TRANSVAAL MEMORIAL INSTITUTE OF CHILD HEALTH AND DEVELOPMENT, DEPARTMENT OF PAEDIATRICS, UNIVERSITY OF WITWATERSRAND. 1990. *Start home teaching programme for families with developmentally delayed children.* Johannesburg: Mike Hylton and Associates.

# 56

# Specific learning problems

## PM LEARY

Most of the people who were alive two hundred years ago were illiterate and had very little use for the written word. Parents were preoccupied not so much with the education of their children as with survival in the face of two ever-present threats: infection and malnutrition. Such circumstances now prevail only in the most underdeveloped regions of the world. Elsewhere, parents are no longer satisfied that their children should simply survive. Good quality of life is also desired and the ability to read and write is perceived as being essential to this end. The advantages of education are recognized by all, and universal literacy has become a goal of most governments.

Doctors are often consulted about children who fail to make adequate progress during their early years of formal schooling. There are many factors – prenatal, perinatal, and postnatal – that can cause or contribute to such problems. The important reasons for school failure are listed in the box below. It is in this area of differential diagnosis that the doctor has a major contribution to make to the management of learning-disabled children.

Children who have grown up in deprived communities are at an educational disadvantage for many reasons. Prenatal factors such

> ## Reasons for school failure
>
> • disadvantage;
> • developmental immaturity;
> • low intelligence;
> • visual defect;
> • hearing defect;
> • chronic ill health;
> • emotional disturbance;
> • undiagnosed seizure disorder;
> • neurological dysfunction; and
> • children in deprived communities.

as smoking, alcohol abuse, and poor maternal nutrition may cause low birthweight. Repeated infections and inadequate diet may impede progress in the early years. Lack of a stimulating environment in the early critical periods may also play a part.

Pre-school education – especially important in such children as a preparation for school – is generally at a premium in such communities, just where it is most urgently needed. Finally, the quality of schooling may be a factor in failure. Overcrowded classes and teachers who are undertrained and lacking in motivation are not conducive to educational success in the pupils.

## DEVELOPMENTAL IMMATURITY

No two children develop at an identical rate. While the majority are ready for formal schooling by the age of six, a significant number are not, and distractibility, inadequate fine motor co-ordination, and perceptual immaturity are likely to retard scholastic progress. Parents of children who show such features are well advised to defer school entry for a year in order to allow for maturation. This natural process is enhanced by the programmes offered at pre-primary schools.

## LOW INTELLIGENCE

Children with IQs in the 80 to 90 bracket will find it difficult to keep abreast of their peers in the classroom. Recognition of their own inadequacies in this context may result in clowning, antisocial behaviour, or depression. The parents of such children frequently fail to recognize the reason for poor scholastic achievement and attempt through home tuition and a variety of other therapies to bring about better results. These efforts are usually resented by the child, and an atmosphere of tension is generated within the home. Psychometric testing is pivotal in the elucidation of a situation of this nature, and the doctor's role is to help parents accept that transfer to a special class is in the child's best interests. Very few parents ever come to regret this move. The advantages to the child soon become evident in terms of reduced anxiety and restored self-esteem. Most children who follow the special class stream ultimately achieve skills that will enable them to take their places in everyday life.

## VISUAL DEFECT

Because of massive ciliary body action, myopia may remain undetected throughout the pre-school years. The child who has never known a normal degree of visual clarity does not complain. However, when reading and writing tasks assume prominence in his or her daily programme, the child is clearly at a disadvantage and scholastic progress inevitably suffers. Routine tests of visual acuity are essential for every child with learning problems, and referral to an ophthalmologist should follow when there is any question of a defect.

## HEARING DEFECT

Whenever deterioration in school work is of recent onset following former satisfactory progress, an acquired hearing defect should be considered. The 30 to 40 decibel hearing loss that accompanies unresolved serous otitis media (glue ear) is not always easy to detect. When spoken to directly, the child will not appear to be deaf, but in the classroom situation will have difficulty in following the teacher. As a consequence, concentration is likely to flag with a fall-off in performance. Audiometry is thus an important component in the assessment of the learning-disabled child.

## CHRONIC ILL HEALTH

Children whose general health is suboptimal can seldom give of their best in the classroom. Inadequately treated asthma and allergic rhinitis will interfere with sleep at night and affect daytime concentration. Chronic pulmonary and renal tract infection, cardiac decompensation, and endocrine disorders will all impair progress. Appropriate treatment must be provided in every case before optimal classroom performance can be expected.

## EMOTIONAL DISTURBANCE

Satisfactory scholastic progress is seldom achieved by children who are emotionally disturbed. Concentration and motivation are usually lacking and little satisfaction is derived from classroom achievement. Most childhood unhappiness stems from domestic circumstances rather than from experiences at school. Factors such as unrealistic parental attitudes, marital disharmony, alcoholism, or sibling rivalry are frequently responsible for sustained misery. Indifferent school performance is likely to persist until the underlying cause has been identified and adjustments have brought about conditions more conducive to happiness and self-assurance. There is often a striking improvement in a child's well-being when a mother who formerly worked full-time changes to spend her afternoons at home.

### UNDIAGNOSED SEIZURE DISORDER

When a seizure occurs during the night, the child's performance throughout the next school day may be impaired or erratic. A history of this nature calls for an EEG investigation, as does a story of recurrent 'blank spells' or daydreaming in class. Such episodes could be unrecognized simple absence attacks. In both situations, marked improvement in classroom performance will follow the administration of appropriate anticonvulsant therapy.

### NEUROLOGICAL DYSFUNCTION

There are some children who lack fine and gross motor control to a degree that is outside an acceptable normal spectrum. The imprecise term 'clumsy' is often applied to such children. Clinical examination reveals mild physical signs in keeping with the syndromes of cerebral palsy, and the term 'minimal cerebral damage', now in disfavour, could perhaps be used with justification. Such children usually require the special facilities and tuition available at a school for children with physical disabilities.

# Specific learning disability

It has come to be accepted that a learning-disabled child is one who fails to make acceptable scholastic progress in reading, writing, and simple arithmetic, despite adequate tuition, intelligence within the normal range, satisfactory emotional adjustment, absence of physical disabilities, and good general health. A degree of learning disability is present in 10 to 15 per cent of the primary school population. A full third of these children will not be able to realize their full potential without skilled remedial teaching. The rest will need some extra tuition over and above what is provided in the regular classroom.

Learning disability must reflect inadequate or disturbed function in those special areas of the cerebral cortex that are concerned with recognition, interpretation, encoding, and reproduction of written symbols, and their transmission into the spoken word. This disturbance in function would appear to come about in a number of different ways. The occurrence of learning disability in successive generations and in siblings suggests a genetic influence. Many children overcome their reading, spelling, and writing difficulties in time, which suggests that their problems reflect immaturity in the cortical areas and not permanent malfunction. A statistical relationship to perinatal morbidity implies that learning disability in some children is a consequence of neuronal damage. This contention gains support from autopsy reports on children with severe learning disability who died in accidents. Detailed studies of brain tissue revealed dysplasia and heterotopia in those areas of the left cerebral cortex that are known to subserve language function and reading. Learning disability experienced by these children may therefore have been a reflection of abnormal neuronal migration during fetal life.

482

## CLINICAL EXAMINATION AND SPECIAL INVESTIGATIONS

Before the learning disability label is applied to any child it is essential that other causes of school failure should be excluded. If this is not done, time, effort, and scarce educational resources will be wasted on children whose real need is for some other form of intervention. In the first instance, clinical examination serves to identify organic disease, gross neurological dysfunction, visual impairment, and hearing loss. In the absence of gross signs, examination of the neurological system is directed towards the elicitation of 'soft signs'. Most of these are indicators of functional immaturity for age rather than of focal pathology. The principal tests used are indicated in Table 56.1 together with norms. The battery includes tests of fine and gross motor

**Table 56.1** Learning disability – principal tests used

| Gross motor functions | Normal development timeframe |
| --- | --- |
| 1  Hop repetitively on one foot on the spot | Achieved by fifth birthday 20 times, with no associated movement by seventh birthday |
| 2  Heel and toe (tandem) straight line walking | No deviations or associated arm movements by seventh birthday |
| 3  Sit up from supine position keeping the arms folded across the chest | From eighth birthday heels do not leave ground |

| Fine motor functions | |
| --- | --- |
| 1  Thread 0,5 cm diameter beads without significant tremor | Achieved before fourth birthday |
| 2  Move protruded tongue rapidly from side to side | From seventh birthday with no associated movements of face or jaw |
| 3  Both hands held up in suppliant gesture with fingers slightly flexed. Fingertips of one hand touched rapidly in succession to thumb × 5. | From seventh birthday no mirror movement in opposite hand |
| 4  Rapid pronation/supernation of hand and forearm arm bent at right angle | From eighth birthday no mirror movements opposite hand |
| 5  Copying tests – see below | |

| Visuomotor functions | |
| --- | --- |
| Catch tennis ball thrown from three metres with both hands | Achieved by sixth birthday |

| Visual function | |
| --- | --- |
| Copy △ | Achieved by 5,5 years |
| Copy ⋈ | Achieved by sixth birthday |
| Copy □ | Achieved by seventh birthday |
| Copy ⋈ | Achieved by eighth birthday |

| Body image | |
| --- | --- |
| Carry out verbal instruction to touch left thumb to right ear etc. on self and tester | Correct on self by seventh birthday<br>Correct on tester by eighth birthday |

function, eye–hand co-ordination, laterality, and visual perception (Levine, 1987). Clinical examination should be completed by the testing of auditory perception and maturity of speech. The Wepman Test of auditory discrimination is useful for this purpose.

Special investigations contribute little to the assessment of healthy well-nourished children with learning disability. Studies have demonstrated an incidence of EEG abnormalities higher than that found in normal controls. However, these abnormalities are largely of non-specific nature and cannot be correlated with the individual child's profile of scholastic weaknesses. Thus, an EEG should not be undertaken in the absence of a history suggestive of seizures. Computer tomography, magnetic resonance imaging, and isotope scanning are not indicated in the absence of focal physical signs.

## MANAGEMENT

Therapeutic intervention for the learning-disabled child is specialized, and should be a team effort spearheaded by the remedial teacher, whose skill lies in identifying a given child's scholastic strengths and weaknesses and in devising a remedial programme that will build on the former and overcome the latter. The doctor's role is supportive. He or she must strive to present the remedial and classroom teachers with a child in the best possible condition to benefit from instruction. Most major centres have school clinics administered by regional education departments. Psychologists attached to these clinics visit individual schools and administer tests to children identified by class teachers. Where indicated, further psychometric and scholastic tests are carried out at the area clinic. Family doctors and paediatricians are well advised to maintain close liaison with these clinics in their approach to children with learning problems. It may fall to the doctor to arrange further referrals.

## Drug therapy

The use of methylphenidate should be considered when it is clear from class teachers' reports that scholastic progress is impaired by excessive motor activity in the classroom or by an inability to sustain concentration. Use of this drug will not diminish the need for remedial teaching. It is most effective in younger children who are developmentally immature for their age and who find the physical constraints of the classroom difficult to endure. The slightly older child with a restless distractible nature will also respond well. The drug should be administered as a dose of 0,3 to 0,5 mg/kg after breakfast on school mornings only. The effect of medication should be evident within a few weeks. Administration should not continue for longer than six months without a two-week period off medication. If there is no significant deterioration in concentration or school work during this trial period, the use of the medication may be stopped. Methylphenidate should not be used when restlessness and distractibility reflect limited intellectual endowment and an inability to cope with classroom demands. Its use is never justified in pre-school children with hyperactive behaviour. When the true cause of classroom failure is severe emotional disturbance, untreated organic disease, impaired hearing, or an unrecognized seizure disorder, it is irresponsible to prescribe the drug.

Other drugs have little place in the management of the healthy child with learning problems. There is no evidence to suggest that tricyclic antidepressants improve scholastic performance in the absence of depressive illness. The arbitrary use of carbamazepine and other anticonvulsant drugs on the basis of non-specific EEG changes is to be condemned. In the absence of a clinical seizure disorder these drugs are likely to induce side effects that in themselves impair classroom performance.

## Dubious measures

Parents are inordinately sensitive to criticism of a child's school achievement. This makes them easy prey to a variety of practitioners who offer interventions totally lacking in scientific foundation or proven effectiveness. One such therapy is the course of 'visual training' offered as a remedy for reading disability by certain optometrists. Reading is essentially a cortical activity and proficiency is not a reflection of eyeball movement. It is naïve to expect that improved reading and scholastic ability will follow a course of eye exercises in a child who has neither squint nor refraction error. This 'therapy' has been widely condemned, but exponents persist and the gullible continue to fall victim.

Another approach of unproven value is dietetic therapy. There can be little doubt that malnutrition is a factor in the poor scholastic achievements of multitudes of underprivileged children. However, there is no evidence (either biochemical or from case studies) to support the contention that massive doses of vitamins (megavitamin therapy) improve the scholastic performance of well-nourished children with learning disability. Neither is there any reliable data to support the theory of trace element deficiency as a cause for learning disability. The role of food additives, such as the colouring agent tartrazine used in cool drinks, foods, and medicines, remains uncertain.

## The therapist and learning problems

Although some specific learning disabilities are only detected at school age (e.g., specific reading, writing, and arithmetic disorders), the majority of children who experience problems with learning and development have evidence of this before school entry. The liaison between the health professional working with the child before school entry and his class teacher and, if available, remedial teacher becomes of paramount importance when decisions about schooling are made. Psychologists, occupational therapists, physiotherapists, and speech therapists are typically involved in assessment and therapy of cognitive, perceptual, motor, and language difficulties related to learning and frequently provide ongoing support to child and family well beyond primary school years.

Various occupational therapy interventions are used in developing appropriate treatment programmes for school-age children, where a problem with sensory and/or motor processing accounts for the learning problem. This is particularly important in sub-standards, where well-developed foundation skills are the building stones for acquisition and development of reading, arithmetic, and writing ability. When problems remain in older children, the focus changes to the development of coping strategies and development of self-actualization in activities where function and skill are sound, thus de-emphasizing dysfunction.

Occupational therapists are frequently involved in determining, with the child and in collaboration with the teacher, which functional and assistive devices could be employed to assist the scholar who is slow with reading and writing.

In environments where the services of occupational therapists are available, the intervention may be provided in various settings; in the child's home, school, or classroom or in a structured therapy treatment facility. The problem in South Africa remains one of access. Many children have special educational needs where not only learning disability affects under achievement, but a variety of other factors necessitates an adapted curriculum (Donald, 1994).

## References and further reading

DONALD D. 1994. Children with special educational needs: The reproduction of disadvantage in poorly served communities. In: A Dawes and D Donald (eds.). *Childhood and adversity. Psychological perspectives from South African research.* Cape Town: David Philip.

ILLINGWORTH RS. 1987. *The normal child,* 9th ed. Edinburgh, London, Melbourne, New York: Churchill Livingstone.

KIRBY R, SWANSON MD, KELLEHER KJ, et al. 1993. Identifying at-risk children for early intervention services. *Journal of Paediatrics.* 22(5): Part i.

LEVINE MD. 1987. Developmental dysfunction in the school-age child. In: RE Behrman & VC Vaughan III (eds.). *Nelson textbook of pediatrics,* 13th ed. Philadelphia: WB Saunders Co.

SHAYWITZ S, SHAYWITZ B, and GROSSMAN HT. 1984. Learning disorders. *Pediatric Clinics of North America.* 31:277–518.

WEISGLAS-KUPERUS N et al. 1993. Effects of biological and social factors on the cognitive development of very low birthweight children. *Paediatrics.* 92(5).

# 57

# Sensory impairment

## Hearing

During the third trimester of pregnancy, a normal fetus will respond to a loud sound with sharp body movements and cardiac acceleration. The neonate responds by blinking, increasing the respiratory rate, or by executing a moro response, depending on the suddenness and loudness of the stimulus. At two months, the normal infant, when awake, will cease activity and listen to sounds. He or she may appear to recognize the maternal voice. By four months, head movements are being made in an effort to locate the source of interesting sounds. Babbling has begun. At seven months, the infant will respond in a special way to his or her own name, and by ten months, it is evident that the association between members of the immediate family and their names is being recognized.

There are many reasons for hearing impairment. Important causes are set out in Table 57.1. The development of language and speech will be affected when hearing loss exceeds 40 decibels in infancy. The inability to comprehend and communicate may evoke great frustration in an affected child, and disturbed behaviour is a common feature of both manifest and covert deafness.

**Table 57.1** Important causes of deafness in childhood

- Congenital malformation of the middle ear, vestibular apparatus, and eighth nerve
- Intra-uterine infections – rubella, syphilis
- Perinatal asphyxia
- Neonatal hyperbilirubinaemia
- Use of ototoxic drugs – streptomycin, kanamycin
- Meningitis
- Hereditary syndromes

### MANAGEMENT

Early diagnosis of deafness is essential if the child is to achieve full potential. Parents can be involved in the early detection of hearing loss. All infants should be tested for hearing at eight to ten months by the distraction test, which can easily be carried out by nurses with appropriate training (see Chapter 21: Health surveillance). Early audiometric screening should be provided for all infants placed in the at-risk category by virtue of maternal gestational illness, premature or difficult birth, hyperbilirubinaemia, neonatal septicaemia, or a family history of congenital deafness. Middle ear infection should be sought and vigorously treated in

487

all ages during infancy and childhood. Infants who show any deviation from the auditory developmental pathway outlined above should be subjected to formal audiometry as soon as suspicion has been aroused. Failure to proceed from the babbling stage of expression to echolalia is of special significance. Specific and long-term management of the hearing-impaired child is best conducted in paediatric audiology departments and schools for the deaf and hard of hearing. Few children are totally deaf, and with the skilled use of modern electronic hearing apparatus and special instruction techniques, most of those with normal intelligence will attain a satisfactory level of communication and comprehensible speech.

# Speech

The human race is the only species on earth capable of articulate speech – most normal children being able to speak in sentences by the age of three years. While the ability to speak is inherent in infants, normal speech development does not occur in the absence of an intellectual endowment which is at least in the trainable category (IQ 50–70), reasonable acuity of hearing, and sustained exposure to the spoken word.

The newborn infant communicates all his or her needs by crying in an undifferentiated manner. However, by the time her baby is six weeks old, the perceptive mother can usually distinguish the cry of hunger from those of insecurity and physical discomfort. At three months, the normal infant has begun to babble. Initially, this consists of repetitive single syllables, but the repertoire expands rapidly as the baby is better able to achieve sound production. Sounds are uttered at random until the age of six or seven months, when echolalia becomes evident. The infant will attempt to repeat vocalizations and words uttered in his or her hearing. Initially, these attempts are

crude but there is rapid progress, culminating round about the first birthday in the first consistently recognizable words. Children with a significant degree of deafness do not progress beyond the babbling stage. Understanding of words precedes by many months the ability to say and use them for communication purposes. By the age of 18 months, the average child is using 20 to 30 words interspersed amongst much jargon. At two years there is a vocabulary of 50 to 100 words and the first attempts are being made at sentence construction. By three years, considerable conversational ability has been acquired. Grammatical errors and articulation immaturities, such as 'lello' for 'yellow', are common and there may be a phase of stammering. Vocabulary and fluency depend to a significant degree on the quality of speech to which the toddler is exposed. Children who live with verbal and highly articulate adults tend to achieve remarkable verbal ability at an early age, while those with limited exposure to good speech during the critical phase may never acquire good language use.

## CAUSES OF DELAYED SPEECH DEVELOPMENT

### Deafness

This may be difficult to detect clinically during infancy, particularly when hearing loss is confined to the higher frequencies as may occur after neonatal hyperbilirubinaemia. Thus, formal audiometry is an essential first step when there is speech delay. It should be instituted during the first year of life if there are any historical circumstances that predispose to deafness.

### Intellectual disability

Diagnosis is relatively easy when there is a delay in the acquisition of speech in a child with global developmental delay. However, many mildly retarded children achieve basic motor milestones at ages within the normal range, and careful history-taking and examination are therefore necessary to demonstrate the child's true developmental level.

## Dysphasia

This term implies dysfunction in the central processing of language at cortical level when there is no record of intellectual disability or peripheral auditory impairment. Such dysfunction may be due to developmental defect or to damage sustained during the perinatal period or subsequently. Dysphasia may be expressive, receptive or a combination of the two. A number of distinct syndromes have been defined, sharing a common denominator of delayed speech development.

## Adverse environment

Infants and toddlers whose exposure to verbal stimulation is restricted will show limited speech development. This is found in the offspring of severely depressed and disturbed parents, in grossly neglected, and in certain institutionalized children. Elective mutism in emotionally disturbed children may masquerade as speech delay.

## Dysarthria

Articulation disorders (dysarthria) and delayed speech development should not be confused, though both may be present in the same child. Dysarthria occurs when there is an abnormality in the anatomy or function of the peripheral organs of speech – the lips, tongue, palate, oropharynx, or larynx. Dysarthria of greater or lesser degree is found in children with cleft lip and palate, palatal palsy, and various syndromes of cerebral palsy. Children with cerebral palsy often present a mixed picture of dysphasia and dysarthria, while those with severe pseudobulbar palsy seldom attain a practical level of articulate speech. *Articulatory apraxia*, akin to manual apraxia, may be found in children who do not show gross signs of cerebral palsy.

*Stammering* (dysfluency) is not uncommon in the pre-school years and does not call for active intervention. Stammering that appears after the age of five is an expression of heightened tension and may accompany such practices as nailbiting or bedwetting. Those affected do not stammer when singing or angry (e.g., swearing). This indicates that there is no intrinsic defect in speech mechanisms.

## MANAGEMENT

A child who is not making two- or three- word sentences by the age of two-and-a-half years should be subjected to investigation. The initial approach should include formal audiometry and a review of the child's sensorimotor, intellectual, and social development. Deafness of any significant degree calls for referral to a consultant skilled in paediatric audiology. When there is unequivocal evidence of global retardation, speech therapy is unlikely to be rewarding in the early years. Speech will be acquired gradually as the child achieves the overall developmental level at which normal children acquire language and speech. When clinical signs of cerebral palsy are present, the child should be referred for further management to a school or centre that provides comprehensive cerebral palsy care. Evidence of understimulation and social pathology call for environmental adjustment in the child's life. Wherever possible, arrangements should be made for the child to attend a pre-school centre or crèche to ensure professionally guided contact with other children of the same age. Referral to a speech therapist is desirable when a child who is otherwise normal shows delayed speech development beyond the age of three. One of the dysphasia syndromes may be responsible and it may be advisable to admit the child to a special nursery school providing intensive speech therapy.

Conventional speech therapy is of limited benefit to stammerers. Attempts to reduce self-consciousness and emotional tension and so increase self-confidence are more likely than speech therapy to bring about an overall improvement than is speech therapy.

# Vision

The optic pathways of the central nervous system are well myelinated at 40 weeks gestation. The full-term newborn baby looks vaguely at objects placed in his or her line of vision and responds to light. At the age of three or four weeks eyes and head will turn to a light source and the child will watch his or her mother intently as she speaks. Objects brought into the line of vision will be followed almost to the midline. At six weeks, conjugate eye movements are evident and the infant will smile at a friendly face. At 12 weeks, an object is followed from one side to a point beyond the midline. Hand regard is practised from this age. By six months, the infant is able to deftly pick up any object within range without hesitation. He or she takes a lively interest in all that goes on in the immediate vicinity. Head and body positions are automatically adjusted to see better any objects that may attract attention. At the time of birth, the normal eye has a relatively short axial length and is hypermetropic by an average of three dioptres. Axial length increases as the eye grows and normal emmetropia is achieved at between three and five years of age.

Some 70 per cent of the total sensory input received by the central nervous system reaches it via visual pathways. Adequate vision is thus an important pre-requisite for overall normal development. The eye is heir to a wide range of congenital and acquired conditions which may impair visual acuity. Mention will be made only of those in which early intervention is important if the effect on visual impairment is to be minimized.

## CORNEAL SCARRING

Corneal ulceration may occur in association with severe conjunctivitis, or it may be caused by trauma. In underprivileged communities with deficient vitamin A intake, extensive corneal ulceration may occur as a complication of measles or in kwashiorkor. It may also result from inadequately treated gonococcal ophthalmia neonatorum. Other causes include the herpes simplex virus and congenital syphilis. Treatment is seldom entirely successful and corneal scarring inevitably impairs visual acuity. An important preventive measure in disadvantaged communities is the oral or intramuscular administration of vitamin A. Prompt treatment of neonatal ophthalmia with parenteral penicillin and irrigations should result in full resolution. The antiviral agent Acyclovir is effective when used locally in herpetic keratitis.

## CATARACTS

These may be hereditary, secondary to systemic disease, post-traumatic or due to ocular disease. Cataracts are a well-recognized feature of the congenital rubella syndrome, and may develop in children who have been treated systemically for more than a year with corticosteroids. Diabetic cataract is uncommon in childhood. Penetrating eye injury is the usual cause of post-traumatic cataract. Many cataracts are obvious to the naked eye and these inevitably impair visual acuity. Active intervention in a specialist centre is indicated. Examination of the newborn should always include elicitation of the red-eye reflex. When this is not positive, the infant should be referred for further ophthalmological investigation.

## STRABISMUS

A *variable squint* is normal in the early months, before binocular vision is established. The most common reason for a persistent squint is failure to develop this normal binocular vision. The remaining aetiologies fall into three groups: neurological disorders – defects in extrinsic eye muscles or paralyses of cranial nerves; eye disease, such as cataract or retinoblastoma; and refractive errors.

A squint may be 'latent', i.e., only revealed when the eye is covered (see Chapter 21: Health surveillance). In an 'alternating squint' either eye can take up fixation. The presence of epicanthic folds may give the erroneous impression that a squint is present ('pseudosquint').

*Paralytic squint* is found in the presence of cranial nerve lesions. It has serious connotations and is an indication that investigation of the central nervous system is required. *Concomitant squint* occurs when there is an imbalance in the strengths of extra-ocular muscles. In consequence, the visual axes of both eyes are not directed at the object of fixation. When the child is viewed full face it is seen that light reflections in the eyes do not correspond. Concomitant strabismus is never acceptable and referral should be made to an ophthalmologist as soon as the condition is identified. Failure to institute early treatment will lead to amblyopia in the squinting eye and failure to develop binocular vision. The cover test for detecting strabismus is described in Chapter 21: Health surveillance.

## REFRACTIVE ERRORS

*Hypermetropia* (long sight) is the most common refractive error. The child has good distance vision but difficulty with close vision. Attempts to focus may induce a convergent squint. *Myopia* (short sight) causes impairment of distance vision. The child may hold objects of interest very close to his or her eyes in order to focus. Children with refractive errors are usually not aware of their own disability and do not complain. As a consequence, school performance may suffer. Hence, routine tests of visual acuity should be performed at regular intervals using Snellen's charts. Children who have any difficulty with these should be referred for formal refraction by an ophthalmologist.

Vision may be affected in cranial dysostoses like Crouzon's disease. Intra-uterine infections like rubella and toxoplasmosis cause a retinopathy that impairs vision. Retinal degenerative conditions, almost always hereditary, lead to progressive loss of vision. This is not amenable to treatment.

Buphthalmos (infantile glaucoma) should be suspected in any child who appears to have enlarged eyes. Early surgery may save vision.

The early treatment of eye infections and injuries and appropriate management for cataracts, squint, and refractive errors will ensure that most of those affected have adequate vision for ordinary school and community life.

## CORTICAL BLINDNESS

Blindness may be of central origin, that is without any ophthalmological abnormality, but most such children have additional problems such as cerebral palsy or severe intellectual disability. These multiple-handicapped children can be extremely difficult to assess. A common situation is the child with hemiplegia who also has a considerable additional disability as a result of hemianopia. The latter is often undetected.

Visually impaired children usually show problems in general development. Motor development is deviant or late, and language acquisition may be characterized by unusual patterns, as symbolic concepts dependent on vision are not easily acquired. Wherever possible, such children should be referred to a multidisciplinary team for full assessment. When vision is worse than 6/60 in the better eye, education as a visually impaired child will generally be required. The child is classified as partially sighted if the sight is 6/24 or worse in the better eye.

When a child is blind or vision is severely limited, referral should be made to one of the special schools for the blind. Education at these institutions promotes the attainment of full potential and opens the way for later placement in appropriate sheltered employment.

## References and further reading

HOSKING G & POWELL R (eds.). 1985. *Chronic childhood disorders*. Bristol: Wright.
POLNAY L & HULL D. 1987. *Community paediatrics*. Edinburgh: Churchill Livingstone.

# 58  Cerebral palsy

## LJ ARENS

Cerebral palsy refers to a group of static encephalopathies that give rise to motor disability. It is defined as a disorder of movement and posture resulting from a non-progressive lesion of the immature brain. Although the lesion is non-progressive, the clinical manifestations often change with neurological maturation. All children with cerebral palsy have motor dysfunction and many, because of the extent of the lesion, will have associated disabilities. Table 58.1 shows some of the motor disorders that should be considered in the differential diagnosis of cerebral palsy.

From a therapeutic viewpoint, it is important to be aware of the rare condition of dopa-responsive dystonia (Segawa syndrome) (Segawa et al., 1976; Gordon, 1996). This is often mistaken for cerebral palsy. The continued oral administration of levodopa gives complete restoration of function in this otherwise progressive condition.

## Prevalence

The prevalence in developed countries is approximately two per thousand (Paneth &

**Table 58.1** Motor disorders

| Site of the lesion | Examples |
| --- | --- |
| *Brain* | |
| Motor cortex and pyramidal tracts | Spastic cerebral palsy |
| Basal ganglia | Dyskinetic cerebral palsy |
| | Torsion dystonia |
| | Dopa-responsive dystonia |
| Cerebellum | Ataxic cerebral palsy |
| | Spino-cerebellar degeneration |
| Multiple lesions | Mixed cerebral palsy |
| *Spinal cord* | Myelomeningocele |
| | Transverse myelitis |
| | Trauma |
| | Tumours |
| *Neuromuscular unit* | |
| Anterior horn cell | Spinal muscular atrophy |
| | Polio |
| Peripheral nerve | Hereditary sensory motor neuropathy |
| Neuromuscular junction | Myasthenia gravis |
| Muscle | Muscular dystrophy |
| | Congenital myopathy |
| *Joints* | Arthrogryposis |
| | Juvenile chronic arthritis |
| *Bones* | Infections, especially tuberculosis |
| | Osteogenesis imperfecta |

Kiely, 1984). In recent years there has been a slight rise in prevalence, especially among very low birthweight infants, concomitant with a parallel fall in infant mortality (Hagberg et al., 1989). The prevalence is unknown in developing countries, but is largely determined by the high incidence of potentially brain-damaging illnesses in poorer communities, and a higher infant mortality rate.

# Aetiology

Some of the factors that may give rise to cerebral palsy are given in Table 58.2. Prenatal causes occur between conception and the onset of labour, and perinatal causes from the onset of labour to the completion of adaptation to extra-uterine life (usually seven days after birth). Pre- and perinatal categories combine to form a congenital group. In the past the perinatal causes (and especially birth asphyxia) have probably been overemphasized. It is now postulated that many of the congenital cases have their origins during pregnancy (Freeman & Nelson, 1988). However, in the developing countries, birth asphyxia continues to be an important aetiological factor among the poorest population (Arens & Molteno, 1996). It must be emphasized that, in most cases, complications of pregnancy and the perinatal period do not result in babies with neurological problems; only a small minority develop cerebral palsy.

*Postnatally acquired* cerebral palsy refers to those cases that result from extraneous causes after birth in a child who was previously normal. In developed countries approximately ten per cent of cases fall into this group, but where poor socio-economic conditions exist, the percentage is much higher. A Cape Town survey (Arens & Molteno, 1989) showed that the prevalence of acquired cerebral palsy among the disadvantaged coloured and black cerebral-palsied children was 24 and 36 per

cent respectively. The sequelae of bacterial meningitis, in particular tuberculous meningitis (Arens et al., 1987), accounts for many of these cases. Another cause directly associated with poor socio-economic conditions is cerebrovenous thrombosis following dehydration resulting from gastroenteritis. Studies from Central and East Africa (Duggan & Mgone, 1982; Makwabe & Mgone, 1984) show even higher figures for postnatally acquired cerebral palsy, with endemic disease, especially cerebral malaria, featuring prominently.

**Table 58.2** Aetiology of cerebral palsy

**Congenital**
*Prenatal*
- Malformations
- Intra-uterine infections
- Intra-uterine growth retardation
- Complications of pregnancy (e.g., eclampsia)
- Multiple pregnancies
- Other causes

*Perinatal*
- Prematurity and associated complications
- Perinatal asphyxia
- Birth trauma
- Bilirubin encephalopathy
- Hypoglycaemia
- Other causes

**Postnatally acquired**
- Cerebral infections
- Trauma (accidental and non-accidental)
- Cerebro-vascular accidents
- Other causes

**Idiopathic**
- Unknown

Cases in which no plausible cause is found, despite adequate history (15 to 20 per cent), are considered *idiopathic* and, where insufficient history or medical data is available, the category of *unknown* is applied.

# Clinical types

A classification of clinical types is given in Table 58.3.

*Spasticity.* This is the commonest type. Spastic cerebral palsy refers to the presence of an upper motor neurone lesion, involving the motor cortex. Spasticity is defined as a velocity-dependent increase of muscle tone. It may be associated with muscle weakness. With growth of the child, fixed joint contractures commonly occur. This group is further subdivided into hemiplegia, quadriplegia, diplegia, triplegia, and monoplegia, depending on the distribution of limb involvement.

The *dyskinetic* (athetoid) group indicates basal ganglion involvement. In this group, abnormal involuntary movements occur. Fixed contractures do not develop. It includes the following:

- *athetosis* – irregular coarse and relatively continuous writhing movements of the extremities;
- *choreo-athetosis* – more abrupt brief and jerking movements; and
- *dystonia* – more sustained spasms of neck, trunk, and extremities resulting in abnormal postures.

*Ataxia* indicates cerebellar dysfunction and is found in less than five per cent of children with cerebral palsy.

*Mixed cases* have signs of involvement of more than one area of the brain.

*Hypotonia.* Most children who present in infancy are *hypotonic*, but in all but one per cent, the picture changes after 12 months of age to one of the other types. One per cent remain hypotonic. Many cases are mixed, indicating involvement of more than one motor area of the brain.

**Table 58.3** Cerebral palsy – clinical types

**Spastic**
- Hemiplegia — one side of the body involved
- Quadriplegia — involvement of whole body musculature
- Tetraplegia — all limbs involved equally or arms more affected than legs
- Diplegia — legs affected more than arms
- Triplegia — one arm uninvolved or only minimally involved
- Monoplegia — very rare; only one arm involved

**Dyskinetic**
- Athetosis
- Choreo-athetosis
- Dystonia

**Ataxic**
**Hypotonic**
**Mixed**

## Associated conditions

Less than ten per cent of cerebral-palsied children have only a motor disability. The remainder have at least one associated condition. These are listed in Table 58.4. Approximately 50 per cent of children with cerebral palsy have an IQ of less than 70. In 30 per cent, the IQ is below 50. About ten per cent of these have severe intellectual disability; often being cortically blind and cortically deaf, and many also have total body involvement. However, stated more positively, half of the children have intellectual abilities within the average or near-average range. Some are highly intelligent. About six per cent have severe visual impairment and about 20 per cent have strabismus. Surely the most devastating disability is the inability to communicate. Impaired speech and delayed language development could be attributed to any of the following:

- intellectual disability;
- deafness;
- dysarthria;
- dysphasia; or
- a combination of these.

Some of these children also have no useful hand function.

Epilepsy, usually partial seizures, occurs in 30 per cent of cases. Significant behaviour problems, especially hyperactivity, occur in 10 per cent of children. Nutritional disorders, either obesity from inactivity or undernutrition associated with sucking and swallowing difficulty, are especially associated with pseudobulbar palsy and special feeding techniques may be necessary. In very severe cases, gastrostomy feeding may be the best solution. Patients who have difficulty in chewing are prone to dental caries and many of the more severely disabled infants suffer from constipation.

**Table 58.4** Cerebral palsy – associated problems

- Intellectual disability
- Visual defects – blindness and visual impairment
- Deafness
- Speech and language disorder
  - dysarthria
  - aphasia (central processing disorder)
  - language delay
- Epilepsy
- Specific learning disabilities including visual perceptual problems
- Behavioural and emotional problems
- Miscellaneous
  - nutritional problems
  - gastro-oesophageal reflex
  - dental caries
  - constipation

## Management

### PREVENTIVE

Reducing the prevalence of cerebral palsy depends upon achieving the highest standards of maternal and child health throughout a community. This involves universal and comprehensive ante- and perinatal care as well as accessible primary health care for all patients. General preventive measures include immunization, nutritional surveillance and health education. Improving socio-economic conditions would lead to a reduction in the high percentage of cases of postnatal origin.

### THERAPEUTIC

Cerebral palsy is not curable but much can be done to alleviate the condition, thus improving the quality of life for each child. This requires a team effort and the co-ordination of services. What follows refers to the situation in large urban centres with good facilities. The concept of community-based rehabilitation, applicable to rural and semi-urban areas, is discussed elsewhere.

Emphasis should be placed on early diagnosis and treatment. Surveillance should detect all children with cerebral palsy within the first year of life. Follow-up programmes for all preterm infants and high- risk infants are of special importance. The diagnosis must be suspected in hypotonic (floppy) infants, and those with delayed motor development, especially if there are persistent primitive reflexes and brisk tendon reflexes. Feeding difficulties and persistent crying are frequently present in affected children. A definitive diagnosis may not be possible in the first few months of life. Abnormal postures (so called 'transient dystonias') sometimes disappear within the first year.

## Specific therapies

Neurodevelopmental therapy, which is applied by physiotherapists, occupational therapists, and speech therapists who have undergone special training, is designed specifically to help children with cerebral palsy (Bobath, 1980). While it is difficult to prove its efficacy, this therapy has much to commend it.

Daily therapy is not feasible in a hospital clinic, but much can be achieved by weekly sessions during which parents are taught how to position and exercise their children. Rural families can attend periodically for a week's intensive treatment. Group therapy has proved useful for the extremely physically and intellectually disabled children, with parents gaining experience in handling and exercising their children correctly while receiving counselling and group support. No child is too disabled to benefit, even if only to facilitate care and minimize the formation of contractures.

Occupational therapists work in several fields, including collaboration with the physiotherapist in treating the motor problems and perceptual training and training for everyday living. They also organize and devise special equipment for use at home and at school.

The speech therapist handles communication problems, improving the speech of the dysarthric child and devising augmentative communication methods for the child who cannot speak (Joleff et al., 1992). These range from sign language to simple communication boards using pictures or symbols (e.g., Blissymbolics) to typewriters and on to the sophisticated 'talking' computer. The speech therapist also deals with sucking and chewing difficulties.

## Therapeutic aids

Therapy equipment includes large balls, rollers, standing frames, walkers, special seats, etc. While excellent equipment can be bought, home-made apparatus is often adequate. For example, three large (750 g) empty coffee tins joined end-to-end, wrapped first in newspaper and then in material, makes a good roller. A wooden toy wagon, weighted with a sandbag, is an excellent walker for a young child. Cardboard cartons can be cut into triangular seats and into tables. A book on disabled children in rural communities provides many other ideas (Werner, 1988).

Orthopaedic appliances and special footwear are often necessary. Appliances such as ankle foot orthoses (AFOs) are made out of lightweight plastic material. Trained orthotists are also valued members of a therapeutic team.

Tricycles are very useful for the non-ambulant, providing good exercise and allowing more freedom than wheelchairs. For the very handicapped quadriplegic, motorized chairs provide a measure of independence.

## Medical treatment

Associated problems (e.g., seizure, visual and auditory disorders) have to be investigated and treated.

Drugs have generally been disappointing in reducing muscle tone in cerebral palsy. At present diazepam is the most widely used. Baclofen is of limited value given orally but has been shown to reduce tone significantly when given as a continual intrathecal infusion, controlled by a programmed pump inserted subcutaneously into the abdominal wall. This is an extremely expensive procedure, requiring maintenance and it has a high complication rate (Albright, 1996).

The intramuscular injection of Botulinum toxin A into muscle groups of both upper and lower limbs of cerebral-palsied children was first introduced in 1993. This is a very effective method of reducing tone, allowing for the development of better function, provided that there is no fixed contracture. However, it is a temporary measure, lasting weeks to months, but it can be repeated. Young children, from one to five years, do particularly well (Boyd & Graham, 1997).

Orthopaedic surgeons deal mainly with the spastic child. Surgery for fixed joint contractures and bone deformities can lead to good functional improvement. However, it is important that the orthopaedic surgeon has knowledge of the dynamics of spasticity and the muscle imbalances of the cerebral palsy child, and that he or she works as part of the team. Post-operative physiotherapy is a prerequisite for successful rehabilitation.

The neurosurgeon also has a role to play. Selective posterior lumbar rhizotomy – the cutting of carefully selected posterior nerve roots – (Peacock et al., 1987; Peter & Arens, 1993) is of value in reducing tone in carefully selected spastic children. Rhizotomy will not alter fixed contractures, so orthopaedic surgery is often also required. A ten-year Cape Town gait analysis study has shown objectively that the favourable results persist (Subramanian et al., 1998).

Community-based rehabilitation is a necessary adjunct to treatment at an urban clinic. Teams are now going out to peri-urban townships and holding clinics there, as well as training staff to care for children at special centres. Many impoverished parents travel from rural areas to the cities to seek help for their disabled children, as therapeutic facilities are still very inadequate in these areas.

# Educational aspects

In South Africa, the educational needs of cerebral-palsied children are being met in urban and in some rural areas in special schools. Many of these have boarding facilities. However, in keeping with world trends in education, the government plans to retain special schools only for those too disabled to attend mainstream schools. Most will be assimilated into 'inclusive' education with the provision of appropriate facilities. While admirable in theory, this may not be as successful as special schooling in meeting the needs of the multiply disabled cerebral-palsied children. In special schools, the therapeutic team are members of the school staff, working closely with the teachers. As all the children have disabilities they do not feel different from their peers. Special sports are available to everyone and all can participate on an equal basis at school functions, the school concert etc. Medical specialists hold clinics at the school.

The general atmosphere in these schools is invariably a happy one. Classes are small and remedial teachers and psychologists are on the staff of most schools. In recent years, more emphasis has been placed on tailoring the education of each child to meet his or her future needs as an adult – ranging from higher education, and the open labour market to semi-sheltered or sheltered employment.

For the child who is 'trainable' but cannot benefit from formal education, training centres with professionally trained staff have been established. However, there is still a shortage of both these centres and care centres for the severely intellectually and physically impaired.

## Supportive management

This rests in the first place with the doctor who makes the diagnosis and it continues with the help of the whole team, including psychologists and social workers. It is an ongoing process as the full picture only becomes clear as the child matures. Parents' questions must be answered honestly as withholding any information requested leads to further distress.

However, most parents need time to accept the full implications of their child's problems, to see the positive factors, and to encourage all aspects of the child's development. The child must also gradually understand and come to terms with his or her disabilities. The development of a pleasant personality will override the physical disabilities. Parents and children are important members of the team.

Help for the cerebral-palsied child should not end with the completion of schooling. Every child should achieve his or her maximum potential, and this should be maintained through adulthood. Where possible, independent living should be aimed at, but a protective environment may be necessary. The general public needs to be educated in their attitudes towards the cerebral palsied, and encouraged to offer them employment in the open labour market. For the more impaired, sheltered workshops are required, while care centres are the only answer for the severely intellectually and physically disabled.

A great deal has been achieved to assist the cerebral palsied but much remains to be done.

## References and further reading

ALBRIGHT AL. 1996. Intrathecal baclofen in cerebral palsy movement disorders. *Journal of Child Neurology.* 11 (Supplement 1): s29–s35.

ARENS LJ & MOLTENO CD. 1989. A comparative study of postnatally acquired cerebral palsy in Cape Town. *Developmental Medicine Child Neurology.* 31:246–57.

ARENS LJ, DEENY JE, MOLTENO CD, and KIBEL MA. 1987. Tuberculous meningitis in children in the Western Cape: Neurological sequelae. *Pediatric Reviews and Communications.* 1:257–75.

ARENS LJ & MOLTENO CD. 1996. Cerebral palsy in Cape Town – Prevalence, etiology and clinical types. *Paediatric Reviews and Communications.* 8:255–63.

BOBATH KA. 1980. A neurophysical basis for the treatment of cerebral palsy. In: *Clinics in Developing Medicine*, No.75. London: William Heinemann.

BOYD R & GRAHAM HK. 1997. Botulinum toxin A in the management of children with cerebral palsy: Indications and outcome. *European Journal of Neurology.* 4 (2): s15–s22.

DUGGAN MB & MGONE CS. 1982. Cerebral palsy in Nigeria – a report from Zaria. *Annals of Tropical Paediatrics.* 2:7–11.

FREEMAN JM & NELSON KB. 1988. Intrapartum asphyxia and cerebral palsy. *Pediatrics.* 82:240–9.

GORDON N. 1996. Dopa-responsive dystonia: A widening spectrum. *Developmental Medicine and Child Neurology.* 38:554–9.

HAGBERG B, HAGBERG G, OLOW I, and VON WENDT L. 1989. The changing panorama of cerebral palsy in Sweden. V. The birth year period 1979–1982. *Acta Paediatrica Scandinavia.* 78:283–90.

JOLEFF N, MCCONACHIE H, WINYARD S, JONES S, WISBEACH A, and CLAYTON C. 1992. Communication aids for children:

Procedures and problems. *Developmental Medicine Child Neurology.* 34:719–30.

MAKWABE CM & MGONE CS. 1984. The pattern and aetiology of cerebral palsy as seen in Dar-es-Salaam, Tanzania. *East African Medical Journal.* 61:896–9.

PANETH N & KIELY J. 1984. The frequency of cerebral palsy: A review of population studies in industrialized nations since 1950. In: F Stanley & E Alberman (eds.). *The Epidemiology of the cerebral palsied. clinics in developing medicine,* No. 87. Oxford: Blackwell Scientific Publications.

PEACOCK WJ, ARENS LJ, and BERMAN B. 1987. Cerebral palsy spasticity. Selective posterior rhizotomy. *Pediatric Neuroscience.* 13:61–66.

PETER JC & ARENS LJ. 1993. Selective posterior lumbosacral rhizotomy for the management of cerebral palsy spasticity: A 10 year experience. *South African Medical Journal.* 83:745–7.

SEGAWA M, HOSAKA A, MIYAGAWA F, NOMURA T, and IMAI H. 1976. Hereditary progressive dystonia with marked diurnal fluctuation. *Advances in Neurology.* 14:215–33.

SUBRAMANIAN N, VAUGHAN CL, PETER JC, and ARENS LJ. 1998. Gait before and 10 years after rhizotomy in children with special palsy spasticity. *Journal of Neurosurgery.* 88: 1014–19.

WERNER D. 1988. *Disabled village children.* Palo Alto, California: The Hesperian Foundation.

# 59

# Chronic disorders

PM LEARY & CD MOLTENO

## Implications for the primary health care provider

Not all children attain Juvenal's gold standard 'mens sana in corpore sano', for in every community there are those whose well-being is impaired by chronic disorder or disease. Doctors and members of various allied professions as well as other health care workers have an obligation to provide these children with treatment and guidance so that each one is maintained in the best possible health, given his or her circumstances. The emphasis today should be placed on these special needs rather than on the children's defects or disabilities.

## Epilepsy

A seizure has been defined as an occasional excessive disorderly discharge of nerve tissue. In infancy and childhood, seizures may be precipitated by anoxia, infection, various metabolic derangements, trauma, and toxin ingestion. The term 'epilepsy' should not be used unless the child's seizures recur over

months and years. Recurrent seizures during infancy and early childhood usually reflect underlying structural brain lesions or one of the specific seizure syndromes, such as Lennox-Gastaut syndrome. Idiopathic epilepsy – recurrent seizures with no demonstrable cause – first manifests in most instances after the age of three years. Family histories of children with idiopathic epilepsy often provide evidence of a genetic influence.

### DIFFERENTIAL DIAGNOSIS

Before applying the epilepsy label to a child it is essential to eliminate other causes of recurrent 'turns'. *Breath-holding* attacks invariably follow minor injury or frustration (see Chapter 50: Behavioural patterns in pre-school children). There is a cry followed by breathholding, cyanosis, and loss of consciousness. Rapid recovery follows the return of respiration.

Reflex anoxic seizures occur when there is momentary cardiac arrest due to surge of vagal tone induced by pain or severe fright. There is immediate loss of consciousness with ashen pallor. Consciousness then returns with resumption of the normal heart beat. *Fainting spells* are uncommon in toddlers, but

501

occur readily in school-age children who are unwell or made to stand for prolonged periods. There is a sensation of increasing malaise followed by loss of consciousness. The child sags to the ground and is noted to be very pale and clammy. The wrist pulse may be impalpable. Full consciousness returns after a few moments in the recumbent posture. Other conditions that must be distinguished from true seizures include *paroxysmal vertigo attacks, infantile masturbation, prolonged QT syndrome* (sudden loss of consciousness on effort due to cardiac arrhythmia), and *simulated attacks* in children with an epileptic relative or acquaintance.

## CLASSIFICATION

The classification of seizures according to clinical form serves a useful purpose, for treatment is determined in some considerable measure by seizure type. The classification system proposed by Dreifuss (1981) (Table 59.1) is of considerable practical value. Special mention must be made of a number of entities peculiar to infancy and childhood.

## FEBRILE SEIZURES

Two to four per cent of young children have one or more fever-associated seizures between the ages of six months and four years. Characteristically these tonic/clonic seizures occur at the onset of an intercurrent ear, throat, or upper respiratory tract infection, and are of short duration. In the great majority, the attacks are quite benign and do not lead to epilepsy later. When the seizure is prolonged (more than 15 minutes), recurs within 24 hours, or has lateralizing features (complex seizures) there is a greater likelihood of underlying neurological disorder and of epilepsy at a later age. Febrile seizures are the most commonly encountered seizure type in pre-school children. Nowadays it is

**Table 59.1** Classification of epileptic seizures

................................................................................

- Partial seizures (focal, local)
  - Simple partial seizures
  - Complex partial seizures
  - Partial seizures becoming secondarily generalized
- Generalized seizures
  - Absence seizures
  - Myoclonic seizures
  - Clonic seizures
  - Tonic seizures
  - Tonic-clonic seizures
  - Atonic seizures
- Unclassified seizures

................................................................................

not general policy to administer anticonvulsants to prevent recurrent 'simple' febrile seizures. Advice should be given on controlling the fever; and parents can be taught to administer diazepam in the event of an incipient or prolonged attack (0,2–0,5 mg/kg, rectally).

## INFANTILE MYOCLONIC EPILEPSY

This condition is characterized by violent myoclonic jerks (salaam spasms) in which the arms extend and the infant is thrown forwards. Onset is in the first year of life and is usually attended by loss of social contact and disappearance of smiling. The EEG pattern of hypsarrhythmia is characteristic. The clinical picture is seen in association with tuberose sclerosis, serious structural abnormality of the brain, and various metabolic derangements. It also occurs without demonstrable cause. Prognosis for intellectual development and control of seizures is poor, except in idiopathic cases treated early with ACTH.

## LENNOX-GASTAUT SYNDROME

This syndrome first manifests in the second year of life. There are recurrent myoclonic seizures that throw the child to the ground, causing scalp and facial injuries. Generalized tonic/clonic seizures also occur and intellectual fall-off becomes evident. The EEG shows a characteristic appearance with paroxysms of two-cycle-per-second spike and wave activity. The attacks are resistant to treatment and most victims become profoundly disabled.

## SIMPLE ABSENCES (PETIT MAL)

This seizure disorder does not manifest before three years and seldom persists beyond the teenage period. Attacks may be subtle and can be interpreted by the teacher as simply daydreaming or inattention. During a seizure, the child stares fixedly and is quite unconscious. There may be eyelid flickering and movement of the brow. No other abnormal motor activity is evident. During the attack, the EEG shows a characteristic pattern of generalized three-cycle-per-second spike and wave activity. When this terminates, usually after 10 to 15 seconds, there is an abrupt return to consciousness. Attacks must be distinguished from complex partial seizures in which motor activity is more prominent.

## BENIGN FOCAL EPILEPSY OF CHILDHOOD

In this condition seizures tend to be nocturnal. Abnormal movements are often confined to the oral region but may be more extensive. Disturbance in consciousness is usually short-lived. The EEG shows a characteristic pattern of spike waves in central leads. Prognosis is excellent. Seizures have usually ceased and the EEG abnormality disappeared by the time the child reaches puberty.

## MANAGEMENT

Anticonvulsant drugs play a major role in the management of children with epilepsy. Their use is governed by a number of general principles. Long-term therapy should seldom, if ever, be instituted after the first seizure. Recurrent seizures justify the use of an anticonvulsant, which should be selected according to seizure type (Table 59.2). It should be borne in mind that all the drugs, with the exception of phenobarbitone, are very expensive in South Africa. The aim of treatment should be control of seizures by one drug with minimal side effects. This can be achieved in most cases by correct dosage and timing of administration. In certain cases, two anticonvulsants may be necessary. When this is so, careful attention must be given to the possibility of drug interaction. The use of three anticonvulsant drugs at the same time will not induce better control than two and can never be justified. A situation of this nature calls for a review of the patient's treatment protocol. In recent years, lamotrigine, vigabatrin, oxcarbazepine, and gabapentin have become available in South Africa as second-line anticonvulsants. These may be effective in certain cases resistant to conventional anticonvulsants, but are expensive and not without side effects. Their use is best left to those with extensive experience in the treatment of childhood seizure disorders.

The quality of life enjoyed by a child with epilepsy will depend on a number of factors. Maintenance of seizure control is clearly of major importance, as is the child's level of intellectual function. When seizures occur infrequently, and intelligence is within the normal range, there is no need for any special provision. Parents should be counselled to avoid overprotection and to treat their child as a normal individual. He or she should attend the school of the parents' choice and be permitted to take part in all school activities. Sensible surveillance should be maintained during swimming activities. A child's need for special schooling is determined more by scholastic progress than by seizures per se. When performance is affected by frequent

**Table 59.2** Appropriate anticonvulsant drugs

| | |
|---|---|
| Febrile seizures | Phenobarbitone |
| | Sodium valproate |
| Tonic-clonic and partial seizures | Phenobarbitone |
| | Phenytoin |
| | Carbamazepine |
| | Sodium valproate |
| | Clonazepam |
| | Primidone |
| Absences | Sodium valproate |
| | Ethosuximide |
| Complex partial seizures | Carbamazepine |
| Myoclonic seizures | Sodium valproate |
| | Clonazepam |
| | Clobazam |
| | Nitrazepam |
| Infantile spasms | ACTH |

seizures, the side effects of anticonvulsants, or by concomitant learning disability, placement in a school for children with epilepsy is advisable. Young children with poorly controlled seizures may do well to attend the nursery and pre-primary classes attached to such schools, if these are available. When there is significant intellectual disability, the child with epilepsy should be placed in an appropriate training centre for children with intellectual disability.

The doctor who treats children with epilepsy should encourage an attitude of optimism both in the child and in parents. In general, seizure control improves with maturation and some 60 per cent of those who have recurrent seizures in childhood are free by their teenage years. When a child on anticonvulsant treatment has been free of attacks for two years and shows EEG improvement, drug dosage may be gradually decreased. If there is no recurrence of seizures, therapy can safely be stopped. Two-thirds of all epileptics lead normal productive lives within the community and need no special provision other than acceptance. The other third, as a conse-

quence of intellectual disability, poor seizure control, or personality problems, have difficulty in making their way in the open market. Their special needs are best met in an environment of sheltered employment.

Community support groups can play an important role in creating awareness and understanding in the community. Useful pamphlets and booklets are available through the South African National Epilepsy League (SANEL).

# Spina bifida

Spina bifida results from a defect in the formation of the neural tube during the latter part of the first month of pregnancy. It presents clinically as spina bifida cystica, in which there is a visible midline defect of the lower end of the spine, or spina bifida occulta, where the defect is hidden but suspicion may be aroused by the presence of an overlying skin dimple, angioma, or tuft of hair. There may also be a lipoma of the underlying soft tissue. A spina bifida occulta can give rise to neural dysfunction because of the malformed neural tissue, to traction from adhesions, or to compression caused by a lipoma. Occasionally an occult lesion is associated with diastematomyelia (division of the cord into two halves), the cord being penetrated and transfixed by a bony or fibrous spur.

Approximately 95 per cent of spina bifida cystica lesions are myelomeningocoeles involving skin, spinal column, and spinal cord with resulting neurological dysfunction. The remaining five per cent are meningocoeles in which the membranes surrounding the cord pouch out, but the cord itself is not involved and consequently there is no neurological deficit.

## PREVALENCE

The birth prevalence of neural tube defects

shows wide geographical and racial variation, as well as fluctuations over time. The prevalence rate for neural tube defects is usually given as between one and two per thousand live births, with approximately two-thirds manifesting as spina bifida. A study in the Western Cape (Buccimazza et al., 1994) reported rates for neural tube defects of 2,56 per 1 000 for whites, 1,05 per 1 000 for coloureds and 0,95 per 1 000 for blacks. There has been a decline in the USA and UK in recent years, but this has not been evident in South Africa.

## AETIOLOGY

The aetiology is multifactorial, involving a genetic predisposition as well as environmental factors (see Chapter 7: Inherited disorders and congenital abnormalities). There is a 5 per cent chance of a neural tube defect if a family member has one, and this rises to 20 per cent if two family members are involved.

## CLINICAL FEATURES

These depend on the degree and type of neurological impairment. Usually the entire cord below the level of the lesion malfunctions, but occasionally an isolated but normally functioning segment is present below the cord. In such a case, the deep tendon reflexes and movements are reflex and not volitional. High lesions involving the lower thoracic segments are usually associated with total paraplegia and little or no deformity. Moderately high lesions result in less severe paralysis but gross deformities, because some muscle groups act on joints while others are paralysed. Hip dislocation occurs when the flexors and adductors are intact, but the extensors and abductors are paralysed (spinal segments L1, 2, and 3 intact; L4 and 5 involved). Loss of plantar flexion at the ankle (required for a 'push off' when walking) occurs when segment S1 is involved. A lesion below this would involve the intrinsic muscles of the foot only. There is usually a loss of skin sensation at a level approximating the motor level. The anaesthesia is always bilateral but may be asymmetrical.

## Sphincter disturbance

Some degree of bladder and bowel incontinence is present as the sphincters are innervated by segments S2, 3, and 4. This presents clinically as loss of bladder control or dribbling incontinence, and constipation or paradoxical diarrhoea.

## Hydrocephalus

Hydrocephalus is almost always present, although the severity may vary. In 70 to 80 per cent of cases it is progressive and will require shunting. It may be associated with an Arnold Chiari malformation of the hind brain, which involves varying degrees of downward displacement of the brain stem, fourth ventricle, and cerebellum towards the foramen magnum. It can result in a compromise of respiratory or bulbar function.

## Spinal deformity

Associated abnormalities of the spine (e.g., hemivertebrae) can give rise to a kyphoscoliosis, and contractures may result from the intra-uterine position of the limbs together with muscle weakness. There may also be abnormalities of other systems.

## MANAGEMENT

The decision to operate on an affected newborn depends on the degree of paralysis, the extent of hydrocephalus, presence or absence of kyphoscoliosis, associated segmental anomalies, and birth injuries or sepsis. The spinal lesion is generally repaired surgically within 24 to 48 hours. If the child is born in an outlying centre, the lesion should be covered with a saline dressing and the infant transferred to an appropriate unit as soon as possible. An open lesion which is draining cerebrospinal fluid requires antibiotic cover and urgent closure of the defect. The presence of a progressive hydrocephalus is determined by serial measurements of the head circumference and brain imaging. If a hydrocephalus is present, a ventriculo-peritoneal shunt should be inserted, usually within the first two months of life.

Ongoing management is best carried out by a multidisciplinary team of specialists experienced in the treatment of children with spina bifida.

## Orthopaedic management

Orthopaedic management aims to prevent or correct deformities, facilitate weightbearing and, where possible, promote ambulation. The techniques available include casting, corrective appliances, and surgery. The new lightweight materials used for orthoses and assistive devices have resulted in greater acceptance of the appliances.

## Urological management

This is aimed at controlling infection and establishing continence. Early investigation determines the state of the kidneys and upper urinary tracts. Kidney damage and/or dilatation of the ureters call for vigorous treatment. Increased urethral resistance requires surgical intervention in the form of transurethral resection of the external sphincter, and occasionally of the bladder neck. Bladder training, including manual compression and abdominal straining is instituted. If this is not successful in eliminating residual urine in the bladder, clean intermittent catheterization is recommended, often with judicious use of pharmacological agents to influence the blad-

der and sphincter tone (anticholinergic agents and adrenergic stimulators or blockers). Urinary diversion procedures using ureteroileostomies are rarely used today.

## Bowel control

Bowel control can be obtained by utilizing the gastro-colic reflex, arranging regular times of defecation, and by taking natural laxatives and foods with a high fibre content. Occasionally enemas, suppositories, or laxatives are needed.

## Other aspects of the management

These include developmental evaluation and intervention, together with recommendations for appropriate school placement. Later on, vocational guidance and employment will need to be addressed. For the more severely handicapped, independent living becomes an issue of great importance. For all patients, self-esteem and peer relationships require attention and, with the approach of puberty, sexuality becomes a matter of major concern to affected children. It is only comparatively recently that these questions have been seriously addressed by the caring professions.

### PREVENTION

Antenatal diagnosis is now possible and recommended when there is a family history of a neural tube defect. Maternal serum alphafeto protein (AFP) is used as a screening test. If elevated, ultrasonography will rule out causes other than myelomeningocele, such as incorrect gestational age, twins, and anencephaly. The sonograph itself may show the myelomeningocele. The final step is to obtain amniotic AFP and acetylcholine levels that are elevated in the presence of a myelomeningocele.

In recent years, randomized controlled trials and community intervention studies have shown that peri-conceptual supplemental folic acid is capable of preventing some, but not all, neural tube defects. The US Public Health Service recommends that all women of childbearing age in the US who are capable of becoming pregnant consume 0,4 mg of folic acid per day to reduce the risk of having a pregnancy affected with a neural tube defect. The introduction of folic acid administration could possibly reduce the prevalence of neural tube defects in South Africa by up to 50 per cent.

# Renal disease

The most common renal disorders in childhood are urinary tract infection and acute post-infectious glomerulonephritis. Prompt diagnosis and vigorous treatment of the former condition will prevent structural damage and ultimate renal failure. The latter condition has become much less common since the introduction of antibiotic treatment for streptococcal throat and skin infections.

The nephrotic syndrome occurs in childhood as an idiopathic condition ('minimal change disease') and also as a consequence of glomerular disease. Idiopathic nephrotic syndrome responds to treatment with prednisone and cyclophosphamide. Relapse may occur but is seldom seen when remission has lasted three years or more. When there is underlying glomerular disease, the nephrotic syndrome represents one stage in a relentless progression towards end stage renal failure. This situation may be brought about by a number of different pathologies. Gross congenital abnormality, persistent renal tract infections, vascular disorders, various glomerular diseases, and some tubular defects all lead eventually to a state of chronic renal insufficiency.

## MANAGEMENT

Early detection and correct treatment of urinary tract infection will serve to prevent chronic renal disease. Every child who presents with acute infection should be subjected to ultrasound or X-ray examination of the renal tract. Those with structural abnormality may require surgical treatment and should be referred to a urologist. Children with nephrotic syndrome and those with evidence of chronic renal failure are best treated by a paediatrician experienced in paediatric nephrology. Optimal management calls for careful attention to fluid and electrolyte intake, calcium and phosphorus metabolism, and acid-base balance. Deteriorating renal function may make essential a restriction in protein intake. Despite this, every effort should be made to achieve an intake of nutrients adequate for growth. Blood pressure must be regularly monitored and intercurrent infection vigorously treated. When glomerular filtration rate falls below 10 ml/minute/1,73m$^2$, dialysis or renal transplantation is necessary to prolong life. Management of this nature can be provided only by specialist renal units.

# Cardiac disease

Chronic heart disease in childhood is usually of congenital origin or a sequel to rheumatic fever. Cyanotic congenital heart disease is clinically evident at birth or in the first months of life. Ventricular septal defect, patent ductus arteriosis and coarctation may not be diagnosed until the patient is several years old, while atrial septal defect may remain undetected until early adulthood. Acute rheumatic fever is uncommon before the age of five years. The consequences of valve damage are encountered in later childhood and the teenage years. Mitral incompetence, mitral stenosis, and aortic incompetence are the most commonly encountered syndromes. Untreated, there is steady progression to cardiac failure and early death. The occurrence of rheumatic fever is reduced when streptococcal throat infections are adequately treated.

Rheumatic heart disease remains one of the most important chronic disorders in South Africa, with a prevalence of six per thousand schoolchildren in some areas (McLaren et al., 1975). Children with established rheumatic heart disease need careful surveillance. Normal schooling should be encouraged in the absence of cardiac failure. The extent of physical exercise should be determined by effort tolerance. Prophylaxis against recurrent streptococcal infection is important. This is best maintained by a monthly injection of benzathine penicillin. Such treatment is available at any clinic, free of charge. Daily oral dosage is less effective. When dental treatment is necessary, amoxycillin should be given one hour before the period of active intervention. Reduced effort tolerance and shortness of breath suggest cardiac decompensation. In such cases use of digitalis and diuretics must be considered. Children with severe rheumatic heart disease can be given a new lease of life by valve replacement surgery. Optimal timing for these operations is important, and so regular review in a paediatric cardiac clinic is an important aspect of long-term management.

Children who have rheumatic valvular damage remain well on regular antibiotic prophylaxis and have good prospects for effective adult life.

*Rheumatic fever and rheumatic heart disease are now notifiable conditions.* Every clinic should maintain a register of cases in the area and ensure that regular prophylaxis is given. A card kept by the child serves as a useful record of injections.

### MANAGEMENT

Optimal management of children with chronic heart disease cannot be achieved without recourse to a specialist paediatric cardiac centre. Neonates and young infants with cyanosis and other signs of serious cardiac dysfunction should be referred at once for definitive diagnosis even when this involves travel over great distances. Older infants and young children with significant murmurs should be seen by a cardiologist without undue delay. It is highly desirable that elective cardiac surgery should be completed well before the start of formal schooling. Patients awaiting surgery require regular monitoring of growth and haemoglobulin levels. Respiratory tract infections must be treated vigorously and antibiotic cover provided during any oral or dental procedures to prevent endocarditis.

# Diabetes

Juvenile onset diabetes mellitus is fortunately uncommon. The condition is found in approximately one child in every 3 000 under the age of 16 years. A disorder of glucose metabolism leads to hyperglycaemia, glycosuria, polyuria, and dehydration. There is ketosis and loss of weight despite an adequate intake of food. The onset of the illness may follow an intercurrent infection or apparently occur spontaneously. There is progressive lassitude and in some instances nocturnal enuresis. Examination of the urine reveals glucose and often ketones as well. The glucose tolerance curve is markedly abnormal. Untreated childhood diabetes is likely to be fatal in a matter of weeks. With rational management the child can look forward to a normal life span, and few restrictions need to be imposed on lifestyle or choice of career. Extensive education in patient self-management is vital. Good compliance ensures normal growth during childhood and deferred development of long-term complications such as atherosclerosis, peripheral neuritis, impaired renal function, and visual loss.

## MANAGEMENT

The initial management of a child with juvenile onset diabetes is best conducted in hospital by a paediatrician with experience in the condition. The administration of appropriate doses of insulin and the correction of dehydration and ketosis are the first priorities. Once stabilization has been achieved, use should be made of further time spent in hospital to educate the child and his or her parents about the diabetic life. Recent standardizations in syringe design and insulin strengths have simplified home management and a child of five or six years can be taught to self-administer the daily doses. Urine testing and blood glucose determination from a finger prick are soon learned and the principles of prudent diet understood. It is important that every diabetic child be taught to recognize the manifestations both of hyperglycaemia and hypoglycaemia and the appropriate steps to be taken should either develop. He or she should never be without a small packet of glucose sweets for use when hypoglycaemia threatens.

After discharge from hospital, the child should resume all normal activities and, if of age, return to school. It is important to ensure that the class teacher has at least elementary information about diabetes. The condition is not a contra-indication to athletic pursuits and international standards have been achieved by diabetics in most games and pastimes. Increased energy consumption during strenuous exercise should be counterbalanced with timely carbohydrate snacks. Successful day-to-day management is the responsibility of the individual concerned and his or her parents. Supervision, ongoing education about diabetes, and support should be provided by a family or clinic doctor who is also available for crisis intervention. The need for continued insulin administration in the face of vomiting or intercurrent infection must be stressed. The potential danger of foot injuries should be understood and appropriate steps taken to prevent these. Skin lesions of any sort should receive prompt treatment to prevent or contain infection.

With appropriate guidance, most diabetic children adapt well to their illness and live full and happy lives. Management may be difficult during times of adolescent identity crises. Understanding and sympathy will assist the young person through these periods and promote a mature approach that will permit healthy and productive adult life.

The South African Diabetic Association plays an important role for such youngsters. Camps for diabetic children are a particularly useful development. Good liaison between the primary care professional and the specialist is of particular importance in diabetes.

# Other chronic disorders

Other conditions run a chronic course during childhood. Some of these have been discussed elsewhere in this book. Children with cystic fibrosis are in constant danger of malabsorption and suffer recurrent respiratory tract infections which impair physical growth and interfere with schooling. Asthma is a major childhood health problem, particularly in the coastal regions of southern Africa and sufferers require to be on prophylactic medications for periods of months and years (see Chapter 45: Childhood asthma).

Major advances in cancer treatment have created a population of survivors who enjoy relatively good health. There is, however, always concern about relapse and many have learning and other problems secondary to radiation therapy.

Children with endocrine disorders may require prolonged replacement therapy and children with rheumatoid arthritis require skilled management over many years.

HIV-infected children form an ever-growing proliferation of those with chronic disorders (see Chapter 39: HIV infection).

In all these conditions, management must include attention to the child's social and educational well-being. Every attempt should be made to promote a normal pattern of activity within the community and at school. Independence and optimism should be cultivated by the medical team, buttressed with assurances of support and appropriate intervention whenever these are necessary.

Finally, the international MedicAlert organization provides an important facility for identifying children with these chronic illnesses in times of emergency.

## References and further reading

BUCCIMAZZA SS, MOLTENO CD, DUNNE TT, and VILJOEN DL. 1994. Prevalence of neural tube defects in Cape Town, South Africa. *Teratology.* 50(3):194–9.

DREIFUSS FE. 1981. A proposal for a revised clinical and electro-encephalographic classification of epileptic seizures. *Epilepsia.* 22:489–501.

HOSKING G & POWELL R (eds.). 1985. *Chronic childhood disorders.* Bristol: John Wright.

MCLAREN MJ, HAWKINS DM, KOORNHOF HJ, et al. 1975. Epidemiology of rheumatic heart disease in black school children in Soweto and Johannesburg. *British Medical Journal.* 3:474–8.

WEBSITE. Guidelines on management of diabetes, including diabetic keto-acidosis (DKA): *www.ispad.org.*

# PART FIFTEEN

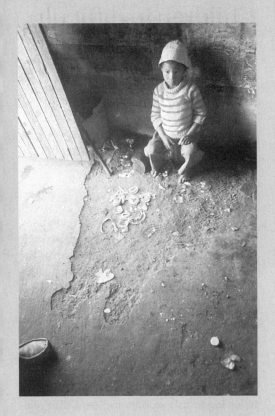

# Children in difficult circumstances

For many millions of children, daily living is a fight for survival. They may be separated from their families and living on the streets, caught up in violence or war, exploited for their labour, in conflict with the law, or suffer from a disability. Awareness of the prevention and management of abused children demands increasing attention. Some issues ensuring the major rights of these children are addressed here, and legislation pertaining to children and health care personnel is outlined.

# 60

# Children in difficult circumstances: An overview

## J LOFFELL & LA WAGSTAFF

Children are classified as being in difficult circumstances when their daily lives constitute a risk to their survival, protection, and development.

---

### Examples of children in difficult circumstances

These include children:
- living on the streets;
- exploited for their labour;
- who are abandoned,
- who are abused or neglected;
- with disabilities;
- who have been separated from their families;
- caught up in or exposed to family or community violence;
- who have been displaced;
- in conflict with the law; and
- affected by AIDS.

---

The concept of 'children in difficult circumstances' has gained recognition and been given special attention within the child rights framework. The basic needs of children are spelt out as survival, protection, development, and participation. South Africa, both in terms of its constitution and as a member of the international community, has made a commitment to address such matters and this is being driven and monitored by the National Programme of Action (NPA).

Many of these issues are discussed in different sections of this book – e.g., psychosocial factors are discussed in Chapter 3: Psychosocial factors in child health, and chapters following in this section also deal with relevant issues. Children in difficult circumstances and those with special needs are frequently overlapping categories related by causes and effects. Difficult circumstances tend to be associated with special needs, and special needs (if unmet) leave the child in difficult circumstances.

The previous section on children with special needs deals with children having special needs consequent on physical and functional disorders. Difficult circumstances, by contrast, generally originate from the child's micro- or macro-environment. Significant poverty is a major underlying factor together with adverse family, social, and political conditions.

Children may be driven to live on the streets because they are 'runaways' from poverty, abuse, overcrowding, and violence. Some have assumed the role of family bread-winners. Girls in these circumstances are often exploited as sex workers. Once embroiled in street culture, reintegration into society becomes increasingly difficult.

Child labour and children in conflict with the law remain very pertinent concerns in South Africa. Finally, HIV/AIDS is an ever-increasing threat to those infected, to children orphaned by the virus, and to society as a whole.

There is a need for strategies and appropriate programmes that will provide protection for children in especially difficult circumstances, and help them to reconstruct their shattered lives. But there is no single 'right' strategy for dealing with the problem: the mission is simple, but the task is not. There is a need for a proliferation of basic services to meet the needs of children on and off the street, and rural children must not be neglected. These services must cater for the maximum number of children, whom we would like to see returning to their communities – able to love, to play, to grow, and to learn.

The experience of readers will enable them to assume their due role as advocates for such children.

## References and further reading

COCKBURN A. 1993. *Street children: Survivors of multiple abuse*. Proceedings of the 2nd African Conference on Child Abuse and Neglect. 50–1.

# 61 Child abuse

WEK LOENING &
L JACKLIN

Only the most callous of individuals will countenance pain and suffering to be inflicted wilfully on a child. The sight, or even the thought of, an infant or young child being subjected to maltreatment naturally repulses people. And yet child abuse and neglect is known to occur in every community. Although not a health problem in the first instance, it is not unusual for health professionals to be the first to identify the true nature of the disorder and to play an essential role in both the treatment of the child and also in the prevention of further abuse by providing medico-legal evidence. Generally, children are not in a position to change the circumstances that control their lives – that control being largely in the hands of the parent or the main caregiver who will decide what the child should wear, eat, or do, even though any of this may be totally against the desires of the child. Similarly, the caregiver decides when and what degree of punishment is required. Furthermore, children usually cannot judge the situation in which they find themselves and thus may assume that they are guilty when in fact they are quite innocent. The child is unlikely to raise any objection for fear of further punishment. Current programmes aimed at preventing child abuse emphasize that it is the responsibility of adults to protect children and that children cannot be made responsible for their own safety. Such programmes do, however, continue to make children aware of their right to safety and control of their own bodies.

The disturbed social and cultural fabric of many communities coupled with disharmony in or disruption of families commonly result in childhood maladjustment. This, in turn, is acted out as unacceptable behaviour, which incurs punishment, ill understood by the child. Failure to identify this problem in the past was partly due to the fact that children were regarded as the property of the parents, an attitude which was reinforced by religious and cultural beliefs and practices. In deprived communities, children may be regarded as a liability adding to life's burdens, or as a resource to be exploited by the parents – as in child labour or prostitution. It was only in June 1969 that the United Nations Declaration of Children's Rights established that children do have the right to protection, love, and security, amongst other essentials, for healthy development. Since then, the United Nations Convention on the Rights of the Child and the

South African Charter of the Rights of the Child have firmly established this ethos.

# Frequency

Reports of prevalence of child abuse vary considerably depending on awareness, on the source of data (e.g., welfare agency, hospital, and police), on definitions applied (maltreatment, physical abuse, and neglect), and whether the abuse is suspected or in fact confirmed. Ignorance of the elementary needs of the developing child results in child abuse being prevalent in *all* communities and levels of society and particularly so when the caregivers themselves are victims of inadequate parenting. Different types of child abuse occur in different cultures but no group is immune to abusing children. It is unquestionably far more common in impoverished communities. Stresses associated with poverty tend to exacerbate and provoke abuse and to heighten the danger of neglect of children. Violence too is also a common feature of disadvantaged and depressed people.

# Definitions and range

Maltreatment covers all types of child abuse (see Table 61.1).

**Table 61.1** Types of child abuse

- Non-accidental injury and physical abuse;
- Sexual abuse;
- Emotional abuse;
- Neglect; and
- Substance abuse.

*Physical abuse and non-accidental injuries* include inappropriate corporal punishment, bites, burns, and fractures, tying up with rope, and poisoning.

*Sexual abuse* has been defined as 'the involvement of dependent, developmentally immature children and adolescents in sexual activities that they do not fully comprehend, are unable to give informed consent to, and that violate the social taboos of family roles'. The activities referred to range from exhibiting genitalia and inappropriate fondling to vaginal and anal intercourse, and they include the use of pornographic material.

*Emotional abuse*, which is commonly associated with other forms of abuse, undermines the dignity and esteem of the child by means of threats, derogatory remarks, and verbal manipulation. Secondary emotional abuse is often inflicted when the child is accused of provoking the perpetrator, just at a time when the victim needs love and security.

*Neglect*, which is undoubtedly the most common form of maltreatment, refers to failure to provide for the child's needs when these are within the means of the caregiver.

It must be emphasized that, in most instances, the child is exposed to a combination of some or all of these forms of abuse.

# Identification of maltreatment

It is important that the abused child is identified and that investigation covers the full extent of the maltreatment. Failure to do this may result in the death of the child as a result of an escalation of violent action or, at the very least, persistent emotional trauma and psychological scarring. Identification must result in some form of intervention. Action is called for even when there is only suspicion of maltreatment. This may include obligatory reporting as mandated in the South African Child Care Act. Proof of abuse often cannot be obtained and this should not be a reason for delaying action. The effective use of the currently underutilized Child Abuse Register managed by the Depart-

515

ment of Welfare could assist in conclusively identifying abused children presenting with suspicious but inconclusive findings to a number of different medical services.

# Circumstances surrounding maltreatment

Apart from the social context, the circumstances surrounding sexual abuse may differ from those that promote other forms of child maltreatment. Socio-economic deprivation, social and cultural upheaval, and isolated families are situations that predispose children to any form of abuse.

Table 61.3 details some of the characteristics that promote an abusing situation and must be considered as presenting *an increased* risk.

**Table 61.2** Factors determining maltreatment

- characteristics of abuser;
- characteristics of non-abusing family members;
- characteristics of abused child;
- social context; and
- situational context.

**Table 61.3** Characteristics promoting an abusing situation

*Characteristics of abuser:*
- childhood deprived of love and nurturance;
- poor self-control;
- unrealistic expectations of child;
- poor empathy with child;
- poor parenting skills; and
- alcohol or substance abuse.

*Characteristics of abuse victim:*
- young child (under 5 years of age);
- stepchild/adopted/fostered;
- disabled;
- hyperactive or behaviour problems; and
- no bond with mother.

*Characteristics of non-abusing family member:*
- other parent ineffectual, dependent, or uncooperative;
- poor cohesion with one with another;
- substance abuser;
- isolated; and
- colluding.

*Characteristics of situational context:*
- life stress event, e.g., loss of job; and
- marital breakdown.

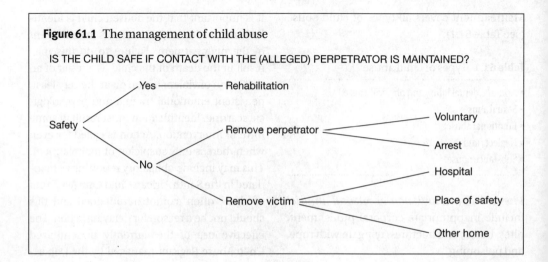

**Figure 61.1** The management of child abuse

IS THE CHILD SAFE IF CONTACT WITH THE (ALLEGED) PERPETRATOR IS MAINTAINED?

Safety
- Yes —— Rehabilitation
- No
  - Remove perpetrator
    - Voluntary
    - Arrest
  - Remove victim
    - Hospital
    - Place of safety
    - Other home

# Principles of management

- Do the nature and severity of the mal-treatment pose a substantial risk for the victim? If yes, an immediate decision must be made to separate the perpetrator and the victim (see Figure 61.1).
- Is the child safe if contact with the (alleged/suspected) perpetrator is maintained? The following considerations will be helpful when assessing the degree of risk:
  - Is the prime caregiver (when not the suspected perpetrator) co-operative and adequate?
  - What was the nature of the incident and the intent of the perpetrator?
  - Were there previous, albeit less serious, events?
  - Can the child protect him- or herself?
  - Generally children are not in favour of changes in environment and commonly resist separation, even in high-risk situations. Hence removal of the alleged perpetrator is preferable, wherever feasible, as removing child victims from their home is frequently regarded by them as further injury or punishment and may reinforce their guilt feelings. Nevertheless, it is the responsibility of the therapist to work through these feelings with the child to avoid deep emotional scars.
- Management should always involve a team with the active participation of at least a social worker, nurse, and doctor. The Child Protection Unit of the South African Police force and the prosecutors are frequently an important part of the team. Where possible an experienced psychologist should be involved. In the absence of any of these professionals, additional skills need to be acquired by others in the team at those centres where expertise is available, by reading around the subject, and by using audio-visual aids.

However, repeated interrogation of the victim by the various team members should be avoided. This is possible if good reports are written and passed on from one team member to the next.

In those cases where prosecution is considered, preparation and support of the child through the court process is now available in some centres. The development of courts dealing exclusively with sexual offences is intended to improve the quality of service to the victims of such crimes.

- All five factors mentioned in Table 61.2 require evaluation and appropriate intervention.
  - The nature and severity of the maltreatment and the degree of prevailing psychopathology determine the management of the perpetrator;
  - Family members frequently require counselling. Every effort should be made to build up the esteem and resources of the non-abusing adult members. Siblings of the victim require emotional support and frequently need to learn skills to protect themselves, particularly in the case of sexual abuse;
  - Over and above meticulous and sensitive medical and nursing care of the victim, psychological assessment is desirable. Cross-cultural issues frequently make this a difficult and complex task;
  - The social context is usually difficult to alter. Upliftment of the morale of the family and community are laudable aims but not easy to attain in the face of oppression and deprivation. Promotion of self-help groups and establishing of contact with church congregations and other non-governmental organisations are starting points. Communities must be encouraged to address moral issues so that values and attitudes can be re-established;

517

– Situational context: marriage coun-selling, assistance with finding employ-ment, and tapping other resources to ease life stress events must be considered.

## Neglect

The commonest form of maltreatment is unquestionably neglect. It refers to persistent failure to provide adequate physical and emo-tional care of the child where the means are available. For example, malnutrition of a child in a family that appears generally well fed must raise the question of neglect. Leaving children alone without adequate care is a seri-ous and frequent act of neglect, which can have disastrous consequences. When avoidable acci-dents occur, several questions must be raised such as: Are the parents fully aware of their responsibilities? Are they exercising their parental duties responsibly? Are they aware of the child's rights, particularly the right to safety? Do they appreciate that the child is vul-nerable and therefore requires special consid-eration and that his or her needs should take priority? Mostly one will be left with no more than an impression of the parents' knowledge in this regard and their attitude towards the child's well-being. Nevertheless, action is called for to improve on the quality of care: some open discussions regarding family values and functions may suffice. The use of parent-ing groups are of value in this respect.

## Physical abuse and non-accidental injuries

Whenever a child is seen with an injury, one must consider the possibility of non-acciden-tal trauma. The younger the child is, and par-ticularly those under one year, the greater is the likelihood of abuse. Table 61.4 lists other factors that increase this probability.

**Table 61.4** Further risk factors of child abuse

- stepchild;
- fostered/adopted child;
- mental or physical abnormality; and
- interference with the mother–child bond during early infancy.

## Features of physical abuse

Linear bruises and abrasions are amongst the most common injuries and are caused by a whipping or hiding with a strap or cane. At times, these ulcerate and become septic. Circular ulcers or scars must raise the suspi-cion of cigarette or other burns. 'Glove' or 'stocking burns' are almost certainly due to the forceful immersion of limbs into a hot liquid.

Eye injuries, especially sub-conjunctival haemorrhage, and a ruptured ear-drum are common signs of facial blows with the hand or an instrument.

Bite, scratch, or pinch marks may be seen, particularly in small children and infants. Complete fractures of long bones and frac-tures of the skull are suspicious and all the more so if they occur in the very young or recur repeatedly. Excessive squeezing of a baby's chest will cause fractures of the ribs. Retinal haemorrhages may result from severe shaking of an infant or small child with possi-ble serious long-term damage. Absence of detectable injuries does not exclude non-accidental trauma: severe pain can be inflict-ed without any visible evidence, particularly where the skin is pigmented.

### ASSOCIATED FEATURES

A 'frozen watchfulness', i.e., an expressionless face with eyes that follow the movements of the caregiver's hands, is often seen in young children who are exposed to repeated injury.

Abused children commonly are withdrawn *or* have poor self-esteem, which can be measured by the fact that they have few friends, little play activity, and poor ambition. Aggressiveness may form part of the acting-out behaviour.

## DIAGNOSIS

The psychosocial factors referred to in Tables 61.2 can be of help in evaluating the situation if non-accidental trauma is suspected. Where the circumstantial evidence is suggestive, one must act on suspicion and not await confirmation. An apparently loving relationship between caregiver and child does not exclude the diagnosis of maltreatment. Examination of the fundi for retinal bleeds is essential in babies where maltreatment is suspected. A skeletal survey may reveal signs of past trauma, which is further supportive evidence. Coagulation studies must be done in children when bruising is one of the manifestations of the maltreatment.

## MANAGEMENT

The principles outlined above form the basis of the management. A decision with regard to the safety of the child (see Figure 61.1) is imperative, as an error at this level may cause the loss of a child's life. Admission to hospital often brings welcome relief to the parents who have inflicted the trauma impulsively or against their better judgement. Where admission is resisted, child care legislation must be invoked. Clinical features must be recorded accurately. Needless to say the best medical/nursing care must be provided and at the same time the emotional trauma must not be overlooked.

# Sexual abuse

## LEGAL TERMS

Doctors who deal with child abuse generally use the term 'sexual abuse' (which is not a term used in law) to include all types of such abuse ranging from fondling, watching pornographic videos, and observing intercourse, to penetrative anal, vaginal, or oral intercourse. Sexual abuse is sometimes sub-classified (by doctors) as penetrative or non-penetrative. However, the legal terminology is different, and the doctor going to court should be familiar with those terms. Current terminology is defined below but is under review and new definitions are to be released in the near future.

*Rape* is unlawful, intentional carnal connection with a person without their consent. A person under 12 years of age cannot give consent; such intercourse is considered statutory rape. Rape (in legal terms) is penetration beyond the labia minora. Anything else falls under the classification of indecent assault, and often a charge of indecent assault will be accepted, when 'rape' cannot be proved. It is important to note that penetration beyond the labia can be assumed to have occurred if the hymen is damaged, since the hymen falls proximal to the labia. In other words, if the hymen is damaged, it is medical proof of legal rape.

*Incest* is the sexual union of two persons who, being related by blood or affinity, may not marry each other.

*Sodomy* is anal penetration of a male; according to the law, such an act perpetrated on a female is indecent assault.

## CIRCUMSTANCES SURROUNDING SEXUAL ABUSE

The circumstances that promote sexual abuse and some of the common factors that put a child at risk of being abused are listed in Table 61.5.

**Table 61.5** Circumstances that promote sexual abuse

● **Characteristics of abuser:**

*Molester:*

– sexually immature;

– no normal adult sexual relationship;

– exclusive preference for children;

– lack of self- control; and

– normal sexual orientation which breaks down at times of stress: marital conflict, substance abuse, loss of job.

*Rapist:*

– power rapist – uses force to dominate; and

– sadist – urge to inflict pain.

● **Characteristics of non-abusing family members:**

● **Little cohesion.**

*Mother:*

– passive, dependent, sexually inhibited;

– promotes/permits daughter taking over her role;

– sexually abused during childhood; and

– pregnant during early adolescence.

● **Characteristics of (potential) victim**

– vary with preference of abuser (see above);

– sexually precocious;

– timid, withdrawn, non-assertive;

– intellectually impaired; and

– oldest girl in family.

● **Social context**

– crowded sleeping facilities;

– children exposed to adult sex act early;

– presence of stepfather; and

– poor family cohesion.

● **Situational context**

– mother absent or incapacitated; and

– poor supervision of the child/lack of after-school care.

It must be appreciated that the family members and the social and situational context may act as, or be built up to act as, a barrier between a perpetrator or potential perpetrator and the child. This is of help in assessing the likelihood of abuse having taken place and may offer treatment opinions.

## PRESENTING FEATURES AND DIAGNOSIS

The child may present with a clear history of sexual interference. Disclosure of abuse may take place during the examination. Such a disclosure is exempt of the 'hearsay' rule and can be *used in court as evidence.* Vaginal discharge or genital sores are indicative of sexual abuse. Often the evidence is more obscure with urinary symptoms (late onset enuresis, dysuria), abdominal or pelvic pain as the presenting complaint. Behaviour out of keeping with the child's personality or precocious sexual behaviour should be regarded with suspicion. The behaviour of the child when examined may give important information as to the likelihood of abuse.

Absence of physical evidence of interference is not uncommon as a great deal of sexual abuse can take place without intercourse. Examples of sexual abuse unlikely to leave physical signs are exposing genitalia, various forms of oral stimulation, masturbation, fondling, and photographing these behaviours.

The child is more often a girl and in cases of incest, usually the oldest daughter in the family, who may have taken on some of the mother's roles in the home. The abuse of boys is thought to be underreported and possibly occurs more commonly in the home than previously thought. The sexually abused boy tends to be the non-assertive, timid type and is most reluctant to report the interference.

A detailed description of the genital and anal abnormalities that can be found in sexual abuse is beyond the scope of this text. However, it is essential that doctors and nurses who examine children must familiarizeise themselves with the range of normal as well as suggestive and definitive features of sexual abuse by means of the available literature and training courses offered.

Good documentation of the physical findings is important, especially as it is likely that the doctor will be required to give evidence in court. A structured format for writing down findings is important. If a charge has been laid down prior to the examination, the doctor will be asked to complete a form called a J88, which represents a request from the law enforcement agency to the doctor to examine the child. It is important that the doctor keep a copy of the report he submits to the police.

If a child is seen within the first 72 hours after the abuse took place, the incident should be managed as a medical emergency. Swabs should be taken for the body fluids and sperm of the offender. If foreign bodies such as hair are present they should be collected. Such specimens should be sent in a Rapekit, which is available from the local police station. Swabs for the purposes of isolating infections are better sent to the local pathology laboratory. Prophylaxis for pregnancy should be given to postpubertal girls, for HIV (in the opinion of the author), and other venereal disease if there are signs of penetration.

In specialized centres in affluent Western countries, colposcopes have been introduced to improve both the examination and the recording of the physical findings.

Sexually transmitted diseases raise a strong suspicion of sexual abuse even in the absence of vaginal penetration. Hence, blood specimens for syphilis and HIV serology should be obtained (blood tests should be repeated six weeks and six months later). Vaginal, urethral, and throat swabs for evidence of gonorrhoea or other sexually transmitted disease are indicated if there are clinical signs of an infection. Examination under general anaesthesia is called for in cases of recent vaginal penetration with subsequent bleeding to establish the full extent of the injury or a vaginal discharge, which does not resolve or recurs after treatment with antibiotics to exclude the presence of a foreign body.

As definite proof of sexual abuse may only be present in 25 per cent of cases, it is important that the examination should be therapeutic for both the child and the parents. Reassurance to the parent and the child when there are no physical signs of trauma or infection and the competent management of medical problems may play an important role in the healing process.

## MANAGEMENT

The principles of management previously detailed also apply to sexual abuse. Protection from further abuse is of paramount importance and separation from the suspected perpetrator is imperative. In some cultures, the abused girl subsequently becomes the victim of severe corporal punishment – either 'to get the truth from her' or to chastise her for her part in the act. This must be forestalled wherever possible and her innocence firmly established, as no child can be held responsible for participating in the sex act, no matter how provocative her behaviour may appear to have been.

Careful psychological assessment and therapy are very important if maladaptive behaviour and disturbance of the personality and sexuality in later years are to be avoided. The available skills and resources will determine the extent to which this can be carried out. Where further referral is not feasible, the local team will need to gather experience elsewhere. This would also apply to the handling of the family where the siblings are also at risk of maltreatment. A decision will need to be made with regard to prosecution of the perpetrator. Sexual abuse is unquestionably an offence for which there are severe penalties, but the strength of the evidence and nature of the case often determine whether prosecution is feasible. Therapy for the offender is even more problematic than therapy for the victim, but it must receive consideration. The situational context may be amenable to alteration. Sleeping arrangements can be adjusted; the victims may be given a 'safe' area where they can lock their doors; shift-times of working parents can be altered; day care by another family or in an after-school centre can sometimes be arranged.

## POISONING

Deliberate administration of poison is not a common form of abuse but it should, nevertheless, be considered whenever a child presents with features of poisoning. It is unfortunate that some parents, and fathers in particular, consider that getting the child 'a little tipsy' with alcohol is amusing. In the author's opinion this 'bit of fun' should be regarded as maltreatment, especially as alcohol may cause potentially lethal metabolic disturbance in the child.

# Child abuse in various cultural settings

The concept of child abuse originated in Eurocentric culture and acceptance of what constitutes child abuse varies in different cultural settings. The rights of the child should nevertheless be applied universally. In disadvantaged communities, and those in cultural transition, there are further complexities that call for special consideration.

Urbanization, crowding, and poverty are amongst the main underlying negative factors. Loss of kinship support and traditional values, in association with poor family cohesion and single and often unplanned parenthood, deprive vast numbers of children of the stability and security that they deserve.

It is especially in these communities that violence abounds – be this political, interfamily, or thuggery – so that there is that added burden of fear and insecurity. No effort

must be spared by all who hold the welfare of the child in high regard to endeavour to correct the underlying wrongs, to improve parenting skills, and to strive for facilities for appropriate nurturing.

There must be a call for commitment to allocate resources in such a manner that the child receives optimal care and is nurtured in a suitable environment.

# Corporal punishment

Children, the next adult generation, should be taught that conflict resolution *can* be achieved without violence. This cannot occur while physical punishment and other forms of shaming children are so widespread in homes and in schools. Recently, more and more educationalists are giving up corporal punishment in favour of more positive methods of enforcing discipline in class. In a number of countries, physical punishment has been banned from school entirely, in keeping with the spirit and letter of the Convention on the Rights of the Child. Namibia was the first African country to do so. The organization EPOCH-WORLDWIDE (End Physical Punishment of Children) has played a leading role in spreading knowledge on the ineffectiveness and dangers of physical methods of punishment and on promoting self-discipline in children through non-abusive child rearing.

## References and further reading

DE VILLIERS FPR. 1992. The doctor as witness in child abuse cases. *South African Medical Journal.* 81:521.

HOLDSTOCK L. 1987. Education for a new nation. Africa Transpersonal Association.

KIBEL MA & NEWELL P. 1995. Ending physical punishment of children in

South Africa. *South African Medical Journal.* 85(2):66–8

PELTON LH (ed.). 1981. *The social context of child abuse and neglect.* New York: Human Sciences Press.

VARIOUS ARTICLES. Child abuse and neglect: *The International Journal.* New York: Pergamon Press.

WALKER CE, BONNER BL, and KAUFMAN KL (eds.). 1988. *The physically and sexually abused child : Evaluation and treatment.* New York: Pergamon Press.

# 62

# Children and legislation in South Africa

## J LOFFELL

Legislation in South Africa has been in a state of flux since the advent of democracy in 1994. Laws affecting children are at present poised to change in what may prove to be quite dramatic ways, as constitutional principles and the impact of national and international child rights agreements make themselves felt.

At the time of writing, lengthy consultative processes concerning proposed new legislation concerning children, steered by the South African Law Commission, are in their final stages. The SA Law Commission has over the past three years appointed project committees to deal with Youth Justice (Project no. 106); Sexual Offences (Project no. 107); and the Review of the Child Care Act (Project no. 110).

The *Child Care Act* of 1983, which has been the law most centrally concerned with formal measures for the care and protection of children, is likely to give way within the next few years to a new comprehensive children's statute, which will concern itself with the broad range of children's needs and rights. The new law will probably incorporate many provisions, which are now scattered between different Acts. New legislation dealing with sexual offences against children and with judicial processes in relation to young

offenders will also come onto the statute books in the near future, either within the comprehensive statute or in separate but extensively cross-referenced laws.

Hence, by the time the reader encounters this chapter, much of what has been said about legislation for children may have changed or may be about to change. An effort will still be made to provide an outline of existing legislation affecting children, particularly those aspects that are more likely to be encountered by health care workers. Some of the newer principles that seem likely to be incorporated into incoming legislation will also be identified. These arise chiefly from the bill of rights in the South African constitution, which in turn reflects central provisions of the United Nations Convention on the Rights of the Child, ratified by South Africa in June 1995. The influence of the African Charter on the Rights and Welfare of the Child, developed by the Organization of African Unity and ratified by this country in January 2000, is also likely to be evident.

All of these legal systems include provisions specifically dealing with, or at least impacting on, children and family relationships. The focus in this chapter is on the common and

## Existing legal framework

The lives of South African children are influenced by various types of law:
- the *constitution* is the supreme law of South Africa. It sets out the principles on which all laws must be based. It includes a bill of rights, which in turn has a section outlining the rights of children;
- the *common law* is the traditional body of legal thinking, based on Roman Dutch and English law, which has emerged over time within the South African courts and is reflected in precedents set by court decisions;
- *statutory law* is comprised of the many Acts passed by the present and past parliaments;
- *regional legislation* exists in the form of provincial laws and local government by-laws, which are passed by the elected legislative bodies at the relevant levels;
- *African customary law* applies in areas and communities where traditional leadership and authority systems are still fully in place. Such law has been handed on through tradition. Customary law varies according to the specific cultural grouping involved;
- *religious law* impacts on people living in certain orthodox religious contexts; and
- *international law* affects South Africans via conventions to which this country is a party. These are used to guide policy and reform, and are referred to in court decisions. They become fully binding if incorporated in South African law.

statutory law; however, it is important to be aware that any specific child may be subject to the rules of, for example, guardianship and custody, parent–child relationship, majority and minority, maintenance, inheritance etc., which arise from customary or religious law, and that these may at times be in tension with the aspects of the formal legal system in South Africa. Also, children may be affected in different ways from region to region by provincial legislation and local government by-laws, which may have an impact on the kinds of services available to them and the way these are regulated. The constitution and the various international conventions concerning children may offer opportunities to promote children's rights beyond what is immediately catered for in other forms of law.

# Constitutional rights of children

Section 28(1) of the constitution provides that all children in South Africa are entitled to: a name and nationality; family or parental care or appropriate alternative care if removed from the family; basic nutrition; shelter; basic heath care services and basic social services; protection from maltreatment, neglect, abuse, and exploitation, including exploitation for their labour; exemption from detention except as a last resort, in which case protective measures must be applied; legal representation at state cost if substantial injustice is otherwise likely to occur; and exclusion from involvement in armed conflict, as well as protection when such conflict occurs. Section 28(2) provides that 'a child's best interest is of paramount importance in every matter concerning the child'. The constitutional right of the child to health care services is the basis for service provision by the Department of Health. The policy that pregnant women and children under six years must receive free health care at state institutions is in partial implementation of this principle.

# Status of children

According to the Constitution, the UN Convention on the Rights of the Child, and the *Child Care Act*, a child is a person under the age of eighteen years, and the protective mechanisms to which these give rise cease at that age, with some exceptions. A person who is over eighteen and unmarried, while not legally a child, remains a 'minor' until legal majority is attained at age twenty-one. However, the young person progressively becomes legally competent to undertake a range of tasks, from opening a savings account at age seven, to obtaining a driver's licence, voting, and setting up a home separate from that of the parents at age eighteen. From age seven to thirteen, a child is considered legally incapable of committing a crime, but this presumption can be rebutted in court. From the age of fourteen, full criminal capacity is considered to exist. A minor requires his or her parents' consent to marry or sign any type of contract before age twenty-one, unless an order of emancipation is obtained from the High Court. A person under eighteen who is legally married automatically has adult status.

There are a number of anomalies in the present law in relation to the age of majority, and young people who are over eighteen but under twenty-one sometimes find themselves in a legal 'twilight zone' where they are not protected from abuse or neglect by the Child Care Act, but also not able to act fully on their own behalf. For example, they may not marry, sign a lease for accommodation, or take up employment without assistance.

# Guardianship

## CHILDREN BORN TO A MARRIED COUPLE

In terms of the *Guardianship Act* 192 of 1993, the mother and father, where they are legally married, are equal guardians of any child born within or prior to their marriage. This is a shift from the previous situation in which guardianship was vested in the father. The guardianship of either parent can be terminated only by adoption or by an order of the High Court, which is the upper guardian of all minors.

## CHILDREN OF UNMARRIED PARENTS

Where the parents of a child are not married, the mother is the legal guardian, unless she is under twenty-one years in which case, in terms of the *Children's Status Act* no. 82 of 1987, her guardian is also the guardian of her child. However, the *Natural Fathers of Children Born out of Wedlock Act* no. 86 of 1997 provides that an unmarried father may apply to the High Court to be granted guardianship or custody of, or access to, his child. An investigation by and recommendation from the Office of the Family Advocate may be requested by the court when considering an application by an unmarried father. The Child Care Act as amended in 1996 includes customary and religious unions within its definition of marriage, thus removing a painful form of discrimination whereby fathers were deprived of legal standing in relation to their children for purposes of this Act.

## CHILDREN BORN THROUGH ASSISTED CONCEPTION AND SURROGACY

The *Human Tissue Act* no. 65 of 1983, and the *Children's Status Act* no. 82 of 1987 spell out the position of a child who is born by means of artificial insemination, *in vitro* fertilization, and related techniques. Such a child is legally the child of the woman who gives birth to him or her and, if applicable, the husband of that woman. There are no legal ties with any sperm or ovum donor who may be involved. In the past, such forms of conception were legally possible only for married women with the written consent of their husbands; however, a 1997 amendment to the regulations under the *Human Tissue Act* gave single women access to these methods. Surrogate childbearing was not an intended focus of either of these Acts; however, the *Children's Status Act* in effect covers the procedures used in most surrogacy arrangements, i.e., the insemination of the surrogate mother with sperm from a would-be father or a donor, and/or the implanting of an ovum from a would-be mother or a donor. In a surrogacy arrangement, a married woman who gives birth to the child and her husband, if he has consented to the pregnancy, will be the child's legal parents. If the surrogate mother is unmarried or has conceived the child from donated gametes without her husband's consent, the infant will legally be regarded as her extramarital child. If she decides, after giving birth, to keep the child, this is her prerogative. It is only through adoption or through a High Court order that guardianship can be transferred to the individual or couple who have sought the services of the surrogate mother. The issue of surrogacy has been the subject of an investigation and recommendations by the SA Law Commission (Project no. 65: Surrogate Motherhood) and more recently by an *ad hoc* parliamentary select committee; however, no finality on this issue has yet been reached.

## Consent to medical treatment

Section 39(4) of the *Child Care Act* no. 74 of 1983, as amended by Act 86 of 1991, empowers a person over eighteen years of age to consent to the performance of an 'operation' on him or herself without assistance from a parent or guardian. A child of fourteen years

or over may consent to 'medical treatment' without adult assistance. The amendment in question was brought about *inter alia* to enable adolescents to obtain contraception without their parents having to be consulted. For an operation on any child, and for medical treatment of a child under fourteen, the consent of a parent or guardian is required. In the case of an unmarried mother aged at least fourteen, her right of consent extends to medical treatment of her child; consent to surgery on her child would, however, have to be given by her (the mother's) guardian.

Where a child is believed by a medical practitioner to be in need of surgery, or of treatment for which the consent of a parent or guardian is required, but the parent or guardian is deceased, cannot be found, is mentally incompetent to give consent, or refuses consent, the following options are available:

- In terms of section 39(1) of the *Child Care Act*, the Minister of Welfare (in practice a senior official in the provincial Department of Welfare), may be approached for consent.
- In a situation in which the performance of the procedure is needed urgently so as to save the child from death or 'serious and lasting disability', and should not be delayed for purposes of seeking the consent of the relevant party, the medical superintendent of the hospital or a medical practitioner acting on his or her behalf may give consent (section 39(2) as amended).
- Where a child has been placed away from home – e.g., in foster care, a children's home, or any other facility – in terms of the *Child Care Act* or the *Criminal Procedures Act*, and a situation of urgency such as described above exists, the foster parent or other official custodian, or the head of the relevant institution may authorize the procedure (section 53(4)).

- The High Court, as upper guardian of all children, can be approached for a decision.

A controversial exception to the requirement of consent for medical procedures on children has been created by the *Choice in Termination of Pregnancy Act* no. 92 of 1996, which allows any woman or girl regardless of age to request termination of pregnancy. Section 5(3) requires that, before such termination is carried out on a minor, 'a medical practitioner or registered midwife ... shall advise her to consult with her parents, guardian, family members or friends'. However, should she choose not to consult any such person, the termination 'shall not be denied ...'. The scarcity of resources in the public health system for counselling of mothers requesting termination is a cause for concern, in particular where the expectant mother is herself a child.

In terms of section 3 of the *Sterilization Act* no. 44 of 1988, a person under eighteen years may be sterilized only with the permission of a parent, spouse, guardian, or curator, and then only if the person has a severe mental disability, his or her physical health is threatened, and there is no other safe and effective means of contraception. A decision as to whether to grant the sterilization must be reached by a panel convened by the person in charge of the hospital, consisting of a psychiatrist or (if no such person is available) a medical practitioner, a psychologist or social worker, and a nurse. If the patient is in custodial care, none of the panel members may be on the staff of the facility concerned.

A gap in the legislation is the absence of any definition of 'operation' and 'medical treatment'. The question of testing of children for HIV is also not adequately covered in the law, although in terms of generally accepted guidelines this should be undertaken only where it is clearly in the best interests of the child concerned and where his or her informed consent has been given. In the case of a younger child, the informed consent of the parent or guardian should be obtained where such a person is available. Pre- and post-test counselling and careful attention to confidentiality are essential. Where a very young child is found to be HIV-positive this will normally indicate that the mother or both parents are infected, and she or they will require support and appropriate referral to deal with the painful realities of their and their child's condition.

There is debate as to whether abandoned babies should be tested for HIV, one view being that such testing is unnecessary where universal precautions against infection are in place, and that testing is used as basis for discrimination whereby children are denied adoption and foster care. The counter-argument is that proper case management as well as honesty with prospective caregivers requires that any abandoned child should be fully medically examined, and that HIV-infection, like any other life-threatening condition, is a critical factor to be taken into account. Some hold that the minister's permission should be sought for HIV testing of abandoned babies as per section 39(1) of the *Child Care Act;* others argue that the test is merely part of the comprehensive evaluation that such children require. This is an issue that will probably be resolved in the new comprehensive children's statute.

# Child abuse and neglect: preventive measures

## MAINTENANCE

Failure on the part of a parent to properly provide for his or her child is one of the causes of child poverty in South Africa. The *Maintenance Act* no. 99 of 1998 strengthens the power of the maintenance courts to ensure that parents who are able to do so provide properly for their children. The court may order direct deductions from the salary of the person concerned. It is now unlawful for children of a later marriage to have preference over children from an earlier relationship – all must be treated equally.

## SOCIAL SECURITY

Social security provision for children within their families is very limited in South Africa, although large numbers benefit from grants that were designed for individual adults, namely the old age pension and the disability grant. In some impoverished rural areas, these grants are the major source of household income, enabling both adults and children to survive. The *Social Assistance Act* no. 59 of 1992 as amended provides for the aforementioned benefits and also for two grants intended specifically for the support of children within their own homes, namely:

- the child support grant – a very small allocation (R100 per month at the time of writing) to the 'primary caregiver' of a child under seven years of age, where the caregiver meets the prescribed means test; and
- the care dependency grant – a monthly amount of R540 for the support of a severely disabled child who requires full-time care and whose parents or guardian meet the means test. The state-employed medical practitioners who assess children to determine whether they qualify for this grant have a most serious responsibility as it seems to be on the basis of their individual judgement that the level of a child's disability is graded. Ill-considered or arbitrary decisions can lead to great misery.

## CHILDREN WHO ARE PRIVATELY PLACED AWAY FROM HOME

In terms of section 10 of the Child Care Act as amended, a child aged less than seven years may not be cared for apart from his or her parents for longer than fourteen days without authorization from the commissioner of child welfare, except by a designated institution including a hospital or a maternity home or a member of the child's extended family. Section 10 also applies to a child of any age whom the caregiver intends to adopt. In this case, an adoption application must be lodged at the children's court within fourteen days of the caregiver's having received the child. The commissioner may in either situation set conditions for the continuation of the care arrangement, such as monitoring by a social worker or a community health nurse. Contravention of section 10 is not a criminal offence but it is grounds for the removal of the child. A major reason for its existence has been to prevent trafficking in infants and young children. It has also been seen as a protective measure against questionable 'private adoptions' brokered by third parties, including, for example, some lawyers and health care workers. Section 10 has come in for criticism *inter alia* because of the large numbers of South African children who live with non-family members for socio-economic reasons. It is likely to be reformulated if it is included in future legislation, possibly by focusing specifically on children destined for adoption.

## CHILDREN OF DIVORCING OR DIVORCED PARENTS

The Family Advocate may be called on by the court to assist in decisions concerning custody and access where these are contested during or after divorce, in terms of the *Mediation in Certain Divorce Matters Act* no. 24 0f 1987. In this way the court seeks to establish what arrangement appears to be in the best interests of the child or children concerned, and as far as possible to promote mediation as a means of reducing trauma for children who are caught up in conflict between their parents. The

Family Advocate's office can call on the assistance of social workers and other practitioners in the community in this process. The Act provides for 'family counsellors' – who at present are seconded by the Department of Welfare – to assist the Family Advocate's office, which is operated by the Department of Justice.

## REGISTRATION OF 'PLACES OF CARE'

A 'place of care' as defined in the *Child Care Act* is 'any building or premises maintained or used, whether for profit or otherwise, for the reception, protection and temporary or partial care of more than six children apart from their parents ...'. (Registered schools are excluded.) It is an offence to receive any child in such a facility if it is not registered with the Department of Welfare in terms of section 30 of the Act. This provision includes all formal and informal pre-school care facilities including child-minder services, as well as afternoon and holiday care centres for school-going children. It is a requirement for registration that the facility be certified as adequate in terms of local government structural and health requirements. All places of care are subject to inspection by persons designated by the Department of Welfare, and local government health care workers frequently monitor places of care within the ambit of the *Child Care Act* and their own regulations. There are regular calls on the one hand for a stricter system in terms of which 'child-minders' dealing with six or fewer children also be required to register and, on the other, for a reduction in burdensome regulation requirements in view of the need to promote self-help in impoverished communities.

## PROHIBITION OF CHILD LABOUR

It is widely recognized that children who enter the labour force prematurely tend to be at risk

of abuse, neglect, and exploitation in a wide range of forms. Such children are frequently caught up in the cycle of poverty that child labour helps to perpetuate, *inter alia* by depriving children of education and promoting adult unemployment. With this in mind, both section 52A of the *Child Care Act* and section 43 of the *Basic Conditions of Employment Act* (BCEA) prohibit the employment of children aged less than 15 years. While the *Child Care Act* allows for the Minister of Welfare to grant exemptions from this ruling, the BCEA allows for none except in the case of advertising, sports, artistic, or cultural activities (section 55(1)), and then only subject to one or more specific 'sectoral determinations', on the basis of which such activities would be regulated. The minimum age is in practice being ignored by many employers. However, the Department of Labour is taking active steps towards its more effective enforcement. The Departments of Health, Education, and Welfare are currently involved, along with labour federations, employer groups, and NGOs, in an intersectoral partnership known as the Child Labour Intersectoral Group (CLIG), which is convened by the Department of Labour, and which aims to deal with child labour in a holistic manner. Health care personnel who encounter child labour can link up with this process through the relevant provincial office of the Department of Labour.

# Child abuse and neglect

## PROTECTIVE MEASURES AND INTERVENTIONS

### Reporting and registration of abuse

Health care professionals encountering actual or suspected child abuse in the course of their duties are required by two separate statutes to report what they have observed.

*Section 42(1) of the Child Care Act* as amended requires that 'every dentist, medical practitioner, nurse, social worker or teacher, or any person employed by or managing a children's home, place of care or shelter, who examines, attends or deals with any child in circumstances giving rise to the suspicion that that child has been ill-treated, or suffers from any injury, single or multiple, the cause of which might probably have been deliberate, or suffers from a nutritional deficiency disease, shall immediately notify the Director-General (of the Department of Welfare) or any officer designated by him or her for the purposes of this section, of those circumstances'. Forms as specified in the regulations under the *Child Care Act* must be completed by the reporter in cases of suspected ill-treatment or deliberate injury (form 25), and nutritional deficiency disease (form 26). Mandatory reporters are protected from legal proceedings arising from any notification made in good faith in fulfilment of their obligations in terms of this Act. The regulations spell out the action to be taken by the Director General, i.e., to initiate steps to ensure the safety of the child and launch a preliminary investigation, and to give instructions for appropriate action thereafter. In addition the regulations provide for the establishment of a national child protection register, to include details of the child concerned and also the perpetrator, where this person has been identified. The regulations allow the Director General, at his or her discretion, to refer a case of which notification has been received to the police for possible prosecution.

Section 4 of the *Prevention of Family Violence Act* no 133 of 1993 is very broad in its scope. In effect it includes as mandatory reporters of child abuse, along with those already bound by section 42(1) of the *Child Care Act*, all paramedical personnel, as well as family and community members who participate in caring for the child. It states as fol-

lows: 'Any person who examines, treats, attends to, advises, instructs or cares for any child in circumstances which ought to give rise to the reasonable suspicion that such child has been ill-treated, or suffers from any injury the cause of which was deliberate, shall immediately report such circumstances ...'. A notification in terms of this Act must be directed to a police official, a commissioner of child welfare, or a social worker employed by a registered welfare organization. This section is still in effect at the time of writing, although almost all the rest of the *Prevention of Family Violence Act* has been repealed by the *Domestic Violence Act* of 1998.

The above two provisions for the reporting of child abuse are not in any way synchronized. There are no regulations to guide reporting in terms of the *Prevention of Family Violence Act*. The reporting system under the *Child Care Act* is now slowly coming into operation after having been stalled for some years, due to delays in the development of the regulations and lack of the necessary infrastructure within the welfare system. Questions have been raised as to the constitutionality of those sections of the regulations which provide for the inclusion of details of alleged (as well as convicted) perpetrators in the register. The question of who should have access to the register has also not been settled, along with numerous other ethical and practical issues. It is likely that the incoming children's statute will replace the current fragmented approach with a single set of provisions surrounding reporting and registration of child abuse.

## Dealing with the perpetrator

The *Domestic Violence Act* no. 116 of 1998 is intended to make the justice system more effective in dealing with domestic violence, and more accessible to those who experience this problem, including children. 'Domestic violence' in terms of the Act includes physical and sexual abuse; emotional, verbal and psychological abuse; economic abuse (the unreasonable withholding of needed resources to which the complainant is entitled by law); disposal of household items or property to which the aggrieved person has a claim; intimidation, harassment and stalking; damage to property; unauthorized entry where the parties do not share a residence; and any other 'controlling or abusive behaviour' that is or may be harmful to the complainant's well-being.

Anyone who is involved in a 'domestic relationship' in which domestic violence is involved is entitled to protection under this Act. A domestic relationship is one in which there are or have been family ties; a present or past marriage or cohabitation, whether heterosexual or homosexual; a present or past engagement or dating or romantic relationship, actual or perceived; or a shared home. Any SA Police Service member called to the scene of an incident of domestic violence is obliged to provide, timeously, whatever help is needed, including help in obtaining shelter and/or medical treatment, and to explain the complainant's options to him or her. A police officer who fails to provide proper assistance can be charged with misconduct. Any peace officer (including a SAPS member) may, without a warrant, arrest someone who he/she reasonably suspects of having committed domestic violence against a complainant.

In terms of section 4, any complainant may approach a magistrate's court or family court to request a protection order. A child may make such an approach without any adult assistance. Section 4(3) provides that the court can be approached by a concerned person such as a health service provider, social worker, teacher, or SAPS member. The written consent of the person affected by the violence is necessary unless he/she is a child, a mentally disabled person, or is unable to give consent for other reasons. Where there is

*prima facie* evidence of domestic violence that is likely to cause undue hardship to the complainant, the court must issue an interim protection order. Thereafter, if the respondent fails to show good reason why this should not be done, a protection order must be issued if evidence is present to justify such a measure. A warrant of arrest is then issued against the respondent. This is suspended as long as he or she refrains from any contravention of the order. If a member of the SAPS has reason to suspect that the terms of the order have been broken, he or she must arrest the respondent forthwith.

A protection order or interim protection order may prohibit the respondent *inter alia* from: committing an act of domestic violence or enlisting the help of a third party to do so; entering the complainant's residence or any part thereof; or entering the complainant's place of employment. The court may also instruct that a weapon in the possession of the respondent be seized, or order the respondent to refrain from any contact with a child, or set conditions for such contact.

## Children's court inquiry

Central to the *Child Care Act* is its provision for the operation of children's courts and its determination of the powers and responsibilities of commissioners of child welfare. Any court can operate as a children's court and every magistrate is *ex officio* a commissioner of child welfare, although, in larger centres, specific courts and magistrates tend to be assigned specifically to this function. The Act provides for the children's court to serve as an informal, non-accusatory forum. Recent changes to the law have removed the concept of an 'unfit parent', which used to be central to its operations, and the focus is now on determining whether a child is at risk and in need of protection by the State. If there is reason to believe that any child is 'in need of care', he or she may be brought

## Children in need of care

The grounds for such a finding would be one or more of the following, as spelled out in Section 14(4):

- the child has no parent or guardian;
- the child has a parent or guardian who cannot be traced; or
- the child
  - has been abandoned or is without visible means of support;
  - displays behaviour that cannot be controlled by his or her parents or the person in whose custody he or she is;
  - lives in circumstances likely to cause or conduce to his or her seduction, abduction, or sexual exploitation;
  - lives in or is exposed to circumstances that may seriously harm the physical, mental, or social well-being of the child;
  - is in a state of physical or mental neglect;
  - has been physically, emotionally or sexually abused, or ill-treated by his or her parents or guardian or the person in whose custody he or she is; or
  - is being maintained in contravention of section 10.

before the local children's court, either by order of the court or on the initiative of a police officer, a social worker employed by the State or a registered welfare organization, an 'authorized officer', a parent or guardian, or a person having custody of the child. The court will then conduct an inquiry to determine whether the child is 'in need of care'.

## Placement options for children in need of care

If the court finds the child to be in need of care, it has several options. The commission-er may place the child back in the care of the parent(s) or guardian(s) or the person in whose custody he or she was before the court proceedings began, under the supervision of a social worker and subject to certain conditions – e.g., the parents and/or the child may be required to undergo treatment or counselling. The commissioner may order that the child be placed in foster care, a children's home, or a school of industries. State grants are available to foster parents and registered children's homes as a contribution towards the costs of providing care. Typically, an order of the children's court lasts for two years, although a shorter period may be set. The order then expires, unless the Minister of Welfare (in practice a designated official) decides, on the basis of a social worker's report, to extend the period of retention. The intention is that services should be delivered to the child and family with a view to helping them overcome their problems and restoring the family unit. Should this prove not to be possible, the child may remain in long-term care, with some social service monitoring and support. Much emphasis is placed in policy documents on achieving 'permanency' for the child either with his or her own family or through, for example, adoption, if the parents' consent is forthcoming or if the court releases the child for this purpose. But shortage of resources for rehabilitation and other factors tend to result in many children growing up in statutory care. Various policy initiatives of the Department of Welfare have been introduced with the aim of enabling these children to move through and out of these placements.

### Adoption

An important option for children whose parents have died or disappeared, or are unable to care for them, is legal adoption, which is provided for in sections 17 to 20 of the *Child Care Act*. This is the placement of choice *inter alia* for abandoned babies. It is vital to facilitate the process whereby such children enter adoption, so as to provide the advantages of bonding within a family environment and to avoid the potentially harmful consequences to very young children of lengthy hospitalization or other forms of institutional care. The steady growth in the numbers of AIDS orphans makes the expansion of adoption as a care alternative a matter of great urgency. South African agencies have in recent years been shifting their policies and revising the arguably unrealistic, Eurocentric standards that adopters have in the past been required to meet. There have been calls for many years for provision in the law for adoption allowances that would enable people who could offer a child a stable home, but cannot afford the costs involved, to adopt. Such an allowance could also make it possible to find adoptive homes for children who at present cannot be placed, owing to disabilities or chronic health conditions that are costly to manage.

Except where a court rules otherwise, a child cannot be adopted without the consent of both parents, if they are married. In the case of a child born extramaritally, consent is required from the mother. In terms of the *Adoption Matters Amendment Act* no. 56 of 1998, a father who is not married to the mother of his child and who 'has acknowledged himself in writing to be the father of the child and has made his identity and whereabouts known ...' must also consent. Where an unmarried mother has consented to the adoption of her child, a natural father who has acknowledged his paternity in this way must be notified that her consent has been given, and be afforded an opportunity to respond. This also applies if the mother confirms that he has acknowledged himself to be the father, and provides details of his identity and whereabouts, or if a social worker provides these details in a report to the court. An unmarried couple may jointly register the birth of their child with the Department of Home Affairs, or the father may apply for an amendment to the birth register to have his name included, provided that the mother gives her consent. If she disputes his claim to paternity, and an adoption is pending, the children's court can make a declaratory order confirming his paternity, presumably on the basis of tissue tests. The court may in terms of section 19 of the *Child Care Act* dispense with the consent of either or both parents to adoption where this is regarded as being in the best interests of the child, if any of a number of grounds exists. These include abandonment or abuse of the child, and the 'unreasonable' withholding of consent.

### State facilities, shelters, children's homes, and other residential facilities for children

The *Child Care Act* empowers the Minister of Welfare to establish and maintain 'places of safety and detention' for the temporary care of children who are awaiting decisions by the children's court or the criminal court. A recent amendment also enables the minister to set up and operate 'secure care facilities' for 'the reception and secure care of children awaiting trial and sentence'. The minister may also operate children's homes; however, these are in practice normally established and run by NGOs.

Any non-governmental facility for the 'reception, care and protection or bringing up' of more than six children away from their families must be registered with the Department of Welfare as a children's home in terms of section 30(1) of the *Child Care Act*. Likewise, a 'shelter' for the 'reception, care, protection and temporary care of more than six children in especially difficult circumstances' must be registered in terms of a recently added clause. Registered children's homes and shelters are required to adhere to a range of standards and requirements prescribed in the regulations under the *Child Care Act*. All such facilities and, in terms of another recent amendment, all state places of safety are subject to inspection in terms of section 31. Inspections can be carried out by 'a social worker, nurse or any other person authorized thereto by the Director General (of the Department of Welfare), or any commissioner ...' who can scrutinize any aspect of the operation of the facility, observe or interview children, and order medical, psychiatric, or psychological examinations. Based on the report of the inspector, the Director General may order various forms of remedial action, or may close down the facility.

## Criminal justice measures to address child abuse and neglect

Section 50 of the *Child Care Act* makes ill-treatment (or the permitting of ill-treatment) or abandonment of a child by his or her parent or guardian a punishable offence. A new section 50A states that not only any person who is involved in the commercial sexual exploitation of a child, but also anyone who owns, manages, or occupies a property where such exploitation takes place and fails to report it, is guilty of an offence. Commercial sexual exploitation as defined in the amended Act means 'the procurement of a child to perform a sexual act for a financial or other reward payable to the child, the parents or guardian of the child ... or any other person'.

Many offences committed against children are common-law crimes. These include homicide, assault, and various sexual offences. The current definition of rape, which extends only to the penetration of a vagina by a penis, is widely considered to be very inadequate and is set to change in a new Act, which is being drafted to replace the *Sexual Offences Act* no. 23 of 1957 as amended. It appears that rape will be redefined to include any form of coerced sexual penetration of either a male or a female, with coercion being considered to be automatically present in the case of penetra-

tion of a child by an older person. In the meanwhile, most sexual offences against children that come before the criminal courts are generally dealt with in terms of the following categories: rape – which includes sexual intercourse, whether coerced or not, with a girl under twelve years; statutory rape – which includes intercourse with a girl who is older than twelve years but still below the age of consent, i.e., sixteen years; and indecent assault.

The *Film and Publications Act* no. 65 of 1996, as amended, prohibits the exposure of children to pornography, and their involvement in its development.

Section 153A of the amended *Criminal Procedures Act* enables the court to put various protective mechanisms in place for a child who is required to give evidence in the criminal trial of an alleged perpetrator of abuse. These include the appointment of an intermediary who can receive questions from defence lawyers and interpret them to the child, thus reducing the trauma caused by hostile cross-examination, and provision for the child to give evidence in a separate room with an audio-visual link-up with the main courtroom. Children, and also older persons with disabilities, may use non-verbal means of communicating in court, such as gestures and demonstrations with dolls. While these measures are significant improvements, their use depends on the court's discretion, and they are in any case not accessible to a great many of the children who need them. The court process remains a traumatic one, calling for intensive support of the child and those close to him or her by all concerned, including the health care workers who become involved.

## Medical examinations of abused and neglected children

Medical assessments of children play a key role in the operation of the justice system as it affects children. In terms of section 14 of the

*Child Care Act*, the children's court may order a medical officer or psychologist to examine the child and produce a report. A medical report as per form 9 is required before a child can be admitted to a children's home or school of industries, and also for the purpose of estimating the child's age where this is not known. The completion of the J88 form required in criminal proceedings in cases of physical assault and sexual abuse, and the associated forensic procedures, are critical to the successful prosecution of these cases. Skilled and sensitive management of medico-legal procedures is vital to the reduction of secondary trauma to abused children. Non-medical members of the child protection team frequently need to have medical findings clearly explained to them so that they can more effectively use these in counselling and planning for the child and family. All provinces now have intersectoral child protection committees, supported by the Department of Health along with other government departments with core child protection responsibilities These committees have co-ordinated the development of provincial protocols to guide all members of the multidisciplinary team dealing with cases of abuse and neglect – i.e., health care workers, social workers, SAPS officers, justice personnel, and community members – and to promote co-ordination between them so as to ensure effective protection and support for abused child and constructive engagement of their families and communities. In some areas, protocols have also been developed at the regional and local levels. Linkages with these processes can be established via the Department of Welfare or local child welfare organizations.

## Refugee and 'undocumented immigrant' children

In terms of various international treaties and conventions to which South Africa is a party,

there is an undertaking by the government to refrain from sending refugees back to situations where they have a well-founded fear of persecution, or where public order is seriously threatened. Child refugees must be afforded special protection. In terms of the *Refugees Act* no. 130 of 1998, a child who is in need of care, including an unaccompanied minor, must be dealt with by the children's court in terms of the provisions of the *Child Care Act*. The court may order that he or she receive special assistance in applying for asylum. A child may be granted refugee status as a dependant of a parent or guardian who is given such status, or may apply in his or her own right. If a removal order is issued with regard to the parents, the child's removal may also be ordered, but only after he or she has been given an opportunity to apply for asylum. In practice, refugee children and, in particular, children who do not have the status of refugees or asylum seekers – for example 'economic refugees' from neighbouring states – are in a very ambiguous position. There is harassment from some officials, and reluctance on the part of some authorities to provide services to non-citizens. It can be argued that, because in the case of children the right to health care and social services is set out in the constitution without reference to nationality, any regulations or policies that exclude immigrant children from health care or social service provision are unconstitutional. Successful implementation of the constitution may require lobbying by service providers and other concerned groups.

## Children with disabilities

This is another particularly vulnerable group of children who have problems in accessing basic services. The constitution prohibits discrimination on the grounds of disability, and entitles children thus affected to basic education and to the various forms of provision due to all. However, most basic services are not planned with disability in mind, and this has the effect of excluding children with disabilities from, for example, appropriate education, recreational and social services, and protective processes. There is thus a need for ongoing advocacy to ensure that proper provision for children with disabilities is built into all basic services, so that the constitutional rights of these children may be translated into reality.

The justice system holds particular difficulties. Children with disabilities tend to be more vulnerable to abuse and neglect. At the same time, they face special obstacles both in the children's court and in the criminal justice system because of problems of accessibility, a lack of personnel who are equipped to assist them, and procedures that do not

take them into account. They may be unjustifiably 'written off' as incompetent to give evidence, leading to the collapse of criminal cases and abusers being left to continue unhindered. Deaf children will normally not be able either to serve as witnesses in court or to understand protection proceedings without the help of sign language interpreters. Support from health and social service workers and legal units is needed to assist such children and their families to negotiate the system, and to lobby for the development of the necessary infrastructure.

## Conclusion

This overview, although far from conclusive, provides a broad idea of the current position of South African children in relation to the

### Possible developments in new legislation

There have been widespread calls in the course of the consultations by the SA Law Commission's Project Committee on the Review of the Child Care Act for a major overhaul of the present legal dispensation for children. While it is not possible to pre-empt the findings of the committee or the decisions of the legislature in this regard, the following are some of the shifts that are likely to be considered:

- a change of emphasis from 'rights' and 'powers' of parents to the idea of a range of parental responsibilities;
- the development of a child-friendly court system that brings together a range of functions affecting children, instead of the current approach in which a single child may be dealt with separately by, for example, the criminal court, the divorce

court, the children's court, the maintenance court, and the magistrate dealing with domestic violence;
- a move towards ongoing involvement of the courts in reviews and decision making concerning children in statutory care, in place of the present system in which all authority is handed over to welfare and education officials after finalization of a children's court inquiry;
- greater attention to cross-border issues, for example, international adoption, trafficking in children, and child immigrants, 'legal' and otherwise;
- increased provision for the exercise of the child's right to participate in decisions concerning him or her; and
- a new emphasis on measures that focus on upholding the constitutional rights of marginalized children, and those in especially difficult circumstances including severe poverty.

law. This is a dynamic and rapidly evolving field, in which all practitioners dealing with children have new opportunities to help shape the emerging dispensation.

## References and further reading

SCHREIER AR & URBAN M. 1995. Legislation affecting children in South Africa. In: MA Kibel & LA Wagstaff. *Child health for all,* 2nd ed. Cape Town: Oxford University Press.

SKELTON A (ed.). 1998, 1999: *Children and the Law* and supplements. Pietermaritzburg, Lawyers for Human Rights.

SA LAW COMMISSION PROJECT 110 – Review of the Child Care Act: Issue Paper and drafts, 1998.

# 63 Care dependency grants

## J HOLLINGSHEAD

With the implementation of the *Social Assistance Act* (no. 59 of 1992) in South Africa in 1996, single care grants were replaced by care dependency grants. The regulations state that a child between the ages of one and 18 years who requires and receives permanent home care due to his/her severe intellectual or physical disability can be regarded as care dependent. Single care grants were originally introduced when there was a severe shortage of accommodation in mental hospitals. The grants were a means of encouraging relatives to care for their children with severe intellectual disability in the community. This practice is in keeping with the concept of community-based rehabilitation and in the knowledge

## Qualifying requirements:

- the parent(s) and the care-dependent child must be South African citizens;
- the applicant and the care-dependent child must be resident in the Republic of South Africa;
- a medical report and functional assessment of the child must be completed by a medical officer who is employed by the State or province;
- the medical report will be evaluated by the Medical Pensions Officer to determine if the child complies with the medical requirements;
- the child must have accommodation, be properly fed and clothed, and receive the

- necessary care and stimulation services and medical and dental care;
- at the age of six, the children must be evaluated as to their educability and trainability for attendance at a school for specialized education;
- only the biological parent(s) or foster parents (legal placement) can apply for a care dependency grant;
- the care-dependent child(ren) shall not be permanently cared for in state institutions; and
- the child(ren) must receive the necessary medical or other treatment, but medical treatment can be refused if it is life threatening.

that many such children are capable of some developmental progress with specialized training. Despite this trend, it must be emphasized that in some instances residential care is essential.

## Means test

A parent is eligible for a care dependency grant if his/her income is less than R48 000 per annum after permissible deductions. This is unlike other grants where there is a sliding scale, depending on income. In the case of a foster parent of a care-dependent child, income is *not* taken into consideration.

Documents required on application include:
- bar-coded identity documents of parent(s);
- an identity document or birth certificate bearing the 13-digit identity number of the child(ren);
- proof of marital status (divorce order, marriage certificate, or death certificate);
- proof of income of the family;
- proof of contribution of other parent; and
- a medical report from a medical officer in respect of the care-dependent child.

The social services branch of the provincial administration then considers funding for the grant.

## Points of debate

Numerous voices have been raised in opposition to many aspects of care dependency grants. Non-governmental organizations at provincial and national level have made representations.

### ELIGIBILITY CRITERIA

This remains a fundamental problem. There is a lobby that all children with disabilities and chronic illnesses should be eligible, as all such families incur extra expenses for visits to health centres, special clothing, assistive devices, and experience loss of income by not being able to work in order to care for such children. Different provinces interpret the regulations differently. There is little consistency at local offices. A working group from the child health policy unit and Western Cape Province Social Services Department is collaborating to rewrite essential criteria.

## ADMINISTRATION

The end of the tricameral system and the removal of these grants from the jurisdiction of magistrates' offices have meant that records and folders have had to be amalgamated at local social services offices. Families who had received single care grants have experienced long delays in transfer of payments because records cannot be found.

Social service offices are understaffed and personnel largely untrained. Lack of clarity about application for the grants has meant that many families are sent from these offices to health centres to social work agencies.

Social work agencies, already dealing with state subsidy cutbacks and diminished services, challenge the need for care-dependent children to be formally placed in foster care with relatives or reliable caregivers where there are no biological parents, before being able to apply for a grant. This is in direct contrast to the child support grant, which can be applied for by caregivers regardless of relationship.

As with other social pensions and grants, payments can be made via a cash point, bank, or post office. Computer system, personnel, and administrative problems have meant that families have experienced payment delays often with serious implications.

The points of debate listed above are by no means exhaustive. The purpose of this chapter is to indicate that welfare legislation does indeed provide social assistance for children with disabilities. Prospective applicants and their relevant health or welfare agencies are, however, cautioned about the many inconsistencies and frustrations in the process.

# PART SIXTEEN

# Communication

'Why then,' asked the Sirian, 'do you quote this Aristotle in Greek?' 'It is,' the learned man replied, 'because it is wiser to quote that which one does not understand at all, in the language that one comprehends least.' Voltaire's eighteenth-century mockery is as pertinent today as it was then. Too often, we resort to scientific jargon as a substitute for true communication with patients, parents, and fellow health workers. Communciation between people widely disparate in culture, level of education, or life experience presents particular difficulties. These and other aspects are addressed in the following part.

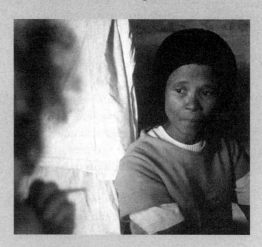

# 64

# Illness from children's and parents' perspectives

## A SCHREIER

Any accident or illness in their child, however minor in the eyes of the health worker, is perceived by parents as a crisis – an event that upsets their everyday pattern of living and generates anxiety. Typical medical definitions of crisis include 'a turning point of disease' and a 'sudden change in the course of an acute illness'. Significantly both these definitions are disease orientated and do not allow for the severe emotional distress that surrounds acute illness or accident. It is apparent that doctors' and parents' perceptions of these events differ.

In an emergency, the parents' main concern is to get the child to a doctor or hospital. Once there, it is assumed or expected that the 'experts' will take responsibility and that the child will recover. Depending on the situation, parents may hope that the doctors will prevent permanent damage or death, yet may fear the worst. Parents are frequently unable to think beyond the immediate emergency situation. Doctors, however, knowing the long-term sequelae of an accident or illness, may view the child's condition in a different light. They may regard it as less serious than do the parents. Alternatively, they may see this as the acute phase of a condition, which may have long-term sequelae and is potentially

chronic. Medical textbooks describe the acute and chronic phases of an injury or illness in objective and coldly scientific terms. The reality for parents is that such an accident or illness is an intensely upsetting event. Even the first episode of a chronic illness (e.g., the first asthmatic attack) is a major crisis. The doctor, confident in his ability to handle the attack and knowing that it is likely to be the precursor of many, may view this as a chronic illness from the outset.

For parents such a realization may take many months, and initially each attack will be a crisis, until they become used to coping with it and know how to prevent the onset. Not only are there differences in the perspectives of the doctors and parents, but children themselves view their illness and hospitalization in a different light. Their perceptions of what is happening to them and the reasons for their condition may be unknown even to the parents. Doctors may regard such relatively common conditions as a broken limb or upper respiratory tract infection as part of their everyday work, not as a crisis. There is a tendency to classify a medical condition in terms of its 'seriousness' and the degree of life threat, and not in terms of its impact on the patient.

# Acute illness

When children become acutely ill or are injured and have to be taken to emergency or casualty departments, both parents and children find the experience extremely stressful. This may be accentuated by any necessary procedures, for example, venepuncture and other investigations and therapeutic interventions such as intravenous cannulation, reduction of fractures, or suture of lacerations.

Unlike the chronically ill, these children have little previous experience with painful procedures. Many parents prefer to be present when blood is taken or intravenous therapy set up but doctors frequently ask them to leave. There is documented evidence of this parental preference and also the presence of a parent supports the child emotionally and facilitates coping with the pain and stress.

Teaching parents how to help their children, by instructing them to sit or stand near the head of the bed, to talk to, touch, or distract the child during the procedure also reduces their own anxiety, and increases their satisfaction with the care received. These behavioural and cognitive approaches may also need to be combined with pharmacological treatment.

Acute illness is defined as symptoms that are severe enough to limit activity or to require a doctor's attention. Acute illness is usually transient and, in contrast to chronic illness, does not usually have any long-term sequelae for the child in terms of interference with normal growth and development.

The incidence of acute illness varies from a lesser frequency in the first six months of life, increasing thereafter until it reaches a peak at three or four years of age. It then decreases with increasing age, although a small peak occurs during the first or second year at school.

The severity, incidence, and types of illness are significantly influenced by socio-economic and environmental factors. While upper respiratory infections are common to all children, malnutrition and some potentially preventable infections are particular afflictions of disadvantaged communities.

The number of non-life-threatening illnesses reported often reflects the ease of access to health care rather than the true morbidity profile. Working mothers may experience difficulty in taking time off and alternative child-minders may not be suitable escorts for sick children.

Acute illness takes up a considerable amount of general practitioners' time and accounts for more than half the patient volume of paediatricians in the United States.

## THE DECISION TO SEEK MEDICAL CARE

The decision to contact the doctor or attend an outpatient clinic appears to be related not only to the child's symptoms but also to how stressed the mother is at the time. It has been noted that mothers frequently attend outpatient clinics or visit the doctor when they are under stress, and use the child's symptoms as a 'cry for help' for other difficulties, for example, marital discord, loneliness, or isolation. In an epidemiological study of illnesses in children, it was found that the probability of telephone calls and visits to emergency and outpatient departments – medical contacts with relatively easy access – is doubled if stress is present. The time when parents actually seek help may be the point at which they can no longer cope. Thus, when they come to the doctor the child may already have improved.

Children of doctors may be at a disadvantage when they become acutely ill. There often seem to be inappropriate delays by doctors as parents in seeking care; problems in communication because of role confusion, (i.e., moving from being the healer to the role of help seeker); and reluctance to address personal, psychological, and behavioural issues. Paediatricians may be hesitant to pursue and uncover the hidden agenda with medical practitioner families, and are less likely to provide early intervention for psychosocial problems. Moreover, there is likely to be decreased continuity of care because of self-referral to specialists.

Although doctors treat their own children, many omit performing physical examinations and laboratory tests, and consequently do not have the data to assist in making an objective treatment plan for their child.

## EFFECT OF THE CHILD'S ILLNESS ON THE FAMILY AND CHILD

The illness, even if of short duration, causes disruption in the daily routine and relationships within the family. Family tension may be created or exacerbated if the father blames the mother for the child's illness. Mothers often see their main task as keeping their children well, and therefore feel that they are at fault if the child becomes ill. It is apparent that a single mother may have a more difficult time because of her lack of support.

For families from the lowest socio-economic strata, illness in a child may be especially disruptive. Difficulties are compounded if working parents have to commute long distances, are away at work for extended hours, and have inadequate help at home for child care and preparation of regular meals.

Overcrowding not only increases the spread of infections, but also may make 'bed' rest an unattainable ideal. Adherence with treatment as well as attendance for follow-up are obviously jeopardized in such circumstances. Once the child seems better there is little incentive to complete a full course of treatment, thus risking relapse or chronic illness. Minor illness can provoke behavioural reactions of anxiety and insecurity in young children, which could have serious emotional repercussions in already insecure or deprived children.

Illness in children often occurs after some crisis or unusual pressure, such as the death of a grandparent, change in residence, near drowning, loss of father's job, or failure at school. Having to adjust to these major environmental changes affects the child emotionally and physically, and this may lower resistance to infection. There is evidence that, although children who come from a home characterized by poverty, overcrowding, and inadequate nutrition are likely to be more prone to illness, poverty-associated factors alone are not the chief causative factors. Children from families disorganized by such factors as alcoholism or maternal inadequacy are more likely to suffer from kwashiorkor, multiple illnesses, recurrent diarrhoea, and infections.

Conversely, even in poor circumstances, parents who are stable role models act as a bulwark against the stresses of the environment. In the absence of good parenting, stress in the family will be magnified, leading to disease and antisocial behaviour.

It can be seen that acute illness, which has mainly physical manifestations and may be of short duration, may have important associated psychosocial factors in its causation and sequelae.

# Chronic and life-threatening illnesses

Chronic illness may be defined as any illness that persists for more than three months. It may be protracted but stable, or progressive and life threatening, or a non-fatal disabling condition.

Parents' reactions to the news of chronic or life-threatening illness are similar. Illnesses such as cystic fibrosis and leukaemia, where children may live for a number of years and then die, may be termed 'chronic and life threatening'. To the young child, admission to hospital for a period longer than ten days will be perceived as a chronic illness, because even a few days appears to be an eternity. Repeated admissions to hospital, even of short duration, will be perceived by the child as an illness that is not getting better. Young children experience high levels of distress when undergoing various procedures. The magnitude of what it means to be told that one's child 'has an illness from which he may die' can be gauged by the fact that the life event judged to be the most severe crisis is the death of a spouse or near relative.

Where childhood mortality rates are low, the death of a child is a rare event. However, even when mortality rates are high, the loss of a child has an enormous impact. Cultural factors, family size, the material investment in the child, or expectations of a future economic asset may have added impact. Where there is only a nuclear family, parents tend to rely to an increasing extent on the medical staff for information and support. This places a greater responsibility on doctors, not only to deal with the physical but also the emotional aspects of caring for the terminally or chronically ill child.

## EFFECTS OF CHRONIC OR TERMINAL ILLNESS

The diagnosis of any life-threatening illness brings with it one of the most deep-seated anxieties, namely separation from a loved one. As with acute minor illness, feelings of inadequacy and failure are aroused and these are far greater when the illness is serious. Breaking bad news is an essential and inescapable task of the doctor. The doctor needs full knowledge of the condition, self-confidence, and sensitivity to handle the interview, which should take place in privacy with both parents present if possible. The help of an interpreter should be requested if the doctor is not conversant with the home lan-

guage of the parents. Not all parents are ready to hear the full truth immediately and due allowance and provision must be made for this. Space and time for parental questioning are of the utmost importance. A follow-up interview and referral to a social worker and/or psychologist may be indicated. The initial reactions of parents to the diagnosis of severe or life-threatening illness have been well documented, and therefore the stages of shock, denial, disbelief, anger, searching for information and cure, and anticipatory mourning will not be dealt with here.

The reactions of the older child with a chronic disabling condition tend to follow three major sequences and characteristics of development. Firstly, there is the realization that 'the disability is not suddenly going to disappear'. This is usually precipitated by separation from peer group members and exposure to other similarly disabled children. This is then followed by a severe depression, which may last from six weeks to an entire year. During this period, the child may speak of the futility of life, refuse to do school work, and may not wish to continue living. The third and final stage is characterized by the gradual development of emotional readiness to accept the physical disability (or chronic illness) as part of the self, and to start tentatively to incorporate it into his or her self image and lifestyle. It is understandable that parents in their own state of turmoil find it extremely difficult to cope with the child's feelings.

The parents' dilemma of simultaneously continuing to care for the child while having to cope with the devastating news imposes tremendous strain on them, their relationship with each other, and with the sick child. They therefore need emotional support, understanding, and reassurance from the medical and nursing staff, who may also find it a stressful situation. The child also needs support, counselling, and explanations from the doctor.

Chronic illness must never be seen in isolation. The meaning of the illness to the family members and its effect on them always has to be considered. Frequent relapses and remissions, sheer fatigue, curtailment of social activities, inability to leave the child or go on holiday, pain, anguish, and isolation, as well as the child's feelings of embarrassment (such as with hair loss due to chemotherapy), are all added stresses.

Siblings, especially those closest in age to the patient, may be neglected or alternatively have to overcompensate for the 'failure' in the family, or have to bear the impact of the guilt and parental disappointment. They may have irrational fears of developing the same condition, which may be attributed to not being informed as well as children's sensitivity to non-verbal communication.

The sick child may experience school difficulties and be teased by peers.

Parents of children and adolescents with chronic illnesses, especially those with likely emergencies, poor prognoses, and visible signs, strongly believe that schoolteachers need medical information about such children and that the doctor is the person to supply this information. Friends and peer groups as well as siblings should also be assisted with appropriate understanding to facilitate desirable interactions.

Chronic illness in a family renders them very vulnerable to any acute stress. This can be precipitated by events such as additional financial expenses, sudden hospitalization, or the death of a familiar child who attends the outpatient clinic. Superimposed on this long-term 'low-level' crisis situation and the accompanying constant strain on the child and family is the medical treatment itself. The child and family may be dependent on the medical services provided by specialist clinics at hospital and use these for their primary care too. They may also use the services of allied health professionals and their general practitioners. Frequently, there may be little co-ordination of these services and no clear pattern as to whose responsibility it is to provide the counselling, co-ordinating, and supportive aspects of care.

Frequent communication between the health team members throughout the child's illness will ensure that a valuable support system is provided for the family. Knowing that they may depend on the medical staff for both 'curative' and palliative care, which includes emotional and psychosocial support, will do much to alleviate anxiety.

It is apparent that acute illness in a child is a stressful event. The diagnosis of a chronic or life-threatening condition is a crisis of much greater magnitude, which may persist over months or years.

## References and further reading

ANDREWS SG. 1991. Informing schools about children's chronic illnesses: Parents' opinions. *Pediatrics.* 88(2):306–11.

BAUCHNER H, VINCI R, and PEARSON C. 1993. Parental presence during procedures: Satisfaction with care. *American Journal of Diseases in Children.* 147:426–7.

BAUCHNER H, VINCI R, and MAY A. 1994. Teaching parents how to comfort their children during common medical procedures. *Archives of Disease in Childhood.* 70: 548–50.

DUSDIEKER LB, MURPH JR, MURPH WE, and DUNGY CI. 1993. Physicians treating their own children. *American Journal of Diseases in Children.* 147:146–9.

MICHELS V. 1989. The physically handicapped child: The parents' child's perspective. *Paediatric Social Work.* 3(2):25–8.

WASSERMAN RC, HASSUK BM, YOUNG PC, and LAND ML. 1989. Health care of physicians' children. *Pediatrics.* 83(3):319–22.

# 65

# Communication guidelines for health workers

F DE VILLIERS &
LA WAGSTAFF

Communication involves the exchange of thoughts, messages, or the like, by speech, signals, or writing, and is thus crucial to health workers. Communication may take the form of scientific publications, formal lectures, and interactions with colleagues, patients and their families, or the broader community. This chapter deals with communicating with individual patients and their caregivers in a health care setting, and communicating with groups for the purpose of health education.

Because communication is a two-way process, health workers need to be proficient not only in *conveying* 'messages' but also in *receiving* them. Too often one hears that the 'doctor' did not listen/hear or did not tell or explain what the health 'problem' was. The fault may lie with the 'sender', the clarity or content of the 'message', or with the 'recipient'.

Health workers are taught the technical aspects of their craft and learn these well. They may be justifiably proud of their clinical skills, diagnostic reasoning, and therapeutic ability, which are undoubtedly of immense importance. However, technical proficiency is not enough to satisfy most patients. They are more impressed by a doctor who communicates with them and appears to have a caring attitude. Doctors who are inadequate communicators have been sued by their patients, and suffer severe psychological and monetary consequences, even when they are eventually professionally vindicated. Good communication skills not only result in patient satisfaction, but also determine adherence to advice and treatment and therefore the quality of care the patient receives. Health workers also need to be *health educators*, and for this and other purposes should have an understanding of issues in *adult education*.

Communication may be verbal or non-verbal. Speech is the verbal medium used by the patient or parent to inform the doctor or other health worker about his or her symptoms and concerns, and by which the health worker responds. Non-verbal communication includes other aspects of behaviour observed by either of the two parties taking part in the communicational transaction. This may include facial expressions, dress, posture, manner (e.g., hurried or pre-occupied), or absence of eye contact it, and sounds indicating attention by either of the two parties.

In paediatric practice, the child usually presents as part of a mother (or mother-substitute)–child dyad. The paediatric consultation requires that attention be given to both members of the dyad, and for the purposes of this discussion they will be referred to as 'the patient'.

# The consultation

During the consultation, the doctor is able to identify and define the nature of the problem and to obtain some understanding of the patient as a person.

The traditional view of the consultation depends on the sections that medical textbooks use to describe illnesses (see Table 65.1). This division is useful for the purpose of the textbook, which describes maladies, but is not very useful during a live consultation.

The practical model of consultation (see Table 65.2) describes what should happen during a consultation (de Villiers, 1982).

## CONDUCTING THE CONSULTATION

Extrinsic factors may contribute to the success or failure of the consultation. Privacy is desirable, while noise and constant interruptions by others or the telephone are obviously disruptive. Pictures and furnishings can help to 'warm' the interview. Toys and books for children should be available in the waiting room and during the consultation. Patients of all ages may need reassurance and all have the right to be treated with dignity. Health workers should introduce themselves. It is important to greet the parent and child with some verbal or non-verbal contact appropriate to age, language, or cultural group. Siblings, if present, should also be similarly recognized.

Seating should preferably be such that the desk is not between the health worker and the patient. Enough chairs should be available for all present, but younger children and infants may prefer to sit on the mothers' laps.

**Table 65.1** Traditional model of the consultation

- History
- Physical examination (including side-room tests)
- Special investigations (laboratory)
- Differential diagnosis
- Diagnosis
- Treatment
- Prognosis

**Table 65.2** Practical model of the consultation

- Statement of the problem by the patient
- Knowledge from previous consultation(s)
- Working hypothesis
- Limited, directed history-taking*
- Physical examination (including side-room tests)
- Selected special investigations
- Working diagnosis
- Management:
  - Reassurance
  - Discuss illness and its causes
  - Discuss related matters (e.g., nutrition, contraception)
  - Discuss special investigations/procedures
  - Treatment (non-drug and medications)
  - How to take the medications
  - Discuss prognosis
  - Discuss next appointment

*Inexperienced examiners may still need to complete a comprehensive history

## HISTORY TAKING

The initial phase comprises a statement of the problem(s) or the statement of the main complaints and the subsidiary complaints, ascertained by open-ended, general questions. Whenever possible, doctors should communicate directly with children in order to obtain information, and they should also be included in the feedback process. These needs were highlighted in a study in which children were found to contribute only four per cent of communication interactions at outpatient visits (van Dulmen, 1998).

A listening posture should be maintained and the parent or patient encouraged and allowed to tell the story. Open-ended general questions such as: 'What brings you here today?' or 'Lerato, how have you been since you were here last?' are used to begin the interview. The child may not give a logical, factual, chronological account (for that matter neither may the accompanying adult) but whatever is said will enable the doctor to understand some of the patient's concerns, and will serve as a start to the interview.

Use open-ended questions most of the time. This helps to obtain accurate, complete information by allowing the parent to respond in detail without being directed to give only specific answers. Children and adolescents may need to be prompted.

Ask brief, simple questions, using the person's own terminology. Do not use negatively phrased questions such as: 'He is not complaining of pain, is he?' or 'You aren't coughing?' The meaning of a 'yes' or 'no' answers to these questions is unclear and such questions suggest to the patient that (s)he should not have those symptoms.

Closed questions such as: 'Has she been taking her feeds well?' limit the probable response to yes or no. An alternative might be: 'How has she been taking her feeds?' Closed questions are however sometimes necessary.

During the elucidation of the main complaint, direct questions are required. These questions should, however, still be open ended. Proceed to direct questions if the response to open-ended questions needs to be clarified. For example, an initial question might be 'Tell me about the cough.' If further information is required, you might say: 'Does anything come up when you cough?'

During the rest of the history taking, (e.g., previous medical and surgical history, family history, history of feeding, immunization, and development), direct questions are also required and closed questions may sometimes be useful. Negatively phrased questions should always be avoided.

Transition statements should be used when seeking additional information, to avoid misunderstandings about the relevance, for example: 'I am just going to ask you some routine questions.' This will help to allay anxiety.

Follow up on cues the parent gives you. This may be done by your body posture (e.g., leaning forward), facial expressions, or nods. Repeating a key phrase indicates that you would like to hear more or you could simply say: 'Tell me more about that.'

Give restricting cues for irrelevant material. This can be done tactfully by saying something like: 'That's fine, let's move on to ...' Remember that even if it seems irrelevant, the parent has some reason for raising the topic.

## ACTIVE LISTENING

This implies that you have heard what was said as evidenced by a response such as the repetition of a few words as an invitation to continue. It facilitates being able to steer the communication without breaking continuity.

When a parent has completed part or all of the history, a brief clarifying summary by the doctor is appropriate. This assures both that the intended message has been conveyed and received.

It is important to find out what the parent is worried about. Understanding this may lead to better communication. There may be a hidden agenda. The child may be used as a possible means to obtain help for some other problem such as domestic difficulty or family abuse. This may be recognized by subtle cues when a parent is reluctant to broach the subject but nevertheless hopes for some helpful intervention.

Silences often give parents an opportunity to tell their story. It is not necessary to break a silence immediately. Doctors tend to feel uncomfortable during a silence, and need to fill the space with another question or statement.

Reasons for obtaining a poor history are seldom that the doctor asked the wrong questions, or that the patient is a 'poor historian'. The most common reason is that the doctor did not listen carefully enough to all the responses, therefore did not understand correctly, and so could not follow up accurately on the cues that were given.

If a parent breaks down and weeps during the interview, allow time for composure to be regained before continuing.

## THE PHYSICAL EXAMINATION

Examination of the child may be either on the parent's lap or on the examination couch, depending on the age and stage of development of the child. Children with stranger-anxiety will respond poorly to removal from the parent. When sitting opposite the parent with your knees touching the parent's, the combined flat surface should be adequate for examination of an infant. The parent will have his or her hands free to hold the child's head steady when necessary.

Explain to the parent and child what you are doing, for example: 'I am going to examine the tummy now.' After doing so, explain what you have found. Demonstrating the procedure (e.g., otoscopy) on yourself or on the mother may allay fear in the younger child. It also helps to familiarize the child with the instruments to be used by allowing him/her to touch them, or to listen with the stethoscope.

## MANAGEMENT

Treatment with medication is only one of the eight steps included under this heading (see Table 65.2). The other seven are all forms of health education and some, or even all, may be necessary.

If such a balance were maintained, the practice of patients expecting, or doctors providing, a medicine for every symptom would be avoided.

## ADVICE AND COUNSELLING DURING THE CONSULTATION

A few simple techniques may make the transfer of information more effective.

The more information imparted to a person at one time, the more (s)he will forget. Health workers frequently ignore this elementary fact and overload the patient with too much information. On the other hand, parents are sometimes dissatisfied with the quality and amount of information provided.

Statements that are repeated, will be remembered more easily. This repetition may occur at one consultation or at consecutive consultations.

Doctors often concentrate on the diagnosis while the patient's main concern is the relief of symptoms. Whatever is communicated first and last will be remembered more easily than what is discussed in the middle despite the relative importance. In most cases, patients do not have sufficient background knowledge to discriminate between important and less important information. Specific instructions will be remembered more clearly than generalizations, for example: 'Drink ten cups of water per day' rather than 'Drink more fluids.'

## THE USE OF TECHNICAL LANGUAGE (JARGON)

It is relatively easy to avoid obvious medical terms such as 'lymphadenopathy', 'hyperthermia', and 'acidosis'. But other words such as 'hypertension', 'femur', and 'thermometer', which are used fairly commonly by lay people, may not be known to all. The health worker should be alert enough to notice when the patient does not understand, and to rephrase the questions.

## REPETITION OF INFORMATION BY THE PATIENT

If patients are able to repeat what the health worker has told them, they will be more likely to remember it. The doctor can also establish whether the patient recalls the most important aspects of the consultation. If the patient misunderstood, the doctor can patiently repeat the correct information.

## WRITTEN INSTRUCTIONS

Written instructions and a patient-held information sheet are very useful in support of verbal information as they can be referred to after leaving the consulting room or clinic. If at all possible, these should be in the patient's home language. When a large amount of information is to be transferred, hand-written instructions are not practical and printed material is desirable. Books and leaflets should be used when obtainable and when the patient is able to use such resources. The South African Medical Association, the Department of Health, Soul City, and various pharmaceutical companies publish such materials at no cost.

If the same information is needed by different patients, a short photocopied pamphlet is useful, relatively cheap, and easy to produce. A further advantage is that the doctor or health worker has control over the contents. Written instructions given to parents must be readily understandable and easily readable.

The way in which the document is presented will determine if and how it is used. If the parent has to pick it up from a pile or if it is handed over without comment, it will usually be discarded unread. If, however, the health worker refers the patient to the document after explaining a particular point, it is much more likely that it will be used to reinforce what the health worker said. Referring to the document again at a subsequent visit will increase the chances that the patient will reread it.

## QUESTIONS FOR THE HEALTH WORKER

Patients frequently have questions they would like to ask the health worker, and they should be encouraged and enabled to do this either at this or a subsequent visit. Before concluding a consultation, always give the patient the opportunity to discuss any other related concerns.

## THE DOCTOR'S ATTITUDE

An autocratic attitude in a doctor may suit some patients, but this approach is unacceptable to many. Lack of time cannot excuse a poor doctor–patient relationship or poorly communicated information during the consultation. Not only is 'a pill for every ill' bad medicine, but it causes patient dependency on the doctor, so that they return frequently for more pills thus worsening the work load and time constraints. Currently there are charters setting out *patients' rights* and these are to be respected.

The patient should feel that the doctor is interested in him or her. The brusque or distant doctor or one who shows boredom or impatience will not be trusted. Such attitudes are most undesirable, and are especially reprehensible when the patient is a child. Dissatisfied patients may 'shop around' from doctor to doctor, thereby increasing costs, and possibly affecting the course of recovery.

## COMPLIANCE AND ADHERENCE

These concepts receive a great deal of attention in many fields of medicine today. The term 'compliance' may be inferred by some to imply a relationship where the patient is a passive follower of the doctor's orders, and where the instructions are largely concerned with drug therapy only. 'Adherence' is held to imply a more equal relationship between doctor and patient, where the patient is involved in decision making. In effect, these terms are synonymous.

Many patients do not adhere to the management plans drawn up for their illnesses. This is a particular problem with chronic diseases and in those requiring complicated drug schedules. When a child is the patient the matter becomes complicated even further. Well-meaning parents and caregivers may be more conscientious in administering therapy to children than to themselves. However, in practice it is frequently more difficult to give medicines and non-drug therapies to children than it is to adults.

The contribution of health education during the consultation to improve compliance should be taken seriously. In a classic study (Korsch et al., 1968), the most critical finding was the extent to which compliance was correlated with patient satisfaction. Mothers frequently feel responsible in some way for their children's illnesses. They want clear explanations of what is wrong with their child and reassurance about the children's future health.

## AWARENESS OF
## NON-VERBAL CUES

Throughout the consultation the doctor should try to understand the feelings of the parent and child through their non-verbal responses. It should be remembered that the parent/patient are also interpreting the doctor's body language. Body language and the spoken word are sometimes inconsistent. For example, a mother may state that she enjoys her baby, but there is little eye contact. The doctor should explore such inconsisten-

cies. When a parent seems to be disturbed but does not say what is wrong, an empathic statement such as: 'Mrs Mkhize, you seem upset about something. Would you like to talk about it?' will enable the parent to talk about her/his worries.

## INTERPRETERS

In a multi-cultural, multi-lingual country, reliance may have to be placed on an interpreter. A skilled interpreter is able to convey the correct message accurately in an understandable and acceptable manner, and does not merely translate words. The doctor should learn some of the common words in the dominant language of that area, so that the interpreter's statements can be understood at least to some extent. The doctor should try to ensure that the correct information has been transmitted both from doctor to patient and from patient to doctor. The doctor and the parent/patient should look at each other rather than at the interpreter; the aim being to have the interpreter intrude as little as possible in the interaction between them. Even though direct verbal communication is not established, the parent should be aware of the doctor's interest.

Ensuring that instructions and explanations regarding medication and treatment are understood is always important, but particular care is needed when a third party is involved. Asking patients to repeat what they understand is useful.

Cultural differences frequently lead to misunderstandings regarding the way feelings are expressed: passivity versus assertiveness; emphasis on different symptoms; expectations of the doctor and/or patient.

## COMMUNICATING
## WITH CHILDREN

The child may be justifiably terrified due to a previous experience with a health care worker who hurt him/her during a procedure, examination, or operation. Children are also traumatized if doctors and health services have been put in a negative light, and those responsible should be reprimanded and advised. Stranger-anxiety is normal and occurs at about 8 to 12 months of age and diminishes at about 15 months of age. If the child is not afraid, it should be easy to obtain his/her co-operation. If getting close to a young child, bend at the knees rather than bending over him or her (this is not relevant in the first year of life, before the child/infant can walk). Smile, greet, or touch the child. Infants and young children will hold a gaze much longer than adults (who consider it rude), and will therefore relate better to an adult if he/she does not look away quickly. Play age-appropriate games with children, and reassure them with gentle touching.

Children who are older than four years can understand everything that is told to them in simple language. It is not necessary to 'talk down' to them or to use 'baby talk'.

Children should be prepared with carefully worded explanations for any procedure. They should be informed how much it will hurt, and told how soon it will be over. Children should never be told not to cry. This is an immature and unworthy response on the part of health workers to protect themselves. It does nothing for the child but serves to reconfirm his/her powerlessness. If there is any way in which the child can be given a choice, for example, which arm should be used for the blood sample, this should be done. A simple offer of a choice returns power (or at least the appearance of power) to the child. Health personnel are often astonished at the maturity children show once given such a choice.

Suitable pain relief should be made available. This may include a mild analgesic (e.g., paracetamol), sedation, local anaesthetic (e.g., EMLA cream), or general anaesthetic. Adequate time should be allowed for these to take effect.

An excellent way to minimize psychological damage due to procedures is to be technically proficient at them. The patient should be properly immobilized for the procedure, and it should be executed quickly and well.

Health services for adolescents and the adolescent interview are discussed in Chapter 18: Health care services for adolescents.

# Health education

Health education is an attempt to modify the views of health or disease held by others. It is hoped that not only views but also behaviours will be modified by health education. Health education may involve individuals or groups and may be formal or informal, structured or unstructured. Much can be learnt from exposure to good role models.

If health education is to be monitored and evaluated, there need to be clear objectives. These may apply to the process (the performance of the educator) or the outcomes (did the learner acquire the intended information and consequently modify related behaviour?). In practice, it is often difficult to apply the necessary measures.

## HEALTH EDUCATORS

The educator should be well informed on the topic and should be genuinely interested in the subject and in those to whom messages are to be communicated.

Audiences judge the credibility of communicators on their perceived trustworthiness and knowledge. A third factor, which often increases during the communication and impacts on audiences, is the goodwill, enthusiasm, and dynamism evidenced.

If health educators have poor reputations, based on the audience's perception of the speaker's abilities, they will have to counteract it before the communication will be effective. If the health educator's socio-economic status is higher than that of the audience, this will generally enhance his/her credibility; if lower, (s)he may encounter obstacles in delivering the communication or may suffer reduced credibility.

The idiom 'good teachers are born, not made' is seldom true and is no excuse for health educators to avoid hard work. Teaching ability is a combination of personality, interest, and hard work. Anyone can improve his/her teaching techniques, and ability and technique are indistinguishable.

## HEALTH LEARNERS

'Congruence' in health education refers to the overlapping of attitudes, knowledge, or beliefs between the 'educator' and the 'learner'. For example, if you are trying to convince someone of the importance of late weaning, and the person has strong beliefs that giving gruel (very thin porridge) to the baby in the first month is beneficial, your message is not congruent with the person's beliefs. The effect of the principle of congruence requires that the health educator should adapt to the health learners and not the other way round. This is an extremely difficult lesson to learn for health workers, who are generally well trained, of higher socio-economic status than their audiences, and may tend to be rigid and authoritarian.

The health educator should know whether the audience consists of men or women, their age groups, their nationality, language and culture, their educational level and occupation, and their social, political, and religious affiliations. Not all of the demographic characteristics will necessarily affect a particular communication.

## COMPREHENSION

The health educator should know what level of difficulty and abstraction can be used in the communication. This will depend on the educational level, the age, prior knowledge of the topic, and the language proficiency of the audience.

Communication also depends on both the underlying and immediate needs of the individual.

## BELIEFS

There are many factors that determine the audience's acceptance of a communication, for example, attitudes, stereotypes, values, interests, motives, opinions, and emotions.

The health educator should concentrate firstly on the health learners' beliefs about the topic, and secondly on their beliefs and attitudes towards the health educator.

## COMMUNICATION PREFERENCES

Some people prefer to receive information visually, and others through auditory means. Furthermore, people have media preferences; some prefer television, others brochures etc.

## PLANNING HEALTH EDUCATION

Timing a health education communication correctly is important. An anxious mother waiting with her sick baby to see the doctor is not a receptive subject for a discussion on routine immunization.

A good time is when the health learner has a strong need for the message. The educator can improve the timing by considering the characteristics of the learner.

## TEMPO

This is the speed with which the communication is delivered. It varies from static to rapid. A static tempo is achieved by using posters, photographs etc. Here the audience may take as much time as they wish over the communication, or none at all. When delivering the health message, the speed can be made faster or slower, for example when speaking or showing a film. But if the delivery is too slow, the audience loses interest; if the delivery is too fast, comprehension is lost. Adjusting speed can be useful. A slower speed is better suited to a complicated point, and vice versa. The tempo chosen should depend on the age (slow for young children), prior knowledge of the topic, level of education, language proficiency, or media preference. Variation in tempo should be considered, especially if it will be a long session. A session should not exceed 15 minutes if the participants are children or if they are uneducated. In the case of educated adults, a session should not exceed 40 minutes.

## STRUCTURE

Health educators will have assembled various facts, opinions, illustrations, or pictures that they wish to communicate to the audience. Certain elements will help to hold the audiences' attention – humour, real-life accounts, and stories. It should be planned where these elements will be most effective.

In the presentation, the most important content may be placed at the beginning, in the middle, or at the end.

## MEDIA

These are used to convey messages, and selection is determined by circumstances. There are variable costs associated with the preparation and use of different media. There is a range from expensive films or television to simple 'home-made' material. In health education the dominant media are the spoken word, or audio-visual illustration. The vast range of available media is becoming increasingly diverse and sophisticated and health educators should be encouraged not to think too narrowly. Using a variety instead of a single format is usually more effective.

Vocal formats include speeches, dialogues, lectures, discussions, and 'health talks'. Article formats include letters, scientific articles, books, editorials, reviews, reports, manuals, memoranda, posters, handouts, and brochures. Story formats include short stories, novels, fables, and many more. Picture formats include picture-stories, advertisements, photo-articles, comics, and cartoons. Three-dimensional formats include models and exhibits as well as 'health demonstrations'. There are also musical and drama formats.

The traditional formats are the 'health talk', the 'health demonstration', posters, handouts, and brochures. New approaches and especially mixtures of presentations should be considered.

If a *spoken medium* is used, the health educator should know how to speak, when to pause, how to use gestures effectively etc. When using a *printed medium* the quality should be controlled, for example, legibility, quality of colour and photographs, and type of paper. If a *projection method* (e.g., film, slides) is chosen, the health educator should ensure that the equipment is reliable and in working order before the communication is delivered. The same applies to *sound media* like tape recorders and radios.

When the presentation is pre-prepared it cannot be changed, unlike verbal presentations. Here the speaker can judge from the audience's reaction whether they understand, are interested, or bored. The health educator should then be able to adjust parts or all of the communication.

## EVALUATION

This may be difficult to obtain but is nevertheless essential. Types of feedback include direct observation (e.g., facial expressions, gestures or remarks made by a person or members of the audience), questionnaires (to determine whether the objectives were realized), tests (e.g., pre- and post-delivery of the communication), changes in behaviour (e.g., fewer antibiotic prescriptions after a lecture), voluntary comments (e.g., after a lecture or sermon; letters to the editor, letters or telephone calls to the radio or TV), and expert evaluation (of both content and presentation).

The health educator, having received feedback, can now evaluate the effectiveness of the communication. This is easy, provided that the objectives have been stated in measurable terms. If the objectives are abstract, evaluation may be more difficult. Nevertheless, if evaluation proves difficult, the educator should consider whether the problem lies with the planning of the objectives, and should in future attempts improve on that aspect of planning.

## TEACHING AIDS AND FACILITIES

### Making teaching aids

Health education often suffers because there is little time and money to design effective campaigns. The health educator can make some teaching aids cheaply, and can learn to use the common ones more effectively. Look for ways to use real objects instead of writing about them or drawing them. Use teaching aids that call for doing things rather than just seeing. Aids that learners can handle are very effective.

### Chalk boards

Keep the audience in mind. Think about the level at which they can understand and read, whether they understand graphs and drawings. Use capital letters. Write only essentials. If you have your back turned to the audience most of the time, they will be bored and your message will have no impact. Complicated or

### Multiple media in action

Here is an outline of a programme that could be used in an informal village campaign:

- *posters* to advertise the subject, using a striking design;
- *songs* related to the subject to start the programme;
- *slides* to convey the main message;
- *demonstration with samples* and specimens to repeat the main message;
- *talk* by a local person to illustrate from his/her experience the value of the ideas presented;
- *discussions* to get the learners involved;
- *leaflets* to give information that is complicated, difficult to remember, or which will be needed long afterwards; and
- *visits to key people* to answer questions about the campaign.

time-consuming drawings, formulae, or writings should be put on the board before the lesson. Do not use the chalkboard if you cannot write legibly.

### Posters

Do not overcrowd. Rather use big, clear writing. If using posters for a presentation, show them one at a time. If they are all in view at the same time, the audience will be reading them and not listening to you.

### Transparencies for overhead projectors

Use note form. Write in big letters, preferably capitals, 1 cm tall. Leave enough space between lines. Do not put more than 10 lines of writing on one transparency. These points apply equally if you are using printed transparencies.

*The uncover technique*: cover the entire transparency with a sheet of paper and gradually uncover the relevant sections.

*The overlay technique*: transparencies can be laid one on top of the other to add more details or labels. Arrange the transparencies in the correct order you are going to use them. (An A4-size magazine is useful to keep them in.) Rehearse using them.

## Slides for slide projectors

Use note form. Use big letters, preferably capitals. Leave enough space between lines. Do not put more than five lines of writing on one slide. If you are using slides from a set, they are presumably of good quality. Illustrations, photographs, and graphs may also be shown on slides. In any event, all slides should be previewed for quality and legibility. Test the projector beforehand, using the slides you are planning to use during the presentation. Incorporate the slides into the presentation to form a seamless whole. The presentation should be rehearsed.

## References and further reading

DE VILLIERS F. 1982. Gesondheidsvoorligting tydens die konsultasie. *South African Medical Journal.* 62:45–7.

DICKSON DA, HARGIE O, and MORROW NC. 1989. *Communication skills training for health professionals.* London: Chapman Hall.

FINLAY F & LUNTS E. 1999. Improving communication between doctors and patients. *Archives of Disease in Childhood.* 80:398.

KAI J. 1996. What worries parents when their preschool children are acutely ill and why. *British Medical Journal.* 313:983–6.

KORSCH BM, GOZZI EK, and FRANCIS V. 1968. Gaps in doctor–patient communications: doctor–patient interaction and satisfaction. *Pediatrics.* 42:855.

KORSCH BM, FREEMAN B, and NEGRETE VF. 1971. Practical implications of doctor–patient interaction: Analysis for pediatric practice. *American Journal of Disease in Childhood.* 121:110–14.

MERYN S. 1998. Improving doctor–patient communication. *British Medical Journal.* 316:1922–30.

ROYAL COLLEGE OF PHYSICIANS. 1997. *Improving communication between doctors and patients.* London: Royal College of Physicians of London.

SLOWIE DF. 1999. Doctors should help patients to communicate better with them. *British Medical Journal.* 319:784.

VAN DULMEN AM. 1998. Children's contributions to pediatric outpatient encounters. *Pediatrics.* 102 (3):563–8.

# Index